Oncogenes

2ND Edition

Volume II

Author

Enrique Pimentel, M.D.

Professor and Director
National Center of Genetics
Institute of Experimental Medicine
Central University of Venezuela
Caracas, Venezuela

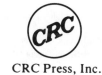

CRC Press, Inc.
Boca Raton, Florida

Information Center
Genetics Institute

Library of Congress Cataloging-in-Publication Data

Pimentel, Enrique.
    Oncogenes / author, Enrique Pimentel. — 2nd ed.
      p. cm.
    Includes bibliographical references.
    ISBN 0-8493-6505-8 (v. 1). — ISBN 0-8493-6506-6 (v. 2)
    1. Oncogenes. 2. Oncogenic viruses. 3. Oncogenic Viruses.
I. Title.
    [DNLM: 1. Cell Transformation, Neoplastic. 2. Oncogenes. QZ 202 P6446]
RC268.42.P56 1989
616.99'4071—dc20
DNLM/DLC
for Library of Congress   89-22100
                                                      CIP

PREFACE

Oncogenes are genes with potential properties for the induction of neoplastic transformation of cells in either natural or experimental conditions. Most oncogenes have been isolated from acute transforming retroviruses, which act as oncogene transducers, although these viruses do not transmit cancer under natural conditions. The viral oncogenes are genes of cellular origin and their normal counterparts, the protooncogenes, are present in the genome of all multicellular animals, including man. Approximately 40 protooncogenes have been detected so far in normal and tumor cells. The normal functions of protooncogenes are related mainly to the transductional mechanisms of cellular signals and to the control of cellular proliferation and differentiation. Structural or functional alterations of protooncogenes are associated with the origin and/or development of malignant diseases. The tumorigenic potential of protooncogenes is counteracted by the effects of tumor suppressor genes or antioncogenes. The available evidence indicates that cancer may be associated with alterations of the normal equilibrium existing between protooncogenes and tumor suppressor genes. The role of protooncogenes and tumor suppressor genes in malignant diseases is at present a subject of very high interest and intensive research work.

Enrique Pimentel, M.D.
May 18, 1989

THE AUTHOR

Enrique Pimentel, M.D., is Professor of General Pathology at the School of Medicine, Central University of Venezuela, Caracas. He was formerly Director of the Institute of Experimental Medicine at the same university and is now Director of the National Center of Genetics in Venezuela.

Born on April 7, 1928 in Caracas, he obtained an M.D. degree from the Universities of Madrid and Caracas. He is a member of the National Academy of Medicine in Venezuela and an honorary, correspondent, or active member of 30 national and international scientific societies. He is Vice President of the International Academy of Tumor Marker Oncology (IATMO).

Dr. Pimentel is the author of more than 100 papers, co-author of 5 books on topics related to endocrinology, genetics, and oncology, and the author of *Hormones, Growth Factors, and Oncogenes* (published by CRC Press, 1987). He is the Editor of a recently created journal (published by CRC Press), *Critical Reviews in Oncogenesis*. On many occasions Dr. Pimentel has been invited to give lectures and seminars at universities and other scientific institutions in North America and Europe. He received several decorations in his country and the Grosse Verdienstkreuz of the Federal Republic of Germany. In 1982, he received the National Award of Science in Venezuela.

TABLE OF CONTENTS

Volume I

Chapter 2
Acute Retroviruses

Chapter 5
DNA Viruses

Chapter 6
Viral and Cellular Oncogenes

Chapter 8

The Rous Sarcoma Virus Oncogene and its Protooncogene Counterpart

Chapter 9
Protooncogenes and Cancer

Chapter 7

FUNCTIONS OF ONCOGENE AND PROTOONCOGENE PROTEIN PRODUCTS

I. INTRODUCTION

The universal presence of protooncogenes in metazoan species, as well as their high conservation in evolution, indicate the biological importance of their protein products. Unfortunately, the normal functions of the protein products of cellular oncogenes are little known. It has been postulated that protooncogenes are involved in the control mechanisms of normal processes of cellular differentiation and proliferation, especially during embryogenesis, and that they would participate in the neoplastic transformation of cells only when they are expressed at inappropriate stages of differentiation.[1,2] Striking degrees of structural and/or functional homologies between the protein products of oncogenes and protooncogenes and a diversity of cellular proteins have been detected.[3] Some of these homologies involve important physiologic agents like hormones and growth factors or their cellular receptors.[4]

Protein kinase activity with remarkable specificity for tyrosine residues is present in several oncogene protein products, including the products of the viral oncogenes *src*, *yes*, *fps*, *fes*, *fgr*, *fms*, *ros*, *erb*-B, *ret*, and *abl*.[5-9] The oncogene v-*kit* may also encode a tyrosine-specific protein kinase.[10] These oncogenes are members of a superfamily of genes with distantly related protein products.[11] Other members of this family are the genes *met*,[12] *neu*,[13] *syn*,[14] *arg*,[15] and *trk*.[16] Tyrosine-specific kinase activity is not, however, an exclusive property of oncogene products. A similar activity is elicited by the binding of several hormones and growth factors to their cell surface receptors, including insulin, IGF-I, EGF, TGF-α, PDGF, and acidic FGF.[4,17,18] Tyrosine-specific protein kinase activity is also associated with the activated receptors for bombesin and the hematopoietic growth factor CSF-1.[19,20] The same type of activity is present in many fetal and adult tissues, including terminally differentiated normal human blood cells.[21] Higher tyrosine-specific protein kinase activity has been detected in resting lymphocytes than in proliferating normal or leukemic blood cells.[22] It seems thus clear that high levels of tyrosine-specific protein kinase activity cannot be considered as characteristic of the action of oncogenes and protooncogenes or the malignant transformation of cells. Protein kinase activity with specificity for serine and threonine residues is frequently present in the same proteins that possess tyrosine kinase activity and may contribute to functional properties of these proteins.

The transforming activity of oncogene products with protein kinase activity may depend on substrate specificity. Each protooncogene-encoded cellular tyrosine protein kinase may be independently regulated and may have a unique substrate specificity. Studies with hematopoietic cells indicate that different protooncogene products with tyrosine protein kinase activity are expressed at distinct stages of differentiation within specific lineages.[23] Cellular substrates for tyrosine protein kinases can be detected by means of antibodies with specificity for phosphotyrosine.[24,25] The molecular mechanisms responsible for substrate specificity of tyrosine protein kinases are not understood. A polypeptide sequence of approximately 100 residues, termed SH2, is shared between all tyrosine-protein kinases which are localized in the cytoplasm or have no transmembrane sequences, including the products encoded by the oncogenes v-*fps/fes*, v-*src*, v-*yes*, v-*abl*, and v-*fgr*.[26] Region SH2 is not essential for catalytic activity but could have a role in directing the cellular actions of the kinase domain by determining interactions of the enzyme with specific cellular components. The tyrosine-specific kinase activity, but not the serine or threonine kinase activity, of oncogene protein products or hormone and growth factor receptors can be inhibited by the isoflavone compound genistein.[27] Synthetic derivatives of 4-hydroxycinnamamide can also act as potential and specific inhibitors of tyrosine protein kinase activity.[28]

These specific inhibitors might be used for elucidating the role of tyrosine phosphorylation in normal or transformed cells.

The protein products of v-*mil*, v-*raf*, and possibly also v-*rel*, possess kinase activity with specificity not for tyrosine but for serine and threonine residues.[29,30] Protein kinase activity is not present in other oncogene protein products, including the products of *myb*, *myc*, *mos*, *ras*, and *sis*. The normal functions of these proteins are only partially understood. The cellular mechanism of action of some oncogene products may be associated with stimulation of phosphoinositide metabolism, which could result in the generation of mitogenic signals through the activation protein kinase C and the intracellular redistribution of calcium ions.[31,32] The predominant nuclear localization of the protein products of some oncogenes and protooncogenes (*myc*, *myb*, *fos*, *ski*, *erb*-A, *jun*, and possibly also *ets*-2) suggests, but does not prove, that they may be involved in the regulation of genomic functions.[33]

II. THE *SIS* ONCOGENE PROTEIN PRODUCT

Simian sarcoma virus (SSV) is a replication-defective, nonhuman primate acute retrovirus that was isolated together with a replication-competent nontransforming virus, the simian sarcoma-associated virus (SSAV), from a spontaneous fibrosarcoma of a pet woolly monkey (*Lagothrix sp*).[34] The genomes of both SSV and SSAV retroviruses were cloned in molecular vectors and their structures were analyzed.[35] The SSV genome contains a region with sequences not shared by SSAV. The SSV/SSAV virus complex induces transformation of cultured primate cells and can induce sarcomas when inoculated into newborn marmoset monkeys.[36,37] Virus-specific proteins are detected in SSV-transformed cells, including a 115,000-Da protein phosphorylated on tyrosine residues.[38] Diploid human skin fibroblasts can be transformed with a recombinant plasmid carrying the v-*sis* oncogene contained in the SSV genome, but the transformed cells do not acquire all the characteristics of fully malignant cells and are nontumorigenic in athymic mice.[39]

The protein product of the v-*sis* oncogene is a 28,000-Da protein, p28^{v-sis}.[40,41] Sequences related to v-*sis* are also transduced by the Parodi-Irgens feline sarcoma virus (PI-FeSV), a virus isolated from a fibrosarcoma of a cat infected with FeLV.[42] The transforming product of PI-FeSV has been identified as a 76-kDa fusion protein containing *gag* and *sis* sequences. The v-*sis* protein has been artificially produced in bacteria. Colonies of bacteria expressing the v-*sis* protein can be detected with monoclonal antibodies made against specific synthetic peptides.[43] A homologous v-*sis* cellular gene, c-*sis*, is present in primates, including humans, as well as in other vertebrate species.[44,45] The human and feline c-*sis* protooncogenes contain coding sequences that are located upstream of the region that was captured in the v-*sis* oncogene of SSV.[42,46]

A. HOMOLOGY BETWEEN *SIS* PROTEIN PRODUCTS AND PLATELET-DERIVED GROWTH FACTOR

A striking degree of structural homology exists between p28^{v-sis} and a cellular growth factor, the platelet-derived growth factor (PDGF), which is present in platelets of normal blood.[47-56] Although the physiological role of PDGF is not completely defined, it is known to be released from platelets during blood clotting and has been recognized as an important mitogen present in serum, being required for the growth of cells of mesenchymal origin maintained in tissue culture.[57-61]

The cellular actions of the v-*sis* gene are mediated by a PDGF-like molecule.[49] SSV-transformed marmoset cells secrete a factor that can mimic the activity of PDGF in all assay systems used.[62] The translational products of v-*sis* are capable of specifically binding PDGF receptors in quiescent fibroblasts, which results in activation of the receptors, stimulation of tyrosine phosphorylation, and induction of DNA synthesis.[63] However, in contrast to PDGF, which is a secretory protein, the vast majority of the v-*sis* protein product remains cell associated.[64]

The SSV transformation-specific polypeptide is antigenically related to PDGF.[25] Antisera produced against a synthetic peptide corresponding to amino acid residues 139 to 155 of the p28[sis] sequence recognize molecules corresponding to different forms of PDGF, and SSV-transformed cells secrete a mitogen which is identical to a form of PDGF.[66,67] Antibodies against PDGF inhibit both cell proliferation and SSV-induced morphological transformation in human diploid fibroblasts.[68] These results, as well as the phenotypic characteristics of SSV-transformed human fibroblast cells, suggest that v-*sis*-induced transformation is due solely to the autocrine action of a PDGF receptor agonist.[69] The specific oncogene product synthesized by v-*sis*-transformed cells is capable of interacting in an autocrine fashion not only with PDGF receptors located on the cell surface but also with receptors located in intracellular compartments, which results in functional activation of the receptors.[70]

Nucleotide sequence analysis identified the human c-*sis* gene as a structural gene for one of the two major polypeptides of the PDGF molecule and it was demonstrated that the c-*sis* gene encodes a precursor of the B chain of PDGF (PDGF-2).[71-75] The human c-*sis*/PDGF-2 gene contains seven exons, but the great majority of the first exon and the entire seventh exon are comprised of noncoding sequences.[75] The oncogene product p28[v-sis] may undergo dimer formation and subsequent processing to a form analogous in structure to that of biologically active human PDGF and it seems likely that the transforming activity of p28[v-sis] is mediated by this processed PDGF-2-like dimer.[50,76,77] The study of deletions in the carboxyl terminal coding region of the v-*sis* oncogene indicates that dimerization of the oncogene protein product is required for neoplastic transformation.[78] The biosynthesis of the v-*sis* gene protein product has been characterized with respect to signal sequence cleavage, glycosylation, and proteolytic processing.[79]

While the entire PDGF-2 sequence is encompassed within the v-*sis* gene product, there are three regions of the predicted v-*sis* protein that are unrelated to PDGF. These regions include the amino terminus of v-*sis*, which is encoded by sequences derived from the viral *env* gene, as well as two v-*sis* cell-derived regions immediately flanking the PDGF-2 homologous sequence.[77] The essential regions for transformation induced by a human c-*sis* cDNA clone correspond to those encoding the amino-terminal sequence, which is presumably a signal sequence for insertion into or across the plasma membrane, and the region of predicted amino acid sequence homology with PDGF.[74] Comparative analysis of the human and feline c-*sis* protooncogenes indicates the existence of 5′ human c-*sis* coding sequences that are not homologous to v-*sis*.[42,46,80]

Several structural differences have been detected between the human c-*sis* protooncogene and woolly monkey-derived v-*sis*, indicating that the predicted amino acid sequences of the human c-*sis* product differ by 6% from that of the woolly monkey-derived v-*sis* product.[71] The p28[v-sis] protein produced by genetically manipulated bacteria inhibits PDGF binding to its cellular receptors, presumably by directly competing for the binding sites, which suggests that the biological activity of the p28[v-sis] protein is the result of its interaction with the PDGF receptor.[81] The p28[v-sis] protein stimulates autocrine growth of SSV-transformed cells through PDGF cell-surface receptors and the rate of tumor growth in athymic nude mice injected with these cells correlates directly with the amounts of p28[v-sis] secreted by the transformed cells in culture.[82] Blockade of PDGF binding to its receptor by suramin indicates that the absence of PDGF receptors in SSV-transformed cells is due to down regulation of the receptor by an autocrine mechanism.[83] The mechanism of SSV-induced transformation does not appear to involve major alterations in phosphorylation of cellular proteins on tyrosine residues.[84]

The oncogenic potential of v-*sis* and c-*sis* genes can be evaluated by transfection of molecular vectors carrying the cloned genes into cultured cells of human or nonhuman origin. Overexpression of a human c-*sis* cDNA cloned in a vector is capable of inducing anchorage-independent growth in human diploid fibroblasts.[83] The v-*sis* oncogene and the c-*sis* protooncogene, as well as the T24 c-H-*ras* gene, are capable of inducing a transformed phenotype upon their transfection into human diploid fibroblasts, but are not capable of conferring infinite lifespan or making such cells tumorigenic.[86] In general, human cells are relatively resistant to malignant transformation induced by cloned oncogenes.

B. EXPRESSION AND FUNCTION OF THE C-*SIS*/PDGF GENE IN NORMAL TISSUES

The primary translational product of the human c-*sis* protooncogene is a 26-kDa protein, p26[c-*sis*].[87] This product is processed to yield a disulfide-linked homodimer, p56[c-*sis*], which is further processed to a 35-kDa dimer, p35[c-*sis*]. Like the v-*sis* oncogene product, the c-*sis*/PDGF-2 precursor undergoes N-linked glycosylation, implying its processing through the endoplasmic reticulum. The human c-*sis*/PDGF-2 product possesses the functional properties of the normal growth factor, PDGF.

Expression of the human c-*sis* coding sequence may induce cell transformation in specific experimental conditions.[76,88] However, under normal conditions the c-*sis* gene protein product is not oncogenic and the c-*sis* gene is normally expressed in a number of tissues. A cDNA clone homologous to the v-*sis* oncogene has been isolated and partially sequenced from human endothelial cells.[89] The c-*sis* gene is expressed in human and bovine endothelial cells in culture as well as *in vivo*.[90] Cultured human endothelial cells express 4.3-kb c-*sis*/PDGF-related RNA transcripts, whose levels are increased in conditions favoring proliferation and decreased in conditions favoring differentiation.[91] Thrombin stimulates c-*sis* gene expression in microvascular endothelial cells.[92] In contrast, modified low-density lipoproteins (LDLs) are able to suppress the production of PDGF-like proteins by cultured endothelial cells.[93] The function of the c-*sis*/PDGF gene product in endothelial cells is unknown but it could have some role in the normal growth and development of the vessel wall. A PDGF-like substance(s) is produced by young rat arterial smooth muscle cells in primary culture. A similar or identical PDGF-like protein is produced by smooth muscle cells derived form adult rats when modulated from contractile to synthetic phenotype, which gives the cells the ability to synthesize DNA and divide when stimulated with serum or growth factors.[95] The possible role of PDGF-like proteins in the development of atherosclerotic lesions is not understood.

The c-*sis* protooncogene is actively transcribed in the first trimester human placenta, especially in the highly proliferative and invasive cytotrophoblastic shell, where it parallels the distribution of c-*myc* transcripts.[96] The translation product of the c-*sis* transcripts in human placenta is a PDGF-like protein, as shown by the release of a PDGF receptor-competing activity into media conditioned by fresh explants of first trimester placenta. Moreover, cultured cytotrophoblasts display abundant high-affinity PDGF receptors and respond to exogenous PDGF by an activation of the c-*myc* gene expression and induction of DNA synthesis.[96] The results suggest that the developing human placenta could represent a case of autocrine growth regulation.

Activated human blood monocytes, but not resting monocytes, release a mediator that attracts smooth muscle cells and cooperates with other mediators to stimulate fibroblast proliferation. This mediator is PDGF or a very similar factor and is apparently produced by transcription of the c-*sis* protooncogene.[97] The results suggest that PDGF/c-*sis* protein product(s) may be involved in the pathogenesis of chronic inflammatory disorders. Similar or identical PDGF-like factors, products of the spontaneous expression of the c-*sis* gene, are secreted by human alveolar and peritoneal macrophages.[98,99] Purified human PDGF and recombinant human c-*sis*/PDGF-2 polypeptide homodimers are equally effective in stimulating fibroblast mitogenesis and chemotaxis or polymorphonuclear leukocytes, monocytes, and fibroblasts *in vitro* and in augmenting wound healing in a rat linear incision model *in vivo*.[100]

C. REGULATION OF C-*SIS* EXPRESSION BY GROWTH FACTORS

Expression of the c-*sis*/PDGF gene may be regulated by particular growth factors. In mouse embryo-derived AKR-2B cells arrested in G_0 phase, c-*sis*/PDGF transcripts appear within 20 min of stimulation with TGF-β and remain elevated thereafter for at least 24 h.[101] Furthermore, two known PDGF-regulated protooncogenes, c-*fos* and c-*myc*, are induced with delayed kinetics by TGF-β in the same system. The results suggest that the mitogenic effects of TGF-β may be mediated by expression of other growth factors like PDGF in an autocrine manner, as well as by the expression of particular protooncogenes.

Expression of c-*sis* transcripts is induced by TGF-β, as well as by thrombin, in cultured human renal microvascular endothelial cells.[102] This induction is blocked by agents that increase the intracellular concentration of cAMP, such as the adrenergic agonists isoproterenol and norepinephrine, or the adenylate cyclase activator, forskolin. Expression of the c-*sis* proto-oncogene in endothelial cells may be thus subjected to bidirectional regulation.

D. EXPRESSION OF THE C-*SIS*/PDGF GENE BY TRANSFORMED CELLS

PDGF-like proteins are synthesized by several transformed cell lines. Human glioblastoma (A172) and fibrosarcoma (HT-1080) cells in culture produce several molecular species of PDGF-like proteins, with sizes ranging from 16 to 140 kDa, and the same lines synthesize a 4.4-kb mRNA that contains sequences from all the six identified exons of the human c-*sis* gene.[103] Mouse neuroblastoma cells (Neuro-2A cells) also express c-*sis* transcripts with concomitant production and secretion of a PDGF-like growth factor.[104] Brain cells cultured from mice treated transplacentally with *N*-ethyl-*N*-nitrosourea (ENU) undergo a sequence of morphological changes characteristic of malignant transformation. Transformed glioma cells from these cultures differ from premalignant glial cells by containing high levels of c-*sis* transcripts and by synthesizing functional PDGF.[105] Since glial cells have PDGF receptors, an autocrine mechanism could play an important role in ENU-induced brain tumorigenesis in mice. However, not all transformed cells express c-*sis* transcripts and protein.

Multiple forms of c-*sis* transcripts and a variety of PDGF-like polypeptides can be detected in certain tumor cell lines, e.g., the U-2 OS human osteosarcoma line, but no c-*sis* mRNA and no PDGF immunoreactivity are detected in other tumor cell lines, e.g., the MG-63 human osteosarcoma line.[106] Although U-2 OS cells exhibit few, if any, cell surface receptors for PDGF, these receptors are present in U-2 OS cells and they can be unmasked by treatment of the cells with the polyanionic compound, suramin.[107] Efficient reversion of SSV-induced transformation and inhibition of growth factor-induced mitogenesis can be obtained by using suramin.[108] These results suggest that U-2 OS cells are capable of autocrine stimulation. High amounts of c-*sis*/PDGF transcripts were found to be constitutively expressed in ten human malignant mesothelioma cell lines.[109] Cytogenetic and restriction enzyme analysis of these cell lines did not reveal a mechanism responsible for the c-*sis* activation.

The transcriptional activity of the c-*sis* oncogene in a ductus deferens smooth muscle tumor cell line is inhibited by glucocorticoids.[110] Phorbol ester induces c-*sis* gene expression in the human leukemia stem cell line K-562.[111] A sevenfold increase in c-*sis*/PDGF-B mRNA expression is also induced by phorbol ester (PMA), but not by DMSO, in the human hematopoietic cell line HEL, which was established from a patient with Hodgkin's disease who later developed erythroleukemia.[112] Since PMA does not induce expression of PDGF-A chain gene in HEL cells, these results indicate that expression of PDGF-A and PDGF-B genes is controlled by independent mechanisms.

The precise role of the expression of the c-*sis*/PDGF gene by particular types of transformed cells is not clear. Studies with somatic cell hybrids of murine origin indicate that PDGF responsiveness may be dissociated from cellular transformation and that cells may be transformed by mechanisms which are apparently independent of PDGF and its v-*sis*-like cellular analogue.[113] Further studies are needed for a better characterization of the structural and functional relationships existing between PDGF and the protein product of the c-*sis*/PDGF gene in normal and neoplastic tissues.

III. THE *ERB*-B ONCOGENE PROTEIN PRODUCT

A particular type of ALV is the avian erythroblastosis virus (AEV), which induces primarily erythroblastosis when injected into susceptible chickens but can also occasionally induce sarcomas or carcinomas.[114] AEV also induces transformation of immature erythroid cells and fibroblasts in culture.[115] The transforming sequences of AEV correspond to the v-*erb* oncogene, whose cellular counterpart, c-*erb*, is present in the genome of all vertebrate species tested, including humans and fish.[116] AEV transduces two different oncogenes, v-*erb*-A and v-*erb*-B, derived from separate, unlinked DNA sequences in the cellular genome.[117] The v-*erb*-A and v-*erb*-B oncogenes can cooperate in the induction of a fully transformed phenotype in erythroblastic and fibroblastic chicken cells.[118] An AEV variant, termed AEV-H, which transduces only the *erb*-B oncogene, is capable of inducing both erythroblastosis and sarcomas in chickens.[119] The *erb*-B gene is frequently transduced by another virus, the Rous-associated virus type 1 (RAV-1), which is also capable of inducing rapid-onset erythroblastosis when inoculated into 1-week-old chickens.[120] Spontaneous differentiation can occur in AEV-transformed avian embryonic erythroid cells transformed by other oncogenes of the same family, e.g., v-*src* and v-*fps*.[121,122]

A. HOMOLOGY BETWEEN *ERB*-B GENE PRODUCTS AND THE EPIDERMAL GROWTH FACTOR RECEPTOR

A striking structural homology has been observed between the transforming protein of the v-*erb*-B oncogene of AEV and the epidermal growth factor (EGF) receptor protein purified from a human epidermoid carcinoma cell line (line A431) and human normal placenta.[123-126] Amplification (approximately 30-fold), rearrangement, and enhanced expression of the EGF receptor gene occurs in A431 cells.[127] Furthermore, both the c-*erb*-B gene and the EGF receptor gene are located in the same region of human chromosome 7,[128,129] which reinforces the suggestion for their identity.

According to the results of a number of studies, the primary translational product of the v-*erb*-B oncogene is a 61-kDa polypeptide, termed p61$^{v\text{-}erb\text{-}B}$, which is glycosylated in AEV-infected cells to yield several species of higher apparent molecular weight.[130] One of these v-*erb*-B product(s) is a 68-kDa glycoprotein, gp68$^{v\text{-}erb\text{-}B}$, which is modified further to a 74-kDa protein, gp74$^{v\text{-}erb\text{-}B}$, the latter being located at the cell surface.[131-134] The orientation of the v-*erb*-B protein product in the plasma membrane was characterized.[135] The use of three different glycoprotein-processing inhibitors has demonstrated that incorrectly glycolsylated v-*erb*-B protein is inserted normally into the plasma membrane and is still capable of exerting its oncogenic activity on susceptible cells. The *erb*-B oncogene product corresponds to a truncated form of the EGF receptor, with deletion of the amino-terminal end, which may explain the absence of cross-reaction between antisera against these two proteins. However, site-specific antibodies to the *erb*-B protein product precipitate EGF receptor.[136] The v-*erb*-B protein contains only the transmembrane attaching part and the cytoplasmic tyrosine-specific kinase domains of the EGF receptor, and lacks most of the extracellular domain responsible for EGF binding.[137] The v-*erb*-B protein corresponds to a growth factor receptor which has lost the regulatory binding domain but has retained the membrane locating and biochemical activating domains. Thus, the v-*erb*-B protein represents a kind of unregulated receptor which is expressed constitutively in the activated state.

The v-*erb*-B 68-kDa protein product is phosphorylated primarily on serine and threonine residues but it contains minor amounts of phosphotyrosine and protein phosphorylation at tyrosine residues is induced by the v-*erb*-B protein *in vivo* and *in vitro*.[138,139] Both the EGF receptor and the v-*erb*-B proteins are tyrosine-specific protein kinases.[140] Site-specific antibodies to the *src*-homologous domain (amino acid residues 373 to 383) of the v-*erb*-B gene product neutralize the tyrosine-protein kinase activity of the EGF receptor.[141] The v-*erb*-B product does not possess intrinsic kinase activity specific for inositol phospholipids.[142]

AEV-transformed chicken embryo fibroblasts show enhanced tyrosine phosphorylation of a number of cellular polypeptides, including 36- and 42-kDa proteins.[139] The major *in vivo* tyrosine autophosphorylation site of the EGF receptor is tyrosine 1173, which is located 14 residues from the carboxy-terminus of the receptor molecule and is not found in the v-*erb*-B protein.[143] The latter protein is fused at the carboxy-terminus to four residues of the viral *env* protein. Therefore, v-*erb*-B represents an oncogene which is terminated prematurely with respect to the cellular EGF receptor sequences from which it is derived.

Antibodies to a synthetic oligopeptide have been used as a probe for the kinase activity of the avian EGF receptor and v-*erb*-B protein.[140] Inhibition of the tyrosine kinase activity of the protein can be achieved by using antibodies generated against a synthetic peptide corresponding to amino acid residues 285 to 296 of the predicted v-*erb*-B protein sequence, which corresponds to the tyrosine-protein kinase domain of both the v-*erb*-B protein and the EGF receptor.[144] The EGF receptor is autophosphorylated on tyrosine residues upon ligand binding but the physiological significance of this modification is not totally clear. A truncated form of the EGF receptor lacking the carboxy-terminal 20,000 Da of the molecule which contain all of the three major autophosphorylation sites is still capable of transducing a mitogenic signal in CHO cells.[145]

A chicken v-*erb*-B probe was used for the isolation of a unique clone of *Drosophila melanogaster* DNA located on chromosome 2, position 57F, and corresponding to the gene coding for a putative EGF receptor protein in the insect.[146] The putative *Drosophila* EGF receptor protein is similar in overall organization to the human homologue, showing three distinct domains: an extracellular putative EGF binding domain, a hydrophobic transmembrane region, and a cytoplasmic kinase domain. The deduced amino acid sequence of a portion of the *Drosophila* EGF receptor that hybridizes with the v-*erb*-B oncogene is 77% homologous to the kinase domain of the human EGF receptor.[147] The general structure of this molecule has been conserved for at least 800 million years.

Complex endogenous and exogenous factors are involved in the regulation of c-*erb*-B/EGF receptor expression in different animal tissues under different physiologic conditions. Hormones and growth factors are importantly involved in this regulation, as discussed in a recent book.[4]

B. STRUCTURAL AND FUNCTIONAL REQUIREMENTS FOR V-*ERB*-B-INDUCED NEOPLASTIC TRANSFORMATION

The structural domains of the v-*erb*-B protein required for fibroblast transformation have been dissected by in-frame insertional mutagenesis procedures.[130] AEV genomes bearing lesions induced within the v-*erb*-B kinase domain exhibit a drastically decreased ability to transform avian fibroblasts. In contrast, mutations in the extracellular domain, between the transmembrane region and the kinase domain, or at the extreme carboxyl terminus of the v-*erb*-B protein have no effect on AEV-mediated fibroblast neoplastic transformation.[130] Mutant v-*erb*-B protein lacking the possible extracellular sites of N-linked glycosylation have unimpaired ability to transform cells to an oncogenic phenotype.[148] The product of a constructed chimeric oncogene containing the transmembrane glycosylated domain of the v-*erb*-B protein linked to the kinase catalytic domain of the v-*src* protein was capable of transforming cultured fibroblasts to an oncogenic phenotype closely resembling that induced by the parent v-*erb*-B oncogene.[149] The chimeric oncogene failed to transform erythroid progenitor cells, which is consistent with evidence indicating that the carboxy-terminal domain of the v-*erb*-B protein is involved in erythroid target cell specificity. Unexpectedly, the transmembrane domain of the v-*erb*-B protein could be deleted without completely abolishing the ability of this protein to transform avian fibroblasts.[150]

A 10-amino acid insertion within the v-*erb*-B protein kinase domain produced a *ts* mutant capable of inducing fibroblast transformation at 36°C but not at 41°C.[130] A single amino acid substitution in the v-*erb*-B product conferred a thermolabile phenotype to *ts* 167 AEV-transformed HD6 erythroid precursor cells.[151] The mutation determined a change from a histidine to an aspartic acid in the *ts* v-*erb*-B polypeptide and is located in the center of the tyrosine-specific protein kinase domain, corresponding to amino acid position 826 of the human EGF receptor sequence. However, the exact relationship between the structural and functional change of the oncogene product could not be ascertained.

The exact relationship between the kinase activity of the v-*erb*-B protein and its ability to induce neoplastic transformation is not clear. Analysis of *ts* mutants and nonconditional host range mutants of AEV demonstrates that there is no simple correlation between auto-phosphorylation activity of the v-*erb*-B protein and the transformation ability of the various AEV mutants.[152] Thus, although the specific kinase activity of the v-*erb*-B protein may be central to AEV-induced transformation, it would be in itself insufficient. Some AEV isolates contain v-*erb*-B oncogenes that lack codons for the immediate carboxyl terminus of the EGF receptor, and the biological properties of these variant viruses are different from those of the prototype virus.[153,154] Thus, differences in the transforming potential of v-*erb*-B-carrying retroviruses correlate with differences in *erb*-B sequences encoding the carboxy-terminal domain of the EGF receptor protein. A chimeric gene construct encoding the extracellular and transmembrane domain of the human EGF receptor joined to sequences coding for the cytoplasmic domain of the v-*erb*-B protein was capable of inducing neoplastic transformation when expressed in Rat 1 cells.[155] The results obtained with this chimeric gene suggest that the carboxy-terminal deletion in the encoded protein (and in the protein encoded by the v-*erb*-B oncogene) may be responsible for its transforming potential.

A constructed *gag*-*erb*-B fused gene coding the v-*erb*-B protein modified at its amino terminus by the large *gag* polypeptide sequence was capable of inducing transformation of CEF cells.[156] This result indicates that modification of the extracellular region of the v-*erb*-B product does not affect its transforming ability and is probably compatible with preservation of the tyrosine-specific kinase activity. A proviral-activated c-*erb*-B gene which lacked the amino-terminal extracellular domain but retained the entire carboxy-terminal sequences possessed leukemogenic but not sarcomagenic properties in chickens.[157]

The tumorigenic potential of the intact EGF receptor protooncogene is indicated by the results of experiments in which the EGF receptor gene was placed in a retrovirus vector. NIH/3T3 cells transfected with this vector or infected with the corresponding rescued retrovirus developed a fully transformed phenotype *in vitro* that required both functional EGF receptor expression and the presence of EGF in the culture medium.[158] Recent evidence suggests that v-*erb*-B-related genomic sequences are involved in tumorigenic processes occurring in *Xiphophorus* fishes.[159]

IV. THE *NEU*/*ERB*-B-2 ONCOGENE PROTEIN PRODUCT

The protooncogene c-*neu* was first isolated from rat neuroblastomas induced with ethylni-trosourea (ENU).[160] The c-*neu* gene is closely related to, but distinct from, the v-*erb*-B oncogene and its normal cellular homologue, the EGF receptor gene.[161] The nucleotide sequence of the cloned rat c-*neu* gene predicts a 1260-amino acid transmembrane protein product similar in overall structure to the EGF receptor.[162] The c-*neu* gene is apparently identical to a protoonco-gene, termed c-*erb*-B-2, detected in the human genome.[163,164] The c-*neu* gene is located on human chromosome region 17q21 and is not coamplified with c-*erb*-B in the A431 human tumor cell line.[165,166] Expression of the human c-*neu*/*erb*-B-2 gene partially depends on regulatory elements contained in the 5' DNA sequences of the gene.[167] The gene HER2, which encodes a receptor with tyrosine-specific protein kinase activity, shows and extensive homology to the EGF receptor and shares chromosomal location with the c-*neu* protooncogene.[168] The c-*neu/erb*-B-2 and HER2 genes appear to be identical. The physiological ligand of the putative receptor encoded by the c-*neu* gene is unknown, but may be represented by an unidentified growth factor.

The product of the human c-*neu/erb*-B-2 gene is a 185-kDa glycoprotein, p185[c-*neu*], which possesses tyrosine-specific kinase activity.[13,169] The amino acid sequence predicted for this protein shows 42 to 52% homology with the sequences of the products of other tyrosine kinase-encoding genes, including *src*, *abl*, *fms*, and the human insulin receptor. The tyrosine kinase domain of the c-*neu/erb*-B-2 protein shows 82% homology to that of the EGF receptor protein.[170] The level of sequence homology of the extracellular domains of the human EGF receptor and the c-*neu/erb*-B-2 protein is 43%, and both molecules have a single putative transmembrane spanning sequence in equivalent positions.[171]

A. PHOSPHORYLATION AND EXPRESSION OF THE C-*NEU* PROTEIN

Phosphorylation of the c-*neu/erb*-B-2 protein in MKN-7 human adenocarcinoma cells is stimulated by both EGF and phorbol ester (TPA), although they act through different mechanisms.[172] EGF induces a rapid increase in phosphotyrosine, followed by relatively gradual increases in phosphoserine and phosphothreonine, whereas the phosphorylations induced by TPA occur exclusively on serine and threonine residues. The action of TPA is apparently mediated by activation of protein kinase C. Since the c-*neu/erb*-B-2 protein does not show detectable EGF-binding activity, its EGF-induced phosphorylation might be catalyzed by the EGF receptor kinase that is activated by EGF binding. Phosphorylation of the c-*neu/erb*-B-2 protein on tyrosine was also observed in SK-BR-3 mammary tumor cells as a direct consequence of the interaction of EGF with its surface receptor.[173]

The c-*neu* gene is widely expressed in normal human adult tissues, as well as in human fetal tissues, where the highest levels of c-*neu* transcripts are found. The use of antibodies specific to the c-*neu* product indicated that the human c-*neu/erb*-B-2 protein is expressed at approximately similar levels in normal and transformed human cells as well as in monkey and rat cell lines.[171] In the intact rat, expression of c-*neu* mRNA and p185[c-*neu*] protein was detected in midgestation embryos in a variety of tissues including nervous system, connective tissue, and secretory epithelium, but not in lymphoid tissue.[174] In the adult rat, c-*neu* mRNA and protein are expressed in secretory epithelial tissues and basal cells of the skin.

B. ONCOGENIC ACTIVATION OF THE C-*NEU* GENE

Cloning of the c-*neu* gene has demonstrated the absence of gross structural alterations in alleles associated with oncogenic processes, as judged by extensive restriction endonuclease mapping.[175] Thus, a minor change in the DNA sequences of c-*neu*, presumably located on the protein-coding region of the gene, would lead to the oncogenic activation of the gene in a way similar to that of particular types of c-*ras* point mutations. Oncogenic activation of the c-*neu* gene may be associated with neurogenic tumors (schwannomas) induced in rats with ENU.[176,177] The tumor cells contain in their DNA a T-A transversion which affects the transmembrane domain of the p185[c-*neu*] protein. The oncogenic potential of unaltered c-*neu* sequences is suggested by the tumorigenic conversion of NIH/3T3 cells induced by transfection of amplified c-*neu* genes.[178] The transforming activity of p185[c-*neu*] crucially depends on its intrinsic tyrosine-specific protein kinase activity, which is modulated by the transmembrane domain of the protein.[179] A single point mutation altering the transmembrane domain of p185[c-*neu*] encoded by the rat c-*neu* gene converts the normal gene into a potent oncogene.

C. REVERSION OF C-*NEU*-INDUCED TRANSFORMATION

Monoclonal antibodies against the p185[c-*neu*] protein can induce reversion of the transformed phenotype in NIH/3T3 cells transformed by transfection of the c-*neu* gene.[180] Moreover, injection of a specific monoclonal antibody into animals bearing tumors composed of c-*neu*-transformed NIH/3T3 cells may result in inhibition of tumor growth and prolonged survival of the tumor-bearing animals.[181] However, in all of these experiments the treated animals eventually died from their tumors.

V. THE *ERB*-A ONCOGENE PROTEIN PRODUCT

The v-*erb*-A oncogene of avian erythroblastosis virus is structurally different from v-*erb*-B. The product of v-*erb*-A is a fusion protein, p75$^{gag\text{-}erb\text{-}A}$, which is predominantly located in the cytoplasm.[131] The oncogene v-*erb*-B is able to transform erythroblasts whereas v-*erb*-A alone induces no transformation. The v-*erb*-A and v-*erb*-B oncogenes can cooperate in the induction of a fully transformed phenotype in chicken erythroblasts and fibroblasts.[118] Apparently, v-*erb*-A potentiates the transforming activity of v-*erb*-B by producing an early blockage of cell differentiation within the erythroid lineages.[182] The four carboxyl terminal amino acids of the v-*erb*-A product are encoded by a c-*erb*-B intron-derived sequence, which demonstrates that AEV acquired a truncated c-*erb*-A gene.[183] The cellular gene is 42 nucleotides longer in the 5′ coding extremity than v-*erb*-A.[184] The c-*erb* A protooncogene has been mapped by high-resolution cytogenetic and molecular analysis to human chromosome 17, at the subband 17q.11.2.[185]

A. HOMOLOGY BETWEEN THE *ERB*-A PROTEIN AND CARBONIC ANHIDRASE

The v-*erb*-A gene product has structural, but not functional, homology with mammalian carbonic anhydrase.[186] The sequence of equine muscle carbonic anhydrase has been determined.[187] The equine enzyme shows strong sequence homology to other mammalian carbonic anhydrases. Carbonic anhydrase is the second most abundant erythrocyte protein and its expression is normally subjected to strict developmental and functional control mechanisms. The enzyme catalyzes the reversible hydration of carbon dioxide and is therefore essential for normal carbon dioxide-bicarbonate exchange. Carbonic anhydrase is ubiquitous in many organs of vertebrates and invertebrates.[188] Carbonic anhydrase is aberrantly and constitutively expressed in human and murine erythroleukemia cells, which may be explained by a change in gene regulation.[189] The biological significance of the homology between the v-*erb*-A protein and carbonic anhydrase is unknown.

B. BIOLOGICAL PROPERTIES OF THE V-*ERB*-A PROTEIN

The biological function of the v-*erb*-A protein product has been studied by using a constructed retrovirus vector able to transfer and express selectively the *gag-erb*-A sequence in chicken cells in culture.[190] Although p75$^{gag\text{-}erb\text{-}A}$ has no transforming activity by itself, it is capable of inducing a strong enhancement of cellular growth *in vitro* and *in vivo*. In contrast to normal fibroblasts (CEF cells), the fibroblasts expressing p75$^{gag\text{-}erb\text{-}A}$ exhibit immediate growth upon replating, and multiply in growth factor-depleted medium at low cell density. Moreover, expression of the viral protein in fibroblasts transformed by v-*erb*-B enhances tumor development and inhibits differentiation of these cells *in vivo*. The v-*erb*-A product specifically suppresses the transcriptional expression of the cellular erythrocyte anion transporter (band 3) gene which is involved in erythroid differentiation.[191] The v-*erb*-A protein exhibits a structural motif consisting in a cysteine-rich region embedded in a domain high in lysine and arginine residues which may represent the DNA-binding region of the protein.[192] An artificial insertion mutation affecting this region abolishes the ability of the v-*erb*-A protein to bind DNA *in vitro* and suppresses the nuclear localization of the protein *in vivo* as well as its capacity to potentiate erythroid differentiation.

C. HOMOLOGY BETWEEN THE *ERB*-A PROTEIN AND STEROID HORMONE RECEPTORS

Domain structures of the human, rabbit, and chicken glucocorticoid, estrogen, and progesterone receptor proteins are related to the v-*erb*-A protein product.[193-201] The v-*erb*-A-homologous domain of the human glucocorticoid receptor is composed of two repeated units containing Cys-Lys-Arg-rich sequences and is the most highly conserved when compared with the v-*erb*-A oncogene and the estrogen receptor. These homologies suggest that steroid receptor genes and the c-*erb*-A protooncogene are derived from a common primordial regulatory gene.

D. HOMOLOGY BETWEEN THE C-*ERB*-A PROTEIN AND THE THYROID HORMONE RECEPTOR

Recently, it has been demonstrated that the c-*erb*-A gene encodes a thyroid hormone receptor and that the c-*erb*-A protein is a high-affinity receptor for thyroid hormone.[202,203] The predicted human thyroid hormone receptor is a protein of 52,000 to 55,000 mol wt with 47% amino acid identity in comparison with the human glucocorticoid receptor and 52% identity when c-*erb*-A is compared with the human estrogen receptor amino acid sequence. The highest degree of similarity is found in a cysteine-rich sequence of 65 amino acids beginning at c-*erb*-A amino acid residue 102, and this region would represent the DNA binding domain of the protein. The v-*erb*-A oncogene product from AEV is unable to bind thyroid hormone and would represent a constitutively active form of the thyroid hormone receptor.[202] The ligand-binding domain of the thyroid hormone receptor is located in an analogous position as compared to steroid receptors.[204] Several mutations in the domain homologous to the ligand-binding region of steroid receptors contribute to the defective ligand binding by $p75^{gag\text{-}erb\text{-}A}$.

There are multiple different molecular forms of the thyroid hormone receptor, which may correspond to the reported existence of multiple c-*erb*-A protooncogenes with different chromosome locations. The thyroid hormone receptor TR-α, isolated from a cDNA clone derived from rat brain mRNA is encoded by a gene, c-*erb*-A-1, located on human chromosome 17.[205] The c-*erb*-A-1 gene was cloned from a human testis cDNA library.[206,207] 2.6-kb RNA transcripts from the c-*erb*-A-1/TR-α gene are expressed at high levels in the central nervous system of the rat as well as in other tissues of the animal such as pituitary and muscle, but are not expressed in the liver. A second thyroid hormone receptor, TR-β, is encoded by a c-*erb*-A-β/TR-β protooncogene located on human chromosome 3 and is expressed in the liver. The protein products of TR-α and TR-β thyroid hormone receptors show limited amino acid sequence homology.[204] The results of these studies suggest that the protein products of c-*erb*-A/thyroid hormone receptor genes may have different functional specificities at both the genome and tissue levels in human cells.

E. REGULATION OF C-*ERB*-A PROTOONCOGENE EXPRESSION

Very little is known about the physiologic factors involved in the regulation of c-*erb*-A protooncogene expression. Exposure of human colon fibroblasts to n-butyrate, a four-carbon aliphatic carboxylic acid, results in an increased accumulation of 2.0-kb c-*erb*-A gene transcripts.[208] It is known that n-butyrate can modify gene expression in eukaryotic cells through a diversity of molecular mechanisms including DNA methylation and acylation of nuclear proteins.

VI. THE PROTEIN PRODUCTS OF THE *RAS* ONCOGENES

The oncogenes v-H-*ras* and v-K-*ras* are present in the genome of the acute retroviruses H-MuSV (Harvey virus) and K-MuSV (Kirsten virus), respectively. H-MuSV and K-MuSV were isolated from solid tumors that appeared in rats injected with the ecotropic chronic mouse retrovirus MuLV.[209,210] Acute retroviruses transducing v-*ras* genes have also been isolated from mouse tumors.[211,212] Another protooncogene from this family, N-*ras*, has not been found in acute transforming retroviruses but was isolated from the genome of human neuroblastoma cells.[213] The c-*ras* genes are present in all vertebrate species studied so far, as well as in many invertebrates and even in yeast.[214-220]

A. STRUCTURE AND EXPRESSION OF C-*RAS* GENES

The c-*ras* protooncogenes are expressed at low levels in most tissues and may belong to the class of housekeeping genes. High levels of c-*ras* gene expression may be observed in actively proliferating normal cells as well as in certain terminally differentiated cells. As in other actively transcribed genes, the promoter region of c-*ras* genes in different cultured human cells of either normal or tumor origin is hypersensitive to DNase I, micrococcal nuclease, endogenous nucleases, and S1 nuclease.[221] The 5' end of the mouse c-K-*ras* gene exhibits features shared by the promoter regions of genes with housekeeping or growth control functions in the cell.[222]

The human c-H-*ras* gene promoter has been localized to a 550 bp fragment located about 1 kb upstream from the *ras* coding sequence.[223] The promoter of the human c-H-*ras* gene lacks TATA and CAAT sequences and contains a GC box at the 3' terminus.[224] The gene appears to contain within the 5' untranslated region both positive- and negative-acting regulatory elements. In addition to the upstream DNA sequences, expression of the c-*ras* gene may be regulated by sequences located downstream of the gene coding sequences. A variable tandem repeat with a 280-kb consensus sequence located approximately 1.5 kb downstream from the 3' terminus of the human c-H-*ras* gene possesses an endogenous enhancer activity.[225,226] Polymorphism of this element in the human population could be responsible for variation in the level of c-H-*ras* expression in normal and transformed cells.

The rat c-H-*ras* gene has peculiar structural characteristics on its 5' flanking region.[227] Promoter activity of the c-H-*ras* gene is contained within the 172-bp 5'-flanking region of the gene.[228] Unlike the human gene, the rat c-H-*ras* promoter region contains a CAAT box in its characteristic position. Both the human and the rat gene share in the same region a number of 10-bp box consensus sequence elements which are important in the regulation of gene expression, but the GC and CAAT boxes in the rat c-H-*ras* gene are related to constitutive, and not regulatory, promoter activity, acting in a coordinate manner. An element with suppressive effect on the c-H-*ras* promoter is located on the 5' flanking region of the c-H-*ras* gene.[229]

B. DETECTION OF P21[RAS] PROTEINS

The products of the *ras* oncogenes (H-*ras*, K-*ras*, and N-*ras*) are proteins of 188 or 189 amino acids and approximate 21,000 mol wt, termed p21[ras] or, more simply, p21 proteins.[230-234] Immunological methods have been widely used for the detection and characterization of p21[ras] proteins. Antisera prepared in mice, rats, and rabbits by immunization with synthetic peptides corresponding to regions of high variability, located near the carboxyl termini of *ras* proteins, have been used for the specific detection of c-H-*ras* and c-K-*ras* proteins in immunoblots and immunoprecipitation reactions.[235,236] Affinity-purified rabbit c-H-*ras* antibody against residues 171 to 189 of the p21 product detects this product in tissue culture cells as well as in tissue sections from normal mouse skin, papillomas, and carcinomas. However, the method does not allow quantitation of the amount of p21 protein present in particular cell populations.

Several types of monoclonal antibodies have been prepared for the study of p21[ras] proteins in murine and human cells. The monoclonal antibody NCC-RAS-004, produced by using recombinant c-H-*ras* p21 protein as immunogen, was found to be extremely sensitive when used in immunoblotting analysis, facilitating semiquantitative detection of c-H-*ras*, c-K-*ras*, and N-*ras* p21 in cell and tissue lysates.[237] In cells carrying a point-mutationally activated c-*ras* gene, the p21 protein with abnormal mobility could be easily detected upon SDS-polyacrylamide gel electrophoresis. Multiple molecular forms of p21 proteins synthesized in human and mouse cells have been resolved by one- and two-dimensional polyacrylamide gel electrophoresis after precipitation with polyclonal or monoclonal antibodies.[238] Quantitative liquid competition radioimmunoassays have been developed for the study of oncogene and protooncogene p21^{ras} products.[239] A photoaffinity labeling procedure with guanosine triphosphate (GTP) cross-linking has been proposed for the specific detection of multiple forms of p21^{ras} proteins in animal tissues.[240] Results obtained with immunologic methods for p21^{ras} detection using polyclonal of monoclonal antibodies should be considered with caution due to the possibility of nonspecific reactions with other cellular proteins.[241]

C. BIOCHEMICAL ASPECTS OF *RAS* GENE PROTEIN PRODUCTS

The v-H-*ras* oncogene encodes a primary protein product, p21$^{v\text{-}ras}$, that is 189 amino acids in length. The protein products of either v-*ras* of c-*ras* genes exhibit biochemical, structural, and functional similarities with vertebrate guanine nucleotide-binding proteins (G proteins).[242-246] Three biochemical activities specific for guanine nucleotides have been identified in *ras* proteins: GTP or GDP binding, autokinase activity, and GTPase activity.

Both viral and cellular p21^{ras} products bind guanine nucleotides and reside at the inner surface of the plasma membrane.[216,247-249] Attachment of p21 proteins to the cell membrane takes place through lipid which is covalently bound to the p21 polypeptide.[250] The p21 proteins are acylated with palmitic acid at a cysteine residue near the carboxyl terminus (cystein-186).[251] Fatty acylation of p21 proteins is a dynamic event that may affect the function of these proteins in a number of ways and in addition to contributing to their association with the cell membrane.[252] In cells transformed by v-K-*ras*, accumulation of p21 occurs preferentially in subcellular locations similar to those where ruffles are observed by phase contrast microscopy and lamellar and villous extensions are observed by scanning electron microscopy.[253]

The p21$^{v\text{-}ras}$ products are susceptible to autophosphorylation at the 59th threonine residue in the presence of GTP, and p21$^{v\text{-}ras}$ products expressed in *Escherichia coli* after cloning of the v-H-*ras* or v-K-*ras* genes in molecular vectors may retain guanine nucleotide binding, GTPase, and autophosphorylating activities.[254-262] The purified v-H-*ras* p21 protein obtained in *E. coli* contains near stoichiometric amounts of noncovalently associated GDP, which acts as a competitive inhibitor of the interaction of added guanine nucleotides with the p21 product.[263] p21 can transfer γ-phosphate from GTP, but not ATP, to the threonine located at position 59th of the molecule. The p21 product of the v-H-*ras* oncogene can be phosphorylated by protein kinase C *in vitro* on serine residues at sites distinct from the site of autophosphorylation.[264]

In contrast to p21$^{v\text{-}ras}$ proteins, p21$^{c\text{-}ras}$ proteins are not phosphorylated due to substitution for the threonine residue with an alanine residue at the major phosphorylating site. The functional properties of p21^{ras} proteins may also be different depending on the viral or cellular origin since p21$^{v\text{-}ras}$ proteins have a half-life of 42 h whereas p21$^{c\text{-}ras}$ have a half-life of only 20 h, thus being much less stable in cells.[265] Normal c-*ras* proteins exhibit a weak GTPase activity and this activity is impaired in the mutant, oncogenic c-*ras* proteins.[266-270] Glycerol and Mn^{2+} strongly stimulate the GTPase activity of *ras* proteins.[271] A GTP-modulated sulfhydryl group of the v-H-*ras* p21 product has been identified as cysteine-80 and is included in a sequence which is highly conserved among various G proteins.[272]

ADP-ribosylation of G proteins by bacterial toxins and cellular ADP-ribosyltransferase stimulates the adenylate cyclase system, and both normal and mutated c-H-*ras* proteins can undergo ADP-ribosylation in the presence of hen liver ADP-ribosyltransferase.[273] The functional consequences of ADP-ribosylation of normal or mutated c-H-*ras* proteins on GTP binding, GTPase activity, or other activities are little understood. ADP-ribosylation of p21 by an NAD:arginine ADP-ribosyltransferase purified from turkey erythrocytes decreases p21 GTPase activity and ability to bind GTP.[274] EGF stimulates guanine nucleotide binding activity and phosphorylation of p21^{ras} products.[74]

Studies with p21-specific antibodies or mutational analysis of *ras* genes may contribute to a better characterization of the biochemical and functional properties of p21 proteins. Two-dimensional proton nuclear magnetic resonance methods have also been applied to the study of highly purified, bacterially expressed p21 product encoded by the c-H-*ras* protooncogene.[275]

1. Studies with p21-Specific Antibodies

The three activities displayed by p21[v-*ras*] proteins (GTP/GDP binding, autophosphorylation, and GTPase) are related and may depend on a single active center within the p21 molecule. The three activities are specifically affected by a monoclonal antibody.[261] The Y13-259 monoclonal antibody specifically neutralizes p21[*ras*] proteins and severely hampers the dissociation rate of guanine exchange reactions.[276] Since Y13-259 has specificity to a carboxy-terminal region of *ras* gene products and inhibits their guanine nucleotide-binding function, these results suggest that this part of the p21 molecule is involved in some way, either directly or indirectly, in guanine nucleotide binding.[277]

Monoclonal antibodies have been used to explore the functional properties of deletion mutants of the v-H-*ras* oncogene product.[278] The results indicate that monoclonal antibodies that are capable of inhibiting GTP binding recognize two major regions of the p21 protein: one region localized from amino acids 5 to 69 and the other region comprising amino acids 107 to 164. Both regions are separated by an amino acid sequence stretch from residues 70 to 106, whose antigenic determinants are not directly involved in GTP binding.

The amino-terminal part of p21[*ras*] proteins is apparently necessary for the transforming capacity of the protein because a transient reversion of v-K-*ras*-transformed cells is observed upon microinjection into the cells of antibodies specific for amino acid 12 of the p21[v-*ras*] protein.[279] An antibody that specifically recognizes the substitution of serine for glycine at position 12 of v-K-*ras* p21 blocks binding of GTP to p21 and, conversely, guanine nucleotides prevent interaction of the antibody with p21.[280] Thus, both the amino-terminal part of p21[*ras*] molecules, involved in guanine nucleotide binding, and the carboxy-terminal region, involved in its localization to the inner aspect of the cell membrane, are apparently required for the expression of transforming capacity of oncogene *ras* proteins (v-*ras* or mutant c-*ras* proteins). Models of the tertiary structure of p21[*ras*] may contribute to a better understanding of the functional properties of the molecule.[233,281]

2. Mutational Analysis of the *ras* Gene

Mutational analysis may contribute to a better definition of the functional domains of p21[*ras*] proteins.[282,283] A chimeric full-length cDNA composed of the v-H-*ras* gene in the amino-terminal region and the N-*ras* gene in the remaining region was constructed, and its expression in *E. coli* resulted in the production of large amounts of the chimeric v-H-*ras*/N-*ras* protein.[284] The study of artificially generated deletions of small sequences from the v-H-*ras* gene and the resulting mutant p21[v-*ras*] proteins expressed in *E. coli* has yielded interesting results.[285] Whereas two small regions located at positions 5 to 23 and 152 to 165 of the p21 product are absolutely required for *in vitro* and *in vivo* activities of the protein, being probably involved in GTP binding, a variable region comprising amino acids 165 to 184 was shown to be dispensable for the same biological activities. It was concluded that GTP binding is required for the transforming activity of p21[*ras*] products and that the variable region at the carboxyl terminal end of the molecule is apparently not required for this activity.[285]

Some particular types of artificial *ras* gene point mutations can abolish the guanine nucleotide binding properties of p21[*ras*] proteins.[286] Mutations of the c-*ras* gene changing asparagine-116 into either a lysine or a tyrosine residue in the p21 protein result in proteins that have lost their ability to bind guanine nucleotides and that do not transform NIH/3T3 cells as do the wild-type gene. On the other hand, amino acid substitutions at position 12 of p21[*ras*] do not modify the GTP or GDP binding ability of the protein, which makes the possibility of a direct contribution of this residue to the binding site unlikely.[287]

Molecular vectors containing either the normal human c-H-*ras* gene or its mutant T24/EJ version have been constructed and expressed in *E. coli*.[266,288] A 576-bp DNA-encoding human c-H-*ras* p21 mutant protein with a valine codon at position 12 has been totally synthesized by chemical methods.[289] A plasmid vector containing the chemically synthetic gene was efficiently expressed in *E. coli* under the control of a tryptophan promoter situated upstream of the gene. The p21 products of both the normal and mutant c-H-*ras* genes expressed in such vectors bind guanine nucleotides in approximately equal amounts but a marked decrease in GTPase activity was observed in the mutant p21 protein. In the absence of Mg^{2+}, GTPase activity of the normal *ras* proteins is about tenfold higher than that of p21 proteins containing amino acid substitutions at position 12.[290] The cytoplasmic GTPase activating protein (GAP) appears to stimulate the GTPase activity of the normal p21, but not that of the oncogenic p21[c-ras] containing a mutation at position 12.[291] Thus, the mutant p21 protein would remain unaltered in the active GTP-bound state. GAP is ubiquitous in the cells of higher eukaryotes and can be essential for p21 biological activity.[292] GAP appears to bind to the effector binding site of mammalian c-*ras* proteins and may translocate from the cytosol to the membrane through association with the GTP-bound form of p21.

Expression vectors have been constructed which encode two truncated forms of the T24 variant protein.[260] One of the truncated proteins was deleted between residues 1 and 23 at the amino terminus and the other truncated protein was deleted for 23 residues at the carboxyl terminus. The full-length c-H-*ras* wild-type and T24 variant proteins produced by the respective vectors in *E. coli* retained guanine nucleotide binding properties in essential equimolar amounts. The carboxyl terminal truncated *ras* protein also retained the ability to bind GTP and, although the extent of binding was somewhat reduced, it was apparent that the carboxy-terminal 23 amino acid residues are not a crucial part of the guanine nucleotide binding site. The carboxy-terminal truncated molecule, however, had lost its transforming capacity, probably as a result of the inability to localize properly to the inner face of the plasma membrane. In contrast, the amino-terminal truncated *ras* protein was completely deficient in guanine nucleotide binding, which suggests that amino acids of this region are part of the nucleotide binding site.[260]

Expression vectors have also been used to construct plasmids which are able to direct the synthesis in *E. coli* of the v-K-*ras* and human c-K-*ras* gene products.[293] After induction, up to 20% of the total bacterial protein may be represented by the *ras* protein and the protein synthesized by the bacteria is active in GTP binding. The products of constructed mutant *ras* genes containing amino acid substitutions at codons 83, 119, or 144 show decreased affinity for GTP by a factor of 25 to 100, primarily as a consequence of increased rates of dissociation of GTP from p21.[294] Nevertheless, these artificial mutant genes induce transformation of NIH/3T3 cells with efficiencies comparable to that of v-H-*ras*. Thus, a role for GTP binding in *ras*-induced oncogenic transformation is not readily apparent on the basis of the results obtained in such experiments. Mutants of p21 with substitutions of threonine-59 exhibit a three- to ninefold higher rate of GDP and GTP release than normal p21 or mutants with other activating lesions.[295] This alteration in the threonine-59 mutant would have the effect of increasing its rate of nucleotide exchange. These findings support a model in which the p21-GTP complex is the biologically active form of the p21 protein.

The 23-kDa (p23) protein product of the human R-*ras* gene has high conservation of amino acids in the region corresponding to the proposed p21 effector region (amino acids 35 to 42). However, this protein cannot be considered as a protooncogene product because it has a function distinct from that of p21[ras] proteins and mutant p23 proteins from the R-*ras* gene do not seem to have oncogenic potential.[296] Analysis of constructed mutant p21 molecules from the H-*ras* gene and p23 molecules from the R-*ras* gene suggests that individual divergences of sequences observed between p21 and p23 proteins may need to be considered within the context of the entire molecule and not as isolated segments of a primary structure.[297]

D. FUNCTIONAL ASPECTS OF P21^{RAS} PROTEINS

The functional properties of p21^{ras} proteins are apparently manifold and remain little characterized. Moreover, the cellular targets for p21^{ras} proteins have not been identified.

1. Relation of p21 Proteins to Cell Cycle Events

Study of human hematopoietic cell lines with a flow cytometric immunofluorescence assay indicates that p21^{c-ras} proteins are equally expressed in all phases of the cell cycle.[298] However, other studies have shown that normal c-*ras* gene activity may increase specifically in late G_1 and that the c-*ras* gene products are required at that time to stimulate cellular events that are needed to initiate DNA replication in serum-stimulated mouse fibroblasts.[299,300] Similar results have been obtained with murine splenic T lymphocytes stimulated with concanavalin A and IL-2, in which the levels of c-H-*ras*-specific RNA are low at early times after stimulation but increase towards the onset of DNA synthesis.[301] The oncogenic p21^{v-ras} product of K-MuSV can stimulate Ca^{2+}- and serum-deprived *ts*K-NRK cells to transit G_1, replicate DNA, and ultimately divide, despite severe Ca^{2+} and serum deficiencies and without help from exogenous growth factors.[302] Thus, at least in some cellular systems the v-K-*ras* protein behaves as a complete mitogen, and this abnormal multifunctional activity may be related to its oncogenic potential.

2. p21 Proteins and the Adenylate Cyclase System

Regulation of the adenylate cyclase system and the intracellular levels of cAMP may be altered by action of v-*ras* proteins,[303,304] which could be due to their homology with G proteins involved in regulation of the adenylate cyclase system. Adenylate cyclase activity is significantly reduced in NIH/3T3 cells expressing the mutant EJ p21^{c-ras} protein.[305] The proteolytic degradation of cAMP-binding proteins is effectively inhibited by c-H-*ras* proteins. This degradation can possibly be carried out by thiol protein kinases.[306] Moreover, the activities of cathepsins B and L are inhibited by c-H-*ras* proteins and there is amino acid homology between c-H-*ras* proteins and thiol proteinase inhibitors such as cystatin.

3. p21 Proteins and Phosphoinositide Metabolism

The physiologic effects of c-*ras* proteins appear to be intimately coupled to phosphoinositide metabolism. The levels of inositol 1,4-bisphosphate and inositol 1,4,5-trisphosphate are elevated in *ras*-transformed NRK cells, in comparison to the nontransformed parental cells.[307] These changes may result in an increased production of 1,2-diacylglycerol and activation of the Ca^{2+}/phospholipid-dependent enzyme, protein kinase C.[308] They could be the consequence of a direct activation of phospholipase C by p21 products. Mutant c-*ras* products would activate the phospholipase C constitutively, thus enhancing the basal level of inositol phospholipid breakdown.[309]

4. Functional Domains of p21 Protein Molecules

Functional domains of p21^{ras} molecules can be characterized by use of chimeric genes.[310] Besides the intramolecular autophosphorylation at threonine-59 of the the viral *ras* proteins, no kinase activity has been detected in p21^{ras} proteins. Apparently, the GTP complex of p21 is required for biological activity and GDP bound to p21 would have to be released and replaced by GTP to activate p21.[263] GTP-binding mutants of p21^{ras} can be isolated by using an *in situ* colony-binding assay.[294] Residues lysine-16 and asparagine-119 play critical roles in the guanine nucleotide binding and biological functions of the H-*ras*-encoded protein.[311] Substitution of an asparagine residue for lysine-16 reduces the affinity of p21^{ras} for GDP and GTP by a factor of 100, and replacement of asparagine-119 with an alanine residue reduces the affinity of p21^{ras} for the same guanine nucleotides by a factor of 20. The c-H-*ras* protein with alanine at position 119 shows enhanced ability to induce transformation in NIH/3T3 cells, as demonstrated in microinjection experiments with the purified protein.[311]

p21^{ras} proteins may contain domains involved in functions which remain still unidentified. Microinjection of a monoclonal antibody, designated Y13-259, which recognizes a shared epitope of p21^{ras} proteins, specifically blocks the serum-induced mitogenic response of tissue culture cells.[300] The Y13-259 antibody does not interact directly with the GTP binding site of p21^{ras} molecule nor interfere with its associated GTPase or autophosphorylation activities.[312] This antibody binds specifically to a small region of around ten amino acid residues at positions 70 to 81 of the p21 coding sequence, which represents a region of the molecule very highly conserved in *ras* proteins from yeast to humans.[312] Protein products of v-H-*ras* deletion mutants lacking at least one codon from the segment encoding amino acid residues 64 to 76 of the p21 product are not immunoprecipitated by monoclonal antibody Y13-259.[313] NIH/3T3 cells transformed by the wild-type v-H-*ras* gene decrease their DNA synthesis and revert to a morphological normal appearance after microinjection with Y13-259. In contrast, cells transformed by deletion mutants not immunoprecipitated by this antibody continue to undergo DNA synthesis and retain the morphological appearance of transformed cells.[313]

E. EXPRESSION OF C-*RAS* PROTEINS IN NORMAL TISSUES

Studies with immunohistochemical methods using specific monoclonal antibodies have shown that p21^{c-ras} proteins are expressed in almost every fetal and adult mammalian tissue, although the levels of expression exhibit wide variations according to the type of cell and its functional state. In some human and rat tissues, expression of p21^{c-ras} proteins correlates with cell proliferation, but in other tissues high levels of these proteins are expressed in fully differentiated cells.[314,315] In many tissues the level of p21^{c-ras} is significantly higher in immature cells than in cells corresponding to later stages of differentiation. Human fetal thymocytes stain strongly for p21^{c-ras}, while cells in adult lymph nodes do not.[314] Fetal and adult stratified epithelia progenitor cells located in the basal and suprabasal layers of tissues like the skin and the gastrointestinal and urinary tracts usually stain more intensely than do cells undergoing terminal differentiation, located in the upper layers.

The study of whole organs may not give accurate information on the expression of p21^{c-ras} proteins at the cellular level. In the rat, the distal tubules of the kidney exhibit high levels of p21 expression, while no detectable levels of this product occur in the glomeruli and proximal tubules.[315] The highest level of p21 expression among mammalian tissues is found in the brain, especially in mature neurons. These observations indicate that p21^{c-ras} proteins may be involved in the control of some specialized cellular functions. The exact nature of these functions is unknown, however. The results further suggest that the high levels of p21 expression found in certain malignant tissues may not be causally associated with the process of neoplastic transformation, but may only reflect the increased rate of cellular proliferation that is characteristically associated with cancer.

F. ROLE OF C-*RAS* PROTEINS IN CELL PROLIFERATION AND CELL DIFFERENTIATION

The functional properties of c-*ras* genes are related to both cell proliferation and cell differentiation as well as to other biological processes which remain poorly characterized. The type of cell and its developmental stage, as well as the predominant environmental conditions, are of great importance in determining the response to p21^{c-ras} proteins.

1. Cell Cycle-Associated Events

The protein products of c-*ras* genes are present in actively proliferating tissues such as hematopoietic cells. The role of c-*ras* proteins in the events associated to the cell cycle remains uncertain, however. Infection of NRK cells with *ts* mutants of K-MuSV suggests that c-*ras* proteins may be required for both G$_1$ progression and G$_2$ transit of cells through the cell cycle.[316] Expression of c-H-*ras* p21 protein is cell cycle dependent in human tumor cell lines, with the levels increasing manifold in G_1 and remaining at increased levels during S and $G_2 + M$.[317] The threshold level of expression of S phase cells was used to subdivide the G_1 cell population into cells with low (G_{1A}) and high (G_{1B}) p21 content. The p21 levels of G_{1B} cells were approximately ten times higher than those in G_{1A} cells. These observations suggested that the levels of p21 are much lower at the onset of the cell cycle than at its end; hence a drop in p21 expression may occur during or immediately after mitotic division.[317] However, a role in regulating the events of cell cycle progression could not be unequivocally assigned to c-H-*ras* p21 protein.

Systematic analysis of the expression of c-*ras* genes (c-H-*ras*, c-K-*ras*, and N-*ras*) in mouse tissues has shown that there are substantial variations in the amounts of mRNA transcripts from these genes among different organs and tissues, especially for N-*ras*.[318] The highest levels of expression of some of these genes, e.g., c-H-*ras*, are found in nonproliferating tissues like muscle and brain. It is thus clear that, although c-*ras* proteins may be in some way involved in the processes related to cell proliferation and cell differentiation, a simple association between the expression of c-*ras* genes and the control mechanisms of cell proliferation and cell differentiation does not appear to exist.

2. Hormone- and Growth Factor-Regulated Processes

The possible involvement of c-*ras* proteins in functions other than the control of cell proliferation is suggested by their presence in neural tissues, including brain.[319,320] Molecular vectors carrying activated c-*ras* genes, or microinjection of an activated (mutated) p21[c-*ras*] protein, can induce differentiation in the rat pheochromocytoma cell line PC12, with neurite outgrowth and cessation of cell division.[321-323] This differentiation can occur in the absence of the specific growth factor (NGF) which is usually required for PC12 cell differentiation. Microinjection of anti-p21[ras] antibody into PC12 cells inhibits neurite formation and produces temporary regression of partially extended neurites, which suggests that p21[ras] is involved in the initiation phase of NGF-induced neurite formation in PC12 cells.[324] The results suggest that p21[ras] proteins may have a role in growth factor-mediated cellular responses associated with cell differentiation and distinct from cell proliferation.

Proteins p21[ras] may have an important role in mediating hormone-induced maturation of amphibian oocytes.[325] Microinjection of monoclonal antibodies against the p21[ras] protein into *Xenopus laevis* oocytes results in acceleration of progesterone-induced germinal vesicle breakdown.[326] The effects of one of these antibodies were correlated with *in vitro* inhibition of adenylate cyclase activity in a concentration-dependent manner. The results suggest that p21[ras] proteins interact with the pathway of normal cell division regulated by progesterone and that regulation of vertebrate cell division by *ras* gene products may also involve regulation of adenylate cyclase activity.[326] On the other hand, microinjection of monoclonal antibody (Y13-259) against p21[ras] proteins markedly reduces *Xenopus* oocyte maturation after induction with insulin.[327] The results suggest that p21[c-*ras*] has a role in the events associated with amphibian oocyte maturation and that insulin induces maturation of oocytes by a different pathway than that of steroid hormones. However, there is evidence that the oocyte maturation effect of both steroid hormones and insulin is mediated by the appearance of a common cytoplasmic meiosis- or maturation-promoting activity (MPF).

Induction of c-*ras* gene expression may be dissociated from the induction of DNA synthesis and cell proliferation in particular systems. In the uterus of ovariectomized mice, estradiol-17 β induces luminal epithelial DNA synthesis which begins 6 to 8 h after administration of the hormone and reaches a maximum at 12 to 15 h, when essentially all cells are engaged in DNA synthesis. By 15 h the cells enter into mitosis and the cell number doubles. Progesterone treatment completely suppresses this proliferative response. At the peak of DNA synthesis, the mRNA levels of c-H-*ras* and ornithine decarboxylase genes are significantly increased, but progesterone treatment, although inhibiting the wave of DNA synthesis, does not greatly influence the levels of these two mRNAs.[328] Thus, in the uterine luminal epithelium estradiol regulates the levels of c-H-*ras* and ornithine decarboxylase expression independently of cell proliferation. These results indicate that the p21 product of the c-H-*ras* gene cannot act as a positive regulator of DNA synthesis and cell proliferation in a way independent of other control mechanisms.[328]

Expression of a normal N-*ras* gene attached to a constructed steroid hormone-inducible transcription unit in NIH/3T3 mouse cells leads to stimulation of DNA synthesis, and this effect is augmented in the presence of EGF.[329] Very high levels of N-*ras* expression in the cells containing the plasmid vector eventually result in the expression of a transformed phenotype. Infection of immune mast cells by H-MuSV results in the enhancement of cell growth and induction of immortalization without affecting differentiation or altering the requirements for the specific growth factor, IL-3.[330] The H-MuSV-infected cells appear to be phenotypically identical to the immune mast cells found in uninfected cultures and, although they express high levels of p21^{v-ras}, they continue to require the growth factor for proliferating *in vitro*.

G. HOMOLOGIES OF THE C-*RAS* PROTEINS

Homology was detected between the human c-*ras* products and the β subunit of mitochondrial and bacterial ATP-synthase.[331] Comparison of amino acid sequences revealed the presence of multiple homologous regions common to all members of the human c-*ras* family and the bacterial elongation factors Tu (EF-Tu) and G (EF-G), which also contain in their aminoterminal region a binding site for GTP.[332,333] Mammalian polypeptide chain elongation factor 2 (EF-2) also shows homology with human c-H-*ras* protein.[334] The α subunit of mammalian G proteins, which are GTP-binding proteins,[335] has striking homology with the c-*ras* proteins, which suggests that both protein families (G proteins and c-*ras* proteins) may be derived from a common ancestor molecule.[336]

In the visual transducing system a G protein analogue, transducin, regulates GMP concentrations in the rod outer segment by inactivating a specific phosphodiesterase and a portion of the amino-terminal peptide sequence of transducin α subunit and bovine brain G protein shows homology to p21^{ras}.[337-339] Transducin functions in the retina to couple the photolysis of rhodopsin to changes in intracellular levels of GMP. In the retina, light stimulates the interaction of transducin with rhodopsin, which results in exchange of GDP, bound to the alpha subunit of transducin, for GTP. The complex formed by transducin-GTP activates a cyclic GMP (cGMP) phosphodiesterase and the process is terminated when the intrinsic GTPase activity of transducin α subunit hydrolyzes the bound GTP, restoring the transducin-GDP complex. The polypeptide sequences of bovine transducin α subunit, as predicted from the respective cDNA, has a 39,971 mol wt and the protein is composed of 350 amino acids.[340] The predicted sequence of transducin α subunit includes four segments, ranging from 11 to 19 residues in length, that exhibit significant homology to sequences of GTP-binding proteins, including the stimulatory (G_s) and inhibitory (G_i) coupling proteins of hormone-sensitive adenylate cyclase, the elongation factors of ribosomal protein synthesis in bacteria, EF-G and EF-Tu, the translation initiation factor IF2, and the c-*ras* proteins of man and yeast.

Although structural similarities suggest similar functions, the functional products of the *ras* and G protein families could be different. Whereas G proteins are involved in control of general cellular functions and metabolism the protein products of c-*ras* genes could be mainly involved in the control of cell proliferation. No direct evidence has been found that p21^{ras} regulates adenylate cyclase activity in a manner similar to G proteins.[341] However, p21 K-*ras* protein stimulates adenylate cyclase activity early in the G_1 phase of the cell cycle of NRK cells.[342] Moreover, the human c-H-*ras* p21 product inhibits the proteolytic cleavage of the regulatory subunit of cAMP-dependent protein kinase, which may be due to thiol proteinase-inhibitor activity of p21 proteins.[343] On the other hand, there is evidence that cAMP and its receptor protein kinase may be involved in a quantitative modulation of *ras* oncogene expression. Treatment of H-MuSV-infected NIH/3T3 cells with two classes of cAMP analogs results in a synergistic inhibition of both p21^{ras} synthesis and phenotypic transformation. Thus, at least some of the effects of cAMP on cell proliferation could be mediated by regulation of p21^{c-ras} synthesis and expression.

H. MECHANISMS OF ACTION AND CELLULAR TARGETS OF *RAS* PROTEINS

The mechanisms of action and cellular targets of p21^{ras} proteins remain poorly characterized but it is known that p21 proteins are associated with the plasma membrane. The p21 protein product of H-MuSV, as well as the oncogene products of RSV and A-MuLV, are tightly bound to cellular lipid on the inner surface of the plasma membrane.[344]

1. Association of p21 Proteins with the Plasma Membrane

The *ras* proteins may play a role in the signal transduction processes across the cell membrane in different biological systems. These proteins are involved in the stimulation of cell surface ruffling and fluid-phase pinocytosis, as demonstrated by the specific inhibition of these processes in cells microinjected with anti-*ras* antibodies.[345] Amino acids located at or near the carboxy terminus of p21 proteins are required for lipid binding, membrane association, and cellular transformation.[346] The study of carboxyl-terminal point mutants of the protein indicates that a simple cysteine residue at position 186 is involved in both the lipid binding and the membrane localization of p21^{v-ras}.[347] A synthetic tetrapeptide of p21 carboxy terminus has been used to identify the acylation site of p21 as cysteine-186 and the lipid moiety of the hydrophobic peptide has been recognized as palmitic acid.[348] The lipid may be bound to p21 through the cysteine-186, probably via a thio-ether or a thiol-ester linkage to diacylglycerol. Since cysteine occupies the same location in all known *ras* oncogene proteins, it may serve a similar function in the other *ras* proteins as well. This function is probably associated with the membrane localization of the *ras* proteins.[250] However, palmitic acid is present in only a minor subpopulation of p21^{v-ras} molecules generated in MuSV-infected cells and other undetected posttranslational modifications of p21^{v-ras} products may be important for the association of these products with the cell membrane.[251] In addition to palmitoylation, *ras* proteins are posttranslationally modified by a methylation reaction.[349] Esterification of *ras* proteins by cellular methyltransferases may contribute to regulate their interaction with plasma components.

2. Guanine Nucleotide Binding

The p21 proteins encoded by v-*ras* oncogenes consist of at least two functional domains, one which specifies the p21 guanine nucleotide binding activity and the other which is involved in the p21-membrane association in transformed cells. Experiments with site-directed mutagenesis indicate that conservation of a functional GTP binding site may be essential for the function of p21 proteins.[286] However, the results of other studies using similar procedures show that p21 proteins with a significant reduction (10- to 5000-fold) in GTP binding activity may have unaltered ability to transform NIH/3T3 cells.[35] In general, there is a lack of correlation between guanine nucleotide binding or GTPase activity and transforming potency of p21 proteins.[351] The portions of G proteins or *ras* proteins that are not directly involved in nucleotide binding or hydrolysis may determine the specificity for interaction with different cellular macromolecules and the respective specific functional properties of these proteins in each tissue.

3. Regulation of Phosphoinositide Metabolism and Interaction with Growth Factor Receptors

The protein products of c-*ras* protooncogenes appear to be involved in the regulation of phosphoinositide metabolism through modification of phospholipase C activity.[352,353] NIH/3T3 cells expressing the mutated EJ c-H-*ras* gene, or elevated levels of the normal human c-H-*ras* gene, exhibit markedly reduced PDGF-stimulated phospholipase C activity and PGE$_2$ biosynthesis. However, the exact relationship between the p21 proteins and the metabolism of phospholipids is not understood at present. Proteins encoded by *ras* genes could induce modifications in the receptors for hormones or growth factors. It has been suggested that the N-*ras* gene encodes a G-like protein, G_p, which couples the receptors for certain growth factors to changes in phosphoinositide metabolism elicited through stimulation of phospholipase C.[354] Expression of the N-*ras* p21 protein would then stimulate cell growth by enhancing cellular sensitivity to growth factors. The p21^{c-ras} proteins possess inhibitory activity against cathepsin L, a protease involved in the degradation of various proteins, including the EGF receptor.[355] The cleavage of EGF receptors by cathepsin L is inhibited by p21 proteins in a dose-dependent fashion. These results raise the possibility that p21 proteins can suppress the degradation of growth-related proteins such as the EGF receptor and thereby affect cell proliferation and/or differentiation. In a set of mouse C3H/10T1/2 cell lines transfected with a mutated T24 c-H-*ras* gene, there was a good correlation between the metastatic potential, the extent of *ras* expression, and the amount of the secreted protease cathepsin L.[356]

4. Modification of Protein Phosphorylation

Although p21^{ras} proteins are devoid of kinase activity for exogenous or endogenous substrates, they may influence the phosphorylation of cellular proteins through indirect pathways. There is evidence that p21 can stimulate or inhibit phosphorylation of specific mitochondrial membrane proteins.[357] A 38-kDa protein present in rat liver plasma membrane is also phosphorylated *in vitro* by the influence of p21^{ras} proteins of either viral or cellular origin.[358] The physiologic significance of p21^{ras}-induced changes in protein phosphorylation is unknown.

5. Alteration of Gene Expression

The p21 proteins encoded by c-*ras* genes may be involved, probably through through indirect pathways, in the control of gene expression in particular types of cells. An activated c-H-*ras* gene, but not a v-K-*ras* oncogene, can induce high levels of expression of metallothionein mRNA in T24 human bladder carcinoma and HS578 mammary carcinosarcoma cell lines.[359] The biological significance of this induction is unknown. Metallothioneins are ubiquitous, cysteine-rich proteins that bind heavy metals such as zinc, copper, and cadmium, but their levels are regulated in relation to cell growth and they may have a role in developmental processes. An activated c-H-*ras* gene can activate the polyoma virus enhancer in a myeloma cell line.[360] Since a similar effect is produced by the phorbol ester TPA, this activation is probably mediated by protein kinase C.

I. MAMMALIAN *RAS*-RELATED GENES

The mammalian genome contain some DNA sequences related to c-*ras* genes. A *ras*-related gene, *ral*, was isolated from a cDNA library of immortalized simian B lymphocytes by the use of a synthetic probe.[361] The *ral* gene codes for a 206-amino acid protein of predicted molecular weight of 23.5-kD that shares more than 50% homology with the c-*ras* gene proteins. The GTP binding region of p21^{ras} and a carboxy-terminal cystein involved in membrane anchoring are also present in the *ral* product, which strongly suggests that this product is a GTP-binding protein with membrane localization.

The 23.4-kDa (p23) protein product of a *ras*-related gene, termed R-*ras*, detected in the human genome by virtue of nucleic acid sequence homology to v-H-*ras*, may have biochemical properties similar to those of the H-, K-, and N-*ras* protooncogenes.[296,297] The predicted R-*ras* p23 protein is 218 amino acids long and its structure is similar to that of p21^{ras} proteins and other members of the GTP-binding protein superfamily. However, p21 and p23 *ras* proteins may have different functions.

J. EVOLUTIONARY ASPECTS OF THE *RAS* GENE FAMILY

DNA sequences homologous to mammalian c-*ras* genes are widely distributed among the animal kingdom. The conservation of these sequences suggest that they are associated with some essential functions. A *ras*-related protein, termed Era, is encoded by the *era* gene of *Escherichia coli*.[362] The bacterial Era protein has GTPase activity and is essential for cell growth.

1. Chicken

In addition to authentic c-*ras* genes, other genes related to *ras* sequences are present in the chicken. A chicken DNA sequence structurally related to the *ras* family (22% identity) is represented by the processed pseudogene CPS1, which contains a polyadenylation signal and an open reading frame that may encode for a 175-amino acid protein.[363] Another DNA sequence, highly related to CPS1, may constitute a gene which is active in the chicken, but only during early development. These facts indicate the general biological importance of the c-*ras* and c-*ras*-related protein products.

2. Mollusks

DNA sequences related to mammalian c-*ras* genes are present in the genome of the marine mollusk *Aplysia californica*, and sequencing of these sequences revealed a putative exon that encodes amino acids sharing 68% homology with residues 5 to 54 of mammalian p21^{c-ras} proteins.[364] The *Aplysia* c-*ras*-like protein is most abundantly expressed in terminally differentiated, nonproliferating neuronal cell bodies and axonal processes.

3. Insects

Three c-*ras* genes expressed in *Drosophila* are subjected to developmental regulation.[365] Each of these genes codes for one large transcript and for one or two smaller transcripts, which may be attributed to differential promotion, splicing, or processing. The larger transcript of each gene is present in a constant abundance at all stages of development, whereas the shorter transcripts are found mainly in embryos.

4. Yeast

Sequences related to *ras* genes are present in yeast,[217,366,367] which suggests that the mechanisms involved in the control of cell division in yeast and vertebrates may be related or similar.[368] Five *ras*-related genes (*RAS*-1, *RAS*-2, *YPT*, *RHO*-1, and *RHO*-2) have been identified in the yeast *Saccharomyces cerevisiae*. The genes *RAS*-1 and *RAS*-2 have been cloned from *S. cerevisiae*, their nucleotide sequences have been determined, and the respective p21 products have been identified.[369-371] These two genes are transcribed in the wild-type yeast cells and they code for polypeptides of 309 and 322 amino acids, respectively. The predicted p21 products of *RAS*-1 and *RAS*-2 are about 70% homologous to mammalian p21^{c-ras}, and the homology is distributed over the first 180 amino acid residues of both *RAS*-1 and *RAS*-2. Transcriptional analysis of mutant yeast *RAS* genes indicates a differential control at the level of their expression.[372] The yeast *ras* genes are functionally homologous to mammalian *ras* genes, being involved in the control of adenylate cyclase, and the *ras*-2 protein exhibit guanine nucleotide binding activity similar to that possessed by mammalian p21^{c-ras}.[373-379] However, a comparison of the amino acid sequences of yeast *ras* proteins with the α subunit of bovine adrenal G$_s$ protein, which is involved in stimulation of adenylate cyclase, shows very little homology.[380] The homology existing between the yeast RAS proteins and the mammalian a subunit of G$_s$ is limited to very short regions that appear to be involved in GTP binding and hydrolysis. A *ras*-like protein present in yeast, termed Sec4, exhibits 325 homology with K-*ras* and is a GTP-binding protein that plays an essential role in controlling a late stage of the yeast secretory pathway.[381]

The *RAS*-2 gene of *S. cerevisiae* is required for gluconeogenic growth and proper response to nutrient limitation.[382] The reserve carbohydrates in yeast are glycogen and trehalose and, as with glycogen in higher cells, their degradative enzymes are activated by cAMP-dependent phosphorylation processes. Consequently, yeast *RAS*-2 mutants are affected in reserve carbohydrates and growth when placed on media with pyruvate or other noncarbohydrate carbon sources.[383] Glucose acts on *S. cerevisiae* to stimulate phosphoinositide turnover, inducing Ca^{2+} mobilization and cAMP formation, which may result in cell proliferation, and *RAS*-encoded proteins are involved in the regulation of these changes in the yeast cell.[384] Yeast cells that lack functional *RAS*-1 and *RAS*-2 genes are ordinarily nonviable,[385,386] but may remain viable if they carry a c-H-*ras* gene of mammalian origin.[374,386,387] These results indicates that yeast *ras* protein products, although more than 50% larger than their mammalian counterparts, have similar functional activities. The amino-terminal domain of the yeast *ras*-1 product binds GTP and GDP and has GTP hydrolytic activity. Moreover, the latter activity is reduced in variant *ras*-1 proteins which are structurally analogous to oncogenic human c-*ras* proteins that also show diminished GTPase activity.[388]

The 23.5-kDa protein encoded by the *YPT* gene of *S. cerevisiae* is essential to growth and is required for cell viability.[389,390] Functional loss of the *ypt* protein product of the *YPT* gene results in distinct microtubule defects. The *ypt* protein of yeast binds GTP specifically, is able to hydrolyze GTP, and a mutant form of the protein with an amino acid substitution within one of the highly conserved protein regions possesses authophosphorylating activity.[391] Moreover, some mutations of the *ypt* protein give rise to distinct lesions of cellular growth. Mutational analysis of the *YPT* gene indicates that two cysteines contained in the carboxy-terminal end of the *ypt* protein are required for full functional activity and that at least one of these two residues is required for palmitic acid binding.[392] Thus, the biochemical and functional properties of the proteins produced by *RAS* and *YPT* genes of yeast and c-*ras* genes of mammalian cells are very similar. Proteins related to *ypt* of yeast are ubiquitous in eukaryotic cells and have been detected in mouse, rat, pig, bovine, and human cell lines.[393] The mouse *ypt*-1 protein has 71% amino acid identity with the protein product with the protein product of the *YPT*-1 gene of *S. cerevisiae*. Screening of a rat brain cDNA library with specific oligonucleotide probes resulted in the isolation of four genes, termed *rab*-1 to *rab*-4, encoding proteins homologous to the yeast *YPT* product.[394] The product of the *rab*-1 gene, which is probably identical to *ypt*-1, exhibited 75% amino acid homology with the product of the yeast *YPT* gene. The genes *rab*-3 and *rab*-4 encode proteins of 230 and 213 amino acids, respectively, that share 39 and 42% homology with the *YPT*-encoded product and around 30% homology with mammalian p21[c-ras] products.[395] The functions of the proteins produced by *RHO* genes of yeast are still little known.

Another yeast species, *Schizosaccharomyces pombe*, possesses a single *ras* gene, *RAS*-1, which encodes a protein 219 amino acids long.[396] The function of the *S. pombe ras*-1 protein product is apparently different from that of *Saccharomyces cerevisiae ras*-1 and *ras*-2 proteins, according to the following aspects: (1) disruption of *Schizosaccharomyces pombe ras*-1 interferes neither with the growth rate nor with the assimilation of carbon sources, but results in the complete loss of the ability to mate, (2) loss of its activity does not stimulate but rather represses sporulation, and (3) loss of *ras*-1 does not affect the intracellular level of cAMP.[396] These results suggest that the target enzymes presumably modulated by *ras* protein in signal transduction across the plasma membrane are apparently not the same for all organisms. The *ras*-1 gene of *S. pombe* seems to act, at least in part, through activation of a closely related gene, *byr*-1, which encodes a putative 340-amino acid product that may function as a protein kinase.[397]

5. Slime Mold

A p21[ras]-related protein is present in the slime mold *Dictyostelium discoideum*, where it is developmentally regulated.[398-400] The *ras*-related protein of *D. discoideum* has an approximate molecular weight of 23,000 (p23). The cellular level of p23 is highest during vegetative growth of the eukaryotic microbe, when the cells divide quickly, and fall rapidly throughout differentiation, with the exception of a transient burst of synthesis coincident with mitosis during the pseudoplasmodium stage of development. The evidence points to an involvement of normal c-*ras* proteins in cell proliferation.

Phenotypic changes may be induced by mutated *ras* genes during the development of *Dictyostelium* transformants.[401,402] The single *ras* gene of *D. discoideum* was cloned and a missense mutation was artificially introduced at position 12 of the gene product, which resulted in threonine at this position instead of the wild-type glycine. While *D. discoideum* amoebae transformed with the wild-type *ras* gene did not exhibit measurable difference with respect to the normal control in spite of expressing fourfold higher levels of the *ras* gene product, amoebae transformed with the mutated *ras* gene showed aberrant developmental anomalies. Further studies with the normal and mutated *ras* genes of *D. discoideum* indicated that the *ras* gene product is involved in the signal transduction leading from the cell surface cAMP to formation of inositol trisphosphate and polyphosphates.[403] Specifically, the *Dictyostelium ras* gene may code for a regulatory protein involved in the inositol phospholipid signal transduction pathway.

K. MECHANISMS OF *RAS*-ASSOCIATED ONCOGENICITY

Viral *ras* genes or mutant c-*ras* genes are much more efficient in inducing transformation than are their normal cellular counterparts. Injection of the purified v-H-*ras* p21 protein into NIH/3T3 cells is sufficient to induce a transformed morphology and to stimulate cell proliferation.[403] On the other hand, transformation of the same cells is not so pronounced when the normal human p21$^{c\text{-}ras}$ counterpart is injected, and higher concentrations of the protein are required in this case to obtain a morphological change. The normal human c-H-*ras* protooncogene can induce oncogenic transformation of murine fibroblasts when it is ligated to a control element (LTR) which determines the production of high amounts of the p21$^{c\text{-}ras}$ product.[404]

Mutation at codon 12, 13, or 69 of c-*ras* genes result in the synthesis of p21 proteins with oncogenic potential in defined cellular systems. Expression of the mutant p21$^{c\text{-}ras}$ proteins in sensitive cells, including human fibroblasts, may result in neoplastic transformation.[405] Moreover, the use of regulatable molecular vectors carrying c-*ras* genes indicates that there may be a continuum of phenotypic changes in cells transfected with these vectors, according to the levels of mutant c-*ras* protein present within the cell.[405] Inhibition of the production of the altered p21 protein in the transfected cells is associated with reversion of the altered phenotype. In contrast, even high levels of the normal, nonmutated c-*ras* protein are ineffective in inducing neoplastic transformation.

Although the mechanisms associated with oncogenic transformation induced by either v-*ras* or mutant c-*ras* proteins are not understood, there is evidence that multistage phenomena are involved in this process, as it is true for oncogenic processes in general.[407] Cultured murine fibroblasts, such as the NIH/3T3 cells, are usually more susceptible than other types of cells to *ras*-induced transformation and many cell types are totally resistant to the transforming potential of the *ras* oncogenes. Probably, NIH/3T3 cells are already premalignant cells. Experiments with transgenic mice support the concepts that tumorigenesis associated with the expression of mutated c-*ras* genes is a multistage process protracted over a long period of time and that additional genetic alterations are crucially required in order for tumor formation to occur. Mammary gland-specific, hormone-dependent expression of an EJ c-H-*ras* gene introduced into the germ line of transgenic mice resulted in the formation of mammary tumors in only a few of the animals and after a long latency period.[408]

The molecular mechanisms by which altered forms of p21$^{c\text{-}ras}$ proteins can induce neoplastic transformation of susceptible cells have not been elucidated. The human c-K-*ras* gene contains two alternative fourth exons, termed 4A and 4B, and can express two distinct p21$^{c\text{-}ras}$ proteins, termed p21$_{4A}$ and p21$_{4B}$, respectively, which differ only in their carboxy termini.[409] Protein p21$_{4b}$ has a basic carboxy terminus which is not closely related to the carboxy terminus of the K-MuSV-encoded protein. In contrast, the p21$_{4A}$ carboxy terminus is virtually identical to the carboxy terminus encoded by the acute retrovirus, K-MuSV. However, the biochemical and transforming properties of p21$_{4A}$ and p21$_{4B}$, carrying a mutation at codon 12, are similar or identical.[410] These results suggest that the effector functions important for transformation reside in the amino-terminal portion of the p21[c-ras] molecules.

p21[ras] proteins display mitogenic action in certain cellular systems. Early passage nonestablished REF cells are much less responsive than the late passage cells to the introduction of the T24 *ras* protein in terms of threshold concentration required to elicit a mitogenic response.[411] c-*ras* proteins are capable of inducing meiosis in *Xenopus* oocytes,[325] and nuclear microinjection of c-H-*ras* DNA into quiescent normal human fibroblasts also results in mitogenic induction.[412] However, the normal and the mutated (EJ/T24) forms of the protooncogene may be equally effective inducers of mitogenesis. The c-H-*ras* gene, either alone or in combination with the adenovirus E1A gene, is incapable to induce DNA synthesis in terminally, nondividing senescent human cells.[412] On the other hand, the v-K-*ras* oncogene product is capable of inducing immortalization of murine B lymphocytes *in vitro*.[413] The immortalized cell lines obtained with this method retain the characteristics of mature B cells, including hapten-specific binding.

Protooncogenes other than c-*ras* may have an important role in determining the response of the cell to *ras* products with oncogenic potential. A cellular phosphoprotein that may be involved in immortalization and/or transformation phenomena is the p53 tumor antigen.[414,415] There is evidence of a cooperation between the gene encoding p53 and *ras* oncogenes in neoplastic transformation.[416] Transfection of a cloned p53 gene into cells of finite lifespan (cultured adult rat chondrocytes) results in cellular immortality and susceptibility to transformation by a mutant T24 c-H-*ras* oncogene.[417] These results suggest that the cellular p53 antigen is involved in the acquisition of an indefinite lifespan, whereas a mutant c-*ras* oncogene can induce transformation of the immortalized cell.

Genes coding for c-*ras* proteins may have a different role in controlling the proliferation of normal and tumor cells. Microinjection of a monoclonal antibody specific against p21[c-ras] proteins into normal cells results in inhibition of cell proliferation, while most tumor cells continue to proliferate following injection.[418] Tumor cells containing a mutant c-*ras* gene exhibit an intermediate phenotype and are only partially inhibited in proliferation by the injected anti-*ras* antibody. These results suggest that genes which act independently of c-*ras* proteins are in large part responsible for tumor cell proliferation.

L. CONCLUSIONS
Oncogenes from the *ras* family encode proteins of 21 kDa (p21) which are known to bind guanine nucleotides (GTP and GDP) and have GTPase activity. In addition, p21[v-ras], but not p21[c-ras] proteins are capable of authophosphorylation and may have a role in the phosphorylation of specific cellular proteins at the level of the mitochondria and the cell membrane. The roles of c-*ras* proteins in cell proliferation and differentiation as well as in neoplastic transformation are little understood. In many normal tissues, expression of c-*ras* genes is more clearly associated with cell differentiation than with cell proliferation, and the highest levels of expression of particular c-*ras* genes are found in nonproliferating adult tissues such as muscle and brain.[318]

The preparation of monoclonal or polyclonal antibodies raised against various synthetic peptides to probe the structural determinants responsible for GDP/GTP binding, GTPase activity, autophosphorylation, membrane association, and transforming activity of the p21[ras] proteins may contribute to a more clear definition of their functions.[419] The results of a systematical mutational analysis of *ras* proteins by linker insertion-deletion mutagenesis suggests that transforming p21[ras] proteins require membrane localization, guanosine nucleotide binding, and an additional undefined function that may consist in the interaction with an unidentified cellular target.[283] In conclusion, it remains to be determined how p21[ras] proteins carry out their normal functions and the metabolic pathway by which they are able to induce neoplastic transformation.

VII. THE *ABL* ONCOGENE PROTEIN PRODUCT

Abelson murine leukemia virus (A-MuLV) is a replication-defective, acute retrovirus that transforms lymphoid cells and fibroblasts *in vitro* and induces lymphoma *in vivo*.[420-423] The virus arose in a glucocorticoid-treated mouse injected with the chronic transforming retrovirus, M-MuLV, probably by recombination of M-MuLV sequences with cellular DNA. The *abl* oncogene is also transduced by the feline (cat) virus HZ2 FeSV.[424]

A. THE V-*ABL* PROTEIN

The protein product of the A-MuLV oncogene, v-*abl*, is p12$^{gag-abl}$, a 120-kDa phosphoprotein, which contains MuLV-derived *gag* polypeptide sequences at the amino-terminal end fused with the sequences coded by the viral oncogene.[425,426] This protein possesses tyrosine-specific protein kinase activity. Antibodies to phosphotyrosine can be isolated by immunization of rabbits with the v-*abl*-encoded protein[84,427,428] These antibodies can detect a variety of tyrosine-phosphorylated proteins in both normal and transformed cells, including receptors for peptide growth factors and other proteins present in v-*abl*-, v-*src*-, and v-*erb*-B-transformed cell lines.[84] Monoclonal antibodies have also been produced against v-*abl*- and c-*abl*-encoded molecules.[429]

Tyrosine-specific kinase activity is associated with the v-*abl* product expressed in bacteria carrying the v-*abl* gene cloned in molecular vectors.[430-433] The tyrosine kinase activity of the p120$^{gag-abl}$ protein is localized to the amino-terminal region of the molecule, corresponding to the first 1.2 kb of the v-*abl* oncogene.[431] This region of the v-*abl* protein is itself phosphorylated on tyrosine residues and, interestingly, the minimal kinase coding region corresponds to the minimal transforming region of the v-*abl* oncogene. Although the tyrosine kinase is completely independent of the large carboxyl terminal portion of the v-*abl* protein, the latter portion could have a role in regulating the kinase activity. Mouse lymphocytes and fibroblasts transformed by the v-*abl* oncogene show alterations in protein phosphorylation at tyrosine residues.[434] Studies performed with *ts* mutants of A-MuLV indicate that the specific tyrosine protein kinase activity of the v-*abl* product is crucially required for transformation induced by the acute retrovirus.[435,436]

The deduced amino acid sequences of v-*abl* and the human protooncogene c-*abl* indicate a structural relatedness to the catalytic chain of the mammalian cyclic AMP-dependent protein kinase.[437] Microinjection of the protein into *Xenopus* oocytes induces phosphorylation of the ribosomal protein S6 on serine, probably by direct or indirect inactivation of an S6 protein kinase and/or inactivation of an S6 protein phosphatase.[438] The widespread correlation existing between S6 phosphorylation and the growth-promoting actions of many different growth factors and oncogene protein products suggests that S6 phosphorylation plays an important role in the regulation of cell proliferation and/or cell transformation. A-MuLV mutants deficient in protein kinase activity have reduced transforming ability.[439] In A-MuLV-infected cells the v-*abl* protein product is mainly localized at the level of the plasma membrane, especially at the points of adhesion between the cell and the substrate.[440]

Although the specific tyrosine protein kinase activity of the p210$^{gag-abl}$ product is strictly required for the induction of neoplastic transformation in A-MuLV-infected cells, it is insufficient by itself for maintaining the transformed state. A-MuLV-infected mouse cells are able to differentiate without a decrease in the amount expressed or the specific enzymatic activity of the v-*abl* oncogene product.[441]

B. THE C-*ABL* PROTOONCOGENE

The c-*abl* protooncogene is the normal cellular homologue of the v-*abl* oncogene.[442] Sequences related to the mammalian c-*abl* gene are present in all the vertebrate genomes tested so far, as well as in *Drosophila*.[443,444] The c-*abl* DNA sequences of *Drosophila* are located near the 5′ end of a gene, *Dash*, which is transcribed to give both long RNAs (5 to 6 kb) and short RNAs (3 kb) by alternative splicing patterns. *Dash*RNAs are most abundant in eggs and early embryos, become rare during larval development, and return in a burst of activity in early pupae.[445] The c-*abl* gene of *Drosophila* consists of 10 exons extending over 26 kb of DNA and encodes a protein of 1520 amino acids which exhibits sequence homology to the human c-*abl* protooncogene product, beginning at the amino terminus and extending 656 amino acids through the region essential for tyrosine kinase activity.[446] The *Drosophila* c-*abl* product appears to possess, as its mammalian homologue, tyrosine-specific protein kinase activity.[447] There is a substantial maternal contribution to c-*abl* transcripts present in *Drosophila* early embryos, and these transcripts are required for the normal development of the insect. Mutant alleles of the *Drosophila* c-*abl* gene may have pleiotropic effects late in development and may result in lethality at the pupal stage. DNA sequences homologous to the v-*abl* oncogene have also been isolated from and characterized in *Caenorhabditis elegans*.[448]

The human c-*abl* protooncogene is located on chromosome 9, at region 9q34.1.[449] Close linkage has been found between the tuberous sclerosis gene and the c-*abl* protooncogene, which would imply that c-*abl* may be useful as a diagnostic marker for tuberous sclerosis.[450] The human c-*abl* protooncogene sequences are dispersed over a region of around 32 kb containing at least 7 introns, and there are 8 regions of highly repetitive DNA sequences in close proximity to the c-*abl* coding sequences.[451] One of the alternative 5' exons of the human c-*abl* gene lies at least 200 kb upstream of the remaining c-*abl* exons, posing formidable problems for transcription regulation and splicing processes.[452] The c-*abl* exon located at the extreme 5' portion includes an unusually long (1276-bp) segment that contains 15 ATG codons and multiple short open ORFs, upstream of the initiation codon for the c-*abl* protein.

C. EXPRESSION OF THE C-*ABL* PROTOONCOGENE

Transcripts of c-*abl* are present, in some cases at high levels, in many tissues of the mouse as well as in most types of cultured cells, either normal or malignant.[453] Four different cDNAs have been derived from mRNAs of 70Z/3 mouse lymphoid cells and these mRNAs differ at their 5' ends.[454] The mechanisms of origin of the different c-*abl* transcripts as well as the respective functions of these transcripts and their translational products have not been characterized, but there is evidence that cells can use alternating addition of 5' exons in c-*abl* mRNA synthesis.

In the mouse, two larger polyadenylated c-*abl* transcripts of 5.5 and 6.5 kb are present in all tissues, and an additional shorter c-*abl* transcript of 4.0 kb is present in the mature, but not immature, testis.[453,455-458] The 4.0-kb c-*abl* transcript is produced in the testis due to the organ-specific premature termination of transcription (3' truncation), related to the use of an alternative polyadenylation site. No consensus polyadenylation signal exists at this site and the mechanism by which this short mRNA is produced as well as the physiological significance of its synthesis are unknown. The c-*abl* protooncogene may be included in the category of genes that exhibit haploid-stage-specific expression. A 2.7-kb transcript of the *HSP*70 gene is also expressed specifically in the germinal cells of the testis, coincidentally with the entry of the cells into the haploid stage.[459] The functional roles of the 4.7-kb c-*abl* transcript and the 2.7-kb *HSP*7O transcript in the germinal cells of the testis are unknown. However, heat shock proteins are synthesized during normal development and differentiation and the genes coding for these proteins are induced in response to particular types of environmental stress, including mildly elevated temperatures. It is well known that mammalian male germ cells are sensitive to increased temperatures and that the germinal compartment of the testis can be readily destroyed by external stresses.

D. PROTEIN KINASE ACTIVITY OF THE *ABL* PROTEIN PRODUCTS

Tyrosine-specific protein kinase activity was initially not detected in the normal c-*abl* gene protein,[460] and it was proposed that an alteration of the human c-*abl* protein in chronic myelogenous leukemia (CML) cells would result in unmasking of the specific kinase activity.[461,462] Activation of the c-*abl* protooncogene by viral transduction or chromosome translocation would result in the generation of altered c-*abl* proteins with similar *in vitro* kinase activity.[463] However, it has been demonstrated more recently that tyrosine kinase activity is present in the normal c-*abl* protein.[454,464] Thus, a qualitative difference in the kinase activity of v-*abl* and c-*abl* products cannot be responsible for the differences observed in the oncogenic potential of these products.

E. MECHANISMS OF V-*ABL*-INDUCED ONCOGENIC TRANSFORMATION

A possible relationship between v-*abl*, protein-associated tyrosine kinase activity, and neoplastic transformation was suggested by the fact that the minimum transforming region of the v-*abl* oncogene corresponds to the sequences encoding tyrosine kinase activity in amino-terminal region of the protein product.[431,465] v-*abl* genes carrying mutations (small deletions and insertions) constructed within the 5′ 1.2-kb sequences are not able to induce transformation of NIH/3T3 cells and in each case mutations which cause a loss of transforming ability cause also a loss of the specific protein kinase activity.[465] More recently, the study of *ts* tyrosine kinase mutants of v-*abl* has demonstrated that the specific kinase activity is crucial to the transforming function of the v-*abl* product.[435] Moreover, the v-*abl* tyrosine-protein kinase activity is required to maintain the transformed phenotype because cells transformed by the *ts* kinase mutants revert back to normal morphology shortly after a shift to the nonpermissive temperature. However, the cellular substrates responsible for the neoplastic transformation induced by the v-*abl* kinase have not been identified.

Mouse cells infected with F-MuLV become independent of their requirement for specific growth factors and acquire tumorigenic properties after superinfection with A-MuLV, but this change does not depend on the endogenous production of any known growth factor required by the cells.[466] A-MuLV can transform growth factor (IL-2 or IL-3)-dependent mast cells, myeloid cells, or lymphoid cells into growth factor-independent, tumorigenic cells but the transformation is also not associated with the endogenous production of specific growth factors.[467-470] These observations argue against an autocrine type of stimulation as a general mechanism responsible for neoplastic cell transformation. However, in other studies the infection of individual multilineage hematopoietic colonies with A-MuLV resulted in formation of cell lines that expressed features characteristic of mast cells and which produced CSF-2 (GM-CSF).[471] The reason for such discrepancy is unknown but it could be attributed to differences in the target cells or in the experimental protocols. In any case, an autocrine mechanism is not universally associated with the abrogation of growth factor requirement by A-MuLV-infected hematopoietic cells.

Expression of the v-*abl* product may not be incompatible with the expression of differentiated cellular functions. A-MuLV-infected immature B precursor cells can differentiate along a normal pathway in spite of the persistent expression of the v-*abl* oncogene.[472] Specific growth factors can stimulate the differentiation of promyelocytic leukemia cell lines derived from A-MuLV-infected mice.[473] It is possible that activation of a number of cellular genes, which may not necessarily be protooncogenes, is required for transformation induced by A-MuLV.[474] Unfortunately, such genes have not yet been characterized, but there is evidence that the v-*abl* product is able to activate embryonic globin gene expression in mouse erythroleukemia cells.[475] A-MuLV potentiates long-term growth of mature B lymphocytes,[476] which requires the activation of specific cellular genes.

VIII. THE *FES/FPS* ONCOGENE PROTEIN PRODUCT

Several independent isolates of feline sarcoma virus (FeSV) containing the v-*fes* oncogene have been described. The genetic differences between these isolates depend on a diversity of recombinational events that occurred between viral sequences and cellular sequences of the protooncogene c-*fes*, which results in the generation of different polyproteins containing v-*fes*-derived sequences.[477] Two isolates of FeSV, the Gardner-Arnstein (GA-FeSV) and Snyder-

Theilen (ST-FeSV) isolates, encode phosphorylated hybrid proteins of around 115,000 mol wt possessing tyrosine-specific protein kinase activity.[478-480] A tyrosine-specific kinase of lower molecular weight, pp85$^{gag-fes}$, produced by ST-FeSV, was purified and characterized.[481] Both GA-FeSV and ST-FeSV are capable of transforming a diversity of cell types *in vitro,* including testes cells from baboons,[482] and can produce fibrosarcomas in a number of mammalian species *in vivo,* including squirrel monkeys.[483] Another FeSV isolate, the Theilen-Pedersen strain of FeSV (TP-FeSV), encodes for a *gag-onc* fusion protein of 83,000 mol wt.[484] The Hardy-Zuckerman 4 isolate of FeSV (HZ4-FeSV) contains a unique oncogene, v-*kit*, which exhibits partial homology with the tyrosine protein kinase gene family.[10] Proteins encoded by different strains of FeSV form stable noncovalent complexes with two cellular proteins termed pp90 and pp50.[485] The same cellular proteins form complexes with the protein product of RSV,[486] but the function of these complexes, if any, is unknown. Specific phosphorylation of cellular substrates by the v-*fes* products could be involved in the transforming action of the viral oncogene product.

An oncogene closely related to v-*fes* is v-*fps*, which is an avian-derived gene contained in the Fujinami sarcoma virus (FSV).[487,488] The chicken v-*fps* oncogene of PRCII ASV and the chicken c-*fps* protooncogene have been cloned in molecular vectors.[489] The chicken c-*fps* sequences span approximately 6 kb, including a number of introns not represented in v-*fps*. The feline c-*fes* gene has also been cloned in a molecular vector and the construction of a chimeric transforming gene containing c-*fes* sequences has been reported.[490] v-*fes* and v-*fps* DNA sequences correspond to a common cellular genetic locus, termed c-*fes/fps*, which has been highly conserved throughout vertebrate evolution.[491] The protein product of the mammalian c-*fes/fps* protooncogene is a 92-kDa protein, p92$^{fes/fps}$, whereas the avian counterpart is a 98 kD protein, p98$^{fes/fps}$.[492] Both the mammalian and the avian proteins possess tyrosine-specific protein kinase activity. A widely distributed cellular protein with tyrosine kinase activity related to, but distinct from, the c-*fes/fps*-encoded protein has been identified with an antipeptide antiserum.[492]

The transforming protein product of FSV is a *gag-fps* hybrid protein of 130 kDa, p130$^{gag-fps}$, which possesses tyrosine-specific protein kinase activity.[487,488,493] Phosphorylation of the p130$^{gag-fps}$ protein at tyrosine 1073 (a residue which is conserved in all tyrosine-specific protein kinases) augments the enzymatic function of the protein.[494] This phosphorylation is sufficient to reactivate a defective kinase encoded by an FeSV variant which is *ts* for transformation. Mutational analysis of the p130$^{gag-fps}$ product in which the codon for tyrosine-1073 was changed for phenylalanine or serine indicated that the latency periods for tumor formation after inoculation with FSV carrying the mutation were significantly larger than those corresponding to inoculation with wild-type FSV.[495] Similarly, in cultured cells the malignancy-related phenotypic characteristics of the mutant FSV-transformed cell line (Rat-2 cells) were intermediate between those of control Rat-2 cells and Rat-2 cells transformed by the wild-type FSV. The results obtained in these studies strongly suggest that the transforming capacity of FSV is intimately associated with the tyrosine-specific kinase activity of its oncogene protein product.

Whereas the normal human c-*fps/fes* gene does not possess transforming capacity even when expressed at high levels, fusion of the *gag* coding region to the protooncogene coding sequences is sufficient to activate the oncogenic potential of the gene.[496] Although the mechanism of this activation is not clear, the specific kinase activity of the fusion *gag*-c-*fps/fes* product is severalfold higher than that of the unaltered protooncogene product.

The biological activity of the v-*fes/fps* product is modulated by specific phosphorylation processes.[497] A noncatalytic domain of approximately 100 residues, located immediately amino-terminal to the kinase domain of the p130$^{gag-fps}$ product, may serve to direct the interaction of the catalytic domain with specific cellular proteins.[498] These proteins may be either substrates for phosphorylation or regulators of kinase activity important for the transforming ability of the p13$^{gag-fps}$ protein. A 140-kDa phosphoprotein, p140$^{gag-fps}$, encoded by the FL-15 clone of FSV, acquire temperature sensitivity in transformation and kinase activity by point mutations affecting either the 3′ kinase domain or the 5′ domain of v-*fps*.[499]

The oncoproteins of different FeSV isolates and the protein product of the c-*fes/fps* protooncogene may have different subcellular locations.[125-127] The p130$^{gag\text{-}fps}$ protein is associated with cellular membranes either directly as a peripheral membrane protein or indirectly via cytoskeletal elements. In contrast, the majority of the protein of the c-*fes/fps* protooncogene is apparently present in the soluble fraction of the cells. The mechanisms responsible for the transforming actions of FeSV oncogene products are not understood. Interaction of the v-*fps* protein with cellular components may depend on sequences determined by the 5′ portion of the v-*fps* oncogene sequences whereas tyrosine-specific protein kinase activity depends on sequences from the 3′ portion of the oncogene. A lysine residue in the ATP-binding site of p130$^{gag\text{-}fps}$ is essentially required for the associated tyrosine kinase activity of the oncogene product.[503] However, both the 5′ and the 3′ portions of the v-*fps* protein are apparently important in determining its transforming capacity.[504] Transfection of a chimeric gene in which the 3′ half of v-*fes* was replaced with homologous c-*fes* sequences resulted in morphological transformation of the transfected cells.[490]

The transforming properties of the p130$^{gag\text{-}fps}$ protein are tightly associated with the tyrosine-specific kinase activity of the oncogene product. In cells from the Chinese hamster lung fibroblast cell line CCL39 transfected with a plasmid vector containing the v-*fps* oncogene, the level of expressed tyrosine kinase activity dictates whether cells retain the ability to enter quiescence, develop an increased response to particular types of growth factors, and become metastatic.[505] The transfected CCL39 cells are hypersensitive to some growth factors and can become metastatic even when their growth factor requirements are not abrogated, but simply reduced.

A. THE C-*FES/FPS* PROTOONCOGENE AND ITS PROTEIN PRODUCT

The entire nucleotide sequences of the human and feline c-*fes/fps* protooncogene have been determined.[506] The human DNA sequences homologous to v-*fes/fps* are dispersed over 11 kbp and consist of at least 19 exon segments. The normal product of the human c-*fes/fps* protooncogene is a protein of 92 kDa, p92$^{c\text{-}fes}$, which possesses tyrosine-specific protein kinase activity.[496] The deduced amino acid sequence of the human c-*fes/fps* protein is highly homologous to the chicken c-*fes/fps* protein. There is also extensive structural homology between the predicted amino acid sequences of the protein product of the human c-*fes/fps* protooncogene and the products encoded by the v-*abl* and v-*fms* oncogenes, the chicken c-*src* protooncogene, the human EGF receptor gene, and the insulin receptor gene.[506,507] All these products have a tyrosine phosphorylation site embedded in remarkably similar surroundings and possess in a similar position a lysine residue which is believed to be part of the ATP binding site. The amino-terminal border of the ATP-binding site defines the start of minimal v-*fps* tyrosine kinase catalytic domain.[505] This minimal domain is competent to bind substrates. More amino-terminal noncatalytic sequences of the v-*fps* protein appear to functionally interact with the catalytic domain. The precise biological role of the c-*fes/fps* protein is unknown.

B. EXPRESSION OF THE C-*FES/FPS* PROTOONCOGENE

The protein product of the c-*fes/fps* protooncogene is expressed in a tissue-specific fashion, being mainly restricted to hematopoietic tissue.[508] In the chicken the c-*fps* protein is preferentially expressed in macrophages and granulocytic cells.[509] Among murine and human tissues the highest levels of c-*fps* expression are found in resident peritoneal macrophages, followed by bone marrow.[492] The c-*fes/fps* protooncogene is also expressed in peripheral blood monocytes and granulocytes but at lower levels than in their bone marrow precursors, suggesting that c-*fes/fps* expression decrease during hematopoietic cell maturation. The human c-*fes/fps* gene is expressed at detectable levels in myeloid (monocyte/macrophage and granulocytic lineages) but not in lymphoid cell populations.[492,510]

The biological significance of differences in c-*fes/fps* expression among different types of cells is unknown. Because the c-*fes/fps* protein product is a tyrosine-specific protein kinase and the expression of the c-*fes/fps* protooncogene apparently correlates with the capacity of myeloid cells to respond to certain hematopoietic growth factors, it is possible that this protooncogene product could have some functional association with myeloid receptors for colony-stimulating growth factors.[492] However, the precise function of the protein product of this protooncogene remains unknown.

C. THE *FUR* GENE

A transcription unit, *fur*, was characterized in the immediately upstream region of the human c-*fes/fps* protooncogene.[511] The *fur* mRNA is characterized by a long noncoding region at its 3′ end. Although the biological role of the putative *fur* protein is unknown, the observation that in man and cat the linkage of the *fur* and c-*fes/fps* transcription units has been conserved during evolution suggests possible functional implications.[511] The nucleotide sequence of a *fur*-specific cDNA isolated from a human cDNA library revealed an ORF of 1498 bp from which the 499 carboxy-terminal amino acids of the primary *fur* translational product can be deduced.[511] Computer analysis indicated that the putative *fur* protein, furin, has receptor-like features with a cysteine-rich region and a transmembrane domain. It is not yet clear whether *fur* and c-*fes/fps* belong to the same locus or represent independent genes.

Analysis of a number of rat tissues for the presence of *fur* transcripts revealed their differential expression, the highest levels being detected in brain, kidney, and thymus. In the African green monkey, the higher levels of *fur* transcripts are present in liver and kidney, and lower levels occur in brain, spleen, and thymus.[512] The *fur* gene is expressed in some established cell lines, including KG-1 and HeLa cells. Analysis of primary human lung tumors of different histological types revealed a highly selective and strong elevation of *fur* gene expression in non-small cell lung carcinomas, but not in small cell lung carcinomas.[512] These results suggest that *fur* expression can be used to discriminate between these two types of human lung cancer.

D. CONTROL OF THE EXPRESSION OF C-*FES/FPS*-ASSOCIATED KINASE

The levels of expression of tyrosine protein kinase activity associated with protooncogene protein products are strictly controlled in different types of cells. Such control would not operate in the case of tyrosine-specific protein kinases associated with the products of viral oncogenes, which would result in the malignant transformation of the cell. Rat-2 cells transfected with a constructed vector carrying the human c-*fes/fpe* protooncogene express approximately 50-fold more human p92^{c-fes} protein than is found in human myeloid cells, but the cells remain morphologically normal and fail to grow in soft agar.[513] Despite the elevated expression of p92^{c-fes}, the transfected cells do not exhibit a substantial increase in cellular phosphotyrosine and the human p92^{c-fes} product is not itself phosphorylated on tyrosine. In contrast, cells transfected with the v-*fes/fps* oncogene exhibit high levels of phosphotyrosine and become readily transformed.

IX. THE *FGR* ONCOGENE PROTEIN PRODUCT

The translation product of the Gardner-Rasheed isolate of FeSV (GR-FeSV) is a hybrid protein of 70 kDa, p70$^{gag-fgr}$, which contains *gag* sequences fused with sequences from the v-*fgr* oncogene.[514-516] From the nucleotide sequences of the GR-FeSV genome it was deduced that an extensive amino acid sequence homology between the v-*fgr* oncogene product and actin, a eukaryotic cytoskeletal protein, existed.[517] However, it has been shown that the human c-*fgr* protooncogene does not contain coding sequences for actin-like protein.[518] A second region of the viral oncogene protein is closely related to the tyrosine-specific protein kinase gene family. Thus, the v-*fgr* oncogene is a tripartite gene which probably arose as a result of recombinational events involving two distant cellular genes, one coding for a structural protein (actin) and the other for an enzyme (protein kinase). The v-*fgr* protein is associated with cytoskeletal structures at or near the cytoplasmic face of the plasma membrane and this association may be mediated by the cytoskeletal matrix.[519] It is not known whether the actin domain of the viral oncogene product has any role in cellular location or transformation. HC14 mouse mammary epithelial cells transformed by the v-*fgr* oncogene are tumorigenic, anchorage independent, have altered growth in collagen, and lose all cytokeratin expression.[520]

A. THE C-*FGR* PROTOONCOGENE AND ITS PRODUCT

The available evidence, including chromosome localization and nucleotide sequence analysis, indicates that the c-*fgr* protooncogene is identical to a c-*src*-related gene which was designated as c-*src*-2.[521] However, the c-*fgr* gene is distinct from the c-*src* protooncogene and is located on human chromosome 1, at region 1p36.1-p36.2.[522] Two c-*fgr* cDNA clones isolated from a cDNA library derived from the human B lymphocyte cell line IM-9 indicated that the gene encodes a polypeptide of 529 amino acids with a calculated molecular weight of 59,478.[523] The c-*fgr* protein is probably a tyrosine-specific protein kinase but its primary structure indicates that it is probably not associated with the plasma membrane. The function of the normal c-*fgr* protein product, p60$^{c\text{-}fgr}$, is unknown.

B. EXPRESSION OF THE C-*FGR* PROTOONCOGENE

In the 12-week-old human fetus, the highest level of c-*fgr* expression has been detected in the liver, which probably reflects the specific role of the c-*fgr* product in the development of normal hematopoietic cells.[523] The major 2.6-kb and the minor 3.5-kb transcripts of the c-*fgr* gene were also detected in smaller amounts in the placenta, lung, and brain. Transcripts of the c-*fgr* gene were not detected with a v-*fgr* probe in several organs of the adult mice (liver, brain, spleen, thymus, heart, and kidney). Expression of the c-*fgr* gene in normal human adult tissues occurs only in mature peripheral blood monocytes and granulocytes and in alveolar macrophages.[524]

Transcripts of the c-*fgr* gene are usually not detectable in human B- or T-cell-derived lymphoid leukemias or in normal PHA-stimulated human peripheral blood T lymphocytes.[23] However, both normal cells committed to the monocyte lineage and leukemia cells with a differentiated myelomonocytic phenotype express c-*fgr* transcripts at later developmental stages. When bone marrow-derived mouse monocytic cells are synchronized and stimulated to proliferate with the specific growth factor, CSF-1, c-*fgr* transcripts (but not transcripts of the highly related genes c-*src* or c-*yes*) begin to rise at 4 h after the addition of CSF-1, are induced to maximal levels (representing a 20-fold induction) 8 h after the addition of CSF-1, and decrease to low levels by 20 h as the monocytic cells enter S phase.[23] The protooncogenes c-*fos* and c-*myc* are also induced, although with different kinetics, in CSF-1-stimulated monocytic cells.

Relatively high levels of c-*fgr* transcripts are present in the human leukemia cell line IM-9, which was derived from a lymphocyte cell established by infection with EBV.[521]

X. THE *FOS* ONCOGENE PROTEIN PRODUCT

The Finkel-Biskis-Jenkins murine osteosarcoma virus (FBJ MuSV) is an acute retrovirus which was initially isolated from a spontaneous osteosarcoma in CF-1 mouse.[525-527] FBJ MuSV can induce bone tumors in mice and arose probably by recombinational events that occurred between a chronic transforming retrovirus, the FBJ murine leukemia virus (FBJ MuLV), and mouse genomic sequences. FBJ MuSV carries the v-*fos* oncogene. The transforming product of this virus is a 55-kDa phosphoprotein, p55$^{v\text{-}fos}$, which contains 381 amino acids and is entirely derived from c-*fos* protooncogene sequences contained in the mouse genome. Another acute retrovirus, FBR MuSV, expresses a 75-kDa *gag-fos* fusion protein, p75$^{gag\text{-}fos}$. The transforming potential of FBR MuSV is generally more pronounced than that of FBJ MuSV, which may be due to the different structures of the v-*fos*-encoded protein. The structure and function of the v-*fos* and c-*fos* genes and their protein products have been discussed recently.[528,529]

The murine v-*fos* oncogene was cloned and its protein product has been expressed in bacteria.[530] Extended lifespan and tumorigenesis may be observed in nonestablished mouse connective tissue cells transformed by MuSV carrying the v-*fos* oncogene.[529] Transcriptional *trans*-activation of cellular genes is elicited by the v-*fos* gene product, as demonstrated in cotransfection experiments using v-*fos*-carrying plasmids.[531] A strongly increased expression of the type III collagen gene is observed in NIH/3T3 cells stably transformed by the v-*fos* oncogene.[532]

An avian transforming virus, NK24, isolated from a chicken nephroblastoma, also contains a v-*fos* oncogene.[533] Unlike the v-*fos* gene products of FBJ and FBR murine retroviruses, the NK24 v-*fos* gene product has the same carboxy-terminal structure as the chicken c-*fos* gene product.

A. STRUCTURE AND SYNTHESIS OF THE V-*FOS* AND C-*FOS* PROTEINS

The protein products of v-*fos* and c-*fos* genes differ at the carboxyl termini due to an out-of-frame deletion of 104 bp.[534-536] The c-*fos* product is a protein of 55 kDa, p55^{c-fos}.[537] This protein is composed of 380 amino acids and undergoes, as the viral product p55^{v-fos}, posttranslational modification related to phosphorylation on serine residues.[538] The enzyme responsible for the phosphorylation of the v-*fos* and c-*fos* proteins has not been identified but it is apparently distinct of protein kinase C.

The functionally indispensable sequences of the murine v-*fos* protein encompasses amino acids 111 to 219, which represent 28% of the entire protein.[539] The functional importance of this domain is emphasized by the evolutionary conservation of this region, which is identical in the mouse and human c-*fos* proteins. A single amino acid change (valine instead of glutamic acid at position 138) in this region activates the immortalizing potential of v-*fos* without affecting its transforming capacity. The presence of additional amino- and carboxy-terminal amino acids is required for efficient expression of a stable protein, and significantly increases its biological activity. In contrast, sequences in the carboxy-terminal half of the v-*fos* protein (between positions 228 and 267) strongly down modulate its transforming activity without decreasing the immortalizing potential.[539]

A cDNA of the chicken c-*fos* gene was obtained from poly(A) RNA derived from serum-stimulated CEF cells.[540] The chicken c-*fos* gene was also isolated and cloned by using a DNA probe from the avian retrovirus NK24.[541] The chicken c-*fos* gene codes for a protein of 367 amino acids which is 79% homologous to murine p55^{c-fos}, excluding several small insertions and gaps. Comparison of the deduced amino acid sequence of the chicken c-*fos* protein to that of mouse and human c-*fos* proteins revealed a highly conserved domain (98% homology between mouse and chicken) in the center of the protein (85 amino acids) which coincides with a region known to be indispensable for transforming activity and which presumably contains contact site for DNA and other proteins as well as a nuclear location signal sequence.[540] In contrast, the domains of the c-*fos* protein between the terminal sequences and the central region show considerable divergence between chicken and mouse.

1. Posttranslational Modification of the c-*fos* Protein

The c-*fos* product is a markedly acidic protein that is extensively modified by posttranslational processes which include phosphorylation and other types of modifications not changing its relative molecular mass (M_r).[542] More than ten different forms of c-*fos* proteins have been identified by two-dimensional analysis in NIH/3T3 cells. The c-*fos* protein present in neoplastically transformed cells is less extensively modified than the protein present in normal cells. Interestingly, the affinity for DNA of less phosphorylated c-*fos* protein complexes is higher than that of the highly modified ones.[542] Phosphorylation could affect the biological activity of c-*fos* protein via a modulation of its direct or indirect DNA binding activity.

2. Nuclear Proteins Complexed with the *fos* Proteins

The v-*fos* and c-*fos* proteins form in the nucleus of fibroblastic cells a noncovalent complex with a 39-kDa protein, p39.[543] While in serum-stimulated rat fibroblasts the c-*fos* protein is mainly associated with p39, in PC12 rat pheochromocytoma cells it is preferentially associated with a 40-kDa protein, p40.[544] In contrast to the c-*fos* protein, p39 is a basic protein that is rendered even more basic by posttranslational modification.[542] Two other forms of p39, the proteins p41 and p43, which differ in specific domains, are complexed with the c-*fos* protein within the nucleus. These complexes can recognize specific oligonucleotide sequences at the genome level, including the consensus binding site for the mammalian transcription factor, the activator protein 1 (AP-1). The p39 protein associated with the c-*fos* protein in fibroblastic cells was identified recently as the product of the c-*jun* protooncogene.[545] The p39/c-*jun* protein product is identical with the AP-1 transcription factor. The c-*jun* protein forms a heterodimeric complex with the c-*fos* protein via a parallel interaction containing a heptad repeat of leucine residues, termed the leucine zipper. The c-*fos*/c-*jun* protein complex recognizes DNA elements containing AP-1 binding sites.[546,547]

3. The r-*fos* Gene

A DNA sequence, r-*fos*, exhibiting homology to c-*fos*, is present, in addition to the c-*fos* gene, in the mouse genome.[548] The r-*fos* gene is structurally related to the third exon, but not to the second and fourth exons, of the c-*fos* protooncogene. Expression of r-*fos* is stimulated in mouse cells by PDGF but the biological significance of this sequence is unknown.

4. The *fra*-1 Gene

A protein that shows extensive structural homology with the c-*fos* product and that is induced by a subset of the agents and conditions which activate c-*fos* expression is encoded by a distinct gene, *fra*-1.[549] The rat *fra*-1 gene was cloned and sequenced. The evidence indicates that *fra*-1 is a member of a family of genes with structural homologies to the authentic c-*fos* protooncogene. The *fra*-1 product, p38^{fra-1}, binds cooperatively with the c-*jun* protein to AP-1 sites in a similar fashion to that observed for p55^{c-fos}. Thus, the *fra*-1 protein contributes to the DNA-binding activity ascribed to transcription factor AP-1.

5. The *egr*-1 Gene

An early growth response gene that is frequently co-stimulated with c-*fos* expression, exhibiting an induction kinetics similar to that of c-*fos* in fibroblasts, epithelial cells, and lymphocytes following mitogenic stimulation, is *egr*-1.[550] This gene maps to human chromosome region 5p23-31 and its sequence analysis predicts a protein with three DNA binding zinc fingers. The *egr*-1 protein is structurally unrelated to the c-*fos* protein but may be localized in the nucleus and may function as a transcriptional regulator in diverse biological systems.

B. EXPRESSION OF THE C-*FOS* GENE

Complex regulatory mechanisms and factors are involved in the regulation of c-*fos* protooncogene expression in different cell types under different physiologic conditions.[551] Expression of c-*fos* transcripts may be regulated by both positive and negative factors at the transcriptional and posttranscriptional levels, depending on the type of cell and the predominant physiological conditions.[552] Transcriptional expression of the c-*fos* protooncogene in differentiating cells is controlled primarily at the level of transcription and is regulated by 5′ flanking sequences that can be specifically cleaved by DNA topoisomerase II *in vitro*.[553] DNase I hypersensitive sites and regulatory upstream sequences of the c-*fos* gene have an important role in the expression of the gene and include a transcriptional enhancer element.[554,555]

Multiple regulatory elements may be contained upstream of the c-*fos* gene, and these elements may exhibit independent responses to different sets of external stimuli.[556,557] The intracellular signaling pathway responsible for c-*fos* induction may depend on *trans*-acting factors that bind to the c-*fos* gene regulatory regions. Specific nuclear proteins would interact with at least three nucleotide sequences located at the 5' flanking region of the c-*fos* gene.[558] One of these regions is a site exhibiting hypersensitivity to DNase I in both human and mouse genes and its deletion eliminates induction of c-*fos* gene expression by serum. This sequence would be necessary for the induction of c-*fos* transcription by hormones and growth factors present in serum. A nucleotide motif contained within the c-*fos* promoter, identified as the serum response element (SRE), is recognized by a specific SRE binding protein of 67 kDa (p67).[559] Other DNA sequences located 5' to the c-*fos* gene would contribute to basal c-*fos* promoter activity *in vivo*. The 3' untranslated region located immediately downstream of the mouse and human c-*fos* gene may contain multiple copies of a 12-bp element that may also be involved in regulation of c-*fos* gene expression.[560]

In addition to regulation at the transcriptional level, the levels of expression of c-*fos* are regulated by mechanisms acting at the posttranscriptional and translational levels. The study of c-*fos* expression in different cell lines demonstrates that the molecular regulatory mechanisms of c-*fos* expression in different types of cells vary according to the cell and the stimulus exerted by different hormones and growth factors.[4,561]

1. Proteins Involved in Regulation of c-*fos* Gene Expression

Expression of the c-*fos* gene depends on complex regulatory mechanisms involving specific protein factors. Short-lived protein repressors appear to be involved in the regulation of c-*fos* expression at the level of transcription. Cultured mouse peritoneal macrophages express c-*fos* transcripts, and arrest of protein synthesis in these cells induced by treatment with cycloheximide results in a very rapid and marked increase in c-*fos* transcription rate.[562] This type of control is apparently specific for c-*fos* since it is not observed with other protooncogenes expressed in macrophages such as the c-*myc* and c-*fms* genes.

Murine fibroblasts (BALB/c 3T3 cells) treated with conditioned medium from v-*sis* oncogene-transformed cells synthesize within 20 min a factor which binds to a sequence approximately 346 bp upstream of the transcription initiation site of the human c-*fos* gene.[556,563] The kinetics of induction of this activity correlates with the transcriptional activity of the c-*fos* gene. Insulin, EGF, and phorbol ester (PMA), which may act as efficient inducers of c-*fos* gene expression, fail to induce this DNA-binding factor, and protein synthesis inhibitors do not block its induction by the conditioned medium. The exact nature and role of this factor are unknown but it may preexist in an inactive form in quiescent cells and its binding activity may be elicited in response to appropriate extracellular inducers. The results of these studies suggest that c-*fos* transcription is controlled by multiple independent enhancer elements, each activated by distinct signals.

Regulation of c-*fos* gene expression by hormones, growth factors, and other external stimuli may be modulated by both positively and negatively acting cellular factors.[564,565] A repressor molecule would block c-*fos* gene expression in unstimulated (serum-starved) cells, and its action would be abrogated or counteracted by a preexisting positively regulating factor when the cell is stimulated by serum, which would thus allow c-*fos* gene transcription. A c-*fos* enhancer-binding protein was purified from HeLa cells nuclear extracts.[566] This protein has a molecular weight of 62 kDa and binds with high affinity to a 20-bp sequence with dyad symmetry located from position -317 to -298 of the c-*fos* gene sequence, relative to the mRNA cap site. This sequence acts as an enhancer element and is required, in addition to other sequences, for induction of c-*fos* gene expression by both EGF and TPA in HeLa cells.[557]

2. Stability of c-*fos* Gene Transcripts

The c-*fos* mRNA is very labile, with a half-life of less than 30 min.[567,568] A portion of the normal 3' untranslated region of c-*fos* mRNA is essential for its rapid degradation. Inhibition of protein synthesis leads to a large accumulation of c-*fos* mRNA which is due, at least partially, to stabilization of this RNA species. Regulation of c-*fos* mRNA accumulation in HeLa cells during heat shock response occurs primarily at the posttranscriptional level.[570]

3. Ion Changes and Regulation of c-*fos* Gene Expression

Changes in voltage-dependent calcium channels are involved in the control of c-*fos* gene expression in the PC12 pheochromocytoma cell line.[571] Activation of the Na^+/H^+ antiporter as well as increased intracellular levels of Ca^{2+} and activation of protein kinase C may lead to c-*fos* gene expression in U937 human monocyte-like leukemia cells.[572] In murine submandibular gland cells, expression of c-*fos* requires the presence of Na^+ and K^+ but not extracellular Ca^{2+}.[573] Whereas bombesin can activate the expression of c-*fos* and c-*myc* genes by pathways that are, at least in part, dependent on phosphoinositide breakdown, mobilization of Ca^{2+}, and activation of protein kinase C, EGF can activate the expression of these protooncogenes through other cellular pathways.[574]

4. Time and Sites of c-*fos* Gene Expression

The c-*fos* protein is expressed in different cell types correlating with either proliferation or differentiation processes.[575-579] From unstimulated human blood cell populations, only granulocytes express c-*fos* transcripts; no such transcripts are present in monocytes and lymphocytes or in alveolar macrophages.[580] Very high levels of c-*fos* transcripts and protein are detected in late gestational mouse and human extraembryonic tissues but smaller amounts are present in all normal fetal and adult tissues tested.[581-583] The very high levels of c-*fos* mRNA detected in mouse extraembryonic membranes during gestation are confined to the amnion.[582] Expression of c-*fos* in amnion cells is apparently regulated by placenta- and embryo-derived factors, but proliferation of the amnion cells is not dependent on a high level of c-*fos* gene expression, which suggests that the c-*fos* product is associated with cellular functions other than proliferation in the differentiated amnion cells.[581] The c-*fos* gene is expressed at high levels during differentiation-dependent growth processes of fetal bone and mesodermal web tissue.[584] Differentially enhanced expression of c-*fos* and TGF-β mRNAs occurs in the growth plates of developing human long bones, suggesting that both genes may have important functions in both skeletal growth and remodeling during embryogenesis as well as in some diseases of bone and cartilage.[585,586] Expression of the c-*fos* gene in the rat brain varies in amount and localization during development.[587] Very low levels of c-*fos* mRNA are detectable during the period of brain development characterized by rapid mitosis, whereas much higher concentrations of this RNA are found in the brain of older neonatal animals. Immunoreactivity specific for c-*fos* is expressed at low basal levels within the nuclei of fully differentiated neurons of the adult rat brain.[589,590] Activation of these neurons leads to expression of high levels of c-*fos* protein within the nucleus.

C. FUNCTIONAL ROLE OF THE C-*FOS* PROTEIN

The c-*fos* protein may play an important role in cellular physiology, but the exact nature of this role remains an enigma. Expression of the c-*fos* gene correlates in certain biological systems with either cell differentiation or cell proliferation. Studies with *fos*-specific antisense RNA and microinjection of *fos*-specific antibodies indicate that the c-*fos* product is required for progression of many types of cells through the cell cycle.[591-593] However, in other cellular systems the expression of c-*fos* does not appear to correlate with either cell differentiation or proliferation.

The v-*fos* and c-*fos* proteins are located in the nucleus and are complexed with a 39-kDa (p39) nuclear protein.[594] This protein was recently identified as the product of the c-*jun* protooncogene.[545] The c-*jun*/p39 product is a sequence-specific transcriptional factor identical with the AP-1 activator of mammalian cells.[595-598] The c-*fos* protein is associated in form of a complex with chromatin and binds to DNA *in vitro*, which suggests that it may be involved in the regulation of gene expression.[599] In certain cells, e.g., the acinar cells of the mouse submandibular salivary gland, the c-*fos* protein has been localized immunohistochemically in both the cytoplasm and the nucleus.[600] Studies with constructed vectors carrying v-*fos* or c-*fos* genes indicate that *fos* proteins can activate the expression of eukaryotic genes from yeast when they are bound to promoter sites positioned upstream of the target genes.[601] A *cis*-acting heptanucleotide consensus DNA sequence (TGACTCA) is recognized by the transcription factors GCN4 in yeast and AP-1 in mammalian cells. The same DNA sequence is recognized by complexes containing the c-*fos* protein. The c-*fos* protein interacts with the c-*jun*/AP-1 protein through the formation of a leucine zipper and the c-*fos*/c-*jun* protein complex recognizes DNA elements containing AP-1 binding sites. Thus, the c-*fos* protein is involved in the regulation of transcriptional processes.[545-547]

1. Role of c-*fos* in Cell Differentiation

Expression of c-*fos* may be observed in processes associated with cell differentiation. Accumulation of c-*fos* transcripts is physiologically linked to terminal differentiation of normal human monocytes and is further maintained when they mature to macrophages.[607] The amount of c-*fos* transcripts in myeloblastic acute leukemias is strongly correlated with the number of cells expressing surface markers specific for mature monocytes and macrophages. A possible role for the c-*fos* protein in the mechanisms of cellular differentiation is suggested by experiments with transfer of mouse or human c-*fos* protooncogenes into F9 teratocarcinoma stem cells, which results in expression of c-*fos* mRNA and protein and appearance of cells with specific markers characteristic of differentiated cells.[603] However, it appears that expression of c-*fos* gene product alone is insufficient to induce the process of differentiation in different types of cell lines and that other cellular events are required to complement the differentiation-promoting properties of c-*fos*.[604] Moreover, differentiation of certain types of cells is associated with suppression of c-*fos* gene expression. Transcripts of c-*fos* and other protooncogenes are abundant in a clonal line of rat myoblasts that retain the capacity to form noncontractile fibers *in vitro*, but the levels of c-*fos* transcripts become rapidly undetectable when these cells differentiate.[605]

2. Role of c-*fos* in Cell Proliferation

There is no simple association between c-*fos* gene expression and cell proliferation. Different mitogenic agents may rapidly stimulate the transcriptional activity of both c-*fos* and c-*myc* genes in murine thymocytes and human lymphocytes, but neither early c-*fos* nor c-*myc* expression is sufficient to commit the cells to DNA synthesis.[606,607] The strong induction of c-*fos* and c-*myc* by phorbol ester (TPA) or calcium ionophore is, however, insufficient by itself to commit the human lymphocytes to DNA synthesis.[607] Anti-Ig-induced cross-linking of surface Ig on murine B cells causes a rapid and transient increase in the levels of c-*fos* mRNA but this effect is associated with inhibition of cell proliferation.[608] These results suggest that c-*fos* expression may be a component of the surface Ig signal transduction mechanism of B lymphocytes but that it is not positively linked to the proliferation of these cells. In certain systems mitogenic stimulation is associated with a decrease in the expression of the c-*fos* gene. For example, a marked decline in the level of c-*fos* mRNA occurs in either T or B lymphocytes within 1.5 h of mitogen stimulation.[609] The levels of c-*fos* mRNA are extremely low, or even undetectable, throughout the cell cycle of actively proliferating NIH/3T3 mouse fibroblasts.[610] High concentrations of a polyclonal serum against c-*fos* protein did not interfere with initiation or continuation of SV40 DNA replication.[611] Thus, it seems that, at least in certain cellular systems, expression of c-*fos* is not part of the normal cell cycle and is not required for DNA synthesis and the continuous cycling and proliferation of cells.

D. EXPRESSION OF C-*FOS* DURING INDUCED CELL DIFFERENTIATION

Induction of differentiation in neoplastic cell lines may be associated with changes in c-*fos* gene expression. Nerve growth factor (NGF) is capable of inducing differentiation in the PC12 rat pheochromocytoma cells and this induction is associated with a rapid increase in c-*fos* gene transcripts.[613,614] The effect of NGF in PC12 cells is characterized by the expression of cellular differentiation (neurite formation) and is not associated with proliferation of these cells. However, the expression of c-*fos* may be unnecessary for NGF-induced differentiation of PC12 cells.[616] Barium is one of the most potent inducers of c-*fos* gene expression in PC12 cells.[617] The mechanism by which barium activates c-*fos* transcription is unclear but it appears that barium enters the cell via voltage-dependent calcium channels. The induction of c-*fos* expression by barium is antagonized by extracellular calcium and dihydrophyrine calcium channel blockers, and it is attenuated in the presence of calcium inhibitors.

The c-*fos* gene may be transiently expressed during the monocytic differentiation of murine and human leukemia cell lines induced by specific growth factors or chemical inducers such as the phorbol ester TPA.[567,618,619] However, the role of c-*fos* expression in the induction of differentiation of leukemic cell lines is not clear. Compounds such as calcitriol and retinoic acid can induce differentiation of HL-60 cells without increasing c-*fos* expression.[619] Induction of macrophage differentiation of HL-60 cells by TPA is accompanied by c-*fos* expression and rising levels or class I MHC levels, whereas induction of granulocyte differentiation by DMSO is not accompanied by c-*fos* expression and is followed by declining MHC levels.[620144] Expression of the c-*fos* gene is neither sufficient nor obligatory for TPA-induced differentiation of HL-60 human leukemia monomyelocytes to macrophages. HL-60 variants resistant to TPA can be induced to differentiate into macrophages in the absence of detectable c-*fos* expression.[567] Induction of differentiation in F9 teratocarcinoma cells by retinoic acid and dibutyryl cAMP is also not accompanied by any large transient increase in c-*fos* gene expression.[582] In mast cell lines derived from murine bone marrow, massive fluctuations of c-*fos* transcripts induced by the addition or absence of the specific growth factor, IL-3, are not associated with detectable changes in the expression of differentiated functions, nor with the accumulation of quiescent, terminally differentiated cells.[621] Thus, there is no clear-cut general correlation between expression of the c-*fos* gene product and cellular proliferation or differentiation.

E. UNSPECIFIC INDUCTION OF C-*FOS* GENE EXPRESSION

A number of apparently unspecific stimuli can induce the expression of c-*fos* to strikingly elevated levels. The mere mechanical disaggregation of neonatal mouse cerebellar tissue followed by its incubation at 37°C induces over 40-fold elevation of c-*fos* mRNA in the absence of any growth factor.[622] Wounding of fibroblast monolayers results in the rapid induction of c-*fos* expression independently of serum growth factors.[623,624] This induction takes place at the pretranslational level. Several known inducers of heat shock response (heat stress, arsenite, and heavy metals) cause a significant elevation of c-*fos* mRNA in HeLa cells.[570] Heat stress results in a time- and temperature-dependent prolonged elevation of c-*fos* mRNA. This elevation is accompanied by increased levels of HSP70 gene expression and occurs primarily through posttranscriptional processes, by stabilization of c-*fos* transcripts.

The c-*fos* gene can be activated when tissue slices or isolated lobes of murine submandibular glands are incubated at 37C in physiologic solutions or in tissue culture media.[625] Dissociation of the cells with collagenase-hyaluronidase treatment also results in increased steady-state levels of c-*fos* mRNA without any additional stimulus. The authors of this interesting study conclude that "this activation is difficult to reconcile with the prevailing view of the role of c-*fos* in development, growth control and differentiation."[625]

F. EXPRESSION OF C-*FOS* IN NEURAL TISSUES

The c-*fos* protein is expressed in the nuclei of neurons throughout the mouse brain, but particularly in the pyriform cortex, anterior olfactory nucleus, and the bed nucleus of the stria terminalis.[626] Physiological stimulation of rat primary sensory neurons caused the expression of c-*fos* protein in nuclei of postsynaptic neurons of the dorsal horn of the spinal cord.[627] Activation of small-diameter cutaneous sensory afferents by noxious heat or chemical stimuli resulted in the rapid appearance of c-*fos*-protein-like immunoreactivity in the superficial layers of the dorsal horn. No induction of c-*fos* occurred in the dorsal root ganglia, gracile nucleus, or ventral horn. The expression of c-*fos* may be due to induction by neurotransmitters. A marked and specific induction of c-*fos* is observed in identifiable neuron populations of the basal brain and cortex *in vivo* after the administration of the convulsivant drug pentylenetetrazole, and this effect is abolished by prior treatment with anticonvulsivant drugs such as benzodiazepine and pentobarbital. Electrically induced seizure activity in rats, which leads to a permanent increase of the brain to future seizures (kindling) rapidly and transiently increases c-*fos* protein immunoreactivity in the nuclei of granule cells in the dentate gyrus.[628] Generalized tonic-clonic seizures in mice are associated with a massive increase of c-*fos* protein expression in the cingulate and piriform cortices and the dentate gyrus 1 h after the injection of pentylenetetrazole.[629] The induction of c-*fos* protein following generalized seizure activity in mice is dependent upon the seizure itself, rather than the method of seizure production. The role of c-*fos* protein expression in brain physiology and pathology is unknown.

G. CONCLUSION

The c-*fos* protein is located primarily within the nucleus. The protein exhibits affinity for gene promoters and is involved in the regulation of transcriptional processes.[529] Complexes between the c-*fos* protein and other cellular proteins may recognize specific oligonucleotide sequences at the genome level, including a consensus binding site for the transcriptional activator AP-1. A 39-kDa protein (p39) which is complexed within the nucleus with the c-*fos* protein has been identified as the product of the c-*jun* protooncogene.[545-547] The p39/c-*jun* protein associated with the c-*fos* protein is the transcriptional activator AP-1 of mammalian cells.[595-598] The c-*fos* protein interacts with the c-*jun*/AP-1 protein through the formation of a leucine zipper and the c-*fos*/c-*jun* protein complex recognizes DNA elements that contain AP-1 binding sites.

Expression of the c-*fos* gene is rapidly and transiently induced in a diversity of cells by a wide variety of external stimuli and it has been suggested that the protein product of this gene may be involved in the control of cell proliferation and/or cell differentiation. Studies using either *fos* antisense RNA or microinjection of *fos*-specific antibodies suggest that the c-*fos* product is required for progression through the cell cycle.[592,593] However, it is dubious that the c-*fos* protein may have a direct role in DNA synthesis. High concentrations of a polyclonal antiserum against c-*fos* protein did not interfere with initiation or continuation of SV40 DNA replication.[611] In certain cellular systems *in vivo,* expression of c-*fos* is correlated neither with cell proliferation nor with cell differentiation but may be associated with the varied responses of organs and tissues to a diversity of physiologic agents such as hormones, growth factors, and neurotransmitters.[600,625] Expression of the c-*fos* gene may also be induced by rather unspecific stimuli, for example, when particular types of cells are mechanically dissociated or wounded or are incubated at physiologic temperature without any known specific stimulus.[622,623,625] The role of the c-*fos* protein in normal and pathologic processes, including neoplastic transformation, is not understood at present.

XI. PROTEIN PRODUCTS OF THE *MYC* ONCOGENE FAMILY

The product of the avian myelocytomatosis virus (AMCV), strain MC29, is a hybrid protein of 110 kDa, p110$^{gag-myc}$.[630-632] This protein contains viral *gag* sequences fused with oncogene *myc* sequences derived from the avian genome. Usually, the protein products of other isolates of ALVs are also hybrid proteins but some viral isolates code for an unlinked v-*myc* protein of 55 kDa, p55^{v-myc}.[633,634] The MC29 AMCV virus proteins occur as monomers or dimers in MC29-transformed cells.[635] The v-*myc* proteins are phosphoproteins and their phosphorylation at specific sites correlates with the transforming ability.[636] Active v-*myc* genes are capable of inducing preneoplastic transformation of bursal lymphocytes in chick embryos but bursal cell DNA containing the activated v-*myc* gene cannot transform NIH/3T3 fibroblasts.[637] Spontaneous nonconditional mutants of the MC29 virus contain internal deletions and generate altered *gag-myc* hybrid proteins of 90 and 100 kDa which are incompletely phosphorylated and have strongly reduced potential to transform hematopoietic cells *in vitro* or to induce tumors in animals but are capable of transforming cultured fibroblasts.[638]

A. STRUCTURE AND TRANSCRIPTION OF THE C-*MYC*, N-*MYC*, AND L-*MYC* GENES

The c-*myc* gene and two structurally related genomic sequences present in the mammalian genome, N-*myc* and L-*myc*, constitute the *myc* gene family. The cellular counterpart of the v-*myc* oncogene is the protooncogene c-*myc*.[639-643] The normal human *myc* proteins exhibit significant homologies in their amino acid sequences, but the lengths of their peptide chains are different: 439 residues for c-*myc*, 456 residues for N-*myc*, and 364 residues for L-*myc*. A novel member of the *myc* gene family, B-*myc*, encodes a protein which exhibits high level of expression in the rat brain.[644]

1. The Human and Murine c-*myc* Protooncogenes

The human c-*myc* protooncogene is located on the distal end of the long arm of chromosome 8, at region 8q24,[645] and comprises three exons, but only exons 2 and 3 would code for the c-*myc* protein.[646-648] However, recent evidence indicates that a non-AUG codon near the 3′ end of c-*myc* exon 1 represents an alternative translation initiation site.[649] The use of this second initiation site, which is a CUG codon, explains the occurrence in human cells of two related c-*myc* encoded proteins differing at their amino termini.

Human c-*myc* transcribes for two mRNA molecular species of 2.2 and 2.4 kb, respectively, starting from alternative promoters (P1 and P2) located within the first exon of the gene.[648,650-652] Cryptic promoters contained within the first intron of the c-*myc* protooncogene are not by themselves sufficient for transcription in microinjected *Xenopus* oocytes.[653] A third promoter of the c-*myc* gene, termed P0, is localized over 500 bp upstream of P1 and P2.[654] P0 RNA is found on ribosomes and released by puromycin, indicating that it functions as an mRNA and can be translated into a polypeptide corresponding to the first ORF of the c-*myc* gene.

The human c-*myc* gene contains at its 5′ flanking region a duplicate set of TATA sequences that serve as promoters and a nonanucleotide that is repeated four times approximately 116 bases 5′ to the first potential transcription initiation site.[648] As demonstrated by microinjection of human c-*myc* genes into frog oocytes, these 5′ sequences are essential elements that act as promoters and are recognized by the transcriptional machinery of frog oocytes.[655] In addition to positive control elements, other elements located in the 5' side of the c-*myc* gene may be involved in regulating its expression. A negative control element of transcription is located upstream of the murine c-*myc* gene.[656] A protein that may be involved in repression of the murine c-*myc* gene expression was identified in plasmacytoma cells.[657] This protein would recognize a single specific binding site located 290 bp 5′ to the transcription start site P1. Studies with transfection into various cell types of constructed hybrid molecules containing part of the human c-*myc* promoter-leader region and the bacterial chloramphenicol acetyltransferase (CAT) gene indicate that the dual promoter of the human c-*myc* gene represents a strong eukaryotic promoter regulated by cooperation of positively and negatively acting cellular transcription factors.[658]

In addition to the transcriptional regulation of c-*myc* expression depending on the upstream regulatory sequences, the dual promoters, and the leader region of the gene, the expression of c-*myc* may depend on other unidentified elements. the c-*myc* gene is frequently truncated in Burkitt's lymphoma cells, with separation of the body of the gene from its physiological promoters and upstream regulatory sequences but, in spite of these alterations, treatment of these cells with the differentiation inducer sodium butyrate results in a rapid decrease of c-*myc* transcripts.[659] Thus, an important, unidentified target site of c-*myc* transcriptional regulation is located outside the upstream regulatory sequences, the dual promoters, and the leader region of the gene.

Topoisomerase II-induced cleavage sites along the human c-*myc* locus correspond to that of DNase I-hypersensitive sites.[660] Several antitumor drugs can block the DNA rejoining reaction of DNA topoisomerase II by stabilizing a reversible enzyme-DNA complex, and it has been shown that these drugs induce DNA breaks *in vivo* within a region located 5' to the first c-*myc* exon.[661]

2. The Chicken c-*myc* Gene

The chicken c-*myc* gene has a complex structure and exhibits several striking dissimilarities in gene organization to the mammalian c-*myc* genes.[662] Protein extracted form chicken erythroid and thymus cell nuclear extracts bind to at least eight sequences upstream of the c-*myc* gene from three chicken cell types: terminally differentiated erythrocytes, 3-week-old chick thymus, and transformed erythroid precursor cells.[663] Although these tissues represent different levels of c-*myc* gene expression, the c-*myc* gene chromatin, even in erythrocyte cells, exists in an active conformation, as evidenced by the presence of DNase I-hypersensitive sites. The chicken c-*myc* locus is variably methylated in all tissues, except blood, where erythrocytic DNA shows no evidence of significant methylation of c-*myc*.[664] The physiologic relevance of this lack of methylation is unknown since chicken erythrocyte DNA is generally considered to be nonfunctional.

3. Transcription of the c-*myc* Protooncogene

The two DNA strands of the c-*myc* protooncogene are transcribed in certain normal and transformed cells.[665] Moreover, transcription of the coding and noncoding strands of the c-*myc* gene may be regulated independently. Changes observed in the transcription of c-*myc* during growth state transitions can be ascribed solely to fluctuations in transcription of the coding strand, while changes in transcription of both strands are observed in the process of differentiation of certain cells, for example, during DMSO-induced differentiation of MEL cells.[665] During mitogen stimulation of splenic T lymphocytes, transcription of the coding strand of the c-*myc* gene undergoes rapid and marked changes, whereas transcription of the noncoding strand is essentially unaltered by these events. Noncoding strand transcription of c-*myc* is also observed in rearranged, truncated c-*myc* genes associated with murine plasmacytomas.[666] The biological significance of these differences is unknown.

4. Degradation of c-*myc* Transcripts

The steady-state levels of specific types of mRNAs are partially determined by their degradation rates. The control of c-*myc* gene expression depends not only on the rate of its transcriptional activity but also on the rate of decay of c-*myc* mRNA.[667] Degradation of c-*myc* mRNA occurs in the 3' to 5' direction, being initiated by shortening of the poly(A) sequence, followed by the generation of short-lived intermediates with progressively shorter 3' sequences.[664] In contrast, the 5' region of the c-*myc* mRNA, which contains the first exon sequences, is relatively stable.

5. Transcription of the N-*myc* Gene

Transcription of the human N-*myc* gene is exceptionally complex.[669] This transcription initiates at numerous sites that may be grouped under the control of two promoters, and the multiplicity of initiation sites combines with alternative splicing to engender two forms of mRNA with different 5' leader sequences. However, both forms of N-*myc* mRNA have identical second and third exons and both encode the identified 65- and 67-kDa products of the human

N-*myc* gene. The c-*myc* and N-*myc* genes display different patterns of expression in developing mouse embryos as well as in murine embryonal carcinoma cells, and they are regulated by partially different mechanisms at the transcriptional and posttranscriptional levels.[670] Posttranscriptional mechanisms, related to the stability of N-*myc* mRNA, are involved in the regulation of N-*myc* expression in human neuroblastoma and retinoblastoma cell lines.[671] Increased levels of N-*myc* transcripts have been observed in rat hepatocytes when growth was stimulated by partial hepatectomy (20-fold increase about 6 h after operation) as well as after the administration of the chemical carcinogen, DENA.[672]

6. Transcription of the L-*myc* Gene

The structure, expression, and transforming capacity of the human and murine L-*myc* genes have been determined.[673] Abundant transcripts of the L-*myc* gene are expressed by the human small-cell lung carcinoma cell line U-1690.[674] Two L-*myc* transcripts (2.2 and 3.8 kb) produced by U-1690 cells have different half-lives. Unlike c-*myc* mRNA in other cells, no significant stabilization of the L-*myc* mRNA occurred when protein synthesis was inhibited in U-1690 cells, suggesting that transcription of the L-*myc* gene may depend on positive control by short-lived proteins. Studies with other small-cell lung carcinoma cell lines indicate the generation of multiple forms of L-*myc* mRNA which are generated by alternative RNA splicing of introns 1 and 2 and by alternative polyadenylation utilization.[675] Some of the mature L-*myc* mRNAs could encode truncated proteins that may lack sequences predicted to be important for nuclear localization and, therefore, may serve a different functional role.

7. Transcription of the B-*myc* Gene

The B-*myc* gene, located on rat chromosome 3, is expressed in the form of 1.3-kb transcripts which are present in most tissues of fetal and adult rats, with the highest levels being observed in the brain.[644]

B. THE PROTEIN PRODUCTS OF THE CELLULAR *MYC* GENES

The major human c-*myc* product is a protein of 64 kDa which differs from the v-*myc* protein by 18 amino acid deletions and 42 additions, being longer by 24 amino acids.[676] The human c-*myc* gene has been cloned and expressed in *Escherichia coli* and *Saccharomyces cerevisiae*.[677] Whereas the *myc* protein produced in *E. coli* has a size of 60 kDa and appears to be unmodified, being identical to the protein synthesized in an *in vitro* system, the manipulated yeast cells synthesize two *myc* proteins of 60 and 62 kDa, respectively. This difference is apparently due to phosphorylation, but both proteins are located predominantly in the nuclear fraction of the yeast cells. The cloned intact human c-*myc* gene is transcribed very efficiently and accurately from its own promoters after microinjection into *Xenopus laevis* oocytes.[678]

1. Detection of *myc* Proteins

The preparation of a rabbit antiserum specific for avian viral and cellular *myc* proteins has been reported.[679,680] Expression of the c-*myc* protein can also be determined specifically by using monoclonal antibodies that have been produced against synthetic oligopeptides corresponding to the predicted amino acid sequence of the human protein.[681] Antisera directed against two polypeptide domains encoded by exons 2 and 3 of the human c-*myc* protein have been prepared by using bacterial expression vectors.[682] Radiolabeled monoclonal antibodies against the c-*myc* protein can be used to study its localization in normal or tumor tissues.[683]

2. Molecular Forms of c-*myc* Proteins

In avian bursal lymphoma cell lines as well as in normal chick embryo cells the phosphorylated c-*myc* proteins detected by specific antisera vary in molecular weight from 58 to 62 kDa and are localized in the cell nucleus.[680] In addition, anti-*myc* antiserum immunoprecipitates a 48-kDa nuclear phosphoprotein that appears to be a breakdown product of the functional c-*myc* protein.

A 48-kDa protein (p48) cross-reactive with an antiserum directed against the 12 carboxyl-terminal amino acids of the human c-*myc* gene-encoded protein has been isolated from a Burkitt's lymphoma cell line.[684] Protein p48 is present in a wide variety of cell types and is evolutionarily conserved at the antigenic level in mouse and human cells. In contrast to the c-*myc* protein, p48 is a basic protein with predominant cytoplasmic localization. Protein p48 is detected at very low levels in normal, resting peripheral blood lymphocytes, but is induced severalfold by a stimulation with either concanavalin A or pokeweed mitogen.[684] The c-*myc*-related cytoplasmic protein, as detected by the use of an antiserum raised in a rabbit against the carboxyl-terminal portion of the human c-*myc* protein, is expressed at high levels in a part of the hepatocytes from human fetuses, but not in the adult human liver, and the same protein was found to be expressed in the proximal convolution cells of the fetal and adult human kidney.[685] The possible functional relationship between p48 and the c-*myc* gene protein product is unknown.

Although it was initially postulated that the first exon of the human c-*myc* gene is a noncoding exon, recent evidence indicates the presence within this exon of an ORF with coding capacity for a 12.5-kDa polypeptide of 188 amino acids.[654,686,687] Transcription of this ORF sequence is controlled by the P0 promoter of the c-*myc* locus, which is located 550 to 650 bp upstream of the P1 c-*myc* promoter. The function(s) of the putative 12.5-kDa protein product of c-*myc* exon 1 is unknown but one possibility is that it could play a role in the regulation of c-*myc* gene expression. However, expression of exon 1 sequences of the c-*myc* gene has no effect on the translational efficiency of c-*myc* mRNA in COS cells.[688] Translation of the first ORF of the human c-*myc* gene *in vitro,* in a rabbit reticulocyte translation system, yielded a 20-kDa protein. Antisera directed against this protein failed to detect any exon 1 product in human cells. Recently, it has been recognized that two different c-*myc* proteins are originated by differential utilization of two initiation codons contained within the exons of the human c-*myc* gene.[649] The smaller and normally more abundant of these two proteins, designated c-Myc-2, is initiated at the first AUG codon in c-*myc* exon 2. The larger and less abundant protein, c-Myc-1, is initiated at a CUG codon located near the 3′ end of exon 1, and differs from c-Myc-2 by 14 or 15 amino-terminal amino acids (depending on whether the initiating amino acid is retained). The physiological significance of the existence of two c-*myc* proteins in human cells is not understood but it seems possible that c-Myc-1 may exert a regulatory effect on the expression of c-Myc-2. As a consequence of structural alterations affecting the c-*myc* gene in tumor cells, protein c-Myc-1 was found to be absent in several Burkitt's lymphoma cell lines.[649]

C. THE N-*MYC* AND L-*MYC* PROTEINS

The proteins encoded by the human N-*myc* and L-*myc* genes have been identified and characterized, or the protein products of these genes have been structurally deduced from the respective coding sequences.[674,690-692] Two human N-*myc* proteins of 65 and 67 kDa have been identified by means of rabbit antisera generated against synthetic oligopeptides as antigens.[693] These two proteins arise from the same mRNA, are phosphorylated, are exceptionally unstable (half-lives of approximately 30 min), are located in the cell nucleus, and bind to both single- and double-stranded DNA *in vitro*. The N-*myc* protein exhibits high homology not only to the c-*myc* protein but also to the c-*fos* protein.[691]

D. CELLULAR LOCALIZATION OF *MYC* PROTEINS

The protein products of viral and cellular *myc* genes are localized in the cell nucleus.[693-695] Mutational analysis of the human c-*myc* gene indicates that amino acid sequences between positions 320 and 368 of the protein may function to direct it to the nuclei of intact cells.[696] Two regions of the human c-*myc* protein are involved in directing the protein to the nucleus.[697] The human protein molecules form oligomeric structures due to interaction of a carboxyl-terminal peptide containing a leucine zipper motif.[698] The *myc* proteins are phosphorylated by casein kinase II.[699]

Multiple nuclear proteins are immunoprecipitated by antisera raised against human c-*myc* peptide antigens.[700] Antisera against the protein product of the human c-*myc* protooncogene precipitate two proteins of 62 to 64 and 66 to 67 kDa, termed p62 or p64 and p66 or p67, respectively, which may be different modified versions of the same gene product and which are associated with the nuclear matrix (nuclear cytoskeleton).[701-703] However, no association of p62[c-myc] with the nuclear matrix was observed in other studies which showed that p62[c-myc] can be extracted from nuclei by mild salt concentration without affecting gross nuclear structure or causing extraction of major chromatin components.[704] Reexamination of this controversial subject suggested that although c-*myc* protein is found in the nuclear cytoskeleton or matrix II fraction, it may be associated with the nuclear matrix I fraction, which is a complex group of proteins implicated in physiological processes within the nucleus.[705] Studies with immunofluorescence and immunoelectron microscopy indicate an association between v-*myc* and c-*myc* proteins and small nuclear ribonuclei particles.[706] According to the results of some studies, the purified c-*myc* protein binds to double- and single-stranded DNA, as measured by a DNA affinity chromatography assay.[699] However, no specific DNA sequences have been recognized as responsible for binding of the c-*myc* protein to DNA and it is possible that chromatin proteins contribute to this binding.[707] Intranuclear degradation of the transforming protein of MC29 retrovirus has been reported.[708]

The c-*myc* proteins are dispersed into the cytoplasm during mitosis and are not associated with chromatin in mitotic cells.[709] In *Xenopus laevi* oocytes a significant portion of the c-*myc* protein is localized not in the nucleus but in the cytoplasm.[710] Predominant cytoplasmic localization of c-*myc* protein was also found in a human hepatoblastoma transplanted in athymic nude mice.[711] The biological significance of cytoplasmic localization of c-*myc* proteins is not understood but one possibility is that c-*myc* protein represents a nuclear component stored in the cytoplasm for future use.

E. PHYSIOLOGICAL ROLE OF THE CELLULAR *MYC* PROTEINS

The physiological role of the cellular *myc* protein products is unknown but expression of this protein may be associated to processes related to either cell proliferation or cell differentiation.

1. Role of the c-*myc* Protein in Cell Proliferation

In different types of cells expression of the c-*myc* protein is positively correlated to cell proliferation.[639,640] In some cultured cell systems the c-*myc* protein may be considered as an intracellular competence factor, i.e., as a factor rendering cells competent for undergoing the G_0-S phase transition in the cell cycle. Quiescent human diploid WI-138 fibroblasts maintained in culture are capable of entering DNA synthesis and proliferate in response to the addition of platelet-poor plasma to the medium as long as they express the c-*myc* protooncogene, but not after this expression is ceased.[712] In stimulated B lymphocytes expression of c-*myc* may be necessary not only for leading to a competence state, rendering quiescent cells able to enter the G_1 phase of the cycle, but also for progression of activated cells to DNA synthesis.[713] Microinjection of the purified c-*myc* protein into nuclei of quiescent Swiss 3T3 fibroblasts exposed to platelet-poor plasma results in stimulation of DNA synthesis.[714] Whereas the presence in the medium of an antibody against PDGF abolishes DNA synthesis induced by microinjected PDGF, the microinjected c-*myc* protein stimulates DNA synthesis even when its own antibody is present in the medium. The addition of affinity-purified polyclonal or monoclonal antibodies against the human c-*myc* protein to nuclei isolated from several types of human cells reversibly inhibits both DNA synthesis and DNA polymerase activity, but not the transcription of RNA.[715] However, this reported inhibition of DNA synthesis by c-*myc* protein-directed antibodies was shown to be due to the presence of an unidentified inhibitor of DNA polymerases α and δ and not to the action on the c-*myc* protein.[611] An antisense oligonucleotide complementary to c-*myc* sequences, capable of inhibiting c-*myc* protein expression, prevents entry of mitogen-stimulated peripheral blood lymphocytes into S phase of the cycle but, interestingly, it does not inhibit G_0 to G_1 transversal as assessed by morphological blast transformation, transcriptional activation of the IL-2 receptor and transferrin receptor genes, or induction of ^{3}H-uridine incorporation into RNA.[716] These results suggest that the c-*myc* protein may participate in some way in the processes of DNA replication. However, the exact role of the c-*myc* protein in these complex processes is unknown.

2. Role of the c-*myc* and N-*myc* Proteins in Cell Differentiation

The proteins of the *myc* protooncogene family may also have some role in the physiological processes related to cell differentiation. Differential expression of the members of the *myc* gene family is observed during murine development.[717] While the expression of c-*myc* is generalized to many tissues and developmental stages, the expression of N-*myc* and L-*myc* is highly restricted with respect to tissue and stage in the developing mouse. The c-*myc* proteins are present in a wide diversity of human cells, which suggests that they have an essential physiological role. The quantity of c-*myc* proteins among different cell lines is highly variable, from the low levels found in normal fibroblasts to approximately tenfold-higher levels found in some tumor cell lines.

The N-*myc* protein may play an important role in neural tissue development. This protein is expressed at high levels in the early human fetal cerebral germinal layer and the primordial human cortex, with lower levels being present in the intermediate layer.[718] After the 20th week, N-*myc* expression declines in the attenuated germinal layer and remains high in the differentiating inner cortex, but declines in the differentiated outer cortex. During this time, expression of the c-*src* protooncogene increases with maturation and differentiation of the neural tissue. The N-*myc* protein is also expressed in some cells of lung and placenta.

3. Mechanisms of Action of the Cellular *myc* Proteins

The molecular mechanisms of action of the cellular *myc* proteins on the processes related to cell proliferation and differentiation remain unknown. There is evidence that the c-*myc* protein may be involved in both the positive and the negative regulation of gene expression, but the exact mechanism of the postulated effect, whether direct or indirect, has not been clarified. The human c-*myc* gene, under the inducible control of the *Drosophila* HSP70 promoter, is capable of inducing G_0/G_1 transition genes in transfected mouse BALB/c 3T3 cells.[719] The c-*myc* gene product can also regulate cellular gene expression at the posttranslational level.[720]

F. EVOLUTIONARY CONSERVATION OF C-*MYC*-RELATED DNA SEQUENCES

The coding sequences of the c-*myc* DNA, as well as the amino acid sequences of the c-*myc* protein, are highly conserved in evolution, which indicates an important biological function. Antisera to specific c-*myc* amino acid sequences precipitate homologous proteins from human, monkey, rat, hamster, and frog cells. The c-*myc* protein from amphibians (*Xenopus laevis*) is highly homologous to both the avian (70% identity) and mammalian (71% identity) c-*myc* proteins, which demonstrates a conserved protooncogene spanning some 380 to 400 million years.[710] The first exon of the human c-*myc* gene, which has been assumed to be a nontranslating exon, is also highly conserved, which indicates its functional importance.[687]

A c-*myc* gene has been isolated, cloned, and sequenced from a lower vertebrate, the rainbow trout (*Salmo gairdneri*), where it is expressed as a single 2.3-kb mRNA species.[721] Genes homologous to c-*myc* have also been detected in invertebrates. c-*myc*-related transcripts are present in *Drosophila* but the transcripts present in early embryos of the insect are of maternal origin.[722] The c-*myc* protein, or a related protein, may be involved in phenomena of physiological adaptation occurring in insects. Heat treatment of *Drosophila* results in dramatic changes in the puffing patterns of polytene chromosomes and transcriptional activation of seven major heat shock protein genes (*HSP* genes).[723-725] The expression of one of these genes, *HSP* 70, may be regulated by a rearranged mouse c-*myc* protooncogene.[726] However, the major mouse *HSP* gene was found to be silent in MPC-11 mouse plasmacytoma cells that produce abundant c-*myc* transcripts.[727] No direct correlation between deregulated c-*myc* expression and the absence of *HSP* gene induction was established in MPC-11 cells.

The biological importance of the c-*myc* protooncogene is indicated by the fact that DNA, RNA, and protein related to this gene is present even in prokaryotic primitive microorganisms like the halophilic archaebacteria *Halobacterium halobium*.[728] A 70-kDa protein of *H. halobium* cross reacts with an antiserum directed against the v-*myc* product of the avian virus MC29. The purified c-*myc*-like protein of *H. halobium* stimulates *in vitro* DNA synthesis carried out by the α-like DNA polymerase of the microorganism.[729]

G. STRUCTURAL HOMOLOGIES OF C-*MYC* PROTEINS

The human c-*myc* protein shows partial sequence homology to β- and γ-crystallins.[730] Crystallins constitute a set of lens-specific proteins of the vertebrate eye. In mammals, the crystallins are classified into three antigenically distinct classes, α-, β-, and γ-crystallins. The classes of β- and γ-crystallins each contain about 6 or 7 polypeptides of related primary structure and it is generally accepted that β- and γ- crystallins have evolved from a common ancestral motif sequence whose successive duplications have created the present mammalian β- and γ-crystallin gene families.[731,732] The c-*myc* protein shows two regions of significant homology with bovine β- and γ-crystallins, especially in two main regions corresponding to amino acid residues 12-197 and 152-337 of the c-*myc* protein.[730] The degrees of homology are between 13 and 19% for the two different crystallins and the different sections of the c-*myc* protein and are unlikely to have arisen by chance. There is no significant homology with α-crystallin.

Significant structural homology has been detected between the mammalian c-*myc* protein and the *AS-C* proteins that are encoded by the *achaeta-scute* gene complex of *Drosophila melanogaster*.[733] These proteins may have a specific function in the process of neuroblast segregation during the embryogenic development of the insect.[734] Structural and functional homologies exist between the c-*myc* protein and the p53 antigen.[161] The biological significance of these homologies is not understood. On the basis of structural homology, it has been suggested that *myc* proteins may act as protein phosphatase inhibitors.[736]

H. EXPRESSION OF THE C-*MYC* GENE

The c-*myc* protooncogene may be one of the housekeeping genes carrying strong promoters which allow constant or constitutive transcription controlled by rather universal transcription factors in a variety of host cell and tissues.[655] However, transcriptional activation of the c-*myc* gene and expression of its protein product are subjected to complex regulatory phenomena, depending on both endogenous signals generated by cell-to-cell contact and other physiological changes, and exogenous signals which include mitogens, hormones, and growth factors.[4,640,641,737] Regulation of c-*myc* expression in cells such as stimulated human lymphocytes takes place at both transcriptional and posttranscriptional levels.[738] Regulation at each of these two levels may involve complex molecular mechanisms. Different types of cells may preferentially employ different modes of regulation of c-*myc* expression under different physiological conditions.[739]

1. Transcriptional Regulation of c-*myc* Expression

Regulation of c-*myc* gene expression at the transcriptional level is apparently very complex. The c-*myc* gene is transcribed at high rate in cells such as G_0-arrested hamster lung fibroblasts and this expression may be regulated at the transcriptional level in response to several physiological stimuli, including the action of hormones and growth factors.[740] Chromatin structural modifications, depending on both alterations in the chromatin-associated proteins and the local physical state of the DNA, may be importantly involved in the regulation of c-*myc* transcriptional activity.[741] The germ-line c-*myc* gene is regulated by specific positive and negative factors that bind to multiple sites near and within the gene.[742] The putative positive regulatory factors bind to two distinct regions near the c-*myc* promoters and the negative factors bind to an upstream site as well as to sites within the c-*myc* gene. Direct interaction of short RNA molecules with specific DNA sites sensitive to S1 nuclease, located within the 5′ end of the human c-*myc* gene sequences induce local alterations in the DNA structure, which could lead to changes in the rate of c-*myc* transcription.[743] In addition to transcription initiation, an important step in the regulation of c-*myc* gene expression may be represented by a block in RNA elongation within the first exon.[744]

2. Turnover of c-*myc* mRNA

The turnover rate of c-*myc* mRNA may show wide variation among different cells. In all human cell lines tested, including normal human embryonic fibroblasts and transformed cell lines of various origins (HeLa cervix carcinoma cells, MCF7 mammary carcinoma cells, Daudi lymphoma cells, and HL60 promyelocytic leukemia cells), c-*myc* mRNA is extremely unstable, with an approximate half-life of 10 to 15 min.[745] In contrast, an extremely long half-life of c-*myc* mRNA is observed in the *Xenopus* egg, in which c-*myc* transcripts of maternal origin are maintained during the whole process of oncogenesis until fertilization, when its degradation is induced.[746]

Changes in the expression of the c-*myc* gene in cultures of aortic smooth muscle cells during the transition from G_0 to G_1 are controlled at the level of c-*myc* mRNA turnover, by stabilization of this RNA.[747] This stabilization could depend on inactivation of a particular ribonucleolytic activity. Polyadenylation of c-*myc* mRNA may contribute to regulate its stability. Two classes of c-*myc* mRNA have been detected in HL-60 human promyelocytic leukemia cells, one which is relatively labile and contains long poly(A) tails that bind to oligo(dT)-cellulose, and the other which is stable and does not contain such tails.[748] These results suggest that the control of c-*myc* expression is regulated, at least in some cellular systems, by posttranscriptional events affecting the degradation of its mRNA.

3. Expression of c-*myc* mRNA and Protein

The synthesis, turnover, and modification of c-*myc* proteins is constant throughout the cell cycle.[749-751] In contrast to authentic cell cycle-dependent genes, in avian and human cells the rate of synthesis (as a fraction of total protein synthesis), turnover, and modification of c-*myc* protein is independent of the cell cycle stage. However, transient increases in level occur upon serum stimulation of resting cells.[639,640,752] Specific antigenic stimulation of resting, hapten-specific B lymphocytes induces elevated levels of c-*myc* mRNA, which could contribute to B cell activation and preparation to growth response.[753] Enhanced c-*myc* gene expression alone does not commit the cell to DNA synthesis since such commitment requires delivery to the activated cells of an additional stimulus. Murine splenic T lymphocytes exhibit maximal c-*myc* gene expression already 3 h after stimulation with concanavalin A, and subsequent down regulation of this expression is observed before the onset of DNA synthesis.[301]

4. Dietary-Induced Changes in c-*myc* Gene Expression

Dietary changes may influence c-*myc* gene expression. Short-time physiological fasting results in a marked decrease of c-*myc* gene expression in the rat liver.[754] This effect does not seem to depend on glucagon, since administration of this hormone leads to an increase in c-*myc* transcripts. Deprivation of dietary protein in rats for several days followed by a meal containing protein results in increased rate of DNA synthesis in the liver. A gradual increase in c-*myc* expression is observed in the liver of rats submitted to protein-deficient diets, and the levels of c-*myc* mRNA are abruptly decreased when the animals are fed a meal containing an appropriate amount of protein.[755] These results demonstrate the occurrence of changes in the expression of a protooncogene during proliferative responses under physiological conditions *in vivo*.

5. Expression of c-*myc* in Senescent Cells

An increased expression of c-*myc* is observed in cultured human fibroblasts derived from patients with progeria (Hutchinson-Gilford syndrome), a genetic disease characterized by premature and accelerated aging.[756] Expression of the c-*myc* gene may decrease during *in vitro* senescence. In cultured human fibroblasts (IMR-90 cells), a significant decrease in c-*myc* mRNA levels occur in late passage when compared to levels found in early passage cells.[757] Cells restimulated with serum after serum restriction also show reduced levels of c-*myc* expression in late passage. Since c-*myc* gene expression also decreases in many types of differentiating cells, these observations give support to the hypothesis which considers senescence as a particular type of cell differentiation. However, senescence of cultured cells *in vitro* is apparently not always associated with decreased expression of c-*myc*. The steady-state levels of c-*myc* transcripts may be unaltered during cellular aging of cultured mouse and rat fibroblasts.[758] Both young and senescent rodent cells can respond to growth factor-induced mitogenic stimulation with a sharp increase in c-*myc* mRNA levels, although the senescent cells do not initiate DNA synthesis after stimulation. The reason for the discrepant results obtained with human and rodent cells in relation to c-*myc* expression during senescence *in vitro* are not clear. Spontaneously (established) immortalized rodent fibroblasts have 3- to 20-fold higher levels of c-*myc* mRNA than their mortal counterparts, but both types of cells respond equally with enhanced c-*myc* expression to growth factor stimulation.[758]

Changes in the tissue-specific patterns of DNA methylation are frequently associated with gene expression and such changes may occur in the c-*myc* gene during aging process of mice.[759] Moreover, these changes are variable among different tissues of the animal. The spleen DNA show hypomethylation as mice age, while hypermethylation occurs in the liver DNA and no change is detected in the brain DNA between young and old mice. Interestingly, there may be an organ-specific regulation of c-*myc* gene expression in relation to aging. Transcripts of the c-*myc* gene, but not of c-*sis* or c-*src* genes, are markedly elevated in the rat liver with age.[760] In contrast, there is no substantial change in transcript levels of any of these protooncogenes in aging brain. The mechanisms and biological significance of increased c-*myc* gene expression in the aging liver are unknown.

I. ASSOCIATION OF C-*MYC* EXPRESSION WITH CELL PROLIFERATION AND DIFFERENTIATION PROCESSES

Although a close association between expression of the c-*myc* gene and cell proliferation and/ or differentiation has been observed in many studies, no simple rules can be deduced in relation to this association. Cerebellar neurons *in vivo*, for example, can accumulate c-*myc* mRNA during proliferation and/or differentiation, perhaps as a cellular response to an external signal.[761]

1. Correlation between Cell Proliferation and c-*myc* Gene Expression

Expression of c-*myc* frequently correlates with the rate of cell proliferation. Transit of cells from G_1 to S phase of the cycle may depend on a threshold level of c-*myc* gene expression.[762] In both nontransformed and transformed cell lines, expression of c-*myc* is frequently correlated with the rate of cell growth.[763] A similar correlation may be observed *in vivo*. Rat cardiac myocytes irreversibly lose their proliferative capacity soon after birth and this loss is associated with a precipitous decrease in the level of c-*myc* gene expression.[764] In contrast, cardiac myocyte hypertrophy, which can be produced in rats by aortic constriction, is associated with increased level of c-*myc* gene expression.[765,766] This hypertrophy is not associated with cell division, but it requires DNA synthesis.

In the human placenta, the c-*myc* protooncogene is expressed predominantly in the cytotrophoblast layer, which is very active in proliferation and possesses invasive properties on the endomentrium.[767,768] In contrast, c-*myc* is not expressed in the syncytiotrophoblast layer, which represents a nonmitotic, terminal derivative or the cytotrophoblast. Interestingly, the syncytiotrophoblast but not the cytotrophoblast express high levels of EGF receptors.

2. Uncoupling between Expression of the c-*myc* Gene and Cell Proliferation

In different types of cells there is no correlation between the expression of c-*myc* and cell division and proliferation. Stimulation of human lymphocytes with either phorbol ester (TPA) or calcium ionophore results in strong induction of c-*fos* and c-*myc* expression but this is not associated with commitment of cells to DNA synthesis.[607,769] Stimulation of human peripheral blood B lymphocytes with the specific growth factor BCGF also induces c-*myc* expression but this expression is not sufficient for cell cycle progression into S phase to occur.[770] In two different human B-cell lines, down regulation of c-*myc* gene expression was not found to be a prerequisite for reduced cell proliferation induced by TNF-α or a monoclonal antibody against an MHC antigen.[771] Quantitation of $p62^{c-myc}$ expression in the nuclei of human hematopoietic cells by flow cytometry using fluorescein-labeled monoclonal antibodies indicates that c-*myc* expression is unrelated to cell proliferation.[772] PCC7 embryonal carcinoma cells do not express c-*myc* transcripts even at an exponential rate of proliferation.[773] Expression of the c-*myc* gene is reduced when C3H 10T1/2 mouse cells are treated with the protease inhibitor antipain.[774] The mechanism responsible for this phenomenon is not understood, but the results indicated that reduction of c-*myc* expression is not necessarily associated with inhibition of cell proliferation.

A striking uncoupling of c-*myc* expression and cell proliferation is observed in the unfertilized *Xenopus* egg, which is a nondividing cell for a very long period but contains about 9 pg of c-*myc* mRNA, i.e., 10^5-fold the content of proliferative somatic cells.[746] This mRNA belongs to the class of stable maternal RNAs which are accumulated from early oogenesis. After fertilization, the c-*myc* mRNA is progressively degraded; nevertheless, its level per cell remains greater that that observed in highly proliferative cells. In the cleaving *Xenopus* embryo c-*myc* transcription is also uncoupled from cell division. In *X. laevis* adult tissues expression of the c-*myc* gene is not restricted to proliferating tissues like the skin, liver, and intestine, but is also found, albeit at lower levels, in tissues with limited proliferative capacity like heart and skeletal muscle.[710]

3. Correlation between c-*myc* Expression and Cell Differentiation

At least in some cellular systems, expression of the c-*myc* gene may be more closely associated, either positively or negatively, with cell differentiation than with cell proliferation. Decreased c-*myc* expression occurs in human HL-60 leukemia cells induced to differentiation by treatment with DMSO and this decrease is apparently caused by the differentiation process itself and not by inhibition of cell proliferation since c-*myc* expression remains elevated in HL-60 growth-inhibited but undifferentiated cells.[775] Differentiation of the pluripotential human teratocarcinoma cell line Tera-2 cl.13 induced by retinoic acid is associated with an initial drop in c-*myc* mRNA levels within the first 3 d, followed by a persistent increase of these levels which lasts until the cells differentiate and cease division.[776] DMSO-induced differentiation of Friend murine erythroleukemia cells is associated with a decrease of c-*myc* mRNA to barely undetectable levels.[777] The c-*myc* gene is down regulated in these cells both at the transcriptional level, presumably by a block in the elongation of primary transcripts, and at the posttranslational level by an increase in the degradation of its mRNA. Expression of a transfected c-*myc* gene inhibits the DMSO-induced terminal differentiation of Friend murine erythroleukemia cells.[778,779]

Explants of the central region of embryonic chicken lens epithelium can be induced to differentiation into lens fiber cells when cultured in the presence of vitreous humor (which contains IGF), fetal calf serum, insulin, or IGF. The levels of c-*myc* transcripts are transiently elevated in the differentiating lens epithelial cells in the absence of mitogenic stimulation, as the cells withdraw from the cell cycle.[780] Not only cell differentiation but also cell dedifferentiation may be associated with increased expression of c-*myc*. Establishment of thyroid follicular cells into monolayer culture results in an acute period of cellular dedifferentiation which is associated with an enhanced expression of mRNAs coding for c-*myc* and β-actin, but not c-*ras*.[781]

4. Uncoupling between Expression of the c-*myc* Gene and Cell Differentiation

Density-dependent arrest of DNA replication is accompanied by decreased levels of c-*myc* mRNA in cultured myogenic but not in differentiation-defective myoblasts.[782] Differentiation of mouse and rat myoblasts into multinucleated myotubes is paralleled by a down regulation of c-*myc* gene transcriptional activity. In myoblast and myotube cultures, decreased levels of c-*myc* transcripts are related to the formation of terminally differentiated myotubes, and not to inhibited DNA synthesis and reduced cell growth. Constitutive expression of an exogenous c-*myc* gene inhibits differentiation of the L_6 rat myoblast cell line.[783] The transcriptional expression of the c-*myc* gene remains inducible by serum in differentiated myogenic cells and the expression of the protooncogene does not suppress the differentiated phenotype.[784] Persistent c-*myc* expression is neither necessary nor sufficient for growth factor-induced suppression of the myogenic phenotype in the nonfusing mouse myogenic cell line BC_3H1.[785] The results of these studies indicate that irreversible expression of c-*myc* is not required for terminal myogenic differentiation to occur and that its expression is insufficient by itself to suppress the differentiated phenotype.

5. Dissociation between c-*myc* Expression and Cell Proliferation and Differentiation

The possible role of c-*myc* in the processes of cell proliferation and cell differentiation is not understood and in particular cases the expression of c-*myc* may be dissociated from both of these processes. For example, inhibition of ornithine decarboxylase (ODC), a key enzyme in polyamine biosynthesis, results in depletion of intracellular spermidine and arrest of proliferation of MEL cells, but this arrest is not associated with detectable changes in c-*myc* expression.[786] Spermidine is required for appearance of the differentiated MEL phenotype, but depletion of this polyamine by ODC inhibition has no detectable effect on the biphasic changes in c-*myc* mRNA observed during MEL cell differentiation. Thus, these biphasic changes in c-*myc* expression are not sufficient for induction of the mature phenotype. These results indicate that, at least in certain conditions, the regulation of c-*myc* expression may be dissociated from both cell proliferation and cell differentiation.

The level of expression of the c-*myc* gene may remain unaltered in differentiating cells. Terminal differentiation of THP-1 human monocytic leukemia cells induced by phorbol ester or retinoic acid is associated with induction of c-*fos* and down regulation of c-*myb*, but no significant changes in the levels of c-*myc* expression are observed in the differentiating THP-1 cells.[787]

Studies with calcitriol suggest that this, and probably other, differentiation-inducing agents may act primarily at the level of inhibition of DNA synthesis. Calcitriol is capable of inducing the differentiation of HL-60 cells into monocyte-like cells and this induction is preceded by a significant decrease in the expression of c-*myc* mRNA.[788,789] When HL-60 human leukemia cells are induced to monocytic differentiation by incubation with calcitriol, there occurs an immediate inhibition of DNA synthesis before any change in c-*myc* gene expression.[790] Moreover, calcitriol is capable of directly inhibiting DNA synthesis in isolated nuclei from HL-60 cells. The delayed inhibition of DNA synthesis in HL-60 cells is accompanied by an elevated expression of the c-*fos* gene which may be related to the monocytic differentiation of HL-60 cells.

6. Conclusion

Expression of the c-*myc* gene, as well as expression of the c-*fos* gene, is frequently associated with cell proliferation or differentiation but the exact role of the protein products of the c-*myc* and c-*fos* genes in these processes remains unknown. Moreover, in certain biological systems *in vitro* and *in vivo,* expression of c-*myc* and c-*fos* protooncogenes is not correlated with either cell proliferation or differentiation.

J. FACTORS INVOLVED IN THE REGULATION OF C-*MYC* EXPRESSION

Expression of the c-*myc* protooncogene may undergo marked changes in response to a diversity of both exogenous and endogenous stimuli. Many different types of intracellular and extracellular signal molecules may be involved in the regulation of c-*myc* expression. The levels of expression of both c-*myc* and N-*myc* genes undergo striking biphasic changes during tissue regeneration, for example, during liver regeneration after partial hepatectomy.[672,791] The level of c-*myc* transcripts may be influenced by variations in the intracellular concentration of cAMP. In PY815 mouse mastocytoma cells grown in cell culture, c-*myc* transcripts increase when the cells are treated with a dibutyryl cAMP analog (which increases the intracellular concentration of cAMP) and the c-*myc* transcripts are relatively more abundant in late G_1 or early S phase of the cell cycle.[792] The role of phosphoinositide metabolism in c-*myc* gene expression is not clear. A correlation between the level of c-*myc* expression and the rate of phosphoinositide turnover was found in two of seven cell lines established from human kidney cancers.[793] The two cell lines showing this correlation expressed high levels of c-*myc* transcripts but in a cell line of hematopoietic origin (HL-60 cells), which also exhibited high level of c-*myc* expression, no correlation between the level of expression of c-*myc* and the rate of phosphoinositide turnover was found. There is evidence, however, that c-*myc* gene expression is stimulated by growth factors, phorbol diesters and other agents that activate protein kinase C.[794] Treatment of human T lymphocytes with phorbol butyrate results in induction of both c-*myc* and IL-2 receptor expression.[795] Strong induction of c-*fos* and, to a lesser extent, of c-*myc* is produced by the phorbol ester TPA and by the calcium ionophore A23187, which supports the hypothesis that protein kinase C may be involved in protooncogene activation by growth factors.[796] The important role of hormones and growth factors in the regulation of c-*myc* expression is discussed in a recent book.[4]

K. CONCLUSION

The protein products of cellular genes of the *myc* family are in some way related to, or associated with, cellular proliferation and/or differentiation. However, no clear-cut general rules or general conclusions can be given at present on this subject and some contradictory results obtained with different cellular systems are difficult to reconcile with a simple general scheme. In certain biological systems, both *in vivo* and *in vitro,* there is no apparent correlation between the expression of c-*myc* and cell proliferation or differentiation. The predominant nuclear localization of *myc* proteins suggest a possible function in genome regulation. The available evidence indicates that in some cellular systems the c-*myc* protein may be involved in the control of DNA synthesis. Studies with monoclonal antibodies specific to *myc* proteins or *myc*-specific antisense RNA may contribute to define the role of *myc* proteins in normal and transformed cells. Studies with a constructed plasmid vector containing antisense *myc* sequences indicate that down regulation of c-*myc* expression in murine F9 teratocarcinoma cells is sufficient and necessary for the induction of differentiation.[797] Further studies are required for a better definition of the exact physiological role of c-*myc* gene expression.

XII. THE *MYB* ONCOGENE PROTEIN PRODUCT

Avian myeloblastosis virus (AMV) is a defective, highly oncogenic retrovirus capable of inducing acute myeloblastic leukemia in birds and transforming myeloid hemapotoietic cells *in vitro.*[798] A *ts* mutant of AMV (strain 6A907/7) is characterized by a reduced capacity to transform myelomonocytic cells, which is associated with a substantial decrease in the amounts of v-*myb* mRNA and protein when the cells are shifted from the permissive to the nonpermissive temperature.[799] Although the *in vitro* transforming potential of AMV is highly restricted to hematopoietic cells, cloned proviral AMV DNA is capable of inducing transformation after transfection into chicken embryo fibroblasts.[800] However, expression of molecular clones of v-*myb* in avian and mammalian cells may be independent of neoplastic transformation.[801] Occasionally, AMV-induced leukemia in chickens may show spontaneous regression.[802]

A. THE V-*MYB* ONCOGENE PROTEIN PRODUCT

Unlike other ALVs, AMV does not express the transforming gene via *gag-onc* fusion protein but as a 45- to 48-kDa protein, p45^{v-myb} or p48^{v-myb}, which is translated from a subgenomic mRNA transcribed from the v-*myb* oncogene located at the 3' end of the viral genome.[803] Transcription regulatory signals corresponding to a cryptic potential promoter are also contained in the v-*myc* oncogene of AMV.[804] Another acute transforming retrovirus, the E26 ALV, contains, in addition to v-*myb*, sequences corresponding to an oncogene termed v-*ets*, and its protein product is a 135-kDa polyprotein termed p135$^{gag-myb-ets}$.[805-808] Monoclonal antibodies have been produced with specificity for v-*myb* oncogene products.[809]

DNA binding activity is associated with the purified proteins of both AMV and E26 ALVs.[810] About two thirds of the p45/p48^{v-myb} product present in AMV-transformed chicken myeloblasts are localized in the nuclear matrix-lamina fraction, a structure which is intimately associated with both DNA replication and transcription.[811] Association of the c-*myb* protein with the nuclear matrix-lamina is preserved if nuclei are isolated and fractionated under isotonic conditions, while hypotonicity leads to disruption of the native nuclear complexes, possibly including nuclear actin.[812] Expression of the viral product p48^{v-myb} may not prevent the expression of the normal endogenous product p75^{c-myb} in the cell nucleus.[813]

B. THE C-*MYB* PROTOONCOGENE AND ITS PRODUCT

The v-*myb* oncogene apparently arose by transduction of several of the exons of a cellular gene, c-*myb*, which is present in the genome of a broad spectrum of metazoan species, including *Drosophila*.[814-816] The c-*myb* protooncogene of *Drosophila* is expressed in early embryos of the insect.[817] DNA sequences related to the c-*myb* gene are present in organisms as primitive as *Archaebacteriae*, which are probably associated with the origin of life in the earth.[818] These observations strongly suggest an essential function for the protein product of this protooncogene. As its viral counterpart, the c-*myc* protein is localized to the cell nucleus. In addition to the c-*myb* protooncogene, the human genome contains two *myb*-related genes, A-*myb* and B-*myb*.[819]

1. The Chicken c-*myb* Protein

The protein products of c-*myb* and v-*myb* genes can be identified by immunoprecipitation with antibodies against a synthetic oligopeptide derived from the known v-*myb* sequence. The chicken c-*myb* product is a 75-kDa protein, termed p75^{c-myb}, and the 45- to 48-kDa v-*myb* product is thus a truncated version of the cellular protein.[820-822] In addition, p45/p48^{v-myb} and p75^{c-myb} differ by the presence of several amino acid substitutions.[823] A constructed recombinant in which the expression of the v-*myb* sequences is under the control of the AMV LTRs produces abnormal *myb*-specific RNA species and *myb*-related polypeptides and is capable of transforming CEF cells upon transfection.[824] Qualitative differences may be responsible for the oncogenic potential of the p45/p48^{v-myb} and p135$^{gag-myb-ets}$ viral oncogene products as compared to the lack of this potential in the normal p75^{c-myb} cellular product. All three proteins are located in the nucleus,[825-827] which indicates that the cellular localization is not sufficient to determine neoplastic transformation.

2. The Murine c-*myb* Protein

cDNA clones have been isolated from a murine pre-B cell library and a composite sequence that includes 3413 bases of the murine c-*myb* mRNA have been generated.[828] The nucleotide sequence of murine c-*myb* mRNA has been determined and S1 nuclease protection analysis provided evidence suggesting an extreme heterogeneity at the 5′ end of the molecule. The predicted translation product of this mRNA contains 636 amino acid residues and is about 71 kDa long.

3. The Human c-*myb* Protein

The protein encoded by the human c-*myb* gene has been identified and characterized.[829] The human c-*myb* product is represented by the 75-kDa protein, p75[c-*myb*], which is expressed within the nucleus in apparent association with the nuclear matrix.[830] Complexation of this protein with a specific antibody resulted in inhibition of the transcriptional activity of cellular genes whose mRNAs may be involved in the regulation of cell proliferation.[831] Several other proteins of higher molecular weight were also precipitated by the anti-*myb* antibody in ML-1 and HL-60 human leukemic cells but their relationship to p75[c-*myb*] remained unknown. The human p75[c-*myb*] protein purified by immunoaffinity chromatography following precipitation by a specific monoclonal antibody binds to double-stranded DNA *in vitro* in a filter-binding assay. Although the c-*myb* protein is a nuclear antigen in the transformed T-lymphocytic cell line Molt-4, in proliferating normal human T cells it was detected almost exclusively in the cytoplasm.[832] This finding suggests a second property of the c-*myb* protein in addition to its interaction with DNA.

C. EXPRESSION OF THE C-*MYB* PROTOONCOGENE PROTEIN PRODUCT

Expression of the c-*myb* protein may be correlated with either cell proliferation or cell differentiation processes. Expression of c-*myb* is downregulated during hematopoietic maturation, which may be mediated by a block to transcription elongation in the first intron of the c-*myb* gene.[833] A similar mechanism of regulation of c-*myb* expression by transcription arrest has been identified in other types of cells.[834] However, the expression of c-*myb* is regulated by complex mechanisms that include, in addition to transcription arrest, transcription initiation and RNA turnover. Different types of cells may predominantly use specific mechanisms for the regulation of c-*myb* expression under different physiologic conditions.

1. Expression of c-*myb* and Cell Proliferation

The c-*myb* protooncogene is expressed at relatively high levels during the proliferation in several types of cells, including hematopoietic cells, chicken embryo fibroblasts, B cells from the bursa of Fabricius, and different types of cell lines.[835] Exposure of normal human hematopoietic cells to c-*myb* antisense oligonucleotides *in vitro* results in a decrease in both colony size and number.[836] In the chicken T cell line MSB-1, induction of c-*myb* expression occurs not only during the initial activation of cells to proliferate by dilution in fresh medium, but also in subsequent cell cycles during exponential growth. The amount of variation in c-*myb* mRNA in the cycle of MSB-1 cells is similar to the variations in mRNA levels reported for several other cell cycle-regulated genes.[835] Variation in c-*myb* mRNA levels during cellular activation and proliferation seems to be predominantly the result of posttranscriptional control. In contrast, high levels of c-*myb* mRNA are maintained in both quiescent and proliferating immature thymocytes as a consequence of increased c-*myb* gene transcription. However, a correlation between c-*myb* expression and cell proliferation is not universally observed. Expression of c-*myb* protein in PHA-stimulated human lymphocytes occurs only after initiation of the S phase of the cell cycle.[837] IL-2-induced proliferation of T cells is not associated with altered c-*myb* gene expression.[612] These results argue strongly against a role for this gene in T cell proliferation. The spleens from mice treated with the hemolytic anemia-promoting agent phenylhydrazine show over the next days after treatment a five- to tenfold increase in weight associated with a reticulocytosis of 30 to 50% and accumulation greater than 95% of cells from erythroid lineage in the organ. In spite of these dramatic changes, c-*myb* and c-*myc* transcripts are not increased over the course of the massive erythroid proliferation that occurs in the spleen of the treated animals.[838]

Mouse c-*myb* gene transcripts display considerable 5′ heterogeneity, probably by a process involving selective utilization of mRNA cap sites.[839] the extent of this heterogeneity is, at least quantitatively, cell type specific, but its physiological significance is unknown.

2. Expression of c-*myb* and Cell Differentiation

In hematopoietic tissues, expression of c-*myb* is restricted mainly to immature cells, which suggests that the c-*myb* protein may have a role in differentiation processes associated with normal hematopoiesis.[840] Immature T cells express relatively high levels of c-*myb* protein and it has been suggested that this protein may have an important function during the processes of T cell differentiation.[841] Expression of c-*myb* (and c-*myc*) is definitely increased in normal human B or T lymphocytes after stimulation with specific mitogens.[609,842] IL-2-induced progression of T cells through the G_1 phase of the cycle is associated with a six- to sevenfold increase in the level of c-*myb* gene expression.[843] Developmental regulation of c-*myb* expression is also observed in normal myeloid progenitor cells. Elevated levels of c-*myb* expression have also been detected at specific stages of differentiation of the macrophage lineage of the myeloid cell population.[844] These levels are similar to those observed in cells transformed by v-*myb*-carrying retroviruses. Although it has been suggested that c-*myb* expression is also elevated during erythroid cell differentiation,[841] these findings were not confirmed in an independent study.[844]

Studies with mice homozygous for the *lpr* gene, which spontaneously develop massive lymphoproliferation and an associated lupus-like autoimmune disease, have indicated an inverse relationship between c-*myb* gene expression and cell proliferation or differentiation.[845] The abnormal lymphocytes from *lpr* mice express increased levels of c-*myb* mRNA, and these levels are decreased after treatment *in vitro* with phorbol ester or calcium ionophore, which is concomitantly associated with activation of IL-2 receptor gene expression and progression of the T cells through the cell cycle. Expression of the c-*myb* gene is regulated mainly at the level of transcription in untreated T cells, but the gene is negatively regulated via posttranscriptional mechanisms in the cells treated with phorbol ester and calcium ionophore.

An early decline in c-*myb* oncogene expression is observed in human myeloblastic leukemia (ML-1) cells induced to differentiation with a phorbol ester (TPA).[846] The 4.3 kb c-*myb* transcript declined at 3 h after induction of differentiation, followed by a decrease in DNA synthesis between 3 and 24 h and an increase in morphological differentiation at about 24 to 48 h. AMV-transformed myeloblasts can, however, be induced to differentiation without affecting the expression of v-*myb*, which demonstrates that, during differentiation, the effect of v-*myb* is suppressed by a mechanism other than altered expression of the viral oncogene.[847]

Changes in c-*myb* expression may occur in nonhematopoietic cells during processes associated with differentiation and development. A transient increase in the levels of c-*myb* transcripts occurs in the rat hyppocampus at 3 d of age, suggesting a role for the c-*myb* protein product at earlier stages of brain development.[848]

XIII. THE *MOS* ONCOGENE PROTEIN PRODUCT

The Moloney murine sarcoma virus (M-MuSV) is a defective, highly oncogenic retrovirus which transforms fibroblasts in culture and induce solid tumors *in vivo*.[849,850] M-MuSV was derived from recombinational events that occurred between a chronic, nondefective retrovirus, the Moloney murine leukemia virus (M-MuLV), and a cellular gene, c-*mos*. M-MuSV contains the oncogene v-*mos*.[851]

A number of proteins of different molecular weights have been identified as translational products of the v-*mos* oncogene of M-MuSV.[852-856] The cytoplasm of M-MuSV-infected cells contains a soluble 37-kDa protein, p37$^{v\text{-}mos}$.[857] A *mos*-specific antiserum generated in rabbits with a peptide predicted from the v-*mos* sequence recognizes, in addition to p37$^{v\text{-}mos}$, the *gag-mos* hybrid proteins p85$^{gag\text{-}mos}$ and p100$^{gag\text{-}mos}$, as well as a protein of 55 kDa (p55), which is present in uninfected mouse cells.[855] The best characterized of these products are the 85-kDa hybrid protein p85$^{gag-mos}$, which is encoded by the *ts*110 variant of M-MuSV, and the *env-mos* hybrid product represented by the soluble cytoplasmic protein, p37^{v-mos}.[857-862] Protein p85$^{gag-mos}$ is translated from a 3.5-kb splice product of a larger 4.0-kb viral RNA. Splicing excises a 431-base intron that contains an out-of-frame *gag-mos* junction, replacing it with a shortened but continuous *gag-mos* ORF.[863]

A. STRUCTURE AND BIOCHEMICAL PROPERTIES OF *MOS* PROTEINS

The amino acid sequences of c-*mos* proteins have been deduced from the cloned cDNAs and their comparative study demonstrated a relatively moderate degree of conservation.[864] The cloned human c-*mos* gene contains an ORF which encodes a protein of 346 amino acids.[865] The chicken c-*mos* protein is composed of 349 amino acids and shows 66% overall homology to mouse and human c-*mos* proteins.

cAMP-independent protein kinase activity specific for serine and threonine residues is associated with both p85$^{gag-mos}$ and p37^{v-mos}.[859] The p37^{v-mos} protein expressed in genetically manipulated yeast cells is capable of undergoing autophosphorylation and possesses protein kinase activity.[866] The *mos* protein expressed in bacteria binds ATP and possesses ATPase activity.[867] A strong correlation exists between the cell transformation activity of various mutant v-*mos* oncogene constructs and the serine/threonine-specific protein kinase activity of the products of these constructs.[868] Histidine to tyrosine substitution at amino acid residue 221 in p37^{v-mos} abolishes both the associated protein kinase activity of the protein and its transforming activity.[869] Exposure of NRK cells infected with the *ts*110 variant of M-MuSV to high concentrations of K$^+$ results in a 90% inhibition of the serine kinase activity associated with the p85$^{gag-mos}$ product and reversion of the transformed phenotype.[870] The effect of K$^+$ on the enzyme may be mediated by the status of enzyme phosphorylation. All the available data support the concept that the specific kinase activity is crucially associated with the transforming ability of the v-*mos* protein, but the molecular mechanism of neoplastic transformation induced by the v-*mos* protein associated kinase activity remains unknown.

The v-*mos* protein binds both DNA and RNA, but only in the presence of ATP or certain other nucleoside triphosphates.[871] The mutant protein p19^{v-mos}, which lacks the amino-terminal half of the v-*mos* product, does not bind DNA, whereas the mutant protein p25^{v-mos}, which lacks the carboxy terminus of the product, binds DNA in the presence of nucleoside trisphosphates. Since the v-*mos* protein is localized mainly in the cytoplasm, the biological significance of its nucleic acid-binding properties is not understood.

B. HOMOLOGIES OF THE *MOS* PROTEIN PRODUCTS

The coding region of the c-*mos* protooncogene is less well conserved between species than most other protooncogenes.[864] However, greater conservation is found in those regions of the protein exhibiting homology to other members of the kinase oncogene family, including residues in the putative ATP-binding domain on the amino-terminal region and residues homologous to the kinase domain on the carboxy-terminal portion.

In contrast to other oncogene products, the v-*mos* and c-*mos* proteins may have identical amino acid sequences. The protein p37^{v-mos} is structurally related to both pp60^{v-src} and the catalytic subunit of mammalian cAMP-dependent protein kinase.[872] A sequence located at amino acids 115 to 128 of the predicted v-*mos* protein sequence shows homology with the ATP-binding site of bovine cAMP-dependent protein kinase as well as with the protein products of the oncogenes v-*abl*, v-*yes,* and v-*fms*, which are members of the *src* oncogene family and which possess intrinsic tyrosine-specific protein kinase activity.[873] In all of these oncogene proteins, including p37^{v-mos}, a group of glycines with the sequence Gly-x-Gly-x-x-Gly lies 16 to 28 residues to the amino-terminal side of a lysine residue implicated in binding of ATP. This lysine residue, located at position 121 in the proposed ATP-binding site of the v-*mos* protein, is required for transformation.[874]

Homology has also been detected between p37$^{v\text{-}mos}$, the predicted protein of the murine c-*mos* protooncogene, and the EGF precursor polypeptide, prepro-EGF.[875] This precursor is a large molecule of 1217 amino acids and the three observed regions of homology together comprise 17% of the pro-EGF and 58% of the c-*mos* sequence. Similarity is greatest between the carboxy-terminal region of the v-*mos* protein (residues 317 to 360) and part of the cytoplasmic domain of prepro-EGF (residues 1127 to 1174). Similarities are also observed between two regions of the murine c-*mos* protein sequence (residues 48 to 134 and 196 to 275) and parts of the extracellular domain of prepro-EGF (residues 565 to 651 and 741 to 817, respectively).[875] Since prepro-EGF has structural homology with the EGF receptor, and since the EGF receptor is structurally related to the c-*erb*-B protein product, these structural homologies suggest that the gene of prepro-EGF, the gene of the EGF receptor, and the c-*mos* protooncogene may have evolved from a common ancestor.

A normal 55-kDa cellular protein, p55, is altered by an enzymatic function associated with the v-*mos* gene product. Although p55 is recognized by an antibody generated against the *env-mos* protein, p37^{mos}, it is not a product of the c-*mos* protooncogene, but is apparently identical to vimentin, a normal cellular protein associated with intermediate filaments.[876] The biological significance of the detected limited homology between the v-*mos* product and the p55 protein is unknown.

C. EXPRESSION OF THE C-*MOS* PROTOONCOGENE

The c-*mos* protooncogene is hypermethylated and appears to be transcriptionally silent in most normal and neoplastic tissues.[877] However, low levels of c-*mos* gene expression have been detected in mouse brain, kidney, placenta, and mammary gland as well as in mouse embryos. The highest levels of c-*mos* expression are found in the gonads.

1. Genomic Sequences Involved in the Control of c-*mos* Expression

In the mouse, c-*mos* activation is prevented by upstream DNA sequences encompassing a region, termed UMS, which is approximately 1 kb in length and is located 0.8 to 1.8 kb upstream from the first ATG in the open reading frame of c-*mos*.[878] However, the rate of nucleotide substitutions in the mammalian c-*mos* protooncogene is comparable to that of many functional genes in DNA genomes, suggesting some important biological function for the c-*mos* protein product.[879] Moreover, sequences upstream of the rat c-*mos* gene that block RNA accumulation in mouse cells do not inhibit this accumulation in human cells and do not inhibit *in vitro* transcription of recombinant plasmids containing a c-*mos* gene.[880] Apparently, UMS-containing transcripts can exist as stable poly(A) RNA and UMS may constitute the polyadenylation/termination region of a gene located upstream from c-*mos*.[881] There is evidence that the UMS is expressed in the same tissues as c-*mos* and that both DNA sequences may share a common transcript.

Rat DNA sequences, termed RIS, located upstream of the c-*mos* gene and functionally equivalent to mouse UMS sequences, may modify c-*mos* expression at the level of RNA processing, possibly by destabilizing the c-*mos* mRNA.[882] An enhancer element acting in a *cis* manner may be responsible for the cell type-specific expression of c-*mos* in the rat. The enhancer is localized close to the RIS repressor sequences and shows species preference. The c-*mos* enhancer DNA segment contains four blocks of nucleotides homologous to the SV40 enhancer core sequence and binds different nuclear proteins. In the human and an Old World monkey, the expression and transforming potential of the c-*mos* gene are regulated not by UMS or RIS sequences but by an upstream overlapping ORF.[883]

2. Expression of c-*mos* in Normal Animal Tissues

By means of a sensitive S1 nuclease assay to screen RNA preparations from mouse tissues, c-*mos*-related transcripts of different sizes have been detected in mouse embryos as well as in mouse testes and ovaries.[884] The c-*mos* transcripts are of different size in the testis (1.7 kb) and in the ovary (1.4 kb), and at least two major c-*mos* transcripts (2.3 kb and 1.3 kb) are present in the mouse embryo. The physiological significance of this variation as well as the function(s) of c-*mos* protein(s) are unknown. The round spermatid, a haploid postmitotic germ cell, is the major source of c-*mos* mRNA in the mouse testis, but grown oocytes contain about 100-fold higher concentrations of c-*mos* mRNA than round spermatids.[885] Testicular c-*mos* mRNA expression correlates with the presence of haploid germ cells in several sterile mouse mutants. In the mouse ovary c-*mos* is expressed in oocytes, but not in somatic cells.[886] Transcripts of c-*mos* are not detectable in primary resting oocytes, but accumulate soon after the oocyte enters the growth phase. High levels of c-*mos* mRNA are present throughout oocyte growth and maturation as well as in ovulated eggs prior to fertilization, declining abruptly thereafter. Direct evidence for a role of the c-*mos* gene product in gametogenesis has been obtained by the demonstration that *mos*-specific antisense oligonucleotides microinjected into *Xenopus laevis* oocytes inhibit meiotic maturation.[887]

Recently, it has been recognized that the c-*mos* gene is expressed not only in mouse gonadal tissues and in late-term embryos but also, albeit at low levels, in adult mouse tissues including brain, kidney, mammary gland, and epidermis.[888] Marked differences are observed in the size of c-*mos* transcripts detected in different tissues, and the expression of c-*mos* in the gonadal tissue exhibits developmental regulation. The results of these studies support the hypothesis that c-*mos* protooncogene protein product has a general function in male and female gametogenesis, but it may also have other functions. As in mice, in the chicken c-*mos* transcripts are most abundant in ovaries and testes.[864] However, c-*mos* gene expression is also present in early (4-d-old) chicken embryos, decreasing in older embryos. Low levels of c-*mos* mRNA are present in adult chicken organs, including heart, kidney, and spleen.

3. Expression of c-*mos* in Neoplastic Cells

The c-*mos* protooncogene has been found to be activated in some mouse mouse myeloma cell lines by the LTR from an IAP virus particle.[889] The biological significance of this activation is unknown. The human c-*mos* gene has a low transforming efficiency for mouse cells even when activated by viral LTR sequences.[890] Transgenic mice expressing high levels of c-*mos* transcripts in a diversity of tissues, as a consequence of embryo injection of a murine c-*mos* gene linked to M-MuSV LTR, do not develop tumors but only exhibit changes in secondary lens fiber differentiation.[891] It is thus clear that the transforming potential of the c-*mos* gene *in vivo* is rather low.

A stage-specific expression of c-*mos* gene transcripts was detected in the pluripotent mouse embryonal carcinoma cell line 311 but not in the quasinullipotent cell line F9.[892] These results suggest that the c-*mos* product is expressed in embryonic cells and that it may play a role in early stages of normal development.

D. BIOLOGICAL EFFECTS OF V-*MOS* ONCOGENE EXPRESSION

Recombinant vectors in which LTR of MMTV have been fused to the coding region of v-*mos* have been constructed to study the biological effects of different levels of p37^{v-mos} expression.[893,894] A certain intracellular basal level of p37^{v-mos} is necessary to produce morphological changes of transformation in cultured cells transfected with the cloned vectors and the results suggest that p37^{v-mos} expression is required for both the initiation and maintenance of v-*mos*-induced transformation. Moreover, there is a direct correlation between the amounts of v-*mos*-specific RNA and p37^{v-mos} protein in the transfected cells and their stage of transformation as defined by several transformation parameters.[894] Persistent expression of the v-*mos* oncogene in M-MuSV-transformed mouse fibroblasts is compatible with their reversion to nonmalignancy after prolonged treatment with IFN.[895] IFN-γ is capable of inducing a virtually complete, but reversible, suppression of the neoplastic properties of mouse NIH/3T3 fibroblasts transformed by a retroviral vector containing the v-*mos* oncogene.[896] This suppression is due to a selective down regulation of the expression of v-*mos* transcripts which are under the control of retroviral promoters. These results indicate that the v-*mos* oncogene product plays a direct role in the expression of a transformed phenotype in NIH/3T3 cells transformed by a retroviral vector carrying the v-*mos* oncogene. Expression of a molecular vector containing the v-*mos* oncogene may not be associated with morphological transformation in other cellular systems.[897]

The mechanisms involved in the biological effects of the v-*mos* product are unknown but the product is able to regulate a collagen gene promoter,[898] and it is known that the synthesis of collagen and fibronectin is reduced in transformed fibroblasts. M-MuSV infection may result in the synthesis and/or activation of cellular proteins. At least three new proteins (60,000 to 66,000 mol wt) can be detected in NRK cells after M-MuSV infection.[899] These proteins, called transformation-associated proteins (TAPs), differ from the known products of M-MuSV, including p85$^{gag-mos}$, in terms of molecular weight, antigenic determinants, and associated kinase activity, which suggests that TAPs may represent cellular factors activated by the M-MuSV genome.

XIV. THE *FMS* ONCOGENE PROTEIN PRODUCT

The Susan-McDonough strain of FeSV (SM-FeSV) transduces the oncogene v-*fms*, whose products are glycoproteins with the protein kinase activity of gp180$^{gag-fms}$, gp140^{v-fms}, and gp120^{v-fms}.[900-902] The cellular DNA sequence from which the v-*fms* oncogene is derived is the protooncogene c-*fms*. The primary translation product of the SM-FeSV genome is a *gag-fms* fusion polyprotein consisting of 536 amino-terminal *gag*-coded residues and 975 carboxy-terminal v-*fms*-coded amino acids.[903] Addition of carbohydrate to the polypeptide chain yields a 180-kDa glycoprotein, termed gp180$^{gag-fms}$. Processing of this glycoprotein results in generation of several products, including a glycoprotein of 140 kDa, gp140^{v-fms}, which represents the mature form of the oncogene product and is located on the cell surface.[904] The amino-terminal domain of v-*fms* oncogene product includes a functional signal peptide that can direct synthesis of a transforming glycoprotein in the absence of FeSV-derived *gag* sequences.[905] A cryptic hydrophobic signal peptide sequence in the v-*fms* protein is unmasked by *gag* deletion, thereby allowing the correct orientation and transport of the v-*fms* product within the cellular membranous organelles. Expression of the gp140^{v-fms} glycoprotein on the cell surface is required for v-*fms*-induced transformation.[906] The gp140^{v-fms} product is phosphorylated in both tyrosine and serine residues on the surface of SM-FeSV-transformed cells.[907] The v-*fms* oncogene encodes a constitutive receptor kinase that can transform both immature and mature hematopoietic cells of the myeloid lineage as well as fibroblasts by a nonautocrine mechanism.[908,909] Site-directed mutagenesis analysis may contribute to a better definition of the functional domains of the v-*fms* protein. Different insertion mutations in the v-*fms* gene affect the capacity of the gene to transform cells *in vitro*, as well as the processing, intracellular distribution, and tyrosine-specific kinase activity of the encoded protein.[910]

An acute transforming feline retrovirus isolate, the Hardy-Zuckerman 4 strain of FeSV (HZ4-FeSV), contains an oncogene, termed v-*kit*, with close homology to v-*fms*.[10,911] The product of v-*kit* corresponds to a carboxy-terminally truncated version of the v-*fms* protein.

A. THE *FMS* PROTEIN PRODUCT AND THE CSF-1 RECEPTOR PROTEIN

The structure and topology of the gp140^{v-fms} protein resembles that of the known cell surface receptors.[904,912] Like the v-*erb*-B product, which is derived from viral transduction of a vertebrate EGF receptor gene, the v-*fms* protein has an amino terminal portion orientated to the cell surface, a membrane-spanning sequence, and a carboxyl-terminal signal transducing function corresponding to the protein kinase domain. Transformation by the v-*fms* oncogene protein depends on glycosylational processing and cell surface expression of the oncogene product.[913] Inhibition of glycosylation of the gp140^{v-fms} product by treatment of SM-FeSV-transformed REF cells with castanospermine results in lack of association of the oncogene product with the plasma membrane and reversion of the cells to a nontransformed phenotype.[914] This reversion occurs in spite of the fact that the tyrosine-specific kinase activity of gp140$^{v\text{-}fms}$ is not affected by treatment with castanospermine. Replacement of carboxy-terminal truncation of v-*fms* with c-*fms* protooncogene sequences markedly reduces transformation potential of the protein product.[915] Conversion of leucine-301 to a serine residue in the extracellular domain of the human c-*fms* gene product is sufficient to unmask its transforming potential.[916] Specific binding occurs between the product of the v-*fms* oncogene and a hematopoietic growth factor, the colony-stimulating factor 1 (CSF-1). It is thus most interesting that the gene coding for the CSF-1 receptor protein is closely related to the c-*fms* protooncogene and that the biosynthesis of the CSF-1 receptor probably depends on the transcription of this protooncogene.[917,918]

B. THE C-*FMS* PROTOONCOGENE AND ITS PROTEIN PRODUCT

The c-*fms* gene has been assigned to human chromosome 5, region 5q34.[919] However, *in situ* hybridization studies map this gene to region 5q31-33.[920] The gene is deleted in patients with the 5q- syndrome. The human c-*fms* product has been characterized as a 140-kDa protein that is expressed in cells of the monocyte-macrophage lineage.[921] The human c-*fms* protein is 972 amino acids long and is composed of an amino-terminal extracellular CSF-1-binding domain, a central membrane-spanning region, and a carboxy-terminal cytoplasmic tyrosine kinase domain. Comparison of the feline and human c-*fms* sequences indicates a high degree of evolutionary conservation, but the two proteins have markedly different carboxyl termini.[922] Antibodies to distal carboxyl-terminal epitopes in the v-*fms*-encoded glycoprotein do not cross-react with the c-*fms* gene product.[923] The product of the cat c-*fms* protooncogene is a normal cellular protein of approximate 170,000 mol wt which serves as a substrate for the associated tyrosine-specific protein kinase activity.[924] A cDNA clone corresponding to the murine c-*fms* gene has been isolated, sequenced, and expressed in mammalian cells.[925] The murine c-*fms* protein, as deduced from the cDNA clone, is composed of 976 amino acids and has 75% general homology with the human c-*fms* protein. The homology between the human and murine proteins is strongest (95%) in the cytoplasmic kinase domain and weakest (63%) in the external domain. The murine c-*fms* protein can specifically bind human CSF-1.

The c-*fms*/CSF-1 receptor protein is phosphorylated on tyrosine *in vivo* and is rapidly degraded in response to CSF-1 binding.[20] Stimulation of the CSF-1 receptor induces immediate phosphorylation of other cellular proteins on tyrosine, which sould mediate biochemical and functional changes occurring in target cells stimulated by CSF-1. In contrast, the mature cell surface gp140 glycoprotein encoded by the v-*fms* oncogene is phosphorylated on tyrosine in the absence of CSF-1 and would function as a ligand-independent, constitutively activated kinase.

C. EXPRESSION OF THE C-*FMS* PROTOONCOGENE

Expression of the c-*fms*/CSF-1 receptor gene is not restricted to mononuclear phagocytes and their precursors. Transcripts of this gene have been detected in a diversity of mammalian organs including spleen, brain, and liver.[924] The c-*fms*/CSF-1 gene is also expressed in the normal placenta and in choriocarcinoma cell lines.[926,927] The possible relationship between the c-*fms* protein and the CSF-1 receptor in cells other than monocyte-macrophages and their precursors is not completely understood. However, the c-*fms*/CSF-1 protein expressed by human chorio-carcinoma cell lines is biochemically indistinguishable from the c-*fms*-coded glycoprotein expressed on the surface of normal peripheral blood mononuclear cells.[927] An enhanced level of expression of the c-*fms*/CSF-1 receptor gene is observed during phorbol ester-induced mon-ocytic differentiation of HL-60 cells.[928]

XV. THE *MIL/MHT/RAF* ONCOGENE PROTEIN PRODUCTS

The v-*mil/mht* oncogene is transduced by the avian carcinoma virus MH2, which also transduces the v-*myc*; a homologous oncogene, v-*raf*, was isolated from the murine sarcoma virus 3611 (MuSV 3611).[929-932]

A. THE V-*MIL*/*MHT* AND V-*RAF* PROTEINS

The highly oncogenic avian retrovirus MH2 transduces two oncogenes, v-*myc* and v-*mil*/*mht*. The latter gene of the MH2 virus is expressed as p100$^{gag-mil}$, a *gag*-related protein which contains amino-terminal sequences encoded by the viral *gag* gene and carboxy-terminal sequences encoded by v-*mil*/*mht*. The v-*mil* oncogene cannot directly transform macrophages, but it induces v-*myc*-transformed macrophages to produce a specific growth factor that stimulates the growth of these cells in an autocrine manner.[933] Furthermore, v-*mil* markedly enhances the capacity of v-*myc* to induce monocytic neoplasms *in vivo*. A spontaneous deletion mutant of the MH2 virus, the PA200-MH2 virus, transduces only the v-*mil* oncogene.[934] PA200-MH2 virus induces morphological transformation of CEF cells in culture but, in contrast to MH2, it is very inefficient in inducing colonies in semisolid medium and is totally unable to induce wing tumors by inoculation into young birds. Although v-*mil* alone is capable of inducing proliferation on cultured chicken neuroretina cells, both the v-*mil* and v-*myc* oncogenes contained in the MH2 retrovirus are required to induce the complete neoplastic transformation of these cells.[935,936] The biological properties of the p100$^{gag-mil}$ product crucially depend on its autophosphorylation on lysine-622, which is located in the ATP-binding domain of the protein, and on the phosphorylation at serine/threonine residues of key cellular substrates.[937] The 35-kDa carboxy-terminal part of the protein, which corresponds to the kinase homologous domain, is sufficient to induce neuroretinal cell proliferation when it is activated by an LTR.[938]

The product of the v-*raf* oncogene contained in the MuSV 3611 genome is a hybrid phosphoprotein, p75$^{gag-raf}$.[939] This protein lacks the amino-terminal region of the normal c-*raf* protooncogene product and is modified by fatty acid acylation (myristylation). Higher molecular weight forms of the p75$^{gag-raf}$ hybrid protein are glycosylated. Deletion of amino-terminal sequences in the c-*raf* gene product is sufficient to confer transforming properties to the protein.[940] Purified recombinant v-*raf* protein expressed in *Escherichia coli* has been used to produce antibodies which are suitable for studying v-*raf* and c-*raf* proteins *in vitro* and *in vivo*.[941]

B. THE *RAF* GENE FAMILY

DNA sequences with homology to avian and murine viral *mil*/*mht*/*raf* oncogenes are present in the cellular genome of all vertebrate species examined so far, including human cells.[929,932,942] At least four v-*raf*-related genes are contained in the human genome: two active genes (c-*raf*-1 and A-*raf*-1) and two inactive pseudogenes (c-*raf*-2 and A-*raf*-2). The general structure of the human c-*raf*-1 gene has been determined and the complete amino acid sequence of the human c-*raf*-1 protein was deduced from the cDNA sequence.[943] The gene A-*raf*-1, also called *pks*, is located on the X chromosome in mouse and man.[944,945] An additional member of the *raf* family, B-raf, was detected recently in the human genome.[946] Two c-*raf* genes, *Draf*-1 and *Draf*-2, are present in the *Drosophila* genome.[947] The *Draf*-1 gene, which is the most closely related to the v-*raf* oncogene, is located on chromosome X and was mapped to position 2F5-6, whereas the *Draf*-2 gene is located on chromosome 2 and was mapped to position 43A2-5.

C. STRUCTURE AND FUNCTION OF C-*RAF* PROTEIN PRODUCTS

The *Drosophila Draf*-1 gene is expressed in form of 3.2-kb transcripts which are most prominent during early embryonic development.[947] Significant steady-state levels of these transcripts persist, albeit at lower levels, throughout the remainder of insect morphogenesis. The protein product of the *Draf*-1 gene shows homology to mammalian serine-threonine kinases and may have a function similar or identical to that of these enzymes.

Two proteins with approximate 71,000 to 73,000 and 210,000 mol wt, respectively, have been detected in normal uninfected chicken cells by using antibodies with specificity for the carboxyl termini of v-*mil* and v-*raf* protein products.[942] The protein of lower molecular weight, p71/73[c-mil], is expressed in a diversity of vertebrate cells including quail fibroblasts and chicken, mouse, rat, and human cell lines. Ehrlich ascites mouse tumor cells and the AMV-transformed chicken myeloblast line BM-2 contain relatively low amounts of the same protein. Chemically transformed or sarcoma virus-transformed quail fibroblasts express p71/73[c-mil] at levels similar to those of untransformed cultured cells from different animal species.[942] Recently, the chicken c-*mil* gene was cloned and the primary structure of the protein product was deduced from the cDNA nucleotide sequence.[948] The chicken c-*mil* protein contains 647 amino acids and has a calculated molecular weight of 73,132. In the protein, 2 domains were recognized: one of 250 amino acids on the carboxy-terminal half exhibiting significant homology to the *src* oncogene product and protein kinase C, and the other on the amino-terminal half containing a cysteine-rich segment which shares significant homology with two similar repetitive domains of protein kinase C. The product of the v-*mil* gene transduced by the MH2 avian retrovirus represents a truncated version of the chicken c-*mil* gene, lacking the amino-terminal portion of the cellular protein. Two distinct, but closely related c-*mil* cDNA clones were isolated from a chicken cDNA library.[949] A study of these clones indicated that a single c-*mil* gene contained in the chicken genome can generate two c-*mil* mRNA species by an alternative splicing mechanism and that these mRNA molecules can be translated into two distinct proteins of 73 and 71 kDa, respectively. The physiologic significance of these two distinct chicken c-*mil* proteins is not understood but the generation of distinct proteins by alternative transcript splicing has been described for other genes, including protooncogenes.

The rat c-*raf*-1 and A-*raf*/*pks* genes have been cloned and the complete nucleotide sequences of the coding regions have been determined.[950,951] The rat c-*raf*-1 product is a 648-amino acid polypeptide of 72,927 putative molecular weight and the rat A-*raf*/*pks* product is a 604-amino acid polypeptide of 67,551 putative molecular weight. Whereas the carboxy-terminal half regions of these polypeptides show high homology with conserved ATP-binding sites and protein kinase catalytic domains, their cysteine-rich amino terminal regions have strong homologies with the cysteine-rich regions present in protein kinase C. These results suggest the existence of important phylogenetic and functional relationships between the *raf* gene family and protein kinase C, including the activities for phosphorylating serine and threonine residues on the protein substrates.

Protein products of the mouse c-*raf*-1 protooncogene have been detected and characterized in murine cell lines by immunoprecipitation analysis with *raf*-specific antisera.[940] A 74-kDa phosphoprotein, p74[c-raf], detected in a spontaneously transformed 3T3 cell line, would represent the full-length product of the murine c-*raf*-1 protooncogene. A 48-kDa phosphoprotein (p48), detected in a cell line transformed by an LTR-activated c-*raf* gene, is a transforming protein which, like the p75[gag-raf] oncogene product of the acute retrovirus MuSV 1316, lacks the amino-terminal portion of the normal c-*raf* protein. The protein encoded by the murine A-*raf*/*pks* gene has 85% amino acid homology with the kinase domain of c-*raf*-1.[945] In contrast to the wide distribution of the c-*raf*-1 protein, expression of A-*raf*/*pks* protein in the mouse is highly restricted in tissue distribution, with highest levels observed in the epididymis, followed by intestine. When incorporated into a MuLV retrovirus, the resulting gag-A-*raf* fusion gene causes transformation of murine fibroblasts *in vitro* and induces tumors after injection into newborn mice. The transformation potential of the recombinant retrovirus is probably related to amino-terminal truncation of the protein product.

The active human c-*raf*-1 gene is located on human chromosome 3, at region 3p25,[952] and the A-*raf*-1/*pks* gene is located on the X chromosome in mouse and man.[944-946] The structure of the human c-*raf*-1 gene has been determined and the complete amino acid sequence of the protein was deduced from the cDNA sequence.[943,953] Full length and truncated versions of the human c-*raf*-1 gene have been expressed as cDNA copies in *Escherichia coli*.[954]

A full length cDNA clone derived from the human A-*raf*-1 gene indicates that it encodes a

606-amino acid protein of 67,530 mol wt.[955] This protein exhibits in the kinase domain 75% amino acid sequence identities with the human c-*raf*-1 product. Whereas the c-*raf*-1 is expressed in a rather generalized fashion, the expression of A-*raf*-1/*pks* is restricted to some tissues in the human, with highest levels in the epididimis. The A-*raf*-1/*pks* gene is is actively transcribed in human hematopoietic cell lines of myeloid and T-cell lineages as well as in mouse-human somatic cell hybrids that retain the human chromosome X.[944] The two transcriptionally active *raf* genes contained in the human genome appear to encode serine/threonine kinases.[946] Expression of c-*raf*-1 in human hematopoietic cells and cell lines is apparently not related to either cell proliferation or differentiation.[956] The normal functions of the c-*raf*-1 and A-*raf*-1/*pks* protein products are unknown.

D. ONCOGENIC POTENTIAL OF C-*RAF* PROTEINS

It has been proposed that the amino-terminal half or the *raf* proteins represents a regulatory domain which if altered or removed would activate the kinase domain and transforming potential of the protein.[955] Hybrid c-*raf*-related rat proteins, in which the 5′ half of the sequence is replaced by an unknown rat sequence, may be produced by DNA rearrangements occurring during the DNA transfection procedure, and the hybrid proteins can display oncogenic capability.[957]

XVI. THE *REL* ONCOGENE PROTEIN PRODUCT

The v-*rel* oncogene is contained in reticuloendotheliosis virus strain T (REV-T), which was isolated from a turkey.[958,959] Apparently, REV-T arose when REV-A, a nondefective helper virus of REV-T, recombined with c-*rel* protooncogene sequences present in the turkey's genome. REV-T is able to transform hematopoietic cells such as avian bone marrow cells.[960] REV-T-transformed cells exhibit lymphoblastoid morphology, acquire infinite growth potential, and are tumorigenic.[961] Cells transformed by REV-T may represent, at least in part, an early stage of lymphoid cell development.[962]

A. THE V-*REL* PROTEIN

The v-*rel* product is a 55- or 59-kDa phosphoprotein, termed p55^{v-rel} or p59^{v-rel}, which is present in REV-T-transformed chicken bone marrow cells and which has a closely associated non-tyrosine-specific protein kinase activity.[30,963,964] In REV-T-transformed chicken spleen cells, p59^{v-rel} is primarily a soluble cytoplasmic protein.[964,965] However, the p59^{v-rel} protein contains sequences that determine its partial localization in the nucleus of REV-T-infected CEF cells.[966] Recently, the v-*rel* protein was purified to near homogeneity by immunoprecipitation with a specific monoclonal antibody.[967] The highly purified p57^{v-rel} protein was found to be complexed with a 40-kDa cellular phosphoprotein in the cytosol of transformed lymphoid cells. The function of the p57^{v-rel}-associated cellular protein is unknown but serine-specific protein kinase activity was detected in the highly purified complex. Transformation of CEF cells by REV-T is associated with a shift of the protein p57^{v-rel} from the nucleus to the cytoplasm.[968]

Transient expression of the v-*rel* oncogene under the control of an SV40 promoter in COS-1 cells results in the synthesis of the v-*rel*-specific protein.[963] The v-*rel* protein has also been expressed in bacteria.[964] There are multiple differences between the primary structures of the predicted translational products of v-*rel* and c-*rel*, which may account for their differential oncogenic potential.[969,970,971] Activation of the c-*rel* protooncogene to a fully transforming gene in REV-T cells requires a series of complex genetic changes that include deletion of the c-*rel* 3′ noncoding sequences, deletion of most of the helper virus-related *env* gene, and alterations of the amino-terminal and central regions of the c-*rel* protein.[972]

B. EXPRESSION OF THE C-*REL* PROTOONCOGENE

There is one large c-*rel* locus in the turkey genome and this locus is transcribed at low levels as a 4.0-kb mRNA in many tissues.[969,970] Levels of c-*rel* transcripts are somewhat higher in hematopoietic tissues than in other tissues. In the normal chicken, c-*rel* transcripts are expressed in all hematopoietic organs.[973] The bursa of Fabricius contains the highest levels of c-*rel* mRNA, followed by liver, bone marrow, spleen, and thymus. Nonhematopoietic organs, such as muscle and brain, contain very low levels of c-*rel* mRNA. In the mouse, relatively high levels of c-*rel* gene transcripts have been observed peripheral B and T lymphocytes, whereas lower levels have been detected in functionally immature thymocytes. High levels of c-*rel* RNA and protein are present in differentiated human lymphoid cells.[974] It seems thus likely that, in contrast to the c-*myb* and c-*ets* proteins, which have been implicated in the earlier stages of hematopoietic differentiation, the c-*rel* protein may have some role in the later stages of lymphocyte differentiation. The exact physiological role of the c-*rel*-encoded protein is unknown, but there is evidence that the product of its viral counterpart, the v-*rel* oncogene, acts as a cell-specific transcriptional activator of certain protmoters.[975] Thus, the c-*rel* protein may be involved in genome regulation. The human genome contains a c-*rel* protooncogene which is located on chromosome 2, region 2p12-p13.[976]

XVII. THE *ROS* ONCOGENE PROTEIN PRODUCT

ASV UR2 is an acute transforming retrovirus capable of inducing sarcomas in chickens *in vivo* and efficiently transform CEF cells in culture.[977] UR2 genome contains 0.8 kb of 5′ leader and *gag* sequences, 1.2 kb of v-*ros* oncogene-specific sequences, and 1.4 kb of *env* and 3′ sequences.[978] UR2 was presumably generated by recombination between the UR2-associated helper virus, UR2AV, and c-*ros* protooncogene sequences, at the expense of part of the *gag* and *env* genes and all of the *pol* gene of UR2AV.[979] Cloned versions of the UR2 virus carrying nonoverlapping deletion mutants within the v-*ros* oncogene have been constructed.[980] Two of these transformation-defective mutants can recombine to produce transforming retrovirus when mixed DNA from both is used to transfect chick embryo fibroblasts along with helper virus DNA.

A. THE V-*ROS* PROTEIN
The UR2 transforming product is a hybrid *gag-ros* protein of 68 kDa, p68$^{gag-ros}$, which is a member of the tyrosine kinase oncogene family.[978] p68$^{gag-ros}$ is a membrane-associated protein whose kinase activity plays a crucial role in UR2-mediated cell transformation. *ts* mutants of UR2 have been isolated and characterized.[981] The *ts* mutant p68$^{gag-ros}$ protein is associated with the cell membrane in mutant-infected cells regardless of the temperature, but is active as protein kinase and cell transformation only at the permissive temperature. Antibodies to the v-*ros* protein product inhibit the tyrosine protein kinase activity of this product in UR2 ASV-transformed rat cells but have no effect on phosphorylation of phosphatidylinositol, suggesting that this activity is not intrinsic to p69$^{gag-ros}$.[982]

Hybrid protein molecules containing v-*ros* sequences fused to discrete portions of the human insulin receptor have been constructed to study the functional properties and transforming potential of the insulin receptor.[983,984] One of these hybrid molecules was capable of transmitting some but not all of the insulin-specific transmembrane signalling. Other hybrid molecules elicited transforming potential in the insulin receptor sequences, apparently by inducing constitutive expression of protein kinase activity.

B. THE C-*ROS* PROTOONCOGENE AND ITS PROTEIN PRODUCT
The c-*ros* protooncogene isolated from a chicken genomic DNA library contains the v-*ros*-homologous sequences distributed among 9 exons ranging in size from 65 to 204 bp.[979] Compared to c-*ros*, the v-*ros* oncogene is truncated at both 5′ and 3′ ends. The predicted c-*ros* protein product shares a striking degree of sequence homology with the insulin and EGF receptor proteins, which suggests that the c-*ros* protein functions as a member of the family of cell surface

receptors possessing tyrosine-specific protein kinase activity. The chicken c-*ros* protein contains at the carboxyl terminus 58 amino acids which are not present in the v-*ros* product.[985] The predicted protein product of the *sevenless* gene of *Drosophila* has 59% amino acid identity with the chicken c-*ros* product in the kinase domain. The *sevenless* product is essential for the development of a specific photoreceptor cell type in the *Drosophila* eye.

The human protooncogene c-*ros*-1, which is the cellular homologue of the v-*ros* oncogene, is composed of 1414 bp spanning 26 kb with 10 exons separated by 1- to 6-kb-long introns.[986-988] This gene is located on human chromosome 6, at region 6q22.[988] Another homologous gene, called c-*ros*-2, *flt*, or *frt*, has been mapped to human chromosome 13, at region 13q12.[988,989] The human c-*ros* gene codes for a molecule with structural features similar to those of growth factor receptors, with an extracellular domain possessing a potential site for N-linked glycosylation, a hydrophobic 24-amino acid stretch which may constitute a transmembrane domain, and a tyrosine kinase domain. Comparison of the human c-*ros*-1 gene and the human insulin receptor gene indicates that the predicted protein molecules are different and that homology between the two proteins in the kinase domain is 48.5%.

C. EXPRESSION OF THE C-*ROS* PROTOONCOGENE

The physiological role of the c-*ros* protein product has not been elucidated as yet. Transcripts of c-*ros* are not detectable in many chicken organs and tissues (spleen, thymus, muscle, heart, liver, and brain), and other tissues (bursa, bone marrow, and kidney) contain only between 1 to 2.5 copies of c-*ros* mRNA per cell.[990] The higher levels of c-*ros* mRNA have been detected in the kidney from 7- to 14-d-old chickens. A c-*ros* transcript of 8.3 kb was detected in normal chicken kidney tissue but not in chicken embryo fibroblasts.[985] No translocation or rearrangement of c-*ros* gene have been detected in various types of human malignancies analyzed.

XVIII. THE *YES* ONCOGENE PROTEIN PRODUCT

The Yamaguchi 73 (Y73) and Esh avian sarcoma viruses were independently isolated from spontaneous tumors in chickens.[991,992] Y73 and Esh ASVs are highly oncogenic, defective retroviruses capable of inducing sarcomas upon inoculation *in vivo* and transformation of CEF cells *in vitro*. The transforming properties of these viruses are associated with the presence of an oncogene, termed v-*yes*, whose product possesses tyrosine-specific protein kinase activity.[993] Y73 and Esh ASVs encode the hybrid proteins p90$^{gag-yes}$ and p80$^{gag-yes}$, respectively.[993,994] The predicted amino acid sequence of p90$^{gag-yes}$ shows significant homology to pp60^{v-src}, especially in the carboxy-terminal region.[995]

A. THE C-*YES* PROTOONCOGENE AND ITS PRODUCT

Clones of c-*yes* cDNA have been derived from poly(A) RNA of human embryo fibroblasts and the sequence analysis of the clones showed that they can encode a human c-*yes* polypeptide consisting of 543 amino acids with a molecular weight of approximately 60 kDa.[996] Comparison of the sequences of c-*yes* and v-*yes* genes revealed that the viral oncogene contains most of the protooncogene coding sequence except the region encoding the extreme carboxyl terminus of the c-*yes* protein. The region missing from v-*yes* protein is the part that is highly conserved in cellular gene products of the protein-tyrosine kinase family.

The chicken c-*yes* protooncogene is expressed in the form of two mRNA transcripts of 3.7 and 3.9 kb which are translated into two proteins of 59 and 62 kDa.[997,998] These proteins are phosphorylated *in vitro* exclusively on tyrosine, whereas *in vivo* their phosphorylation takes place predominantly on serine and to a much less extent on tyrosine. It is not known whether the two c-*yes* transcripts and proteins are generated by different splicing of RNA transcribed from a single c-*yes* gene or as the result of expression of two different c-*yes* genes that would be present in the chicken genome.

B. EXPRESSION OF C-*YES* PROTEINS

The product of the c-*yes*-1 gene (which is a homologue of the Y73 ASV v-*yes* oncogene product) belongs to the nonreceptor types of proteins from the protein-tyrosine kinase family.[996] High levels of expression of c-*yes* proteins have been detected in various chicken tissues, including brain (telencephalon), retina, kidney, and liver, whereas expression of these proteins in muscle, heart, bone marrow, and spleen is apparently very low.[998] The physiological role of the c-*yes* proteins is unknown but immunofluorescence analysis with *yes*-specific antipeptide antibodies indicate that hybrid *gag-yes* proteins are located at several cytoplasmic sites as well as in adhesion plaques and cell-cell junctions in cells infected with Y73 or Esh ASVs.[999]

XIX. THE *KIT* ONCOGENE PROTEIN PRODUCT

The Hardy-Zuckerman 4 strain of feline sarcoma virus (HZ4-FeSV), which was isolated from a cat fibrosarcoma, contains the oncogene v-*kit*.[10] The product of v-*kit* is a hybrid protein of 80 kDa, p80$^{gag-kit}$, whose oncogene-related sequences exhibit homology with the tyrosine kinase family of proteins, especially with the product of the v-*fms* oncogene. The normal counterpart of the v-*kit* oncogene is the protooncogene c-*kit*. The human c-*kit* protooncogene has been mapped to chromosome 4, at region 4q11-q12.[1000] The c-*kit* protein product is a transmembrane protein-tyrosine kinase.[911]

XX. THE *CRK* ONCOGENE PROTEIN PRODUCT

The avian sarcoma virus CT10 contains the oncogene v-*crk*, which exhibits structural similarities to genes of the *src* family as well as to phospholipase C, an enzyme involved in the metabolism of phosphoinositides.[1001,1002] The product of the v-*crk* oncogene is a 47-kDa hybrid protein, p47$^{gag-crk}$, which is composed of 208 amino acids of the viral *gag* sequence fused to 232 amino acids of a protooncogene sequence, c-*crk*. The function of the domain common to v-*src* and phospholipase C is uncertain.

XXI. THE *ETS* ONCOGENE PROTEIN PRODUCT

The acute retrovirus AMV E26 contains, in addition to the oncogene v-*myb*, the oncogene v-*ets*.[1003] Cellular DNA sequences homologous to v-*ets* of AMV E26 are split into two stretches (6.0 and 18.0 kbp, respectively) separated by about 40.0 kbp of the v-*ets*-unrelated DNA.[1004] The v-*myb* and v-*ets* oncogenes of AMV E26 are expressed as part of a 135-kDa polyprotein, p135$^{gag-myb-ets}$, which contains retroviral *gag* sequences at its amino-terminal portion.[1005] This product is localized mainly in the nucleus.[825] The v-*ets* oncogene shows two major stuctural differences in comparison to the normal chicken c-*ets* protooncogene: truncation of sequences present at both the 5′ and 3′ ends of c-*ets* and acquisition of noncoding c-*ets* sequences into the virus.[1006]

A. THE C-*ETS* PROTOONCOGENES AND THEIR PRODUCTS

The chicken c-*ets* protooncogene is a typical eukaryotic gene, with nine viral homologous coding regions separated by introns of varying size, each defined by consensus splice-donor/ acceptor signals.[1006] The products of the chicken c-*ets* gene are a major 54-kDa protein (p54^{c-ets}) and a minor 56-kDa protein (p56^{c-ets}), both proteins being present in the cytoplasm.[1007] These proteins are expressed at high level in the thymocytes and share common antigenic determinants with proteins of 60, 62, and 64 kDa that are expressed at high levels in the macrophages.[1008] This second set of proteins recognized by the anti-*ets* serum are highly related to each other but display only a limited domain of homology with p54^{c-ets} and p135$^{gag-myb-ets}$ and are encoded by a distinct gene, c-*ets*-2, which is partially related to the classic gene, c-*ets*-1.[1009] A major 4.0-kb transcript of the c-*ets*-2 gene is expressed in the cell nuclei from most chicken tissues. The c-*ets*-

1 and c-*ets*-2 genes encode highly conserved proteins and *ets*-related coding sequences are present not only in mammals and birds but also in *Xenopus laevis*, the sea urchin, and *Drosophila melanogaster*.[1010]

There are two c-*ets* protooncogenes in the human genome, one located on chromosome 11 (c-*ets*-1) and the other on chromosome 21 (c-*ets*-2), and both of these human loci are transcriptionally active.[1011] The human c-*ets*-1 gene product was identified as a 51-kDa protein, p51[c-ets-1], which is located mainly in the cytoplasm, and the product of c-*ets*-2 as a 56-kDa protein, p56[c-ets-2], which is located in the nucleus.[1012] Comparison of the predicted amino acid sequences of human c-*ets*-1 and c-*ets*-2 products with their viral counterparts demonstrates 98 and 95% homology, respectively.[1013] The viral p135 v-*ets* hybrid protein and the human c-*ets*-2 gene product are predicted to have different carboxyl termini.

Molecular heterogeneity of the protein products of c-*ets*-1 and c-*ets*-2 is mainly due to posttranslational modification related to phosphorylation on serine and, to a lesser extent, on threonine residues.[1014] These phosphorylations are rapidly stimulated by the calcium ionophore A23187 and are abolished by lowering the extracellular calcium concentration. Mitogenic doses of concanavalin A stimulate the phosphorylation of the c-*ets*-1 protein in thymocytes, suggesting that this product may mediate early events linked to T-cell activation.[1014]

B. HOMOLOGIES OF THE *ETS* ONCOGENE PROTEIN PRODUCT

The protein product of the *ets* oncogene shows significant primary sequence homology with the predicted translational products of two cell division cycle (*CDC*) genes, *CDC4* and *CDC36*, which are involved in the control of cell proliferation in yeast.[93] The nucleotide sequences of four *CDC* yeast genes (*CDC28*, *CDC36*, *CDC37*, and *CDC39*) have been determined.[1015] A portion of the *CDC4* gene product bears highly significant structural homology with the β subunit of bovine transducin.[1016] Another gene (*CDC28*) involved in the control of cell proliferation in yeast is a member of the *src* family and its product is associated with protein kinase activity.[1017,1018] Still another *CDC* gene of *Saccharomyces cerevisiae*, *CDC7*, operates late in the G_1 phase of the cell cycle and is required for the initiation of mitotic DNA synthesis.[1019] The protein product of the *CDC7* gene has regions of homology with *CDC28* as well as with oncogene protein kinases, and may also possess protein kinase activity.

C. EXPRESSION OF C-*ETS* GENES

The human and chicken c-*ets*-1 protooncogenes are preferentially expressed in lymphoid cells and may be involved in regulating the growth of these cells.[1017-1020] Expression of the c-*ets* genes has been studied in detail in the mouse.[1021] The results of this study demonstrated the following: (1) both c-*ets*-1 and c-*ets*-2 loci are transcriptionally active, (2) the c-*ets*-2 locus encodes a major 3.5-kb mRNA that is expressed in most of the mouse tissues examined, whereas the c-*ets*-1 locus encodes a major 5.3-kb mRNA species that is expressed at highest levels in the thymus, (3) both the c-*ets*-1 and the c-*ets*-2 mRNAs are abundant in young proliferating tissues and are greatly reduced in terminally differentiated tissues, except thymus, (4) compensatory growth of liver after partial hepatectomy induces c-*ets*-2 mRNA before DNA synthesis, but after c-*fos* and c-*myc* induction, and (5) c-*ets*-2 mRNA, but not c-*ets*-1 mRNA, is stabilized in the absence of protein synthesis (i.e., in the presence of cycloheximide) during hepatic regeneration. These results indicate that expression of c-*ets*-2 gene is intrinsically linked with cell proliferation. During hepatic regeneration, c-*ets*-1 and c-*ets*-2 loci are subject to differential regulation.[1021] In the adult human brain c-*ets*-1 and c-*ets*-2 are expressed in astrocytes, but not in neurons.[1022] Since, unlike neurons, astrocytes are glial cells able to divide, this expression suggests that the products of c-*ets* genes are involved in the regulation of cell proliferation.

Phorbol ester-induced differentiation of AMV-transformed avian myeloblasts, as well as HL-60 and U937 human leukemia cells, into macrophages is accompanied by an increased synthesis of 68-, 62-, and 58-kDa proteins encoded by the c-*ets* protooncogene or a c-*ets*-related gene.[1009] These proteins may be involved in the induction or maintenance of macrophage differentiation or function.

D. THE *ERG* GENE

The gene *erg*, identified in the human colon carcinoma cell line COLO 320, is closely related to the v-*ets* oncogene and encodes a protein of 462 amino acids whose function is unknown.[1023] The *erg* gene has been assigned to human chromosome 21, which also contains the c-*ets*-2 gene.

XXII. THE *JUN* ONCOGENE PROTEIN PRODUCT

The oncogene v-*jun*, transduced by the acute retrovirus ASV-17,[1024] encodes a protein that possesses DNA-binding domains and is functionally homologous to yeast GCN4 transcriptional activator proteins.[1025,1026] The c-*jun* protooncogene is located on human chromosome 1, at region 1p31-p32.[1027] Both the v-*jun* oncoprotein and the normal product of the human c-*jun* protooncogene are nuclear proteins exhibiting enhancer binding properties similar to that of the mammalian transcription factor AP-1.[595-598] The AP-1 protein is a positive-acting transcription factor which binds to and activates a *cis*-acting DNA sequence involved in controlling the expression of a diversity of genes, particularly those controlled by the tumor promoter phorbol ester, TPA. The AP-1 factor and the product of the c-*jun* protooncogene are identical proteins. The AP-1/c-*jun* protein and the v-*fos* and c-*fos* proteins can recognize the consensus DNA heptanucleotide sequence TGACTCA.[597] Cooperation between c-*jun* and c-*fos* proteins in the regulation of the *cis*-acting heptanucleotide DNA consensus sequence could involve the formation of specific protein complexes between these two proteins and/or other cellular proteins. A 39-kDa protein (p39) that is associated in form of a complex with the c-*fos* protein within the nucleus of fibroblastic cells was identified as the product of the c-*jun* protooncogene. The c-*fos* protein interacts with the c-*jun*/AP-1 protein through the formation of a leucine zipper and the c-*fos*/c-*jun* protein complex recognizes DNA elements containing AP-1 binding sites. Thus, the c-*fos* and c-*jun* proteins are involved in the regulation of transcriptional processes.[545-547]

XXIII. THE *MET* GENE PROTEIN PRODUCT

A putative protooncogene, *met*, was isolated and cloned from the MNNG-HOS cell line, a human osteogenic sarcoma cell line transformed after prolonged exposure to the carcinogen, MNNG.[1028,1029] DNA from the MNNG-HOS cell line is capable of inducing transformation in the NIH/3T3 DNA transfection assay. The *met* gene is contained within 25-35 kb of human DNA and is located on human chromosome 7q31-q32.[1029] This gene is closely homologous to the tyrosine kinase family of genes, including a number of protooncogenes as well as the insulin receptor gene. The product of the normal human *met* gene is a protein of 140 kDa, p140^{met}, which possesses tyrosine-specific protein kinase activity.[1030,1031] Nucleotide sequence of *met* cDNA revealed an ORF with capacity for coding 1408 amino acids with features characteristic of the growth factor tyrosine protein kinase family. The putative ligand of this receptor has not been identified as yet. The p140^{met} protein is located on the cell surface and is phosphorylated on serine and threonine residues.

The gene contained in MNNG-HOS cells is composed of DNA sequences rearranged in the form of a hybrid between the *met* gene and a translocated promoter region (*tpr*) located on human chromosome 1. The product of the fused *tpr-met* gene is a hybrid protein of 65 kDa, p65$^{trp-met}$, which is phosphorylated on both serine and tyrosine residues.[1031] The amino-terminal end of the p65$^{trp-met}$ product exhibits 35% amino acid homology to laminin B1, a glycoprotein that is present in the extracellular matrix.[1032]

A. EXPRESSION OF THE *MET* GENE

The human *met* gene expresses a 9.0-kb transcript, which is predominantly present in fibroblast and epithelial cell lines. The activated protooncogene present in both MNNG-HOS cells and *met* NIH/3T3 transformants expresses a novel 5.0-kb hybrid transcript, which has 5′ sequences derived from the *tpr* locus which maps to human chromosome 1, and 3′ sequences derived from the *met* gene on human chromosome 7.[1033-1035] 10.0-kb *tpr* transcripts are expressed in all human cell lines tested so far.[1033] The possible role of *tpr-met* hybrid transcripts in cell neoplastic transformation is unknown but amplification and overexpression of the *met* gene have been detected in spontaneously transformed NIH/3T3 cells.[1036]

XXIV. OTHER PUTATIVE PROTOONCOGENES FROM THE *SRC* FAMILY

Putative protooncogenes of the *src* family are the genes *fyn/syn/slk*, *lck/lsk/tck*, *hck*, *lyn*, *tkl*, and *arg*. These genes code for proteins with tyrosine-specific kinase activity which are expressed in particular types of cells. Viral counterparts of these genes have not been identified.

A. THE *FYN/SYN/SLK* GENE PROTEIN PRODUCT

The *fyn* gene, also called *syn* or *slk*, is located on human chromosome 6q21 and encodes for a 537-amino acid protein closely related to the tyrosine kinases of other members of the family (*src*, *yes*, and *fgr*).[14,1037,1038] The gene is expressed as a 2.8-kb transcript in various human cell lines. The product of the human and mouse *fyn* gene is a 59-kDa protein, p59^{fyn}, which has covalently attached myristic acid.[1039] The p59^{fyn} protein is phosphorylated both *in vivo* and *in vitro* on serine and tyrosine residues and possesses tyrosine-specific kinase activity. The protein product of the human *fyn* gene is 86% identical to the chicken pp60^{c-src} protein over a stretch of 191 amino acids at its carboxy terminus. In contrast, only 6% amino acid homology exists within the amino-terminal 82 residues of these two proteins. The *fyn* gene can acquire transforming activity by substituting approximately two thirds of its coding sequence for an analogous region of the v-*fgr* oncogene, and the resulting hybrid protein molecule expressed in transformed cells exhibits tyrosine-specific protein kinase activity.[1038]

B. THE *LCK/LSK/TCK* GENE PROTEIN PRODUCT

The gene *lck*, also called *lsk* or *tck*, was detected and identified in the LSTRA cell line, a line which was originally derived from a mouse infected with the retrovirus M-MuLV and which contains an elevated level of tyrosine-specific protein kinase activity.[1040-1042] The product of this gene is a 56-kDa tyrosine protein kinase, p56^{lck}, which is normally expressed at low levels in most murine and human cells.[1043-1045] The kinase activity of p56^{lck} appears to correlate with its state of autophosphorylation.[1046] Studies on *lck* expression in thymocytes, peripheral T cells, and leukemia T-cell lines, arrested at different stages of differentiation, suggest that the *lck* gene is developmentally regulated during the maturation of normal human T lymphocytes and may play a role in the proliferation and differentiation of T cells.[1047] Stimulation of resting T lymphocytes is associated with a prompt decline in the levels of p56^{lck} mRNA and protein expression, which coincides with the maximal induction of lymphokine (IL-2 and IFN) production by the stimulated cells.[1048] In addition, the *lck* gene, as well as the *fyn* and c-*yes*-1 genes, is expressed at relatively high levels in some human colon carcinoma cell lines.[1049]

The *lck* gene is located at the distal end of mouse chromosome 4 and on human chromosome 1, at position 1p32-35, near a site of frequent structural abnormalities in human lymphomas and neuroblastomas.[1042] DNA sequences located 5′ to the murine *lck* gene, containing AUG codons, significantly reduce the *in vivo* efficiency of p56^{lck} translation from the normal mRNA.[1050] Translational activation of the *lck* gene may occur when the 5′ translational control region of the gene is deleted or rearranged, for example, by insertion of an M-MuLV provirus.

High levels of p56^{lck} expression occurring on LSTRA cells are probably responsible for the elevated level of tyrosine protein kinase activity observed in these cells. Moreover, LSTRA cells express a p56[lck] protein that has enhanced kinase activity as a consequence of hypophosphorylation at a regulatory tyrosine residue (tyrosine-505) located on the carboxy-terminal region of the molecule.[1051] The expression of a transformed phenotype by LSTRA cells may be the consequence of the alterations occurring in the *lck* gene and the p56[lck] protein. In LSTRA DNA an internally rearranged M-MuLV genome is interposed between two distinct promoters that normally generate *lck* transcripts differing only in 5′ untranslated regions.[1052] The viral intercalation permits the generation of M-MuLV LTR-*lck* fusion transcripts by using a normal splice acceptor site.

C. THE *HCK/BMK* GENE PROTEIN PRODUCT

A gene termed *hck* has been isolated and characterized using a murine *lck* probe to screen a cDNA library from mitogen-stimulated human leukocytes.[1053,1054] The *hck* gene encodes a 505-residue, 57-kDa polypeptide that is closely related to the p56[lck] gene product and which possesses tyrosine-specific protein kinase activity. The *hck* gene is a member of the *src* family and its product is expressed in blood cells, especially in terminally differentiated granulocytes. The *hck* protein is likely to be a surface membrane protein and might represent a receptor for some hematopoietic growth factor. The *hck* gene has been mapped to human chromosome region 20q11-12, which is not far from the c-*src* locus. That the *lck* gene is maximally expressed in nonproliferating lymphoid cells and the *hck* gene is mainly expressed in peripheral blood granulocytes whose lifespan is less than 12 h clearly indicates that the expression of tyrosine-specific protein kinases is not always correlated with cell proliferation.

A murine homolog of the human *hck* gene has been described under the name of *bmk*.[1055] This gene is expressed in mouse organs characterized by active hematopoiesis, predominantly in cells of the myeloid and B lineages. The B-cell line W279.1 was found to coexpress the *lck* and *hck/bmk* genes. Coexpression of these genes was also detected in A-MuLV-transformed thymic mouse cells.

D. THE *LYN* GENE PROTEIN PRODUCT

The *lyn* gene has been cloned from a human cDNA library and its product is a protein of 58.5 kDa and 512 amino acids.[1056] The *lyn* gene is transcribed into a 3.2-kb mRNA which is expressed in a variety of tissues of the human fetus, with particularly high levels in the liver, but is not expressed in cultured human embryo fibroblasts.

E. THE *TKL* GENE PROTEIN PRODUCT

A cDNA clone isolated from chicken spleen coded for a 457-amino acid protein which is a member of the *src*/tyrosine protein kinase family.[1057] The gene, termed *tkl*, is highly homologous to *lck* and *lyn*, and has a lesser degree of homology to *yes*, *src*, and *syn*. A 3.8-kb transcript of the *tkl* gene was detected in cultured CEF cells as well as in chicken spleen and brain. Chicken spleen transcripts assigned in previous studies to the c-*src* protooncogene may rather correspond to the *tkl* gene.

F. THE *ARG* GENE PROTEIN PRODUCT

The protein product of a gene, termed *arg*, may also possess tyrosine-specific protein kinase activity.[15] This gene is located on human chromosome region 1q24-25 and consists of two exons. The *arg* gene is highly homologous to the v-*abl* and c-*abl* oncogenes and is expressed in normal human cells (brain tissue and fibroblasts) as well as in some human tumor cell lines.

XXV. OTHER PUTATIVE PROTOONCOGENES

Other genes which may be considered as putative protooncogenes have been identified by means of the DNA transfection/transformation assays or other techniques. The putative protooncogenes *int* and *pim* are frequently activated by insertional mechanisms in mice infected by chronic retroviruses and are discussed in Chapter 3.

A. THE *HST* GENE PROTEIN PRODUCT

A putative protooncogene, termed *hst*, with transforming ability in the NIH/3T3 DNA transfection assay, was identified in 2 of 21 samples of primary or metastatic human stomach cancers as well as in a noncancerous portion of the stomach mucosa from one of these two patients.[1058,1059] A gene similar or identical to *hst* was found to be active in the transfection assay with DNA from Kaposi's sarcoma.[1060]

The protein encoded by the *hst* gene, as predicted from the DNA sequence, is 206 amino acids long and exhibits significant homology to fibroblast growth factors (FGFs), especially to basic FGF.[1061] The *hst* protein, expressed in genetically manipulated mouse fibroblasts, stimulates cell proliferation. The product of the *int*-2 gene, which is frequently activated by an insertional mechanism in MMTV-induced mouse mammary tumorigenesis,[1062] also exhibits structural homology to basic FGF.[1063] The *hst* gene product may thus be considered as a growth factor from the FGF family. FGFs could have a role in tumor growth by an autocrine or paracrine mechanism. Transfection into mouse NR6 cells of a recombinant plasmid expressing acidic FGF results in loss of contact inhibition and induction of tumorigenic capability.[1064]

Oncogenic activation of the *hst* gene may occur by DNA rearrangement during or after DNA transfection procedures.[1065] The possible role of this gene in human tumorigenic processes, if any, is not understood. Of 8 primary human melanomas, 1 contained an amplification of *hst* as well as *int*-2 sequences.[1066] Both genes are located on the same human chromosomal band, 11q13. They may derive from a common ancestor by duplication.

B. THE *RIG* GENE PROTEIN PRODUCT

A gene, termed *rig*, was found to be transcriptionally activated in insulinomas induced in rats by a combined treatment with streptozotocin and nicotinamide and in hamsters by inoculation with BK virus.[1067] The same gene is expressed in human insulinomas but not in normal pancreatic islets or in regenerating islets of Langerhans. The *rig* gene was also found to be expressed in a variety of human tumors such as neuroblastomas, esophageal cancer, and colon cancers, as well as in normal rat embryo fibroblasts. The *rig* gene was cloned form hamster and human insulinoma cDNA libraries and the nucleotide sequences were determined.[1067] Both hamster and human homologues contain an ORF of 435 nucleotides capable of coding a 145-amino acid polypeptide. The deduced amino acid sequences of the *rig* protein product has remained invariant in hamster, human, and rat cells, indicating the physiological importance of the *rig* protein. This protein may have DNA binding properties but its function is unknown.

C. THE *DBL* GENE PROTEIN PRODUCT

The *dbl* gene was initially isolated as a 45-kbp DNA sequence contained in a human diffuse B-cell lymphoma which gave positive results in the NIH/3T3 transfection/transformation assay. An independent isolate of *dbl* was obtained following transfection of NIH/3T3 cells with DNA of a human nodular poorly differentiated lymphoma.[1069] Oncogenic activation of the *dbl* gene is due to structural rearrangements affecting its 5′ end, but these changes seem to occur during the DNA transfection procedure *in vitro*. A biologically active cDNA clone of the human *dbl* gene was isolated and sequenced.[1070] Expression of a constructed vector carrying the cloned human *dbl* gene in NIH/3T3 cells resulted in neoplastic transformation with an efficiency comparable to that of the v-H-*ras* oncogene.

The normal human *dbl* gene encodes a 66-kDa protein, p66^{dbl}, which is phosphorylated on serine residues and lacks tyrosine-specific protein kinase activity.[1071] The p66^{dbl} *dbl* product is equally distributed within cytosol and crude membrane fractions and lacks detectable homology with known retroviral oncogenes. The normal function of this product is unknown.

D. THE *BCL*-2 GENE PROTEIN PRODUCT

A putative protooncogene, termed *bcl*-2, was detected in a cell line derived from the tumor cells of a patient with acute B-cell leukemia carrying a t(14;18) translocation.[1072] This type of translocation occurs frequently in patients with follicular lymphoma. Analysis of the structure, transcripts, and protein products of the *bcl*-2 gene have been reported.[1073] The study of the cloned human *bcl*-2 gene indicates that it consists of at least two exons and that it codes for two protein products, bcl-2 α and bcl-2 β, the first of 239 amino acids and the second of 205 amino acids, differing at the carboxyl terminus. The *bcl*-2-encoded products do not seem to be secreted proteins and their functions are unknown. Subcellular fractionation and immunoprecipitation analyses indicate that the *bcl*-2 α protein most likely resides in the cell membrane althouth it does not have a transmembrane domain and is probably not a receptor-like protein.[1074] The membrane association of the *bcl*-2 α protein suggest that *bcl*-2 proteins may be involved in signal transduction during B-cell proliferation. Apparently, the *bcl*-2 proteins produced in follicular lymphoma cells with t(14;18) translocation are identical to the normal *bcl*-2 protein products.

Transcripts of the *bcl*-2 gene are expressed in normal human and mouse B and T lymphocytes stimulated with appropriate mitogens.[1075] Equivalent transcripts are expressed in mouse B cell lymphomas, but only in tumors consisting of pre-B and follicular center mature B cells, not in pro-B or plasma cell tumors, which suggests that the product of the *bcl*-2 gene represents a differentiation marker that is expressed only in committed B cells, but is shut off in end stage plasma cells.[1076] Regulation of *bcl*-2 gene expression takes place mainly at the transcriptional level and is apparently subjected to both positive and negative control mechanisms.[1075]

E. THE *LYM* GENE PROTEIN PRODUCTS

The cellular *lym* genes are putative protooncogenes that have been detected by means of the NIH/3T3 DNA transfection/transformation assay. Genes of this type, termed B-*lym*-1 and T-*lym*-I, are active at specific stages of differentiation of mouse and human B-cell and T-cell lymphoid lineages, as well as in chicken, mouse, and human lymphoid neoplasms.[1077-1081] These genes may have a normal function at specific stages of differentiation within discrete lymphoid cell lineages. The protein product of the B-*lym*-1 gene has 58 amino acids (compared to 65 for chicken B-*lym*-1) and shares partial homology with the amino-terminal region of members of the transferrin family of proteins.[1081-1083] Recently, it has been shown that mouse B-*lym*-1 is a portion of mouse LINES repetitive elements and that human B-*lym*-1 is 50 to 60% homologous to the mouse sequence but shows no significant homology to human LINES elements.[1084] The human B-*lym*-1 gene contains an *Alu* sequence repeat. The functional role of B-*lym*-1 in normal cells is not understood and further studies are required for a better characterization of the role of these genes in human lymphomas.[1085]

XXVI. THE P53 GENE PROTEIN PRODUCT

Antigen p53 is a cell-encoded phosphoprotein that was initially identified in association with large T antigen in SV40-transformed cells. Antigen p53 is expressed at elevated levels in a wide variety of transformed cells and is capable of complementing the action of protooncogenes such as c-*ras* and c-*abl* in particular types of experimental systems for the expression of a transformed phenotype.[1086-1091] For these reasons, p53 has been considered as a protooncogene product.

A. THE P53 GENE

The mouse genome contains a single functional p53 gene, which is located on chromosome 11.[1092,1093] The mouse p53 gene has been cloned and the predicted 389-amino acid sequence showed no obvious general homology with any known oncogene but contained a putative tyrosine kinase acceptor site.[1094,1095] The 5′ region of the p53 gene has been well conserved in evolution and there is evidence for a negative regulatory element located within this region.[1096]

A functional gene homologous to the mouse p53 gene is present in human cells, from where it has been cloned and expressed.[1097-1100] The gene coding for p53 is located on the short arm of human chromosome 17, at region 17p13.[1101] The human p53 gene is split into 11 exons that are distributed over 20 kb of DNA.[1102] A gene coding for p53 protein has been cloned and isolated from *Xenopus laevis*.[1103] The nucleotide sequence of the *Xenopus* p53 gene shows a high degree of homology with the human (68%) and murine (70%) p53 coding sequences. The clone derived from *Xenopus* contained a single ORF coding for a protein of 363 amino acids which exhibited 51% homology to human p53 protein and 57% homology to murine p53 protein. Moreover, there is at least one epitope in common between the *Xenopus* and human p53 protein.

B. THE P53 PROTEIN

The human p53 protein comprises 393 amino acid residues and shows 81% homology with mouse p53, although the conservation of homology is not equally distributed along the molecule.[1099,1100] In mouse cells, p53 is phosphorylated on serine-389 and serine-312, and these residues, as well as adjoining amino acid sequences, are conserved in both mouse and human p53, which suggests that they may have an important functional role.[1104] Interestingly, serine-389 may contain a phosphodiester linkage to RNA. Six major tryptic phosphopeptides from p53 have been identified in NIH/3T3 cells, and transformation of these cells with SV40 results in a specific increase in phosphorylation at p53 serine residues 310 and/or 312.[1105] Monoclonal antibodies have been produced against different epitopes present in the murine p53 protein.[1098,1106] Protein p53 is predominantly located in the nucleus in both transformed and nontransformed cells.[1107] A monoclonal antibody (PAb1620) which was originally reported to recognize the nuclear large T antigen of SV40 is, in fact, directed against the p53 protein which is frequently complexed with the large T antigen in SV40-transformed cells.[1108]

Two different forms of p53 have been detected by monoclonal antibodies in nondividing and dividing lymphocytes, which suggests the possibility that they represent different functional forms of the protein.[1109] The two forms of p53 may be originated by posttranslational modification and may be selectively present in particular types of transformed cell lines.[1110] However, the two forms of p53 may be originated by gene polymorphism, as demonstrated by nucleic acid analysis which suggested the existence of at least two alleles coding for p53 protein in human cells.[1111]

Several different mutant forms of mouse p53 protein have been isolated. While wild-type mouse p53 binds predominantly to large T antigen in SV40 infected cells, the mutant p53 proteins complex to cellular heat shock proteins HSP 72/73 in SV40-transformed COS cells.[1112] The biological significance of such complexes is unknown.

C. FUNCTIONAL ROLE OF THE P53 PROTEIN

The p53 protein could be involved in the regulation of cellular growth. Cooperation between p53 and platelet-poor plasma may result in the induction of cellular DNA synthesis.[1113] The p53 gene has been considered as a cell cycle-dependent gene whose expression can be regulated by different mitogens in different cell types, including human peripheral blood lymphocytes.[1114] In nontransformed, mitogen-stimulated 3T3 fibroblasts, synthesis and steady-state levels of p53 protein and mRNA increase prior to DNA synthesis in late G_1 phase of the cell cycle, which suggests a role for p53 in the progression of cells from a growth-arrested state to an actively dividing state.[1115] Microinjection into the nucleus of a monoclonal antibody directed against the p53 protein at or around the time of serum stimulation of quiescent Swiss 3T3 mouse cells inhibits the subsequent entry of the cells into the S phase of the cycle.[1116]

The physiological role of the p53 antigen remains unknown. Antigen p53 may be expressed at a constant level during the cell cycle in actively growing normal cells, for example, in FR 3T3 rat cells.[1117] It is thus unlikely that p53 is directly involved in cell cycle regulation. Expression of p53 in normal and leukemic cells is more correlated with cell growth than with entrance to

TABLE 1
Homologies between Oncogene Protein Products and other Cellular Proteins

Oncogene protein	Cellular protein
sis	Platelet-derived growth factor (PDGF)
erb-B	Epidermal growth factor (EGF) receptor
mos	Epidermal growth factor (EGF) precursor
src family	Insulin receptor and catalytic chain of mammalian cAMP-dependent protein kinase
ras	α subunit of GTP-binding proteins (G proteins)
erb-A	Thyroid hormone receptor
myc	β and γ crystallins
fms	Mononuclear-phagocyte colony-stimulating factor 1 (CSF-1) receptor
jun	Transcription factor AP-1
int-2 and *hst*	Fibroblast growth factors (FGFs)
crk	Phospholipase C
mas	Angiotensin receptor

the cell cycle or progression through particular phases of the cycle.[1118] In exponentially growing cells there is a concordant relationship between RNA, total protein, and p53, and a parallel decrease in their content is observed in quiescent cells. The notion that p53 is essential for cell proliferation is supported by the observation that introduction of DNA constructs encoding p53-specific antisense RNA into transformed and nontransformed mouse cells results in the complete cessation of cell proliferation.[1119] DNA binding is an intrinsic property of p53.[1120] Recent evidence obtained with the study of human colorectal carcinomas suggests that the p53 gene may act, at least in some cases, as a tumor suppressor gene.[1121] However, the precise function of p53 remains unknown.

XXVII. CONCLUSIONS

The normal functions of oncogene protein products are not well understood but several of these products have mechanisms of action related to those of hormones and growth factors, especially in the regulatory phenomena associated with cell differentiation and cell proliferation. However, it is still unknown whether specific modulations in protooncogene expression are critically required for cell cycle progression or for terminal differentiation.

Tyrosine-specific protein kinase activity is present in some oncogene products, in particular in the products of the *src* family. However, this activity is not an exclusive property of oncogene products since it is also present in the activated receptors of a number of hormones and growth factors, including the receptors for insulin, IGF-I, EGF, TGF-α, PDGF, acidic FGF, bombesin, and growth hormone. Some oncogene products possess kinase activity for nontyrosine (serine/threonine) residues. Other oncogene products are devoid of kinase activity and display different functions at the level of the plasma membrane, the cytoplasm, or the nucleus.

Striking degrees of structural and/or functional homologies exist between oncogene protein products and a diversity of cellular proteins which include hormones and growth factors as well as their cellular receptors (Table 1). Several protooncogenes encode for growth factor components or for the cellular receptors of hormones or growth factors: c-*sis* encodes the B chain of PDGF, c-*erb*-B codes for the EGF receptor, c-*fms* for the CSF-1 receptor, and c-*erb*-A for the thyroid hormone receptor. Recently, it has been recognized that the *mas* oncogene encodes an angiotensin receptor.[1122] The predominant subcellular localization of oncogene protein products may give some clues about their normal functions. The v-*ras*, v-*src*, v-*erb*-B, v-*fms*, v-*yes*, and v-*abl* proteins are localized on the plasma membrane, the v-*raf* and v-*mos* proteins are soluble in the cytosol, and the v-*fos*, v-*myc*, v-*myb*, v-*ski*, v-*jun*, and v-*erb*-A proteins are localized in the nucleus. The product of v-*rel* is localized in both the cytoplasm and the nucleus. The cellular (protooncogene) counterparts of these products have usually the same location. The cellular p53 antigen is predominantly located in the nucleus. The predominant localization of oncogene protein products in the membrane, the cytoplasm, or the nucleus can give clues about the mechanisms of malignant transformation induced by these products. However, changes occurring at cellular sites other than the predominant localization of oncogene products may be involved in the origin and/or development of neoplastic transformation.

REFERENCES

1. Bishop, J.M., Enemies within: the genesis of retrovirus oncogenes, *Cell,* 23, 5, 1981.
2. Bishop, J.M., The molecular genetics of cancer, *Science,* 235, 305, 1987.
3. Adamson, E.D., Oncogenes in development, *Development,* 99, 449, 1987.
4. Pimentel, E., *Hormones, Growth Factors, and Oncogenes,* CRC Press, Boca Raton, FL, 1987.
5. Cooper, J.A. and Hunter, T., Regulation of cell growth and transformation by tyrosine-specific protein kinases: the search for important cellular substrate proteins, *Curr. Top. Microbiol. Immunol.,* 107, 125, 1983.
6. Hunter, T. and Cooper, J.A., Protein-tyrosine kinases, *Annu. Rev. Biochem.,* 54, 895, 1985.
7. Sefton, B.M., Oncogenes encoding protein kinases, *Trends Genet.,* 1, 306, 1985.
8. Sefton, B.M., The viral tyrosine protein kinases, *Curr. Top. Microbiol. Immunol.,* 123, 39, 1986.
9. Hanks, S.K., Quinn, A.M., and Hunter, T., The protein kinase family: conserved features and deduced phylogeny of the catalytic domains, *Science,* 241, 42, 1988.
10. Besmer, P., Murphy, J.E., George, P.C., Qiu, F., Bergold, P.J., Lederman, L., Snyder, H.W., Jr., Brodeur, D., Zuckerman, E.E., and Hardy, W.D., A new acute transforming feline retrovirus and relationship of its oncogene v-*kit* with the protein kinase gene family, *Nature,* 320, 415, 1986.
11. Shilo, B.-Z., Evolution of cellular oncogenes, *Adv. Viral Oncol.,* 4, 29, 1984.
12. Dean, M., Park, M., Le Beau, M.M., Robins, T.S., Diaz, M.O., Rowley, J.D., Blair, D.G., and Vande Woude, G.F., The human *met* oncogene is related to the tyrosine kinase oncogenes, *Nature,* 318, 385, 1985.
13. Stern, D.F., Hefferman, P.A., and Weinberg, R.A., p185, a product of the *neu* proto-oncogene, is a receptorlike protein associated with tyrosine kinase activity, *Mol. Cell. Biol.,* 6, 1729, 1986.
14. Semba, K., Nishizawa, M., Miyajima, N., Yoshida, M.C., Sukegawa, J., Yamanashi, Y., Sasaki, M., Yamamoto, T., and Toyoshima, K., *yes*-related proto-oncogene, *syn*, belongs to the protein-tyrosine kinase family, *Proc. Natl. Acad. Sci. U.S.A.,* 83, 5459, 1986.
15. Kruh, G.D., King, C.R., Kraus, M.H., Popescu, N.C., Amsbaugh, S.C., McBride, W.O., and Aaronson, S.A., A novel gene closely related to the *abl* proto-oncogene, *Science,* 234, 1545, 1986.
16. Martin-Zanca, D., Hughes, S.H., and Barbacid, M., A human oncogene formed by the fusion of truncated tropomyosin and protein tyrosine kinase sequences, *Nature,* 319, 743, 1986.
17. Heldin, C.-H. and Westermark, B., Growth factors: mechanism of action and relation to oncogenes, *Cell,* 37, 9, 1984.
18. Feige, J.-J. and Chambaz, E.M., Membrane receptors with protein-tyrosine kinase activity, *Biochimie,* 69, 379, 1987.
19. Cirillo, D.M., Gaudino, G., Naldini, L., and Comoglio, P.M., Receptor for bombesin with associated tyrosine kinase activity, *Mol. Cell. Biol.,* 6, 4641, 1986.
20. Downing, J.R., Rettenmier, C.W., and Sherr, C.J., Ligand-induced tyrosine kinase activity of the colony-stimulating factor 1 receptor in a murine macrophage cell line, *Mol. Cell. Biol.,* 8, 1795, 1988.
21. Tuy, F.P.D., Henry, J., Rosenfeld, C., and Kahn, A., High tyrosine kinase activity in normal nonproliferating cells, *Nature,* 305, 435, 1983.
22. Piga, A., Taheri, M.R., Yaxley, J.C., Wickremashinghe, R.G., and Hoffbrand, A.V., Higher tyrosine protein kinase activity in resting lymphocytes than in proliferating normal or leukaemic blood cells, *Biochem. Biophys. Res. Commun.,* 124, 766, 1984.
23. Willman, C.L., Stewart, C.C., Griffith, J.K., Stewart, S.J., and Tomasi, T.B., Differential expression and regulation of the c-*src* and c-*fgr* protooncogenes in myelomonocytic cells, *Proc. Natl. Acad. Sci. U.S.A.,* 84, 4480, 1987.
24. Seki, J., Owada, M.K., Sakato, N., and Fujio, H., Direct identification of phosphotyrosine-containing proteins in some retrovirus-transformed cells by use of anti-phosphotyrosine antibody, *Cancer Res.,* 46, 907, 11986.

25. Di Renzo, M.F., Ferracini, R., Naldini, L., Giordano, S., and Comoglio, P.M., Immunological detection of proteins phosphorylated at tyrosine in cells stimulated by growth factor or transformed by retroviral-oncogene-coded tyrosine kinases, *Eur. J. Biochem.*, 158, 383, 1986.

26. Sadowski, I., Stone, J.C., and Pawson, T., A noncatalytic domain conserved among cytoplasmic protein-tyrosine kinases modifies the kinase function and transforming activity of Fujinami sarcoma virus P130$^{gag-fps}$, *Mol. Cell. Biol.*, 6, 4396, 1986.

27. Akiyama, T., Ishida, J., Nakagawa, S., Ogawara, H., Watanabe, S., Itoh, N., Shibuya, M., and Fukami, Y., Genistein, a specific inhibitor of tyrosine-specific protein kinases, *J. Biol. Chem.*, 262, 5592, 1987.

28. Shiraishi, T., Domoto, T., Imai, N., Shimada, Y., and Watanabe, K., Specific inhibitors of tyrosine-specific protein kinase, synthetic 4-hydroxycinnamamide derivatives, *Biochem. Biophys. Res. Commun.*, 147, 322, 1987.

29. Moelling, K., Heimann, B., Beimling, P., Rapp, U.R., and Sander, T., Serine- and threonine-specific protein kinase activities of purified gag-mil and gag-raf proteins, *Nature*, 312, 558, 1984.

30. Rice, N.R., Copeland, T.D., Simek, S., Oroszlan, S., and Gilden, R.V., Detection and characterization of the protein encoded by the v-*rel* oncogene, *Virology*, 149, 217, 1986.

31. Berridge, M.J., Growth factors, oncogenes and inositol lipids, *Cancer Surv.*, 5, 413, 1986.

32. Berridge, M.J., Inositol lipids and cell proliferation, *Biochim. Biophys. Acta*, 907, 33, 1987.

33. Eisenman, R.N. and Thompson, C.B., Oncogenes with potential nuclear function: *myc*, *myb* and *fos*, *Cancer Surv.*, 5, 309, 1986.

34. Theilen, G.H., Gould, D., Fowler, M., and Dungworth, D.L., C-type virus in tumor tissues of a woolly monkey (*Lagothrix ssp*) with fibrosarcoma, *J. Natl. Cancer Inst.*, 47, 881, 1971.

35. Gelmann, E.P., Wong-Staal, F., Kramer, R.A., and Gallo, R.C., Molecular cloning and comparative analyses of the genome of simian sarcoma virus and its associated helper virus, *Proc. Natl. Acad. Sci. U.S.A.*, 78, 3373, 1981.

36. Wolfe, L.G., Deinhardt, F., Theilen, G.H., Rabin, H., Kawakami, T., and Bustad, L.K., Induction of tumors in marmoset monkey by simian sarcoma virus type 1 (*Lagothrix*): a preliminary report, *J. Natl. Cancer Inst.*, 47, 1115, 1971.

37. Wolfe, L.G., Smith, R.F., and Deinhardt, F., Simian sarcoma virus, type I (Lagothrix): focus assay and demonstration of nontransforming associated virus, *J. Natl. Cancer Inst.*, 48, 1905, 1972.

38. Born, M., von der Helm, K., and Deinhardt, F., Virus-specific phosphoproteins in simian sarcoma virus-transformed primate cells, *EMBO J.*, 1, 1029, 1982.

39. Fry, D.G., Milam, L.D., Maher, V.M., and McCormick, J.J., Transformation of diploid human fibroblasts by DNA transfection with the v-*sis* oncogene, *J. Cell. Physiol.*, 128, 313, 1986.

40. Wong-Staal, F., Dalla Favera, R., Gelmann, E.P., Manzari, V., Szala, S., Josephs, S.F., and Gallo, R.C., The v-*sis* transforming gene of simian sarcoma virus is a new *onc* gene of primate origin, *Nature*, 294, 273, 1981.

41. Robbins, K.C., Devare, S.G., Reddy, E.P., and Aaronson, S.A., *In vivo* identification of the transforming gene product of simian sarcoma virus, *Science*, 218, 1131, 1982.

42. van den Ouweland, A.M.W., Breuer, M.L., Steenbergh, P.H., Schalken, J.A., Bloemers, H.P.J., and Van de Ven, W.J.M., Comparative analysis of the human and feline c-*sis* proto-oncogenes. Identification of 5′ human c-*sis* coding sequences that are not homologous to the transforming gene of simian sarcoma virus, *Biochim. Biophys. Acta*, 825, 140, 1985.

43. Kennett, R.H., Leunk, R., Meyer, B., and Silenzio, V., Detection of *E. coli* colonies expressing the v-sis oncogene product with monoclonal antibodies made against synthetic peptides, *J. Immunol. Methods*, 85, 169, 1985.

44. Wong-Staal, F., Dalla-Favera, R., Franchini, G., Gelmann, E.P., and Gallo, R.C., Three distinct genes in human DNA related to the transforming genes of mammalian sarcoma retroviruses, *Science*, 213, 226, 1981.

45. Dalla Favera, R., Gelmann, E.P., Gallo, R.C., and Wong-Staal, F., A human *onc* gene homologous to the transforming gene (v-*sis*) of simian sarcoma virus, *Nature*, 292, 31, 1981.

46. Van den Ouweland, A.M.W., Roebroek, A.J.M., Schalken, J.A., Claesen, C.A.A., Bloemers, H.P.J., and Van de Ven, W.J.M., Structure and nucleotide sequence of the 5′ region of the human and feline c-*sis* proto-oncogenes, *Nucleic Acids Res.*, 14, 765, 1986.

47. Waterfield, M.D., Scrace, G.T., Whittle, N., Stroobant, P., Johnsson, A., Wasteson, A., Westermark, B., Heldin, C-H., Huang, J.S., and Deuel, T.F., Platelet-derived growth factor is structurally related to the putative transforming protein p28^{sis} of simian sarcoma virus, *Nature*, 304, 35, 1983.

48. Doolittle, R.F., Hunkapiller, M.W., Hood, L.E., Devare, S.G., Robbins, K.C., Aaronson, S.A., and Antoniades, H.N., Simian sarcoma *onc* gene, v-*sis*, is derived from the gene (or genes) encoding a platelet-derived growth factor, *Science*, 221, 275, 1983.

49. Deuel, T.F., Huang, J.S., Huang, S.S., Stroobant, P., and Waterfield, M.D., Expression of a platelet-derived growth factor-like protein in simian sarcoma virus transformed cells, *Science*, 221, 1348, 1983.

50. Robbins, K.C., Antoniades, H.N., Devare, S.G., Hunkapiller, M.W., and Aaronson, S.A., Structural and immunological similarities between simian sarcoma virus gene product(s) and human platelet-derived growth factor, *Nature*, 305, 605, 1983.

51. Stiles, C.D., The biological role of oncogenes — insights from platelet-derived growth factor, *Cancer Res.,* 45, 5215, 1985.
52. Deuel, T.F., Kimura, A., Maehama, S., and Tong, B.D., Platelet-derived growth factor: roles in normal and v-sis transformed cells, *Cancer Surv.,* 4, 633, 1985.
53. Ross, R., Raines, E.W., and Bowen-Pope, D.F., The biology of platelet-derived growth factor, *Cell,* 46, 155, 1986.
54. Williams, L.T., The *sis* gene and PDGF, *Cancer Surv.,* 5, 233, 1986.
55. Deuel, T.F., Pierce, G.F., Yeh, H.-J., Shawver, L.K., Milner, P.G., and Kimura, A., Platelet-derived growth factor/sis in normal and neoplastic cell growth, *J. Cell. Physiol.,* Suppl. 5, 95, 1987.
56. Ross, R., Platelet-derived growth factor, *Annu. Rev. Med.,* 38, 71, 1987.
57. Antoniades, H.N. and Williams, L.T., Human platelet-derived growth factor: structure and function, *Fed. Proc. Fed. Am Soc Exp. Biol.,* 42, 2630, 1983.
58. Stiles, C.D., The molecular biology of platelet-derived growth factor, *Cell,* 33, 653, 1983.
59. Deuel, T.F. and Huang, J.S., Platelet-derived growth factor: structure, function, and roles in normal and transformed cells, *J. Clin. Invest.,* 74, 669, 1984.
60. Antoniades, H.N., Platelet-derived growth factor and malignant transformation, *Biochem. Pharmacol.,* 33, 2823, 1984.
61. Heldin, C.-H., Wasteson, A., and Westermark, B., Platelet-derived growth factor, *Mol. Cell. Endocrinol.,* 39, 169, 1985.
62. Johnsson, A., Betsholtz, C., von der Helm, K., Heldin, C.-H., and Westermark, B., Platelet-derived growth factor agonist activity of a secreted form or the v-*sis* oncogene product, *Proc. Natl. Acad. Sci. U.S.A.,* 82, 1721, 1985.
63. Leal, F., Williams, L.T., Robbins, K.C., and Aaronson, S.A., Evidence that the v-*sis* gene product transforms by interaction with the receptor for platelet-derived growth factor, *Science,* 230, 327, 1985.
64. Robbins, K.C., Leal, F., Pierce, J.H., and Aaronson, S.A., The v-*sis*/PDGF-2 transforming gene product localizes to cell membranes but is not a secretory protein, *EMBO J.,* 4, 1783, 1985.
65. Thiel, H.-J. and Hafenrichter, R., Simian sarcoma virus transformation-specific glycopeptide: immunological relationship to human platelet-derived growth factor, *Virology,* 136, 414, 1984.
66. Niman, H.L., Antisera to a synthetic peptide of the *sis* viral oncogene product recognize human platelet-derived growth factor, *Nature,* 307, 180, 1984.
67. Owen, A.J., Pantazis, P., and Antoniades, H.H., Simian sarcoma virus-transformed cells secrete a mitogen identical to platelet-derived growth factor, *Science,* 225, 54, 1984.
68. Johnsson, A., Betsholtz, C., Heldin, C.-H., and Westermark, B., Antibodies against platelet-derived growth factor inhibit acute transformation by simian sarcoma virus, *Nature,* 317, 438, 1985.
69. Johnsson, A., Betsholtz, C., Heldin, C.-H., and Westermark, B., The phenotypic characteristics of simian sarcoma virus-transformed human fibroblasts suggest that the v-*sis* gene product acts solely as a PDGF receptor agonist in cell transformation, *EMBO J.,* 5, 1535, 1986.
70. Keating, M.T. and Williams, L.T., Autocrine stimulation of intracellular PDGF receptors in v-*sis*-transformed cells, *Science,* 239, 914, 1988.
71. Chiu, I.-M., Reddy, E.P., Givol, D., Robbins, K.C., Tronick, S.R., and Aaronson, S.A., Nucleotide sequence analysis identifies the human c-*sis* proto-oncogene as a structural gene for platelet-derived growth factor, *Cell,* 37, 123, 1984.
72. Johnson, A., Heldin, C.-H., Wasteson, A., Westermark, B., Deuel, T.F., Huang, J.S., Seeburg, P.H., Gray, A., Ullrich, A., Scrace, G., Stroobant, P., and Waterfield, M.D., The c-*sis* gene encodes a precursor of the B chain of platelet-derived growth factor, *EMBO J.,* 3, 921, 1984.
73. Josephs, S.F., Ratner, L., Clarke, M.F., Westin, E.H., Reitz, M.S., and Wong-Staal, F., Transforming potential of human c-*sis* nucleotide sequences encoding platelet-derived growth factor, *Science,* 225, 636, 1984.
74. Ratner, L., Josephs, S.F., Jarrett, R., Reitz, M.S., Jr., and Wong-Staal, F., Nucleotide sequence of transforming human c-*sis* cDNA clones with homology to platelet-derived growth factor, *Nucleic Acids Res.,* 13, 5007, 1985.
75. Rao, C.D., Igarashi, H., Chiu, I.-M., Robbins, K.C., and Aaronson, S.A., Structure and sequence of the human c-*sis*/platelet-derived growth factor 2 (*SIS/PDGF2*) transcriptional unit, *Proc. Natl. Acad. Sci. U.S.A.,* 83, 2392, 1986.
76. Gazit, A., Igarashi, H., Chiu, I.-M., Srinivasan, A., Yaniv, A., Tronick, S.R., Robbins, K.C., and Aaronson, S.A., Expression of the normal human *sis*/PDGF-2 coding sequence induces cellular transformation, *Cell,* 39, 89, 1984.
77. King, C.R., Giese, N.A., Robbins, K.C., and Aaronson, S.A., *In vitro* mutagenesis of the v-*sis* transforming gene defines functional domains of its growth factor-related product, *Proc. Natl. Acad. Sci. U.S.A.,* 82, 5295, 1985.
78. Hannink, M., Sauer, M.K., and Donoghue, D.J., Deletions in the C-terminal region of the v-*sis* gene: dimerization is required for transformation, *Mol. Cell. Biol.,* 6, 1304, 1986.
79. Hannink, M. and Donoghue, D.J., Biosynthesis of the v-*sis* gene product: signal sequence cleavage, glycosylation, and proteolytic processing, *Mol. Cell. Biol.,* 6, 1343, 1986.

80. Van den Ouweland, A.M.W., van Groningen, J.J.M., Hendriksen, P.J.M., Bloemers, H.P.J., and Van de Ven, W.J.M., Nucleotide sequence of the DNA region immediately upstream of the human c-*sis* proto-oncogene, *Nucleic Acids Res.,* 15, 4349, 1987.

81. Wang, J.Y.J. and Williams, L.T., A v-*sis* oncogene protein produced in bacteria competes for platelet-derived growth factor binding to its receptor, *J. Biol. Chem.,* 259, 10645, 1984.

82. Huang, J.S., Huang, S.S., and Deuel, T.F., Transforming protein of simian sarcoma virus stimulates autocrine growth of SSV-transformed cells through PDGF cell-surface receptors, *Cell,* 39, 79, 1984.

83. Garrett, J.S., Coughlin, S.R., Niman, H.L., Tremble, P.M., Giels, G.M., and Williams, L.T., Blockade of autocrine stimulation in simian sarcoma virus-transformed cells reverses down-regulation of platelet-derived growth factor receptors, *Proc. Natl. Acad. Sci. U.S.A.,* 81, 7466, 1984.

84. Wang, J.Y.J., Isolation of antibodies for phosphotyrosine by immunization with a v-*abl* oncogene-encoded protein, *Mol. Cell. Biol.,* 5, 3640, 1985.

85. Stevens, C.W., Brondyk, W.H., Burgess, J.A., Manoharan, T.H., Häne, B.G., and Fahl, W.E., Partially transformed, anchorage-independent human diploid fibroblasts result from overexpression of the c-*sis* oncogene: mitogenic activity of an apparent monomeric platelet-derived growth factor 2 species, *Mol. Cell. Biol.,* 8, 2089, 1988.

86. Fry, D.G., Hurlin, P.J., Maher, V.M., and McCormick, J.J., Transformation of diploid human fibroblasts by transfection with the v-*sis*, *PDGF2*/c-*sis*, or T24 H-*ras* genes, *Mutat. Res.,* 199, 341, 1988.

87. Igarashi, H., Rao, C.D., Siroff, M., Leal, F., Robbins, K.C., and Aaronson, S.A., Detection of PDGF-2 homodimers in human tumor cells, *Oncogene,* 1, 79, 1987.

88. Clarke, M.F., Westin, E., Schmidt, D., Josephs, S.F., Ratner, L., Wong-Staal, F., Gallo, R.C., and Reitz, M.S., Jr., Transformation of NIH 3T3 cells by a human c-*sis* cDNA clone, *Nature,* 308, 464, 1984.

89. Tong, B.D., Levine, S.E., Jaye, M., Ricca, G., Drohan, W., Maciag, T., and Deuel, T.F., Isolation and sequencing of a cDNA clone homologous to the v-*sis* oncogene from human endothelial cells, *Mol. Cell. Biol.,* 6, 3018, 1986.

90. Barrett, T.B., Gajdusek, C.M., Schwartz, S.M., McDougall, J.K., and Benditt, E.P., Expression of the *sis* gene by endothelial cells in culture and *in vivo*, *Proc. Natl. Acad. Sci. U.S.A.,* 81, 6772, 1984.

91. Jaye, M., McConathy, E.M., Drohan, W., Tong, B., Deuel, T., and Maciag, T., Modulation of the *sis* gene transcript during endothelial cell differentiation *in vitro*, *Science,* 228, 882, 1985.

92. Daniel, T.O., Gibbs, V.C., Milfay, D.F., Garovoy, M.R., and Williams, L.T., Thrombin stimulates c-*sis* gene expression in microvascular endothelial cells, *J. Biol. Chem.,* 261, 9582, 1986.

93. Fox, P.L. and DiCorleto, P.E., Modified low density lipoproteins suppress production of a platelet-derived growth factor-like protein by cultured endothelial cells, *Proc. Natl. Acad. Sci. U.S.A.,* 83, 4774, 1986.

94. Seifert, R.A., Schwartz, S.M., and Bowen-Pope, S.M., Developmentally regulated production of platelet-derived growth factor-like molecules, *Nature,* 311, 669, 1984.

95. Nilsson, J., Sjölund, M., Palmberg, L., Thyberg, J., and Heldin, C.-H., Arterial smooth muscle cells in primary culture produce a platelet-derived growth factor-like protein, *Proc. Natl. Acad. Sci. U.S.A.,* 82, 4418, 1985.

96. Goustin, A.S., Betsholtz, C., Pfeiffer-Ohlsson, S., Persson, H., Rydnert, J., Bywater, M., Holmgren, G., Heldin, C.-H., Westermark, B., and Ohlsson, R., Coexpression of the *sis* and *myc* proto-oncogenes in developing human placenta suggests autocrine control of trophoblast growth, *Cell,* 41, 301, 1985.

97. Martinet, Y., Bitterman, P.B., Mornex, J.-F., Grotendorst, G.R., Martin, G.R., and Crystal, R.G., Activated human monocytes express the c-*sis* proto-oncogene and release a mediator showing PDGF-like activity, *Nature,* 319, 158, 1986.

98. Shimokado, K., Raines, E.W., Madtes, D.K., Barrett, T.B., Benditt, E.P., and Ross, R., A significant part of macrophage-derived growth factor consists of at least two forms of PDGF, *Cell,* 43, 277, 1985.

99. Mornex, J.-F., Martinet, Y., Yamauchi, K., Bitterman, P.B., Grotendorst, G.R., Chytil-Weir, A., Martin, G.R., and Crystal, R.G., *J. Clin. Invest.,* 78, 61, 1986.

100. Pierce, G.F., Mustoe, T.A., Senior, R.M., Reed, J., Griffin, G.L., Thomason, A., and Deuel, T.F., *In vivo* incisional wound healing augmented by platelet-derived growth factor and recombinant c-*sis* gene homo-dimeric proteins, *J. Exp. Med.,* 167, 974, 1988.

101. Leof, E.B., Proper, J.A., Goustin, A.S., Shipley, G.D., DiCorleto, P.E., and Moses, H.L., Induction of c-sis mRNA and activity similar to platelet-derived growth factor by transforming growth factor beta: a proposed model for indirect mitogenesis involving autocrine activity, *Proc. Natl. Acad. Sci. U.S.A.,* 83, 2453, 1986.

102. Daniel, T.O., Gibbs, V.C., Milfay, D.F., and Williams, L.T., Agents that increase cAMP accumulation block endothelial c-*sis* induction by thrombin and transforming growth factor-beta, *J. Biol. Chem.,* 262, 11893, 1987.

103. Pantazis, P., Pelicci, P.G., Dalla-Favera, R., and Antoniades, H.N., Synthesis and secretion of proteins resembling platelet-derived growth factor by human glioblastoma and fibrosarcoma cells in culture, *Proc. Natl. Acad. Sci. U.S.A.,* 82, 2404, 1985.

104. van Zoelen, E.J.J., van de Ven, W.J.M., Franssen, H.J., van Oostwaard, T.M.J., van der Saag, P.T., Heldin, C.-H., and de Laat, S.W., Neuroblastoma cells express c-*sis* and produce a transforming growth factor antigenically related to the platelet-derived growth factor, *Mol. Cell. Biol.,* 5, 2289, 1985.

105. Lens, P.F., Altena, B., and Nusse, R., Expression of c-*sis* and platelet-derived growth factor in *in vitro*-transformed glioma cells from rat brain tissue transplacentally treated with ethylnitrosourea, *Mol. Cell. Biol.*, 6, 3537, 1986.

106. Graves, D.T., Owen, A.J., Barth, R.K., Tempst, P., Winoto, A., Fors, L., Hood, L.E., and Antoniades, H.N., Detection of c-*sis* transcripts and synthesis of PDGF-like proteins by human osteosarcoma cells, *Science*, 226, 972, 1984.

107. Graves, D.T., Owen, A.J., and Antoniades, H.N., Demonstration of receptors for a PDGF-like mitogen on human osteosarcoma cells, *Biochem. Biophys. Res. Commun.*, 129, 56, 1985.

108. Betsholtz, C., Johnsson, A., Heldin, C.-H., and Westermark, B., Efficient reversion of simian sarcoma virus-transformation and inhibition of growth factor-induced mitogenesis by suramin, *Proc. Natl. Acad. Sci. U.S.A.*, 83, 6440, 1986.

109. Versnel, M.A., Hagemeijer, A., Bouts, M.J., van der Kwast, T.H., and Hoogsteden, H.C., Expression of c-*sis* (PDGF B-chain) and PDGF A-chain genes in ten human malignant mesothelioma cell lines derived from primary and metastatic tumors, *Oncogene*, 2, 601, 1988.

110. Norris, J.S., Cornett, L.E., Hardin, J.W., Kohler, P.O., MacLeod, S.L., Srivastava, A., Syms, A.J., and Smith, R.G., Autocrine regulation of growth. II. Glucocorticoid inhibit transcription of c-*sis* oncogene-specific RNA transcripts, *Biochem. Biophys. Res. Commun.*, 122, 124, 1984.

111. Colamonici, O.R., Trepel, J.B., Vidal, C.A., and Neckers, L.M., Phorbol ester induces c-*sis* gene transcription in stem cell line K-562, *Mol. Cell. Biol.*, 6, 1847, 1986.

112. Weich, H.A., Herbst, D., Schairer, H.U., and Hoppe, J., Platelet-derived growth factor: phorbol ester induces the expression of the B-chain but not the A-chain in HEL cells, *FEBS Lett.*, 213, 89, 1987.

113. Scher, C.D., Engle, L.J., Eberenz, W.M., Ganguly, K., and Wharton, W., Dissociation of cellular transformation from platelet-derived growth factor independence, *J. Cell. Physiol.*, 126, 333, 1986.

114. Graf, T. and Beug, H., Avian leukemia viruses: interaction with their target cells *in vivo* and *in vitro*, *Biochim. Biophys. Acta*, 516, 269, 1978.

115. Gazzolo, L., Samarut, J., Bouabdelli, M., and Blanchet, J.P., Early precursors in the erythroid lineage are the specific target cells of avian erythroblastosis virus *in vitro*, *Cell*, 22, 683, 1980.

116. Saule, S.S., Roussel, M., Lagrou, C., and Stehelin, D., Characterization of the oncogene (*erb*) of avian erythroblastosis virus and its cellular progenitor, *J. Virol.*, 38, 409, 1981.

117. Graf, T. and Beug, H., Role of the v-*erbA* and v-*erbB* oncogenes of avian erythroblastosis virus in erythroid cell transformation, *Cell*, 34, 7, 1983.

118. Jansson, M., Beug, H., Gray, C., Graf, T., and Vennström, B., Defective v-*erbB* genes can be complemented by v-*erbA* in erythroblast and fibroblast transformation, *Oncogene*, 1, 167, 1987.

119. Yamamoto, T., Hihara, H., Nishida, T., Kawai, S., and Toyoshima, K., A new avian erythroblastosis virus, AEV-H, carries *erbB* gene responsible for the induction of both erythroblastosis and sarcomas, *Cell*, 34, 225, 1983.

120. Miles, B.D. and Robinson, H.L., High-frequency transduction of c-*erbB* in avian leukosis virus-induced erythroblastosis, *J. Virol.*, 54, 295, 1985.

121. Kahn, P., Adkins, B., Beug, H., and Graf, T., *src*- and *fps*-containing avian sarcoma viruses transform chicken erythroid cells, *Proc. Natl. Acad. Sci. U.S.A.*, 81, 7122, 1984.

122. Jurdic, P., Bouabdelli, M., Moscovici, M.G., and Moscovici, C., Embryonic erythroid cells transformed by avian erythroblastosis virus may proliferate and differentiate, *Virology*, 144, 73, 1985.

123. Downward, J., Yarden, Y., Mayes, E., Scrace, G., Totty, N., Stockwell, P., Ullrich, A., Schlessinger, J., and Waterfield, M.D., Close similarity of epidermal growth factor receptor and v-*erb-B* oncogene protein sequences, *Nature*, 307, 521, 1984.

124. Hayman, M.J., *erb*-B: growth factor receptor turned oncogene, *Trends Genet.*, 2, 260, 1986.

125. Carpenter, G., Receptors for epidermal growth factor and other polypeptide mitogens, *Annu. Rev. Biochem.*, 56, 881, 1987.

126. Maihle, N.J. and Kung, H.-J., c-*erbB* and the epidermal growth-factor receptor: a molecule with dual identity, *Biochem. Biophys. Acta*, 948, 287, 1989.

127. Merlino, G.T., Xu, Y.-H., Ishii, S., Clark, A.J.L., Semba, K., Toyoshima, K., Yamamoto, T., and Pastan, I., Amplification and enhanced expression of the epidermal growth factor receptor gene in A431 human carcinoma cells, *Science*, 224, 417, 1984.

128. Kondo, I. and Shimizu, N., Mapping of the human gene for epidermal growth factor receptor (EGFR) on the p13-q22 region of chromosome 7, *Cytogenet. Cell Genet.*, 35, 9, 1983.

129. Spurr, N.K., Solomon, E., Jansson, M., Sheer, D., Goodfellow, P.N., Bodmer, W.F., and Vennstrom, B., Chromosomal localisation of the human homologues to the oncogenes *erbA* and B, *EMBO J.*, 3, 159, 1984.

130. Ng, M. and Privalsky, M.L., Structural domains of the avian erythroblastosis virus *erbB* protein required for fibroblast transformation: dissection by in-frame insertional mutagenesis, *J. Virol.*, 58, 542, 1986.

131. Hayman, M.J., Ramsey, G., Savin, K., Kitchener, G., Graf, T., and Beug, H., Identification and characterization of the avian erythroblastosis virus *erbB* gene product as a membrane glycoprotein, *Cell*, 32, 579, 1983.

132. Beug, H. and Hayman, M.J., Temperature-sensitive mutants of avian erythroblastosis virus: surface expression of the *erbB* product correlates with transformation, *Cell,* 36, 963, 1984.
133. Hayman, M.J. and Beug, H., Identification of a form of the avian erythroblastosis virus *erb-B* gene product at the cell surface, *Nature,* 309, 460, 1984.
134. Privalsky, M.L. and Bishop, J.M., Subcellular localization of the v-*erb*-B protein, the product of a transforming gene of avian erythroblastosis virus, *Virology,* 135, 356, 1984.
135. Schatzman, R.C., Evan, G.I., Privalsky, M.L., and Bishop, J.M., Orientation of the v-*erb*-B gene product in the plasma membrane, *Mol. Cell. Biol,* 6, 1329, 1986.
136. Akiyama, T., Yamada, Y., Ogawara, H., Richert, N., Pastan, I., Yamamoto, T., and Kasuga, M., Site-specific antibodies to the *erbB* oncogene product immunoprecipitate epidermal growth factor receptor, *Biochem. Biophys. Res. Commun.,* 123, 797, 1984.
137. Ullrich, A., Coussens, L., Hayflick, J.S., Dull, T.J. Gray, A., Tam, A.W., Lee, J., Yarden, Y., Libermann, T.A., Schlessinger, J., Downward, J., Mayes, E.L.V., Whittle, N., Waterfield, M.D., and Seeburg, P.H., Human epidermal growth factor receptor cDNA sequence and aberrant expression of the amplified gene in A431 epidermoid carcinoma cells, *Nature,* 309, 418, 1984.
138. Decker, S.J., Phosphorylation of the erbB gene product from an avian erythroblastosis virus-transformed chick fibroblast cell line, *J. Biol. Chem.,* 260, 2003, 1985.
139. Gilmore, T., De Clue, J.E., and Martin, G.S., Protein phosphorylation at tyrosine is induced by the v-*erbB* gene product *in vivo* and *in vitro, Cell,* 40, 609, 1985.
140. Kris, R.M., Lax, I., Gullick, W., Waterfield, M.D., Ullrich, A., Fridkin, M., and Schlessinger, J., Antibodies against a synthetic peptide as a probe for the kinase activity of the avian EGF receptor and v-erbB protein, *Cell,* 40, 619, 1985.
141. Akiyama, T., Kadooka, T., Ogawara, H., and Sakakibara, S., Characterization of the epidermal growth factor receptor and the *erbB* oncogene product by site-specific antibodies, *Arch. Biochem. Biophys.,* 245, 531, 1986.
142. Kato, M., Kawai, S., and Takenawa, T., Altered signal transduction in erbB-transformed cells — implication of enhanced inositol phospholipid metabolism in erbB-induced transformation, *J. Biol. Chem.,* 262, 5696, 1987.
143. Downward, J., Parker, P., and Waterfield, M.D., Autophosphorylation sites on the epidermal growth factor receptor, *Nature,* 311, 483, 1984.
144. Gentry, L.E. and Lawton, A., Characterization of site-specific antibodies to the *erbB* gene product and EGF receptor: inhibition of tyrosine kinase activity, *Virology,* 152, 421, 1986.
145. Clark, S., Cheng, D.J., Hsuan, J.J., Haley, J.D., and Waterfield, M.D., Loss of three major auto phosphorylation sites in the EGF receptor does not block the mitogenic action of EGF, *J. Cell. Physiol.,* 134, 421, 1988.
146. Livneh, E., Glazer, L., Segal, D., Schlessinger, J., and Shilo, B.-Z., The *Drosophila* EGF receptor gene homolog: conservation of both hormone binding and kinase domains, *Cell,* 40, 599, 1985.
147. Wadsworth, S.C., Vincent, W.S., III, and Bilodeau-Wentworth, D., A *Drosophila* genomic sequence with homology to human epidermal growth factor receptor, *Nature,* 314, 178, 1985.
148. Bassiri, M. and Privalsky, M.L., Mutagenesis of the avian erythroblastosis virus *erbB* coding region: an intact extracellular domain is not required for oncogenic transformation, *J. Virol.,* 59, 525, 1986.
149. Privalsky, M.L., Creation of a chimeric oncogene: analysis of the biochemical and biological properties of a v-*erbB/src* fusion polypeptide, *J. Virol.,* 61, 1938, 1987.
150. Bassiri, M. and Privalsky, M.L., Transmembrane domain of the AEV *erb* B oncogene protein is not required for partial manifestation of the transformed phenotype, *Virology,* 159, 20, 1987.
151. Choi, O.-R., Trainor, C., Graf, T., Beug, H., and Engel, J.D., A single amino acid substitution in v-*erbB* confers a thermolabile phenotype to *ts*167 avian erythroblastosis virus-transformed erythroid cells, *Mol. Cell. Biol.,* 6, 1751, 1986.
152. Hayman, M.J., Kitchener, G., Knight, J., McMahon, J., Watson, R., and Beug, H., Analysis of the auto-phosphorylation activity of transformation defective mutants of avian erythroblastosis virus, *Virology,* 150, 270, 1986.
153. Tracy, S.E., Woda, B.A., and Robinson, H.L., Induction of angiosarcoma by a c-*erb*B transducing virus, *J. Virol.,* 54, 304, 1985.
154. Gamett, D.C., Tracy, S.E., and Robinson, H.L., Differences in sequences encoding the carboxyl-terminal domain of the epidermal growth factor receptor correlate with differences in the disease potential of viral *erbB* genes, *Proc. Natl. Acad. Sci. U.S.A.,* 83, 6053, 1986.
155. Riedel, H., Schlessinger, J., and Ullrich, A., A chimeric, ligand-binding verbB/EGF receptor retains transforming potential, *Science,* 236, 197, 1987.
156. Kawai, S., Nishizawa, M., Yamamoto, T., and Toyoshima, K., Cell transformation by a virus containing a molecularly constructed *gag-erbB* fused gene, *J. Virol.,* 61, 1665, 1987.
157. Pelley, R.J., Moscovici, C., Hughes, S., and Kung, H-J., Proviral-activated c-*erbB* is leukemogenic but not sarcomagenic: characterization of a replication-competent retrovirus containing the activated c-*erbB*, *J. Virol.,* 62, 1840, 1988.

158. Velu, T.J., Beguinot, L., Vass, W.C., Willingham, M.C., Merlino, G.T., Pastan, I., and Lowy, D.R., Epidermal growth factor-dependent transformation by a human EGF receptor proto-oncogene, *Science,* 238, 1408, 1987.

159. Zechel, C., Schleenbecker, U., Anders, A., and Anders, F., v-*erb*B related sequences in *Xiphophorus* that map to melanoma determining Mendelian loci and overexpress in a melanoma cell line, *Oncogene,* 3, 605, 1988.

160. Shih, C., Padhy, L.C., Murray, M., and Weinberg, R.A., Transforming genes of carcinomas and neuroblastomas introduced into mouse fibroblasts, *Nature,* 290, 261, 1981.

161. Schechter, A.L., Stern, D.F., Vaidyanathan, L., Decker, S.J., Drebin, J.A., Green, M.I., and Weinberg, R.A., The *neu* oncogene: an *erb*-B-related gene encoding a 185,000 M_r tumour antigen, *Nature,* 312, 513, 1984.

162. Bargmann, C.I., Hung, M.-C., and Weinberg, R.A., The *neu* oncogene encodes an epidermal growth factor receptor-related protein, *Nature,* 319, 226, 1986.

163. King, C.R., Kraus, M.H., and Aaronson, S.A., Amplification of a novel v-*erb*B-related gene in a human mammary carcinoma, *Science,* 229, 974, 1985.

164. Semba, K., Kamata, N., Toyoshima, K., and Yamamoto, T., A v-*erbB*-related protooncogene, c-*erbB*-2, is distinct from the c-*erbB-1*/epidermal growth factor-receptor gene and is amplified in a human salivary gland adenocarcinoma, *Proc. Natl. Acad. Sci. U.S.A.,* 82, 6497, 1985.

165. Schechter, A.L., Hung, M.-C., Vaidyanathan, L., Weinberg, R.A., Yang-Feng, T.L., Francke, U., Ullrich, A., and Coussens, L., The *neu* gene: an *erb*B-homologous gene distinct from and unlinked to the gene encoding the EGF receptor, *Science,* 229, 976, 1985.

166. Fukushige, S.-I., Matsubara, K.-I., Yoshida, M., Sasaki, M., Suzuki, T., Semba, K., Toyoshima, K., and Yamamoto, T., Localization of a novel v-*erbB*-related gene, c-*erbB*-2, on human chromosome 17 and its amplification in a gastric cancer cell line, *Mol. Cell. Biol.,* 6, 955, 1986.

167. Tal, M., King, C.R., Kraus, M.H., Ullrich, A., Schlessinger, J., and Givol, D., Human HER2 (*neu*) promoter: evidence for multiple mechanisms for transcriptional initiation, *Mol. Cell. Biol.,* 7, 2597, 1987.

168. Coussens, L., Yang-Feng, T.-L., Liao, Y.-C., Chen, E., Gray, A., McGrath, J., Seeburg, P.H., Libermann, T.A., Schlessinger, J., Francke, U., Levinson, A., and Ullrich, A., Tyrosine kinase receptor with extensive homology to EGF receptor shares chromosomal location with *neu* oncogene, *Science,* 230, 1132, 1985.

169. Akiyama, T., Sudo, C., Ogawara, H., Toyoshima, K., and Yamamoto, T., The product of the human c-*erbB*-2 gene: a 185-kilodalton glycoprotein with tyrosine kinase activity, *Science,* 232, 1644, 1986.

170. Yamamoto, T., Ikawa, S., Akiyama, T., Semba, K., Nomura, N., Miyajima, N., Saito, T., and Toyoshima, K., Similarity of protein encoded by the human c-*erb*-B-2 gene to epidermal growth factor receptor, *Nature,* 319, 230, 1986.

171. Gullick, W.J., Berger, M.S., Bennett, P.L.P., Rothbard, J.B., and Waterfield, M.D., Expression of the c-*erbB*-2 protein in normal and transformed cells, *Int. J. Cancer,* 40, 246, 1987.

172. Akiyama, T., Saito, T., Ogawara, H., Toyoshima, K., and Yamamoto, T., Tumor promoter and epidermal growth factor stimulate phosphorylation of the c-*erbB*-2 gene product in MKN-7 human adenocarcinoma cells, *Mol. Cell. Biol.,* 8, 1019, 1988.

173. King, C.R., Borrello, I., Bellot, F., Comoglio, P., and Schlessinger, J., EGF binding to its receptor triggers a rapid tyrosine phosphorylation of the *erb*B-2 protein in the mammary tumor cell line SK-BR-3, *EMBO J.,* 7, 1647, 1988.

174. Kokai, Y., Cohen, J.A., Drebin, J.A., and Greene, M.I., Stage- and tissue-specific expression of the *neu* oncogene in rat development, *Proc. Natl. Acad. Sci. U.S.A.,* 84, 8498, 1987.

175. Hung, M.-C., Schechter, A.L., Chevray, P.-Y.M., Stern, D.F., and Weinberg, R.A., Molecular cloning of the *neu* gene: absence of gross structural alteration in oncogenic alleles, *Proc. Natl. Acad. Sci. U.S.A.,* 83, 261, 1986.

176. Bargmann, C.I., Hung, M.-C., and Weinberg, R.A., Multiple independent activations of the *neu* oncogene by a point mutation altering the transmembrane domain of p185, *Cell,* 45, 649, 1986.

177. Perantoni, A.O., Rice, J.M., Reed, C.D., Watatani, M., and Wenk, M.L., Activated *neu* oncogene sequences in primary tumors of the peripheral nervous system induced in rats by transplacenta exposure to ethylnitrosourea, *Proc. Natl. Acad. Sci. U.S.A.,* 84, 6317, 1987.

178. Hudziak, R.M., Schlessinger, J., and Ullrich, A., Increased expression of the putative growth factor receptor p185[HER2] causes transformation and tumorigenesis of NIH 3T3 cells, *Proc. Natl. Acad. Sci. U.S.A.,* 84, 7159, 1987.

179. Bargmann, C.I. and Weinberg, R.A., Increased tyrosine kinase activity associated with the protein encoded by the activated *neu* oncogene, *Proc. Natl. Acad. Sci. U.S.A.,* 85, 5394, 1988.

180. Drebin, J.A., Link, V.C., Stern, D.F., Weinberg, R.A., and Greene, M.I., Down-modulation of an oncogene protein product and reversion of the transformed phenotype by monoclonal antibodies, *Cell,* 41, 695, 1985.

181. Drebin, J.A., Link, V.A., Weinberg, R.A., and Greene, M.I., Inhibition of tumor growth by a monoclonal antibody reactive with an oncogene-encoded tumor antigen, *Proc. Natl. Acad. Sci. U.S.A.,* 23, 9129, 1986.

182. Graf, T. and Beug, H., Role of the v-*erbA* and v-*erbB* oncogenes of avian erythroblastosis virus in erythroid cell transformation, *Cell,* 34, 7, 1983.

183. Henry, C., Coquillaud, M., Saule, S., Stehelin, D., and Debuire, B., The four C-terminal amino acids of the v-*erbA* polypeptide are encoded by an intronic sequence of the v-*erbB* oncogene, *Virology,* 140, 179, 1985.

184. Zahroui, A. and Cuny, G., Nucleotide sequence of the chicken proto-oncogene c-*erbA* corresponding to domain 1 of v-*erbA*, *Eur. J. Biochem.*, 166, 63, 1987.

185. Mitelman, F., Manolov, G., Manolova, Y., Billström, R., Heim, S., Kristoffersson, U., Mandahl, N., Ferro, M.T., and San Roman, C., High resolution chromosome analysis of constitutional and acquired t(15;27) maps c-*erbA* to subband 17q11.2, *Cancer Genet. Cytogenet.*, 22, 95, 1986.

186. Debuire, B., Henry, C., Benaissa, M., Biserte, G., Claverie, J.M., Saule, S., Martin, P., and Stehelin, D., Sequencing the *erbA* gene of avian erythroblastosis virus reveals a new type of oncogene, *Science*, 224, 1456, 1984.

187. Wendorff, K.M., Nishita, T., Jabusch, J.R., and Deutsch, H.F., The sequence of equine muscle carbonic anhydrase, *J. Biol. Chem.*, 260, 6129, 1985.

188. Maren, T.H., Carbonic anhydrase, *N. Engl. J. Med.*, 313, 179, 1985.

189. Frankel, S.R., Walloch, J., Hirata, R.K., Bondurant, M.C., Villanueva, R., and Weil, S.C., Carbonic anhydrase is aberrantly and constitutively expressed in both human and murine erythroleukemia cells, *Proc. Natl. Acad. Sci. U.S.A.*, 82, 5175, 1985.

190. Gandrillon, O., Jurdic, P., Benchaibi, M., Xiao, J.-H., Ghysdael, J., and Samarut, J., Expression of the v-*erbA* oncogene in chicken embryo fibroblasts stimulates their proliferation *in vitro* and enhances tumor growth *in vivo*, *Cell*, 49, 687, 1987.

191. Zenke, M., Kahn, P., Disela, C., Vennström, B., Leutz, A., Keegan, K., Hayman, M.J., Choi, H.-R., Yew, N., Engel, J.D., and Beug, H., v-*erbA* specifically suppresses transcription of the avian erythrocyte anion transporter (band 3) gene, *Cell*, 52, 107, 1988.

192. Boucher, P., Konink, A., and Privalsky, M.L., The avian erythroblastosis virus *erbA* oncogene encodes a DNA-binding protein exhibiting distinct nuclear and cytoplasmic subcellular localizations, *J. Virol.*, 62, 534, 1988.

193. Weinberger, C., Hollenberg, S.M., Rosenfeld, M.G., and Evans, R.M., Domain structure of human glucocorticoid receptor and its relationship to the v-*erb-A* oncogene product, *Nature*, 318, 670, 1985.

194. Greene, G.L., Gilna, P., Waterfield, M., Baker, A., Hort, Y., and Shine, J., Sequence and expression of human estrogen receptor complementary DNA, *Science*, 231, 1150, 1986.

195. Green, S., Walter, P., Kumar, V., Krust, A., Bornert, J.-M., Argos, P., and Chambon, P., Human oestrogen receptor cDNA: sequence, expression and homology to v-*erb-*A, *Nature*, 320, 134, 1986.

196. Krust, A., Green, S., Argos, P., Kumar, V., Walter, P., Bornert, J.-M., and Chambon, P., The chicken oestrogen receptor sequence: homology with v-*erbA* and the human oestrogen and glucocorticoid receptors, *EMBO J.*, 5, 891, 1986.

197. Jeltsch, J.M., Krozowski, A., Quirin-Stricker, C., Gronemeyer, H., Simpson, R.J., Garnier, J.M., Krust, A., Jacob, F., and Chambon, P., Cloning of the chicken progesterone receptor, *Proc. Natl. Acad. Sci. U.S.A.*, 83, 5424, 1986.

198. Giguère, V., Hollenberg, S.M., Rosenfeld, M.G., and Evans, R.M., Functional domains of the human glucocorticoid receptor, *Cell*, 46, 645, 1986.

199. Loosfelt, H., Atger, M., Misrahi, M., Guiochon-Mantel, A., Meriel, C., Logeat, F., Benarous, R., and Milgrom, E., Cloning and sequence analysis of rabbit progesterone-receptor complementary DNA, *Proc. Natl. Acad. Sci. U.S.A.*, 83, 9045, 1986.

200. Bishop, J.M., Oncogenes as hormone receptors, *Nature*, 321, 112, 1986.

201. Weinberger, C., Giguère, V., Hollenberg, S., Rosenfeld, M.G., and Evans, R.M., Human steroid receptors and *erbA* proto-oncogene products: members of a new superfamily of enhancer binding proteins, *Cold Spring Harbor Symp. Quant. Biol.*, 51, 759, 1986.

202. Sap, J., Muñoz, A., Damm, K., Goldberg, Y., Ghysdael, J., Leutz, A., Beug, H., and Vennström, B., The c-*erb-A* protein is a high-affinity receptor for thyroid hormone, *Nature*, 324, 635, 1986.

203. Weinberger, C., Thompson, C.C., Ong, E.S., Lebo, R., Gruol, D.J., and Evans, R.M., The c-*erb-A* gene encodes a thyroid hormone receptor, *Nature*, 324, 641, 1986.

204. Muñoz, A., Zenke, M., Gehring, U., Sap, J., Beug, H., and Vennström, B., Characterization of the hormone-binding domain of the chicken c-*erbA*/thyroid hormone receptor protein, *EMBO J.*, 7, 155, 1988.

205. Thompson, C.C., Weinberger, C., Lebo, R., and Evans, R.M., Identification of a novel thyroid hormone receptor expressed in the mammalian central nervous system, *Science*, 237, 1610, 1987.

206. Benbrook, D. and Pfahl, M., A novel hormone receptor encoded by a cDNA clone from a human testis library, *Science*, 238, 788, 1987.

207. Pfahl, M. and Benbrook, D., Nucleotide sequence of cDNA encoding a novel human thyroid hormone receptor, *Nucleic Acids Res.*, 15, 9613, 1987.

208. Bahn, R.S., Zeller, J.C., and Smith, T.J., n-Butyrate increases c-*erb* A oncogene expression in human colon fibroblasts, *Biochem. Biophys. Res. Commun.*, 150, 259, 1988.

209. Harvey, T.T., An unidentified virus which causes rapid production of tumors in mice, *Nature*, 204, 1104, 1964.

210. Kirsten, W.H. and Mayer, L.A., Morphologic responses to a murine erythroblastosis virus, *J. Natl. Cancer Inst.*, 39, 311, 1967.

211. Andersen, P.R., Tronick, S.R., and Aaronson, S.A., Structural organization and biological activity of molecular clones of the integrated genome of a BALB/c mouse sarcoma virus, *J. Virol.*, 40, 431, 1981.

212. Fredrickson, T.N., O'Neill, R.R., Rutledge, R.A., Theodore, T.S., Martin, M.A., Ruscetti, S.K., Austin, J.B., and Hartley, J.W., Biologic and molecular characterization of two newly isolated *ras*-containing murine leukemia viruses, *J. Virol.,* 61, 2109, 1987.

213. Shimizu, K., Goldfarb, M., Suard, Y., Perucho, M., Li, Y., Kamata, T., Feramisco, J., Stavnezer, E., Fogh, J., and Wigler, M.H., Three human transforming genes are related to the viral *ras* oncogenes, *Proc. Natl. Acad. Sci. U.S.A.,* 80, 2112, 1983.

214. Langbeheim, H., Shih, T.Y., and Scolnick, E.M., Identification of a normal vertebrate cell protein related to the p21 *src* of Harvey murine sarcoma virus, *Virology,* 106, 292, 1980.

215. Shilo, B. and Weinberg, R.A., DNA sequences homologous to vertebrate oncogenes are conserved in *Drosophila melanogaster, Proc. Natl. Acad. Sci. U.S.A.,* 78, 6789, 1981.

216. Ellis, R.W., DeFeo, D., Shih, T.Y., Gonda, M.A., Young, H.A., Tsuchida, N., Lowy, D.R., and Scolnick, E.M., The p21 *src* genes of Harvey and Kirsten sarcoma viruses originate from divergent members of a family of normal vertebrate genes, *Nature,* 292, 506, 1981.

217. DeFeo-Jones, D., Scolnick, E.M., Koller, R., and Dhar, R., *ras*-related gene sequences identified and isolated from *Saccharomyces cerevisiae, Nature,* 306, 707, 1983.

218. Neuman-Silberberg, F.S., Schejter, E., Hoffmann, F.M., and Shilo, B.-Z., The *Drosophila ras* oncogenes: structure and nucleotide sequence, *Cell,* 37, 1027, 1984.

219. Temeles, G.L., DeFeo-Jones, D., Tatchell, K., Ellinger, M.S., and Scolnick, E.M., Expression and characterization of *ras* mRNAs from *Saccharomyces cerevisiae, Mol. Cell. Biol.,* 4, 2298, 1984.

220. Fukui, Y. and Kaziro, Y., Molecular cloning and sequence analysis of a *ras* gene from *Saccharomyces cerevisiae, EMBO J.,* 4, 687, 1985.

221. Jordano, J. and Perucho, M., Chromatin structure of the promoter region of the human c-K-ras gene, *Nucleic Acids Res.,* 14, 7361, 1986.

222. Hoffman, E.K., Trusko, S.P., Freeman, N., and George, D.L., Structural and functional characterization of the promoter region of the mouse c-Ki-*ras* gene, *Mol. Cell. Biol.,* 7, 2592, 1987.

223. Trimble, W.S. and Hozumi, N., Deletion analysis of the c-Ha-*ras* oncogene promoter, *FEBS Lett.,* 219, 70, 1987.

224. Honkawa, H., Masahashi, W., Hashimoto, S., and Hashimoto-Gotoh, T., Identification of the principal promoter sequence of the c-H-*ras* transforming oncogene: deletion analysis of the 5′-flanking region by focus formation assay, *Mol. Cell. Biol.,* 7, 2933, 1987.

225. Spandidos, D.A. and Holmes, L., Transcriptional enhancer activity in the variable tandem repeat DNA sequence downstream of the human Ha-*ras*1 gene, *FEBS Lett.,* 218, 41, 1987.

226. Cohen, J.B., Walter, M.V., and Levinson, A.D., A repetitive sequence element 3′ of the human c-Ha-*ras*1 gene has enhancer activity, *J. Cell. Physiol.,* Suppl. 5, 75, 1987.

227. Damante, G., Filetti, S., and Rapoport, B., Nucleotide sequence and characterization of the 5′ flanking region of the rat Ha-*ras* protooncogene, *Proc. Natl. Acad. Sci. U.S.A.,* 84, 774, 1987.

228. Damante, G., Filetti, S., and Rapoport, B., Studies on the promoter region of the c-Ha-*ras* gene in FRTL5 rat thyroid cells, *Mol. Endocrinol.,* 1, 279, 1987.

229. Damante, G. and Rapoport, B., A suppressor of transcriptional activity is present upstream from the rat c-Ha-ras promoter, *J. Mol. Biol.,* 200, 213, 1988.

230. Gibbs, J.B., Sigal, I.S., and Scolnick, E.M., Biochemical properties of normal and oncogenic *ras* p21, *Trends Biochem. Sci.,* 10, 350, 1985.

231. Levinson, A.D., Normal and activated ras oncogenes and their encoded products, *Trends Genet.,* 2, 81, 1986.

232. Lowy, D.R. and Willumsen, B.M., The *ras* gene family, *Cancer Surv.,* 5, 275, 1986.

233. Sigal, I.S., Smith, G.M., Jurnak, F., Marsico-Ahern, J.D., D'Alonzo, J.S., Scolnick, E.M., and Gibbs, J.B., Molecular approaches towards an anti-*ras* drug, *Anti-Cancer Drug Design,* 2, 107, 1987.

234. Barbacid, M., *ras* genes, *Annu. Rev. Biochem.,* 56, 779, 1987.

235. Bizub, D., Heimer, E.P., Felix, A., Chizzonite, R., Wood, A., Skalka, A.M., Slater, D., Aldrich, T.H., and Furth, M.E., Antisera to the variable region of *ras* oncogene proteins, and specific detection of H-*ras* expression in an experimental model of chemical carcinogenesis, *Oncogene,* 1, 131, 1987.

236. Ishihara, H., Nakagawa, H., Ono, K., and Fukuda, A., Antibodies against synthetic carboxy-terminal peptides distinguish H-*ras* and K-*ras* oncogene products of p21, *J. Immunol. Methods,* 103, 131, 1987.

237. Kanai, T., Hirohashi, S., Noguchi, M., Shimoyama, Y., Shimosato, Y., Noguchi, S., Nishimura, S., and Abe, O., Monoclonal antibody highly sensitive for the detection of *ras* p21 in immunoblotting analysis, *Jpn. J. Cancer Res.,* 78, 1314, 1987.

238. Polonis, V.R., Anderson, G.R., and Doyle, D., Two-dimensional polyacrylamide gel electrophoresis analysis for phosphorylated, membrane-localized *ras* p21 proteins, *Arch. Biochem. Biophys.,* 254, 541, 1987.

239. Caruso, A., Schlom, J., Vilasi, V., Weeks, M.O., and Hand, P.H., Development of quantitative liquid completion radioimmunoassays for the *ras* oncogene and proto-oncogene p21 products, *Int. J. Cancer,* 38, 587, 1986.

240. Basu, A. and Modak, M.J., An affinity labeling of *ras* p21 protein and its use in the identification of *ras* p21 in cellular and tissue extracts, *J. Biol. Chem.,* 262, 2369, 1987.

241. Wick, M.R., Immunohistologic detection of *ras* oncogene products — specific or spruious?, *Arch. Pathol. Lab. Med.*, 113, 13, 1989.

242. Bourne, H.R. and Sullivan, K.A., Mammalian G proteins: models for *ras* proteins in transmembrane signalling?, *Cancer Surv.*, 5, 257, 1986.

243. Stryer, L. and Bourne, H.R., G proteins: a family of signal transducers, *Annu. Rev. Cell Biol.*, 2, 391, 1986.

244. Spiegel, A.M., Signal transduction by guanine nucleotide binding proteins, *Mol. Cell. Endocrinol.*, 49, 1, 1987.

245. Litosch, I., Regulatory GTP-binding proteins: emerging concepts on their role in cell function, *Life Sci.*, 41, 251, 1987.

246. Casey, P.J. and Gilman, A.G., G protein involvement in receptor-effector coupling, *J. Biol. Chem.*, 263, 2577, 1988.

247. Willingham, M.C., Pastan, I., Shih, T.Y., and Scolnick, E.M., Localization of the *src* gene product of the Harvey strain of MSV to plasma membrane of transformed cells by electron microscopic immunocytochemistry, *Cell*, 19, 1005, 1980.

248. Papageorge, A., Lowy, D., and Scolnick, E.M., Comparative biochemical properties of the p21 *ras* molecules coded for by viral and cellular *ras* genes, *J. Virol.*, 44, 509, 1982.

249. Hoshino, M., Clanton, D.J., Shih, T.Y., Kawakita, M., and Hattori, S., Interaction of *ras* oncogene product p21 with guanine nucleotides, *J. Biochem.*, 102, 503, 1987.

250. Grand, R.J.A., Smith, K.J., and Gallimore, P.H., Purification and characterization of the protein encoded by the activated human N-*ras* gene and its membrane localisation, *Oncogene*, 1, 305, 1987.

251. Buss, J.E. and Sefton, B.M., Direct identification of palmitic acid as the lipid attached to p21^{ras}, *Mol. Cell. Biol.*, 6, 116, 1986.

252. Magee, A.I., Gutierrez, L., McKay, I.A., Marshall, C.J., and Hall, A., Dynamic fatty acylation of p21^{N-ras}, *EMBO J.*, 6, 3353, 1987.

253. Myrdal, S.E. and Auersperg, N., p21^{ras} heterogeneous localization in transformed cells, *Exp. Cell Res.*, 159, 441, 1985.

254. Shih, T.Y., Papageorge, A.G., Stokes, P.E., Weeks, M.O., and Scolnick, E.M., Guanine nucleotide-binding and autophosphorylating activities associated with the p21^{src} protein of Harvey murine sarcoma virus, *Nature*, 287, 686, 1980.

255. Shih, T.Y., Stokes, P.E., Smythers, G.W., Dhar, R., and Oroszlan, S., Characterization of the phosphorylation sites and surrounding amino acid sequences of the p21 transforming proteins coded for by the Harvey and Kirsten strains of sarcoma viruses, *J. Biol. Chem.*, 257, 11767, 1982.

256. Lautenberger, J.A., Ulsh, L., Shih, T.Y., and Papas, T.S., High-level expression in *Escherichia coli* of enzymatically active Harvey murine sarcoma virus p21^{ras} protein, *Science*, 221, 858, 1983.

257. Stein, R.B., Robinson, P.S., and Scolnick, E.M., Photoaffinity labeling with GTP of viral p21 *ras* protein expressed in *Escherichia coli*, *J. Virol.*, 50, 343, 1984.

258. Lacal, J.C., Santos, E., Notario, V., Barbacid, M., Yamazaki, S., Kung, H., Seamans, C., McAndrew, S., and Crowl, R., Expression of normal and transforming H-*ras* genes in *Escherichia coli* and purification of their encoded proteins, *Proc. Natl. Acad. Sci. U.S.A.*, 81, 5305, 1984.

259. Manne, V., Yamazaki, S., and Kung, H.-F., Guanosine nucleotide binding by highly purified Ha-*ras*-encoded p21 protein produced in *Escherichia coli*, *Proc. Natl. Acad. Sci. U.S.A.*, 81, 6953, 1984.

260. Gross, M., Sweet, R.W., Sathe, G., Yokoyama, S., Fasano, O., Goldfarb, M., Wigler, M., and Rosenberg, M., Purification and characterization of human H-*ras* proteins expressed in *Escherichia coli*, *Mol. Cell. Biol.*, 5, 1015, 1985.

261. Hattori, S., Ulsh, L.S., Halliday, K., and Shih, T.Y., Biochemical properties of a highly purified v-*ras*^{H} p21 protein overproduced in *Escherichia coli* and inhibition of its activities by a monoclonal antibody, *Mol. Cell. Biol.*, 5, 1449, 1985.

262. Tamaoki, T., Mizukami, T., Perucho, M., and Nakano, H., Expression of intact Ki-*ras* p21 protein in *Escherichia coli*, *Biochem. Biophys. Res. Commun.*, 132, 126, 1985.

263. Poe, M., Scolnick, E.M., and Stein, R.B., Viral Harvey *ras* p21 expressed in *Escherichia coli* purifies as a binary one-to-one complex with GDP, *J. Biol. Chem.*, 260, 3906, 1985.

264. Jeng, A.Y., Srivastava, S.K., Lacal, J.C., and Blumberg, P.M., Phosphorylation of *ras* oncogene product by protein kinase C, *Biochem. Biophys. Res. Commun.*, 145, 782, 1987.

265. Ulsh, L.S. and Shih, T.Y., Metabolic turnover of human c-*ras*^{H} p21 protein of EJ bladder carcinoma and its normal cellular and viral homologs, *Mol. Cell. Biol.*, 4, 1647, 1984.

266. McGrath, J.P., Capon, D.J., Goeddel, D.V., and Levinson, A.D., Comparative biochemical properties of normal and activated human *ras* p21 protein, *Nature*, 310, 644, 1984.

267. Sweet, R.W., Yokoyama, S., Kamata, T., Feramisco, J.R., Rosenberg, M., and Gross, M., The product of *ras* is a GTPase and a T24 oncogenic mutant is deficient in this activity, *Nature*, 311, 273, 1984.

268. Gibbs, J.B., Sigal, I.S., Poe, M., and Scolnick, E.M., Intrinsic GTPase activity distinguishes normal and oncogenic *ras* p21 molecules, *Proc. Natl. Acad. Sci. U.S.A.*, 81, 5704, 1984.

269. Manne, V., Bekesi, E., and Kung, H.-F., Ha-*ras* proteins exhibit GTPase activity: point mutations that activate Ha-*ras* gene products result in decreased GTPase activity, *Proc. Natl. Acad. Sci. U.S.A.*, 82, 376, 1985.

270. Geis, A.M., Nicolson, M., and Goldman, R.A., Biochemical and biological activities of N-ras proteins, *Biochem. Biophys. Res. Commun.,* 139, 771, 1986.

271. Manne, V. and Kung, H., Effect of divalent metal ions and glycerol on the GTPase activity of H-*ras* proteins, *Biochem. Biophys. Res. Commun.,* 128, 1440, 1985.

272. Hattori, S., Yamashita, T., Copeland, T.D., Oroszlan, S., and Shih, T.Y., Reactivity of a sulfhydryl group of the *ras* oncogene product p21 modulated by GTP binding, *J. Biol. Chem.,* 261, 14582, 1986.

273. Kawamitsu, H., Miwa, M., Tanigawa, Y., Shimoyama, M., Noguchi, S., Nishimura, S., Ohtsuka, E., and Sugimura, T., A hen enzyme ADP-ribosylates normal human and mutated c-Ha-*ras* oncogene products synthesized in *Escherichia coli, Proc. Jpn. Acad.,* 62B, 102, 1986.

274. Tsai, S.-C., Adamik, R., Moss, J., Vaughan, M., Manne, V., and Kung, H., Effects of phospholipids and ADP-ribosylation on GTP hydrolysis by *Escherichia coli*-synthesized Ha-*ras*-encoded p21, *Proc. Natl. Acad. Sci. U.S.A.,* 82, 8310, 1985.

275. Schlichting, I., Wittinghofer, A., and Rösch, P., Proton NMR studies of the GDP.Mg^{2+} complex of the Ha-ras oncogene product p21, *Biochem. Biophys. Res. Commun.,* 150, 444, 1988.

276. Hattori, S., Clanton, D.J., Satoh, T., Nakamura, S., Kaziro, Y., Kawakita, M., and Shih, T.Y., Neutralizing monoclonal antibody against *ras* oncogene product p21 which impairs guanine nucleotide exchange, *Mol. Cell. Biol.,* 7, 1999, 1987.

277. Srivastava, S.K., Lacal, J.C., Reynolds, S.H., and Aaronson, S.A., Antibody of predetermined specificity to a carboxy-terminal region of H-*ras* gene products inhibits their guanine nucleotide binding function, *Mol. Cell. Biol.,* 5, 3316, 1985.

278. Lacal, J.C. and Aaronson, S.A. *ras* p21 deletion mutants and monoclonal antibodies as tools for localization of regions relevant to p21 function, *Proc. Natl. Acad. Sci. U.S.A.,* 83, 5400, 1986.

279. Feramisco, J.R., Clark, R., Wong, G., Arnheim, N., Milley, R., and McCormick, F., Transient reversion of *ras* oncogene-induced cell transformation by antibodies specific for amino acid 12 of *ras* protein, *Nature,* 314, 639, 1985.

280. Clark, R., Wong, G., Arnheim, N., Nitecki, D., and McCormick, F., Antibodies specific for amino acid 12 of the *ras* oncogene product inhibit GTP binding, *Proc. Natl. Acad. Sci. U.S.A.,* 82, 5280, 1985.

281. de Vos, A.M., Tong, L., Milburn, M.W., Matias, P.M., Jancarik, J., Noguchi, S., Nishimura, S., Miura, K., Ohtsuka, E., and Kim, S.-H., Three dimensional structure of an oncogene protein: catalytic domain of human c-H-*ras* p21, *Science,* 239, 888, 1988.

282. Sigal, I.S., Gibbs, J.B., D'Alonzo, J.S., and Scolnick, E.M., Identification of effector residues and a neutralizing epitope of Ha-*ras*-encoded p21, *Proc. Natl. Acad. Sci. U.S.A.,* 83, 4725, 1986.

283. Willumsen, B.M., Papageorge, A.G., Kung, H.-F., Bekesi, E., Robins, T., Johnsen, M., Vass, W.C., and Lowy, D.R., Mutational analysis of a *ras* catalytic domain, *Mol. Cell. Biol.,* 6, 2646, 1986.

284. Matsui, T., Hirano, M., Naoe, T., Yamada, K., and Kurosawa, Y., Production of chimeric protein coded by the fused viral H-*ras* and human N-*ras* genes in *Escherichia coli, Gene,* 52, 215, 1987.

285. Lacal, J.C., Anderson, P.S., and Aaronson, S.A., Deletion mutants of Harvey *ras* p21 protein reveal the absolute requirement of at least two distant regions for GTP-binding and transforming activities, *EMBO J.,* 5, 679, 1986.

286. Clanton, D.J., Hattori, S., and Shih, T.Y., Mutations of the *ras* gene product p21 that abolish guanine nucleotide binding, *Proc. Natl. Acad. Sci. U.S.A.,* 83, 5076, 1986.

287. Lacal, J.C., Srivastava, S.K., Anderson, P.S., and Aaronson, S.A., *ras* p21 proteins with high or low GTPase activity can efficiently transform NIH/3T3 cells, *Cell,* 44, 609, 1986.

288. Robins, T., Jhappan, C., Chirikjian, J., and Vande Woude, G.F., Molecular cloning of the intronless EJ *ras* oncogene using a murine retrovirus shuttle vector, *Gene Anal. Tech.,* 3, 12, 1986.

289. Miura, K., Inoue, Y., Nakamori, H., Iwai, S., Ohtsuka, E., Ikehara, M., Noguchi, S., and Nishimura, S., Synthesis and expression of a synthetic gene for the activated human c-Ha-*ras* protein, *Jpn. J. Cancer Res.,* 77, 45, 1986.

290. Satoh, T., Nakamura, S., Nakafuku, M., and Kaziro, Y., Studies on *ras* proteins. Catalytic properties of normal and activated *ras* proteins purified in the absence of protein denaturants, *Biochim. Biophys. Acta,* 949, 97, 1988.

291. Trahey, M. and McCormick, F., A cytoplasmic protein stimulates normal N-*ras* p21 GTPase, but does not affect oncogenic mutants, *Science,* 238, 542, 1987.

292. Adari, H., Lowy, D.R., Willumsen, B.M., Der, C., and McCormick, F., Guanosine triphosphatase activating protein (GAP) interacts with the p21 *ras* effector binding domain, *Science,* 240, 518, 1988.

293. Nakano, E.T., Rao, M.M., Perucho, M., and Inouye, M., Expression of the Kirsten *ras* viral and human proteins in *Escherichia coli, J. Virol.,* 61, 302, 1987.

294. Feig, L.A., Pan, B.-T., Roberts, T.M., and Cooper, G.M., Isolation of *ras* GTP-binding mutants using an *in situ* colony-binding assay, *Proc. Natl. Acad. Sci. U.S.A.,* 83, 4607, 1986.

295. Lacal, J.C. and Aaronson, S.A., Activation of *ras* p21 transforming properties associated with an increase in the release rate of bound guanine nucleotide, *Mol. Cell. Biol.,* 6, 4214, 1986.

296. Lowe, D.G. and Goeddel, D.V., Heterologous expression and characterization of the human R-*ras* gene product, *Mol. Cell. Biol.,* 7, 2845, 1987.

297. Lowe, D.G., Ricketts, M., Levinson, A.D., and Goeddel, D.V., Chimeric proteins define variable and essential regions of Ha-*ras*-encoded protein, *Proc. Natl. Acad. Sci. U.S.A.,* 85, 1015, 1988.

298. Andreeff, M., Slater, D.E., Bressler, J., and Furth, M.E., Cellular *ras* oncogene expression and cell cycle measured by flow cytometry in hematopoietic cell lines, *Blood,* 67, 676, 1986.

299. Campisi, J., Gray, H.E., Pardee, A.B., Dean, M., and Sonenshein, G.E., Cell-cycle control of c-*myc* but not c-*ras* expression is lost following chemical transformation, *Cell,* 36, 241, 1984.

300. Mulcahy, L.S., Smith, M.R., and Stacey, D.W., Requirement for *ras* proto-oncogene function during serum-stimulated growth of NIH 3T3 cells, *Nature,* 313, 241, 1985.

301. Schneider-Schaulies, J., Hünig, T., Schipl, A., and Wecker, E., Kinetics of cellular oncogene expression in mouse lymphocytes. I. Expression of c-myc and c-ras^{Ha} in T lymphocytes induced by various mitogens, *Eur. J. Immunol.,* 16, 312, 1986.

302. Durkin, J.P. and Whitfield, J.F., Characterization of G$_1$ transit induced by the mitogenic-oncogenic viral Ki-*ras* gene product, *Mol. Cell. Biol.,* 6, 1386, 1986.

303. Saltarelli, D., Fischer, S., and Gacon, G., Modulation of adenylate cyclase by guanine nucleotide and Kirsten sarcoma virus mediated transformation, *Biochem. Biophys. Res. Commun.,* 127, 318, 1985.

304. Franks, D.J., Whitfield, J.F., and Durkin, J.P., Viral *p21* Ki-ras protein: a potent intracellular mitogen that stimulates adenylate cyclase activity in early G$_1$ phase of cultured cells, *J. Cell. Biochem.,* 33, 87, 1987.

305. Tarpley, W.G., Hopkins, N.K., and Gorman, R.R., Reduced hormone-stimulated adenylate cyclase activity in NIH-3T3 cells expressing the EJ human bladder *ras* oncogene, *Proc. Natl. Acad. Sci. U.S.A.,* 83, 3703, 1986.

306. Hiwasa, T., Yokoyama, S., Ha, J.-M., Noguchi, S., and Sakiyama, S., c-Ha-*ras* gene products are potent inhibitors of cathepsins B and L, *FEBS Lett.,* 211, 23, 1987.

307. Fleischman, L.F., Chahwala, S.B., and Cantley, L., *ras*-transformed cells: altered levels of phosphatidylinositol-4,5-bisphosphate and catabolytes, *Science,* 231, 407, 1986.

308. Wolfman, A. and Macara, I.G., Elevated levels of diacylglycerol and decreased phorbol ester sensitivity in *ras*-transformed fibroblasts, *Nature,* 325, 359, 1987.

309. Wakelam, M.J.O., Houslay, M.D., Davies, S.A., Marshall, C.J., and Hall, A., The role of N-*ras* p21 in the coupling of growth factor receptors to inositol phospholipid turnover, *Biochem. Soc. Trans.,* 15, 45, 1987.

310. Schejter, E.D. and Shilo, B.-Z., Characterization of functional domains of p21 *ras* by use of chimeric genes, *EMBO J.,* 4, 407, 1985.

311. Sigal, I.S., Gibbs, J.B., D'Alonzo, J.S., Temeles, G.L., Wolanski, B.S., Socher, S.H., and Scolnick, E.M., Mutant *ras*-encoded proteins altered nucleotide binding exert dominant biological effects, *Proc. Natl. Acad. Sci. U.S.A.,* 83, 952, 1986.

312. Lacal, J.C. and Aaronson, S.A., Monoclonal antibody Y13-259 recognizes an epitope of the p21 *ras* molecule not directly involved in the GTP-binding activity of the protein, *Mol. Cell. Biol.,* 6, 1002, 1986.

313. Papageorge, A.G., Willumsen, B.M., Johnsen, M., Kung, H.-F., Stacey, D.W., Vass, W.C., and Lowy, D.R., A transforming *ras* gene can provide an essential function ordinarily supplied by an endogenous *ras* gene, *Mol. Cell. Biol.,* 6, 1843, 1986.

314. Furth, M.E., Aldrich, T.H., and Cordon-Cardo, C., Expression of *ras* proto-oncogene proteins in normal human tissues, *Oncogene,* 1, 47, 1987.

315. Tanaka, T., Ida, N., Waki, C., Shimoda, H., Slamon, D.J., and Cline, M.J., Cell type-specific expressions of c-ras gene products in the normal rat, *Mol. Cell. Biochem.,* 75, 23, 1987.

316. Durkin, J.P. and Whitfield, J.F., The viral Ki-*ras* gene must be expressed in the G$_2$ phas if *ts* Kirsten sarcoma virus-infected NRK cells are to proliferate in serum-free medium, *Mol. Cell. Biol.,* 7, 444, 1987.

317. Czerniak, B., Herz, F., Wersto, R.P., and Koss, L.G., Expression of Ha-*ras* oncogene p21 protein in relation to the cell cycle of cultured human tumor cells, *Am. J. Pathol.,* 126, 411, 1987.

318. Leon, J., Guerrero, I., and Pellicer, A., Differential expression of the *ras* gene family in mice, *Mol. Cell. Biol,* 7, 1535, 1987.

319. Scolnick, E.M., Weeks, M.O., Shih, T.Y., Ruscetti, S.K., and Dexter, T.M., Markedly elevated levels of an endogenous *sarc* protein in a hematopoietic precursor cell line, *Mol. Cell. Biol.,* 1, 66, 1981.

320. Scheinberg, D.A. and Strand, M., A brain membrane protein similar to the rat *src* gene product, *Proc. Natl. Acad. Sci. U.S.A.,* 78, 55, 1981.

321. Bar-Sagi, D. and Feramisco, J.R., Microinjection of the *ras* oncogene protein into PC12 cells induces morphological differentiation, *Cell,* 42, 841, 1985.

322. Noda, M., Ko, M., Ogura, A., Liu, D., Amano, T., Takano, T., and Ikawa, Y., Sarcoma viruses carrying *ras* oncogenes induce differentiation-associated properties in a neuronal cell line, *Nature,* 318, 73, 1985.

323. Guerrero, I., Wong, H., Pellicer, A., and Burstein, D.E., Activated N-ras gene induces neuronal differentiation of PC12 rat pheochromocytoma cells, *J. Cell. Physiol.,* 129, 71, 1986.

324. Hagag, N., Halegoua, S., and Viola, M., Inhibition of growth factor-induced differentiation of PC12 cells by microinjection of antibody to *ras* p21, *Nature,* 319, 680, 1986.

325. Birchmeier, C., Broek, D., and Wigler, M., RAS protein can induce meiosis in *Xenopus* oocytes, *Cell,* 43, 615, 1985.

326. Sadler, S.E., Schechter, A.L., Tabin, C.J., and Maller, J.L., Antibodies to the *ras* gene product inhibit adenylate cyclase and accelerate progesterone-induced cell division in *Xenopus laevis* oocytes, *Mol. Cell. Biol.,* 6, 719, 1986.

327. Deshpande, A.K. and Kung, H.-F., Insulin induction of *Xenopus laevis* oocyte maturation is inhibited by monoclonal antibody against p21 *ras* proteins, *Mol. Cell. Biol.,* 7, 1825, 1987.

328. Cheng, S.V.Y. and Pollard, J.W., c-*ras*[H] and ornithine decarboxylase are induced by oestradiol-17 beta in the mouse uterine luminal epithelium independently of the proliferative status of the cell, *FEBS Lett.,* 196, 309, 1986.

329. McKay, I.A., Marshall, C.J., Calés, C., and Hall, A., Transformation and stimulation of DNA synthesis in NIH-3T3 cells are titrable function of normal p21[N-ras] expression, *EMBO J.,* 5, 2617, 1986.

330. Rein, A., Keller, J., Schultz, A.M., Holmes, K.L., Medicus, R., and Ihle, J.N., Infection of immune mast cells by Harvey sarcoma virus: immortalization without loss of requirement for interleukin-3, *Mol. Cell. Biol,* 5, 2257, 1985.

331. Gay, N.J. and Walker, J.E., Homology between human bladder carcinoma oncogene product and mitochondrial ATP-synthase, *Nature,* 301, 262, 1983.

332. Halliday, K.R., Regional homology in GTP-binding proto-oncogene products and elongation factors, *J. Cyclic Nucleot. Prot. Phosphoryl. Res.,* 9, 435, 1983-1984.

333. Jurnak, F., Structure of the GDP domain of EF-Tu and location of the amino acids homologous to *ras* oncogene proteins, *Science,* 230, 32, 1985.

334. Kohno, K., Uchida, T., Ohkubo, H., Nakanishi, S., Nakanishi, T., Fukui, T., Ohtsuka, E., Ikehara, M., and Okada, Y., Amino acid sequence of mammalian elongation factor 2 deduced from the cDNA sequence: homology with GTP-binding proteins, *Proc. Natl. Acad. Sci. U.S.A.,* 83, 4978, 1986.

335. Gilman, A.G., G proteins and dual control of adenylate cyclase, *Cell,* 36, 577, 1984.

336. Sullivan, K.A., Liao, Y.-C., Alborzi, A., Beiderman, B., Chang, F.-H., Masters, S.B., Levinson, A.D., and Bourne, H.R., Inhibitory and stimulatory G proteins of adenylate cyclase: cDNA and amino acid sequences of the alpha chains, *Proc. Natl. Acad. Sci. U.S.A.,* 83, 6687, 1986.

337. Hurley, J.B., Simon, M.I., Teplow, D.B., Robishaw, J.D., and Gilman, A.G., Homologies between signal transducing G proteins and *ras* gene products, *Science,* 226, 860, 1984.

338. Lochrie, M.A., Hurley, J.B., and Simon, M.I., Sequence of the alpha subunit of photoreceptor G protein: homologies between transducin, *ras*, and elongation factors, *Science,* 228, 96, 1985.

339. Tanabe, T., Nukada, T., Nishikawa, Y., Sugimoto, K., Suzuki, H., Takahashi, H., Noda, M., Haga, T., Ichiyama, A., Kangawa, K., Minamino, N., Matsuo, H., and Numa, S., Primary structure of the alpha-subunit of transducin and its relationship to *ras* proteins, *Nature,* 315, 242, 1985.

340. Medynski, D.C., Sullivan, K., Smith, D., Van Dop, C., Chang, F.-H., Fung, B.K.-K., Seeburg, P.H., and Bourne, H.R., Amino acid sequence of the alpha subunit of transducin deduced from the c-DNA sequence, *Proc. Natl. Acad. Sci. U.S.A.,* 82, 4311, 1985.

341. Beckner, S.K., Hattori, S., and Shih, T.Y., The *ras* oncogene product p21 is not a regulatory component of adenylate cyclase, *Nature,* 317, 71, 1985.

342. Franks, D.J., Whitfield, J.F., and Durkin, J.P., The mitogenic/oncogenic p21 Ki-ras protein stimulate adenylate cyclase activity early in the G_1 phase of NRK rat kidney cells, *Biochem. Biophys. Res. Commun.,* 132, 780, 1985.

343. Hiwasa, T., Sakiyama, S., Noguchi, S., Ha, J.-M., Miyazawa, T., and Yokoyama, S., Degradation of a cAMP-binding protein is inhibited by human c-Ha-*ras* gene products, *Biochem. Biophys. Res. Commun.,* 146, 731, 1987.

344. Sefton, B.M., Trowbridge, I.S., Cooper, J.A., and Scolnick, E.M., The transforming proteins of Rous sarcoma virus, Abelson sarcoma virus, and Harvey sarcoma virus contain tightly-bound lipid, *Cell,* 31, 465, 1982.

345. Bar-Sagi, D., McCormick, F., Milley, R.J., and Feramisco, J.R., Inhibition of cell surface ruffling and fluid-phase pinocytosis by microinjection of anti-*ras* antibodies into living cells, *J. Cell. Physiol.,* Suppl. 5, 69, 1987.

346. Willumsen, B.M., Christensen, A., Hubbert, N.L., Papageorge, A.G., and Lowy, D.R., The p21 *ras* C-terminus is required for transformation and membrane association, *Nature,* 310, 583, 1984.

347. Willumsen, B.M., Norris, K., Papageorge, A.G., Hubbert, N.L., and Lowy, D.R., Harvey murine sarcoma virus p21 *ras* protein: biological and biochemical significance of the cysteine nearest the carboxy terminus, *EMBO J.,* 3, 2581, 1984.

348. Chen, Z.-Q., Ulsh, L.S., DuBois, G., and Shih, T.Y., Posttranslational processing of p21 *ras* proteins involves palmitylation of the C-terminal tetrapeptide containing cysteine-186, *J. Virol.,* 56, 607, 1985.

349. Clarke, S., Vogel, J.P., Deschenes, R.J., and Stock, J., Posttranslational modification of the Ha-*ras* oncogene protein: evidence for a third class of protein carboxyl methyltransferases, *Proc. Natl. Acad. Sci. U.S.A.,* 85, 4643, 1988.

350. Der, C.J., Pan, B.-T., and Cooper, G.M., *ras*[H] mutants deficient in GTP binding, *Mol. Cell. Biol.,* 6, 3291, 1986.

351. Trahey, M., Milley, R.J., Cole, G.E., Innis, M., Paterson, H., Marshall, C.J., Hall, A., and McCormick, F., Biochemical and biological properties of the human N-*ras* p21 protein, *Mol. Cell. Biol.,* 7, 541, 1987.

352. Benjamin, C.W., Tarpley, W.G., and Gorman, R.R., Loss of platelet-derived growth factor-stimulated phospholipase activity in NIH-3T3 cells expressing the EJ-*ras* oncogene, *Proc. Natl. Acad. Sci. U.S.A.,* 84, 546, 1987.

353. Olinger, P.L. and Gorman, R.R., NIH-3T3 cells expressing high levels of the c-*ras* proto-oncogene display reduced platelet derived growth factor-stimulated phospholipase activity, *Biochem. Biophys. Res. Commun.,* 150, 937, 1988.

354. Wakelam, M.J.O., Davies, S.A., Houslay, M.D., McKay, I., Marshall, C.J., and Hall, A., Normal p21$^{\text{N-}ras}$ couples bombesin and other growth factor receptors to inositol phosphate production, *Nature,* 323, 173, 1986.

355. Hiwasa, T., Sakiyama, S., Yokoyama, S., Ha, J.-M., Fujita, J., Noguchi, S., Bando, Y., Kominami, E., and Katanuma, N., Inhibition of cathepsin L-induced degradation of epidermal growth factor receptors by c-Ha-*ras* gene products, *Biochem. Biophys. Res. Commun.,* 151, 78, 1988.

356. Denhardt, D.T., Greenberg, A.H., Egan, S.E., Hamilton, R.T., and Wright, J.A., Cysteine proteinase cathepsin L expression correlates closely with the metastatic potential of H-*ras*-transformed murine fibroblasts, *Oncogene,* 2, 55, 1987.

357. Backer, J.M. and Weinstein, I.B., Proteins encoded by *ras* oncogenes stimulate or inhibit phosphorylation of specific mitochondrial membrane proteins, *Biochem. Biophys. Res. Commun.,* 135, 316, 1986.

358. Hedge, A.N. and Das, M.R., *ras* proteins enhance the phosphorylation of a 38 kDa protein (p38) in rat liver plasma membrane, *FEBS Lett.,* 217, 74, 1987.

359. Schmidt, C.J. and Hamer, D.H., Cell specificity and an effect of *ras* on human metallothionein gene expression, *Proc. Natl. Acad. Sci. U.S.A.,* 83, 3346, 1986.

360. Wasylyk, C., Imler, J.L., Perez-Mutul, J., and Wasylyk, B., The c-Ha-*ras* oncogene and a tumor promoter activate the polyoma virus enhancer, *Cell,* 48, 525, 1987.

361. Chardin, P. and Tavitian, A., The *ral* gene: a new *ras* related gene isolated by the use of a synthetic probe, *EMBO J.,* 5, 2203, 1986.

362. March, P.E., Lerner, C.G., Ahnn, J., Cui, X., and Inouye, M., The *Escherichia coli* Ras-like protein (Era) has GTPase activity and is essential for cell growth, *Oncogene,* 2, 539, 1988.

363. Alsip, G.R. and Konkel, D.A., A processed chicken pseudogene (CPS1) related to the *ras* oncogene superfamily, *Nucleic Acids Res.,* 14, 2123, 1986.

364. Swanson, M.E., Elste, A.M., Greenberg, S.M., Schwartz, J.H., Aldrich, T.H., and Furth, M.E., Abundant expression of *ras* proteins in *Aplysia* neurons, *J. Cell Biol.,* 103, 485, 1986.

365. Lev, Z., Kimchie, Z., Hessel, R., and Segev, O., Expression of *ras* cellular oncogenes during development of *Drosophila melanogaster*, *Mol. Cell. Biol.,* 5, 1540, 1985.

366. Wheals, A.E., Oncogene homologues in yeast, *BioEssays,* 3, 108, 1985.

367. Tamanoi, F., Yeast *RAS* genes, *Biochim. Biophys. Acta,* 948, 1, 1988.

368. Peterson, T.A., Yochem, J., Byers, B., Nunn, M.F., Duesberg, P.H., Doolittle, R.F., and Reed, S.I., A relationship between the yeast cell cycle genes *CDC4* and *CDC36* and the *ets* sequence of oncogenic virus E26, *Nature,* 309, 556, 1984.

369. Papageorge, A.G., DeFeo-Jones, D., Robinson, P.S., Temeles, G., and Scolnick, E.M., *Saccharomyces cerevisiae* synthesizes proteins related to the p21 gene product of *ras* genes found in mammals, 4, 23, 1984.

370. Dhar, R., Nieto, A., Koller, R., DeFeo-Jones, D., and Scolnick, E.M., Nucleotide sequence of two *ras*^{H}-related genes isolated from the yeast *Saccharomyces cerevisiae*, *Nucleic Acids Res.,* 12, 3611, 1984.

371. Temeles, G.L., DeFeo-Jones, D., Tatchell, K., Ellinger, M.S., and Scolnick, E.M., Expression and characterization of *ras* mRNAs from *Saccharomyces cerevisiae*, *Mol. Cell. Biol.,* 4, 2298, 1984.

372. Breviario, D., Hinnebusch, A., Cannon, J., Tatchell, K., and Dhar, R., Carbon source regulation of *RAS1* expression in *Saccharomyces cerevisiae* and the phenotypes of *ras2*$^-$ cells, *Proc. Natl. Acad. Sci. U.S.A.,* 83, 4152, 1986.

373. Tamanoi, F., Walsh, M., Kataoka, T., and Wigler, M., A product of yeast *RAS2* gene is a guanine nucleotide binding protein, *Proc. Natl. Acad. Sci. U.S.A.,* 81, 6924, 1984.

374. Kataoka, T., Powers, S., Cameron, S., Fasano, O., Goldfarb, M., Broach, J., and Wigler, M., Functional homology of mammalian and yeast RAS genes, *Cell,* 40, 19, 1985.

375. Toda, T., Uno, I., Ishikawa, T., Powers, S., Kataoka, T., Broek, D., Carmeron, S., Broach, J., Matsumoto, K., and Wigler, M., In yeast, RAS proteins are controlling elements of adenylate cyclase, *Cell,* 40, 27, 1985.

376. De Vendittis, E., Vitelli, A., Zahn, R., and Fasano, O., Suppression of defective *RAS1* and *RAS2* functions in yeast by an adenylate cyclase activated by a single amino acid change, *EMBO J.,* 5, 3657, 1986.

377. Robinson, L.C., Gibbs, J.B., Marshall, M.S., Sigal, I.S., and Tatchell, K., *CDC25*: a component of the *RAS*-adenylate cyclase pathway in *Saccharomyces cerevisiae*, *Science,* 235, 1218, 1987.

378. Marshall, M.S., Gibbs, J.B., Scolnick, E.M., and Sigal, I.S., Regulatory function of the *Saccharomyces cerevisiae* RAS C-terminus, *Mol. Cell. Biol.,* 7, 2309, 1987.

379. Gibbs, J.B., Schaber, M.D., Marshall, M.S., Scolnick, E.M., and Sigal, I.S., Identification of guanine nucleotides bound to *ras*-encoded proteins in growing yeast cells, *J. Biol. Chem.,* 262, 10426, 1987.

380. Robishaw, J.D., Russell, D.W., Harris, B.A., Smigel, M.D., and Gilman, A.G., Deduced primary structure of the alpha subunit of the GTP-binding stimulatory protein of adenylate cyclase, *Proc. Natl. Acad. Sci. U.S.A.,* 83, 1251, 1986.

381. Salminen, A. and Novick, P.J., A *ras*-like protein is required for a post-Golgi event in yeast secretion, *Cell,* 49, 527, 1987.

382. Tatchell, K., Robinson, L.C., and Breitenbach, M., *RAS2* of *Saccharomyces cerevisiae* is required for gluconeogenic growth and proper response to nutrient limitation, *Proc. Natl. Acad. Sci. U.S.A.,* 82, 3785, 1985.

383. Fraenkel, D.G., On *ras* gene function in yeast, *Proc. Natl. Acad. Sci. U.S.A.,* 82, 4740, 1985.

384. Kaibuchi, K., Miyajima, A., Arai, K., and Matsumoto, K., Possible involvement of *RAS*-encoded proteins in glucose-induced inositolphospholipid turnover in *Saccharomyces cerevisiae*, *Proc. Natl. Acad. Sci. U.S.A.,* 83, 8172, 1986.

385. Kataoka, T., Powers, S., McGill, C., Fasano, O., Strathern, J., Broach, J., and Wigler, M., Genetic analysis of yeast *RAS1* and *RAS2* genes, *Cell,* 37, 437, 1984.

386. Tatchell, K., Chaleff, D.T., DeFeo-Jones, D., and Scolnick, E.M., Requirement of either a pair of *ras*-related gene of *Saccharomyces cerevisiae* for spore viability, *Nature,* 309, 523, 1984.

387. DeFeo-Jones, D., Tatchell, K., Robinson, L.C., Sigal, I.S., Vass, W.C., Lowy, D.R., and Scolnick, E.M., Mammalian and yeast *ras* gene products: biological function in their heterologous systems, *Science,* 228, 179, 1985.

388. Temeles, G.L., Gibbs, J.B., D'Alonzo, J.S., Sigal, I.S., and Scolnick, E.M., Yeast and mammalian *ras* proteins have conserved biochemical properties, *Nature,* 313, 700, 1985.

389. Gallwitz, D., Donath, C., and Sander, C., A yeast gene encoding a protein homologous to the human c-*has/bas* proto-oncogene product, *Nature,* 306, 704, 1983.

390. Schmitt, H.D., Wagner, P., Pfaff, E., and Gallwitz, D., The *ras*-related *YPT1* gene product in yeast: a GTP-binding protein that might be involved in microtubule organization, *Cell,* 47, 401, 1986.

391. Wagner, P., Molenaar, C.M.T., Rauh, A.J.G., Brökel, R., Schmitt, H.D., and Gallwitz, D., Biochemical properties of the *ras*-related *YPT* protein in yeast: a mutational analysis, *EMBO J.,* 6, 2373, 1987.

392. Molenaar, C.M.T., Prange, R., and Gallwitz, D., A carboxyl-terminal cysteine residue is required for palmitic acid binding and biological activity of the *ras*-related yeast *YPT1* protein, *EMBO J.,* 7, 971, 1988.

393. Haubruck, H., Disela, C., Wagner, P., and Gallwitz, D., The *ras*-related *ypt* protein is an ubiquitous eukaryotic protein: isolation and sequence analysis of mouse cDNA clones highly homologous to the yeast *YPT1* gene, *EMBO J.,* 6, 13, 1987.

394. Touchot, N., Chardin, P., and Tavitian, A., Four additional members of the *ras* gene superfamily isolated by an oligonucleotide strategy: molecular cloning of YPT-related cDNAs from a rat brain library, *Proc. Natl. Acad. Sci. U.S.A.,* 84, 8210, 1987.

395. Zahraoui, A., Touchot, N., Chardin, P., and Tavitian, A., Complete coding sequences of the *ras* related *rab 3* and 4 cDNAs, *Nucleic Acids Res.,* 16, 1204, 1988.

396. Fukui, Y., Kozasa, T., Kaziro, Y., Takeda, T., and Yamamoto, M., Role of a *ras* homolog in the life cycle of *Schizosaccharomyces pombe, Cell,* 44, 329, 1986.

397. Nadin-Davis, S.A. and Nasim, A., A gene which encodes a predicted protein kinase can restore some functions of the *ras* gene in fission yeast, *EMBO J.,* 7, 985, 1988.

398. Pawson, T. and Weeks, G., Expression of *ras*-encoded proteins in relation to cell growth and differentiation, in *Genes and Cancer,* Alan R. Liss, New York, 1984, 461.

399. Pawson, T., Amiel, T., Hinze, E., Auersperg, N., Neave, N., Sobolewski, A., and Weeks, G., Regulation of a *ras*-related protein during development of *Dictyostelium discoideum, Mol. Cell. Biol.,* 5, 33, 1985.

400. Reymond, C.D., Nellen, W., and Firtel, R.A., Regulated expression of *ras* gene constructs in *Dictyostelium* transformants, *Proc. Natl. Acad. Sci. U.S.A.,* 82, 7005, 1985.

401. Reymond, C.D., Gomer, R.H., Nellen, W., Theibert, A., Devreotes, P., and Firtel, R.A., Phenotypic changes induced by a mutated *ras* gene during the development of *Dictyostelium* transformants, *Nature,* 323, 340, 1986.

402. Van Haastert, P.J.M., Kesbeke, F., Reymond, C.D., Firtel, R.A., Luderus, E., and Van Driel, R., Aberrant transmembrane signal transduction in *Dictyostelium* cells expressing a mutated *ras* gene, *Proc. Natl. Acad. Sci. U.S.A.,* 84, 4905, 1987.

403. Stacey, D.W. and Kung, H.-F., Transformation of NIH 3T3 cells by microinjection of Ha-*ras* p21 protein, *Nature,* 310, 508, 1984.

404. Chang, E.H., Furth, M.E., Scolnick, E.M., and Lowy, D.R., Tumorigenic transformation of mammalian cells induced by a normal human gene homologous to the oncogene of Harvey murine sarcoma virus, *Nature,* 297, 479, 1982.

405. Hurlin, P.J., Maher, V.M., and McCormick, J.J., Malignant transformation of human fibroblasts caused by expression of a transfected T24 HRAS oncogene, *Proc. Natl. Acad. Sci. U.S.A.,* 86, 187, 1989.

406. Reynolds, V.L., Lebovitz, R.M., Warren, S., Hawley, T.S., Godwin, A.K., and Lieberman, M.W., Regulation of a metallothionein-*ras* T24 fusion gene by zinc results in graded alterations in cell morphology and growth, *Oncogene,* 1, 323, 1987.

407. Balmain, A., Transforming *ras* oncogenes and multistage carcinogenesis, *Br. J. Cancer,* 51, 1, 1985.

408. Andres, A.-C., Schönenberger, C.-A., Groner, B., Hennighausen, L., LeMeur, M., and Gerlinger, P., Ha-*ras* oncogene expression directed by a milk protein gene promoter: tissue specificity, hormonal regulation, and tumor induction in transgenic mice, *Proc. Natl. Acad. Sci. U.S.A.,* 84, 1299, 1987.

409. McCoy, M.S., Bargmann, C.I., and Weinberg, R.A., Human colon carcinoma Ki-*ras*2 oncogene and its corresponding proto-oncogene, *Mol. Cell. Biol.,* 4, 1577, 1984.
410. McCoy, M.S. and Weinberg, R.A., A human Ki-*ras* oncogene encodes two transforming proteins, *Mol. Cell. Biol.,* 6, 1326, 1986.
411. Sullivan, N.F., Sweet, R.W., Rosenberg, M., and Feramisco, J.R., Microinjection of the *ras* oncogene protein into nonestablished rat embryo fibroblasts, *Cancer Res.,* 46, 6427, 1986.
412. Lumpkin, C.K., Knepper, J.E., Butel, J.S., Smith, J.R., and Pereira-Smith, O.M., Mitogenic effects of the proto-oncogene and oncogene forms of c-H-*ras* DNA in human diploid fibroblasts, *Mol. Cell. Biol.,* 6, 2990, 1986.
413. Lichtman, A.H., Reynolds, D.S., Faller, D.V., and Abbas, A.K., Mature murine B lymphocytes immortalized by Kirsten sarcoma virus, *Nature,* 324, 489, 1986.
414. Dippold, W.G., Jay, G., DeLeo, A.B., Khoury, G., and Old, L.J., p53 transformation-related protein: detection by monoclonal antibody in mouse and human cells, *Proc. Natl. Acad. Sci. U.S.A.,* 78, 1695, 1981.
415. Eliyahu, D., Raz, A., Gruss, P., Givol, D., and Oren, M., Participation of p53 cellular tumour antigen in transformation of normal embryonic cells, *Nature,* 312, 646, 1984.
416. Parada, L.F., Land, H., Weinberg, R.A., Wolf, D., and Rotter, V., Cooperation between gene encoding p53 tumour antigen and *ras* in cellular transformation, *Nature,* 312, 649, 1984.
417. Jenkins, J.R., Rudge, K., and Currie, G.A., Cellular immortalization by a cDNA clone encoding the transformation-associated phosphoprotein p53, *Nature,* 312, 651, 1984.
418. Stacey, D.W., DeGudicibus, S.R., and Smith, M.R., Cellular *ras* activity and tumor cell proliferation, *Exp. Cell Res.,* 171, 232, 1987.
419. Kung, H.-F., Smith, M.R., Bekesi, E., Manne, V., and Stacey, D.W., Reversal or transformed phenotype by monoclonal antibodies against Ha-*ras* p21 proteins, *Exp. Cell Res.,* 162, 363, 1986.
420. Abelson, H.T. and Rabstein, L.S., Influence of prednisolone on Moloney leukemogenic virus in BALB/c mice, *Cancer Res.,* 30, 2208, 1970.
421. Goff, S.P., The Abelson murine leukemia virus oncogene, *Proc. Soc. Exp. Biol. Med.,* 179, 403, 1985.
422. Risser, R. and Green, P.L., Abelson virus: current status of a viral oncogene, *Proc. Soc. Exp. Biol. Med.,* 188, 235, 1988.
423. Rosenberg, N. and Witte, O.N., The viral and cellular forms of the Abelson (abl) oncogene, *Adv. Virus Res.,* 35, 39, 1988.
424. Besmer, P., Hardy, W.D., Jr., Zuckerman, E.E., Bergold, P., Lederman, L., and Snyder, H.W., Jr., The Hardy-Zuckerman 2-FeSV, a new feline retrovirus which oncogene homology to Abelson-MuLV, *Nature,* 303, 825, 1983.
425. Witte, O.N., Rosenberg, N., Paskind, M., Shields, A., and Baltimore, D., Identification of an Abelson murine leukemia virus-encoded protein present in transformed fibroblasts and lymphoid cells, *Proc. Nat. Acad. Sci. U.S.A.,* 75, 2488, 1978.
426. Reddy, E.P., Smith, M.J., and Srinivasan, A., Nucleotide sequence of Abelson murine leukemia virus genome: structural similarity of its transforming gene product to other *onc* gene products with tyrosine-specific kinase activity, *Proc. Natl. Acad. Sci. U.S.A.,* 80, 3623, 1983.
427. Witte, O.N., Dasgupta, A., and Baltimore, D., Abelson murine leukaemia virus protein is phosphorylated *in vitro* to form phosphotyrosine, *Nature,* 283, 826, 1980.
428. Sefton, B.M., Hunter, T., and Raschke, W.C., Evidence that the Abelson virus protein functions *in vivo* as a protein kinase that phosphorylates tyrosine, *Proc. Natl. Acad. Sci. U.S.A.,* 78, 1552, 1981.
429. Schiffmaker, L., Burns, M.C., Konopka, J.B., Clark, S., Witte, O.N., and Rosenberg, N., Monoclonal antibodies specific for v-*abl*- and c-*abl*-encoded molecules, *J. Virol.,* 57, 1182, 1986.
430. Wang, J.Y.J., Queen, C., and Baltimore, D., Expression of an Abelson murine leukemia virus-encoded protein in *Escherichia coli* causes extensive phosphorylation of tyrosine residues, *J. Biol. Chem.,* 257, 13181, 1982.
431. Wang, J.Y.J. and Baltimore, D., Localization of tyrosine kinase-coding region in v-*abl* oncogene by the expression of v-*abl*-encoded proteins in bacteria, *J. Biol. Chem.,* 260, 64, 1985.
432. Ferguson, B., Pritchard, M.L., Feild, J., Rieman, J., Rieman, D., Greig, R.G., Poste, G., and Rosenberg, M., Isolation and analysis of an Abelson murine leukemia virus-encoded tyrosine-specific kinase produced in *Escherichia coli, J. Biol. Chem.,* 260, 3652, 1985.
433. Foulkes, J.G., Chow, M., Gorka, C., Frackelton, A.R., Jr., and Baltimore, D., Purification and characterization of a protein-tyrosine kinase encoded by the Abelson murine leukemia virus, *J. Biol. Chem.,* 260, 8070, 1985.
434. Saggioro, D., Ferracini, R., DiRenzo, M.F., Naldini, L., Chieco-Bianchi, L., and Comoglio, P.M., Protein phosphorylation at tyrosine residues in v-*abl* transformed mouse lymphocytes and fibroblasts, *Int. J. Cancer,* 37, 623, 1986.
435. Kipreos, E.T., Lee, G.J., and Wang, J.Y.J., Isolation of temperature-sensitive tyrosine kinase mutants of v-*abl* oncogene by screening with antibodies for phosphotyrosine, *Proc. Natl. Acad. Sci. U.S.A.,* 84, 1345, 1987.
436. Takemori, T., Miyazoe, I., Shirasawa, T., Taniguchi, M., and Graf, T., A temperature-sensitive mutant of Abelson murine leukemia virus confers inducibility of IgM expression to transformed lymphoid cells, *EMBO J.,* 6, 951, 1987.

437. Groffen, J., Heisterkamp, N., Reynolds, F.H., Jr., and Stephenson, J.R., Homology between phosphotyrosine acceptor site of human c-*abl* and viral oncogene products, *Nature,* 304, 167, 1983.

438. Maller, J.L., Foulkes, J.G., Erikson, E., and Baltimore, D., Phosphorylation of ribosomal protein S6 on serine after microinjection of the Abelson murine leukemia virus tyrosine-specific protein kinase into *Xenopus* oocytes, *Proc. Natl. Acad. Sci. U.S.A.,* 82, 272, 1985.

439. Rosenberg, N.E., Clark, D.R., and Witte, O.N., Abelson murine leukemia virus mutants deficient in kinase activity and lymphoid cell transformation, *J. Virol.,* 36, 766, 1980.

440. Rohrschneider, L.R. and Najita, L.M., Detection of the v-*abl* gene product at cell-substratum contact sites in Abelson murine leukemia virus-transformed fibroblasts, *J. Virol.,* 51, 547, 1984.

441. Hines, D.L., Viral oncogene expression during differentiation of Abelson virus-infected murine promonocytic leukemia cells, *Cancer Res.,* 48, 1702, 1988.

442. Rosson, D. and Reddy, E.P., Activation of the *abl* oncogene and its involvement in chromosomal translocations in human leukemia, *Mutat. Res.,* 195, 231, 1988.

443. Goff, S.P., Gilboa, E., Witte, O.N., and Baltimore, D., Structure of the Abelson murine leukemia virus genome and the homologous cellular gene: studies with cloned viral DNA, *Cell,* 22, 777, 1980.

444. Schalken, J.A., van den Ouweland, A.M.W., Bloemers, H.P.J., and van de Ven, W.J.M., Characterization of the feline c-*abl* proto-oncogene, *Biochim. Biophys. Acta,* 824, 104, 1985.

445. Telford, J., Burckhardt, J., Butler, B., and Pirrotta, V., Alternative processing and developmental control of the transcripts of the *Drosophila abl* oncogene homologue, EMBO J., 4, 2609, 1985.

446. Henkemeyer, M.J., Gertler, F.B., Goodman, W., and Hoffmann, F.M., The *Drosophila* Abelson proto-oncogene homolog: identification of mutant alleles that have pleiotropic effects late in development, *Cell,* 51, 821, 1987.

447. Henkemeyer, M.J., Bennett, R.L., Gertler, F.B., and Hoffmann, F.M., DNA sequence, structure, and tyrosine kinase activity of the *Drosophila melanogaster* Abelson proto-oncogene homolog, *Mol. Cell. Biol.,* 8, 843, 1988.

448. Goddard, J.M., Weiland, J.J., and Capecchi, M.R., Isolation and characterization of Caenorhabditis elegans DNA sequences homologous to the v-*abl* oncogene, *Proc. Natl. Acad. Sci. U.S.A.,* 83, 2172, 1986.

449. Jhanwar, S.C., Neel, B.G., Hayward, W.S., and Chaganti, R.S.K., Localization of the cellular oncogenes *ABL,* *SIS,* and *FES* on human germ-line chromosomes, *Cytogenet. Cell Genet.,* 38, 73, 1984.

450. Connor, J.M., Pirrit, L.A., Yates, J.R.W., Fryer, A.E., and Ferguson-Smith, M., Linkage of the tuberous sclerosis locus to a DNA polymorphism detected by v-*abl, J. Med. Genet.,* 24, 544, 1987.

451. Heisterkamp, N., Groffen, J., and Stephenson, J.R., The human v-*abl* cellular homologue, *J. Mol. Appl. Genet.,* 2, 57, 1983.

452. Bernards, A., Rubin, C.M., Westbrook, C.A., Paskind, M., and Baltimore, D., The first intron in the human c-*abl* gene is at least 200 kilobases long and is a target for translocations in chronic myelogenous leukemia, *Mol. Cell. Biol.,* 7, 3231, 1987.

453. Wang, J.Y.J. and Baltimore, D., Cellular RNA homologous to the Abelson murine leukemia virus transforming gene: expression and relationship to the viral sequence, *Mol. Cell. Biol.,* 3, 773, 1983.

454. Ben-Neriah, Y., Bernards, A., Paskind, M., Daley, G.Q., and Baltimore, D., Alternative 5′ exons in c-*abl* mRNA, *Cell,* 44, 577, 1986.

455. Müller, R., Slamon, D.J., Tremblay, J.M., Cline, M.J., and Verma, I.M., Differential expression of cellular oncogenes during pre- and postnatal development of the mouse, *Nature,* 299, 640, 1982.

456. Ponzetto, C. and Wolgemuth, D.J., Haploid expression of a unique c-*abl* transcript in the mouse male germ line, *Mol. Cell. Biol.,* 5, 1791, 1985.

457. Oppi, C., Shore, S.K., and Reddy, E.P., Nucleotide sequence of testis-derived c-*abl* cDNAs: implications for testis-specific transcription and *abl* oncogene activation, *Proc. Natl. Acad. Sci. U.S.A.,* 84, 8200, 1987.

458. Meijer, D., Hermans, A., von Lindern, M., van Agthoven, T., de Klein, A., Mackenbach, P., Gootegoed, A., Talarico, D., Della Valle, G., and Grosveld, G., Molecular characterization of the testis specific c-*abl* mRNA in mouse, *EMBO J.,* 6, 4041, 1987.

459. Zaheri, Z.F. and Wolgemuth, D.J., Developmental-stage-specific expression of the hsp70 gene family during differentiation of the mammalian male germ line, *Mol. Cell. Biol.,* 7, 1791, 1987.

460. Ponticelli, A.S., Whitlock, C.A., Rosenberg, N., and Witte, O.N., In vivo tyrosine phosphorylations of the Abelson virus transforming protein are absent in its normal cellular homolog, *Cell,* 29, 953, 1982.

461. Konopka, J.B., Watanabe, S.M., and Witte, O.N., An alteration of the human c-*abl* protein in K562 leukemia cells unmasks associated tyrosine kinase activity, *Cell,* 37, 1035, 1984.

462. Kloetzer, W., Kurzrock, R., Smith, L., Talpaz, M., Spiller, M., Gutterman, J., and Arlinghaus, R., The human cellular *abl* gene product in the chronic myelogenous leukemia cell line K562 has an associated tyrosine protein kinase activity, *Virology,* 140, 230, 1985.

463. Davis, R.L., Konopka, J.B., and Witte, O.N., Activation of the c-*abl* oncogene by viral transduction or chromosome translocation generates altered c-*abl* proteins with similar *in vitro* kinase properties, *Mol. Cell. Biol.,* 5, 204, 1985.

464. Konopka, J.B. and Witte, O.N., Activation of the *abl* oncogene in murine and human leukemias, *Biochim. Biophys. Acta*, 823, 1, 1985.

465. Prywes, R., Foulkes, J.G., and Baltimore, D., The minimum transforming region of v-*abl* is the segment encoding protein-tyrosine kinase, *J. Virol.*, 54, 114, 1985.

466. Oliff, A., Agranovsky, O., McKinney, M.D., Murty, V.V.V.S., and Bauchwitz, R., Friend murine leukemia virus-immortalized myeloid cells are converted into tumorigenic cell lines by Abelson leukemia virus, *Proc. Natl. Acad. Sci. U.S.A.*, 82, 3306, 1985.

467. Cook, W.D., Metcalf, D., Nicola, N.A., Burgess, A.W., and Walker, F., Malignant transformation of a growth factor-dependent myeloid cell line by Abelson virus without evidence of an autocrine mechanism, *Cell*, 41, 677, 1985.

468. Pierce, J.H., Di Fiore, P.P., Aaronson, S.A., Potter, M., Pumphrey, J., Scott, A., and Ihle, J.N., Neoplastic transformation of mast cells by Abelson-MuLV: abrogation of IL-3 dependence by a nonautocrine mechanism, *Cell*, 41, 685, 1985.

469. Mathey-Prevot, B., Nabel, G., Palacios, R., and Baltimore, D., Abelson murine leukemia virus abrogation of interleukin 3 dependence in a lymphoid cell line, *Mol. Cell. Biol.*, 6, 4133, 1986.

470. Cook, W.D., Fazekas de St. Groth, B., Miller, J.F.A.P., MacDonald, H.R., and Gabathuler, R., Abelson virus transformation of an interleukin 2-dependent antigen-specific T-cell line, *Mol. Cell. Biol.*, 7, 2631, 1987.

471. Chung, S.W., Wong, P.M.C., Shen-Ong, G., Ruscetti, S., Ishizaka, T., and Eaves, C.J., Production of granulocyte-macrophage colony-stimulating factor by Abelson virus-induced tumorigenic mast cell lines, *Blood*, 68, 1074, 1986.

472. Maeda, T., Owada, M.K., Sugiyama, H., Miyake, S., Tani, Y., Ogawa, H., Oka, Y., Komori, T., Soma, T., Kishimoto, S., Seki, J., Sakato, N., and Hakura, A., Differentiation of an Abelson virus-transformed immature B precursor cell line under the expression of tyrosine kinase activity of v-abl oncogene product, *Cell Different.*, 20, 263, 1987.

473. Hines, D.L., Differentiation of Abelson murine leukemia virus-infected promonocytic leukemia cells, *Int. J. Cancer*, 36, 233, 1985.

474. Lane, M.-A., Neary, D., and Cooper, G.M., Activation of a cellular transforming gene in tumours induced by Abelson murine leukaemia virus, *Nature*, 300, 659, 1982.

475. Lopez, A.R., Barker, J., and Deisseroth, A.B., v-*abl* activates embryonic globin gene expression in mouse erythroleukemia cells, *Proc. Natl. Acad. Sci. U.S.A.*, 83, 2041, 1986.

476. Serunian, L.A. and Rosenberg, N., Abelson virus potentiates long-term growth of mature B lymphocytes, *Mol. Cell. Biol.*, 6, 183, 1986.

477. Reynolds, F.H., Jr., Van de Ven, W.J.M., and Stephenson, J.R., Feline sarcoma virus polyprotein P115 binds a host phosphoprotein in transformed cells, *Nature*, 286, 409, 1980.

478. Reynolds, F.H., Jr., Van de Ven, W.J.M., and Stephenson, J.R., Feline sarcoma virus P115-associated protein kinase phosphorylates tyrosine: identification of a cellular substrate conserved during evolution, *J. Biol. Chem.*, 255, 11040, 1980.

479. Snyder, H.W., Jr., Biochemical characterization of protein kinase activities associated with transforming gene products of Snyder-Theilen and Gardner-Arnstein strains of feline sarcoma virus, *Virology*, 117, 165, 1982.

480. Reynolds, F.H., Jr., Oroszlan, S., Blomberg, J., and Stephenson, J.R., Tyrosine phosphorylation sites common to transforming proteins encoded by Gardner and Snyder-Theilen FeSV, *Virology*, 122, 134, 1982.

481. Schmitz, M., Käbisch, A., Niemann, H., Bauer, H., and Tamura, T., Purification and characterization of the feline sarcoma virus tyrosine-specific kinase pp85$^{gag\text{-}fes}$, *Virology*, 148, 23, 1986.

482. Melnick, J.L., Altenburg, B., Arnstein, P., Mirkovic, R., and Tavethia, S.S., Transformation of baboon cells with feline sarcoma virus, *Intervirology*, 1, 386, 1973.

483. Rabin, H., Theilen, G.H., Sarma, P.S., Dungworth, D.L., Nelson-Rees, W.A., and Cooper, R.W., Tumor induction in squirrel monkeys by the ST strain of feline sarcoma virus, *J. Natl. Cancer Inst.*, 49, 441, 1972.

484. Ziemicki, A., Hennig, D., Gardner, L., Ferdinand, F.-J., Friis, R.R., Bauer, H., Pedersen, N.C., Johnson, L., and Theilen, G.H., Biological and biochemical characterization of a new isolate of feline sarcoma virus: Theilen-Pedersen (TP1-FeSV), *Virology*, 138, 324, 1984.

485. Ziemicki, A., Characterization of the monomeric and complex-associated forms of the *gag-onc* fusion proteins of three isolates of feline sarcoma virus: phosphorylation, kinase activity, acylation, and kinetics of complex formation, *Virology*, 151, 265, 1986.

486. Brugge, J.S., Interaction of the Rous sarcoma virus protein pp60^{src} with the cellular proteins pp50 and pp90, *Curr. Top. Microbiol. Immunol.*, 123, 1, 1986.

487. Feldman, R.A., Hanafusa, T., and Hanafusa, H., Characterization of protein kinase activity associated with the transforming gene product of Fujinami sarcoma virus, *Cell*, 22, 757, 1980.

488. Pawson, T., Guyden, J., Kung, T.-H., Radke, K., Gilmore, T., and Martin, G.S., A strain of Fujinami sarcoma virus which is temperature-sensitive in protein phosphorylation and cellular transformation, *Cell*, 22, 767, 1980.

489. Hammond, C.I., Vogt, P.K., and Bishop, J.M., Molecular cloning of the PRCII sarcoma viral genome and the chicken proto-oncogene c-*fps*, *Virology*, 143, 300, 1985.

490. Verbeek, J.S., van den Ouweland, A.M.W., Schalken, J.A., Roebroek, A.J.M., Onnekink, C., Bloemers, H.P.J., and van de Ven, W.J.M., Molecular cloning of the feline c-*fes* proto-oncogene and construction of a chimeric transforming gene, *Gene,* 35, 33, 1985.

491. Groffen, J., Heisterkamp, N., Shibuya, M., Hanafusa, H., and Stephenson, J.R., Transforming genes o, esian (v-*fps*) and mammalian (v-*fes*) retroviruses correspond to a common cellular locus, *Virology,* 125, 480, 1983.

492. Feldman, R.A., Gabrilove, J.L., Tam, J.P., Moore, M.A.S., and Hanafusa, H., Specific expression of the human cellular *fps/fes*-encoded protein NCP92 in normal and leukemic myeloid cells, *Proc. Natl. Acad. Sci. U.S.A.,* 82, 2379, 1985.

493. Weinmaster, G. and Pawson, T., Protein kinase activity of FSV (Fujinami sarcoma virus) p13$^{gag-fps}$ shows a strict specificity for tyrosine residues, *J. Biol. Chem.,* 261, 328, 1986.

494. Meckling-Hansen, K., Nelson, R., Branton, P., and Pawson, T., Enzymatic activation of Fujinami sarcoma virus *gag-fps* transforming proteins by autophosphorylation at tyrosine, *EMBO J.,* 6, 659, 1987.

495. Auersperg, N., Pawson, T., Worth, A., and Weinmaster, G., Modifications of tumor histology by point mutations in the v-*fps* oncogene: possible role of extracellular matrix, *Cancer Res.,* 47, 6341, 1987.

496. Feldman, R.A., Vass, W.C., and Tambourin, P.E., Human cellular *fps/fes* cDNA rescued via retroviral shuttle vector encodes myeloid cell NCP92 and has transforming potential, *Oncogene Res.,* 1, 441, 1987.

497. Weinmaster, G., Zoller, M.J., Smith, M., Hinze, E., and Pawson, T., Mutagenesis of Fujinami sarcoma virus: evidence that tyrosine phosphorylation of P130$^{gag-fps}$ modulates its biological activity, *Cell,* 37, 559, 1984.

498. DeClue, J.E., Sadowski, I., Martin, G.S., and Pawson, T., A conserved domain regulates interactions of the v-fps protein-tyrosine kinase with the host cell, *Proc. Natl. Acad. Sci. U.S.A.,* 84, 9064, 1987.

499. Chen, L.-H., Hatada, E., Wheatley, W., and Lee, W.-H., Single amino acid substitution, from Glu^{1025} to Asp, of the *fps* oncogenic protein causes temperature sensitivity in transformation and kinase activity, *Virology,* 155, 106, 1986.

500. Woolford, J. and Beemon, K., Transforming proteins of Fujinami and PRCII avian sarcoma viruses have different subcellular locations, *Virology,* 135, 168, 1984.

501. Moss, P., Radke, K., Carter, V.C., Young, J., Gilmore, T., and Martin, G.S., Cellular localization of the transforming protein of wild-type and temperature-sensitive Fujinami sarcoma virus, *J. Virol.,* 52, 557, 1984.

502. Young, J.C. and Martin, G.S., Cellular localization of c-*fps* gene product NPC98, *J. Virol.,* 52, 913, 1984.

503. Weinmaster, G., Zoller, M.J, and Pawson, T., A lysine in the ATP-binding site of p130$^{gag-fps}$ is essential for protein-tyrosine kinase activity, *EMBO J.,* 5, 69, 1986.

504. Arizumi, K. and Shibuya, M., Construction and biological analysis of deletion mutants of Fujinami sarcoma virus: 5'-*fps* sequence has a role in the transforming activity, *J. Virol.,* 55, 660, 1985.

505. Sadowski, I., Pawson, T., and Lagarde, A., v-*fps* protein-tyrosine kinase coordinately enhances the malignancy and growth factor responsiveness of pre-neoplastic lung fibroblasts, *Oncogene,* 2, 241, 1988.

506. Roebroek, A.J.M., Schalken, J.A., Verbeek, J.S., Van den Ouweland, A.M.W., Onnekink, C., Bloemers, H.P.J., and Van de Ven, W.J.M., The structure of the human c-*fes/fps* proto-oncogene, *EMBO J.,* 4, 2897, 1985.

507. Roebroek, A.J.M., Schalken, J.A., Leunissen, J.A.M., Onnekink, C., Bloemers, H.P.J., and Van de Ven, W.J.M., Evolutionary conserved close linkage of the c-*fes/fps* proto-oncogene and genetic sequences encoding a receptor-like protein, *EMBO J.,* 5, 2197, 1986.

508. Mathey-Prevot, B., Hanafusa, H., and Kawai, S., A cellular protein is immunologically crossreactive with and functionally homologous to the Fujinami sarcoma virus transforming protein, *Cell,* 28, 897, 1982.

509. Samarut, J., Mathey-Prevot, B., and Hanafusa, H., Preferential expression of the c-*fps* protein in chicken macrophages and granulocytic cells, *Mol. Cell. Biol.,* 5, 1067, 1985.

510. Ferrari, S., Torelli, U., Selleri, L., Donell, A., Venturelli, D., Moretti, L., and Torelli, G., Expression of human c-*fes onc*-gene occurs at detectable levels in myeloid but not in lymphoid cell populations, *Br. J. Haematol.,* 59, 21, 1985.

511. Roebroek, A.J.M., Schalken, J.A., Bussemakers, M.J.G., van Heerikhuizen, H., Onnekink, C., Debruyne, F.M.J., Bloemers, H.P.J., and Van de Ven, W.J.M., Characterization of human c-fes/fps reveals a new transcription unit (fur) in the immediately upstream region of the proto-oncogene, *Mol. Biol. Rep.,* 11, 117, 1986.

512. Schalken, J.A., Roebroek, A.J.M., Oomen, P.P.C.A., Wagenaar, S.S., Debruyne, F.M.J., Bloemers, H.P.J., and Van de Ven, W.J.M., *fur* gene expression as a discriminating marker for small cell and nonsmall cell lung carcinomas, *J. Clin. Invest.,* 80, 1545, 1987.

513. Greer, P.A., Meckling-Hansen, K., and Pawson, T., The human c-*fps/fes* gene product expressed ectopically in rat fibroblasts is nontransforming and has restrained protein-tyrosine kinase activity, *Mol. Cell. Biol.,* 8, 578, 1988.

514. Rasheed, S., Barbacid, M., Aaronson, S., and Gardner, M.B., Origin and biological properties of a new feline sarcoma virus, *Virology,* 117, 238, 1982.

515. Naharro, G., Tronick, S.R., Rasheed, S., Gardner, M.B., Aaronson, S.A., and Robbins, K.C., Molecular cloning of integrated Gardner-Rasheed feline sarcoma virus: genetic structure of its cell-derived sequence differs from that of other tyrosine kinase-coding *onc* genes, *J. Virol.,* 47, 611, 1983.

516. Naharro, G., Dunn, C.Y., and Robbins, K.C., Analysis of the primary translation product and integrated DNA of a new feline virus, GR-FeSV, *Virology,* 125, 502, 1983.

517. Naharro, G., Robbins, K.C., and Reddy, E.P., Gene product of v-*fgr onc*: hybrid protein containing a portion of actin and a tyrosine-specific protein kinase, *Science,* 223, 63, 1984.

518. Nishizawa, M., Semba, K., Yamamoto, T., and Toyoshima, K., Human c-*fgr* gene does not contain coding sequence for actin-like protein, *Jpn. J. Cancer Res.,* 76, 155, 1985.

519. Manger, R., Rasheed, S., and Rohrschneider, L., Localization of the feline sarcoma virus *fgr* gene product (P70$^{gag-actin-fgr}$): association with the plasma membrane and detergent-insoluble matrix, *J. Virol.,* 59, 66, 1986.

520. Ball, R.K., Ziemicki, A., Schönenberger, C.A., Reichmann, E., Redmond, S.M.S., and Groner, B., v-*myc* alters the response of a cloned mouse mammary epithelial cell line to lactogenic hormones, *Mol. Endocrinol.,* 2, 133, 1988.

521. Nishizawa, M., Semba, K., Yoshida, M.C., Yamamoto, T., Sasaki, M., and Toyoshima, K., Structure, expression, and chromosomal location of the human c-*fgr* gene, *Mol. Cell. Biol.,* 6, 511, 1986.

522. Tronick, S.R., Popescu, N.C., Cheah, M.S.C., Swan, D.C., Amsbaugh, S.C., Lengel, C.R., DiPaolo, J.A., and Robbins, K.C., Isolation and chromosomal localization of the human *fgr* protooncogene, a distinct member of the tyrosine kinase gene family, *Proc. Natl. Acad. Sci. U.S.A.,* 82, 6595, 1985.

523. Inoue, K., Ikawa, S., Semba, K., Sukegawa, J., Yamamoto, T., and Toyoshima, K., Isolation and sequencing of cDNA clones homologous to the v-*fgr* oncogene from a human B lymphocyte cell line, IM-9, *Oncogene,* 1, 301, 1987.

524. Ley, T.J., Connolly, N.L., Katamine, S., Cheah, M.S.C., Senior, R.M., and Robbins, K.C., Tissue-specific expression and developmental regulation of the human *fgr* proto-oncogene, *Mol. Cell. Biol.,* 9, 92, 1989.

525. Finkel, M.P., Biskis, B.O., and Jinkins, P.B., Virus induction of osteosarcomas in mice, *Science,* 151, 698, 1966.

526. Finkel, M.P. and Biskis, B.O., Experimental induction of osteosarcomas, *Prog. Exp. Tumor Res.,* 10, 72, 1968.

527. Curran, T., Peters, G., van Beveren, C., Teich, N.M., and Verma, I.M., FBJ murine osteosarcoma virus: identification and molecular cloning of biologically active proviral DNA, *J. Virol.,* 44, 674, 1982.

528. Müller, R., Cellular and viral *fos* genes: structure, regulation of expression and biological properties of their encoded products, *Biochim. Biophys. Acta,* 823, 207, 1986.

529. Cohen, D.R. and Curran, T., The structure and function of the *fos* proto-oncogene, *Crit. Rev. Oncogenesis,* 1, 65, 1989.

530. MacConnell, W.P. and Verma, I.M., Expression of FBJ-MSV oncogene (*fos*) product in bacteria, *Virology,* 131, 367, 1983.

531. Setoyama, C., Frunzio, R., Liau, G., Mudryj, M., and de Crombrugghe, B., Transcriptional activation encoded by the v-*fos* gene, *Proc. Natl. Acad. Sci. U.S.A.,* 83, 3213, 1986.

532. Setoyama, C., Hatamochi, A., Peterkofsky, B., Prather, W., and de Crombrugghe, B., v-*fos* stimulates expression of the α₁(III) collagen gene in NIH 3T3 cells, *Biochem. Biophys. Res. Commun.,* 136, 1042, 1986.

533. Nishizawa, M., Goto, N., and Kawai, S., An avian transforming retrovirus isolated from a nephroblastoma that carries the *fos* gene as the oncogene, *J. Virol.,* 61, 3733, 1987.

534. Curran, T. and Teich, N.M., Candidate product of the FBJ murine osteosarcoma virus oncogene: characterization of a 55,000-dalton phosphoprotein, *J. Virol.,* 42, 114, 1982.

535. van Beveren, C., van Straaten, F., Curran, T., Muller, R., and Verma, I.M., Analysis of FBJ-MuSV provirus and c-*fos* (mouse) gene reveals that viral and cellular *fos* gene products have different carboxy terminus, *Cell,* 32, 1241, 1983.

536. van Straaten, F., Muller, R., Curran, T., van Beveren, C., and Verma, I.M., Complete nucleotide sequence of a human c-*onc* gene: deduced amino acid sequence of the human c-*fos* protein, *Proc. Natl. Acad. Sci. U.S.A.,* 80, 3183, 1983.

537. Curran, T., Miller, A.D., Zokas, L., and Verma, I.M., Viral and cellular *fos* proteins: a comparative analysis, *Cell,* 36, 259, 1984.

538. Barber, J.R. and Verma, I.M., Modification of *fos* proteins: phosphorylation of c-*fos*, but not v-*fos*, is stimulated by 12-tetradecanoyl-phorbol-13-acetate and serum, *Mol. Cell. Biol.,* 7, 2201, 1987.

539. Jenuwein, T. and Müller, R., Structure-function analysis of *fos* protein: a single amino acid change activates the immortalizing potential of v-*fos*, *Cell,* 48, 647, 1987.

540. Mölders, H., Jenuwein, T., Adamkiewicz, J., and Müller, R., Isolation and structural analysis of a biologically active chicken c-*fos* cDNA: identification of evolutionarily conserved domains in *fos* protein, *Oncogene,* 1, 377, 1987.

541. Fujiwara, K.T., Ashida, K., Nishina, H., Iba, H., Miyajima, N., Nishizawa, M., and Kawai, S., The chicken c-*fos* gene: cloning and nucleotide sequence analysis, *J. Virol.,* 61, 4012, 1987.

542. Müller, R., Bravo, R., Müller, D., Kurz, C., and Renz, M., Different types of modification in c-*fos* and its associated protein p39: modulation of DNA binding by phosphorylation, *Oncogene Res.,* 2, 19, 1987.

543. Curran, T., Van Beveren, C., Ling, N., and Verma, I.M., Viral and cellular *fox* proteins are complexed with a 39,000-dalton cellular protein, *Mol. Cell. Biol.,* 5, 167, 1985.

544. Franza, B.R., Jr., Sambucetti, L.C., Cohen, D.R., and Curran, T., Analysis of Fos protein complexes and Fos-related antigens by high-resolution two-dimensional gel electrophoresis, *Oncogene,* 1, 213, 1987.

545. Rauscher, F.J., III, Cohen, D.R., Curran, T., Bos, T.J., Vogt, P.K., Bohmann, D., Tjian, R., and Franza, R.B., Jr., Fos-associated protein p39 is the product of the *jun* proto-oncogene, *Science,* 240, 1010, 1988.

546. Sassone-Corsi, P., Ransone, L.J., Lamph, W.W., and Verma, I.M., Direct interaction between fos and jun nuclear oncoproteins: role of the leucine zipper domain, *Nature,* 336, 692, 1988.

547. Gentz, R., Rauscher, F.J., III, Abate, C., and Curran, T., Parallel association of fos and jun leucine zippers juxtaposes DNA binding domains, *Science,* 243, 1695, 1989.

548. Cochran, B.H., Zullo, J., Verma, I.M., and Stiles, C.D., Expression of the c-*fos* gene and of an *fos*-related gene is stimulated by platelet-derived growth factor, *Science,* 226, 1080, 1984.

549. Cohen, D.R. and Curran, T., *fra*-1: a serum-inducible, cellular immediate-early gene that encodes a Fos-related antigen, *Mol. Cell. Biol.,* 8, 2063, 1988.

550. Sukhatme, V.P., Cao, X., Chang, L.C., Tsai-Morris, C.-H., Stamenkovich, D., Ferreira, P.C.P., Cohen, D.R., Edwards, S.A., Shows, T.B., Curran, T., Le Beau, M.M., and Adamson, E.D., A zinc finger-encoding gene coregulated with c-*fos* during growth and differentiation, and after cellular depolarization, *Cell,* 53, 37, 1988.

551. Verma, I.M. and Sassone-Corsi, P., Proto-oncogene *fos*: complex but versatile regulation, *Cell,* 51, 513, 1987.

552. Sariban, E., Luebbers, R., and Kufe, D., Transcriptional and posttranscriptional control of c-*fos* gene expression in human monocytes, *Mol. Cell. Biol.,* 8, 340, 1988.

553. Darby, M.K., Herrera, R.E., Vosberg, H.P. and Nordheim, A., DNA topoisomerase II cleaves at specific sites in the 5' flanking region of c-*fos* proto-oncogenes *in vitro*, *EMBO J.,* 5, 2257, 1986.

554. Deschamps, J., Meijlink, F., and Verma, I.M., Identification of a transcriptional enhancer element upstream from proto-oncogene *fos*, *Science,* 230, 1174, 1985.

555. Renz, M., Neuberg, M., Kurz, C., Bravo, R., and Müller, R., Regulation of c-*fos* transcription in mouse fibroblasts: identification of DNase I-hypersensitive sites and regulatory upstream sequences, *EMBO J.,* 4, 3711, 1985.

556. Hayes, T.E., Kitchen, A.M., and Cochran, B.H., A rapidly inducible DNA-binding activity which binds upstream of the c-*fos* proto-oncogene, *J. Cell. Physiol.,* Suppl. 5, 63, 1987.

557. Fisch, T.M., Prywes, R., and Roeder, R.G., c-*fos* sequences necessary for basal expression and induction by epidermal growth factor, 12-*O*-tetradecanoyl phorbol-13-acetate, and the calcium ionophore, *Mol. Cell. Biol.,* 7, 3490, 1987.

558. Gilman, M.Z., Wilson, R.N., and Weinberg, R.A., Multiple protein-binding sites in the 5'-flanking region regulate c-*fos* expression, *Mol. Cell. Biol.,* 6, 4305, 1986.

559. Schröter, H., Shaw, P.E., and Nordheim, A., Purification of intercalator-released p67, a polypeptide that interacts specifically with the c-fos serum response element, *Nucleic Acids Res.,* 15, 10145, 1987.

560. Renan, M.J., Conserved elements in the 3' untranslated regions of c-*fos* and actin mRNAs, *Biosci. Rep.,* 6, 819, 1986.

561. Liboi, E., Di Francesco, P., Gallinari, P., Testa, U., Rossi, G.B., and Peschle, C., TGF beta induces a sustained c-fos expression associated with stimulation or inhibition of cell growth in EL2 or NIH 3T3 fibroblasts, *Biochem. Biophys. Res. Commun.,* 151, 298, 1988.

562. Collart, M.A., Belin, D., Vassalli, J.-D., and Vassalli, P., Modulations of functional activity in differentiated macrophages are accompanied by early and transient increase or decrease in c-*fos* gene transcription, *J. Immunol.,* 139, 949, 1987.

563. Hayes, T.E., Kitchen, A.M., and Cochran, B.H., Inducible binding of a factor to the c-*fos* regulatory region, *Proc. Natl. Acad. Sci. U.S.A.,* 84, 1272, 1987.

564. Sassone-Corsi, P. and Verma, I.M., Modulation of c-*fos* gene transcription by negative and positive cellular factors, *Nature,* 326, 507, 1987.

565. Fort, P., Rech, J., Vie, A., Piechaczyk, M., Bonnieu, A., Jeanteur, P., and Blanchard, J.-M., Regulation of c-*fos* gene expression in hamster fibroblasts: initiation and elongation of transcription and mRNA degradation, *Nucleic Acids Res.,* 15, 5657, 1987.

566. Prywes, R. and Roeder, R.G., Purification of the c-*fos* enhancer-binding protein, *Mol. Cell. Biol.,* 7, 3482, 1987.

567. Mitchell, R.L., Henning-Chubb, C., Huberman, E., and Verma, I.M., c-*fos* expression is neither sufficient nor obligatory for differentiation of monomyelocytes to macrophages, *Cell,* 45, 497, 1986.

568. Milbrandt, J., Nerve growth factor rapidly induces c-fos mRNA in PC12 rat pheochromocytoma cells, *Proc. Natl. Acad. Sci. U.S.A.,* 83, 4789, 1986.

569. Rahmsdorf, H.J., Schönthal, A., Angel, P., Liftin, M., Rüther, U., and Herrlich, P., Posttranscriptional regulation of c-fos mRNA expression, *Nucleic Acids Res.,* 15, 1643, 1987.

570. Andrews, G.K., Harding, M.A., Calvet, J.P., and Adamson, E.D., The heat shock response in HeLa cells is accompanied by elevated expression of the c-*fos* proto-oncogene, *Mol. Cell. Biol.,* 7, 3452, 1987.

571. Morgan, J.I. and Curran, T., Role of ion flux in the control of c-*fos* expression, *Nature,* 322, 552, 1986.

572. Shibanuma, M., Kuroki, T., and Nose, K., Inhibition of proto-oncogene c-*fos* transcription by inhibitors of protein kinase C and ion transport, *Eur. J. Biochem.,* 164, 15, 1987.

573. Barka, T., van der Noen, H., and Shaw, P.A., Proto-oncogene *fos* (c-*fos*) expression in the heart, *Oncogene,* 1, 439, 1987.

574. Bravo, R., Macdonald-Bravo, H., Müller, R., Hübsch, D., and Almendral, J.M., Bombesin induces c-*fos* and c-*myc* expression in quiescent Swiss 3T3 cells: comparative study with other mitogens, *Exp. Cell Res.,* 170, 103, 1987.

575. Müller, R., Müller, D., and Guilbert, L., Differential expression of c-*fos* in hematopoietic cells: correlation with differentiation of monomyelocytic cells *in vitro, EMBO J.,* 3, 1887, 1984.

576. Mitchell, R.L., Zokas, L., Schreiber, R.D., and Verma, I.M., Rapid induction of the expression of proto-oncogene *fos* during human monocytic differentiation, *Cell,* 40, 209, 1985.

577. Corral, M., Tichonicky, L., Guguen-Guilluzo, C., Corcos, D., Raymondjean, M., Paris, B., Kruh, J., and Defer, N., Expression of c-*fos* oncogene during hepatocarcinogenesis, liver regeneration and in synchronized HTC cells, *Exp. Cell Res.,* 160, 427, 1985.

578. Deschamps, J., Mitchell, R.L., Meijlink, F., Kruijer, W., Schubert, D., and Verma, I.M., Proto-oncogene *fos* is expressed during development, differentiation, and growth, *Cold Spring Harbor Symp. Quant. Biol.,* 50, 733, 1985.

579. Verma, I.M., Proto-oncogene *fos*: a multifaceted gene, *Trends Genet.,* 2, 93, 1986.

580. Heidorn, K., Kreipe, H., Radzun, H.J., Müller, R., and Parwaresch, M.R., The protooncogene c-*fos* is transcriptionally active in normal human granulocytes, *Blood,* 70, 456, 1987.

581. Müller, R., Verma, I.M., and Adamson, E.D., Expression of c-*onc* genes: c-*fos* transcripts accumulate to high levels during development of mouse placenta, yolk sac and amnion, *EMBO J.,* 2, 679, 1983.

582. Mason, I., Murphy, D., and Hogan, B.L.M., Expression of c-fos in parietal endoderm, amnion and differentiating F9 teratocarcinoma cells, *Differentiation,* 30, 76, 1985.

583. Adamson, E.D., Meek, J., and Edwards, S.A., Product of the cellular oncogene, c-*fos*, observed in mouse and human tissues using an antibody to a synthetic peptide, *EMBO J.,* 4, 941, 1985.

584. Dony, C. and Gruss, P., Proto-oncogene c-*fos* expression in growth regions of fetal bone and mesodermal web tissue, *Nature,* 328, 711, 1987.

585. Sandberg, M., Vuorio, T., Hirvonen, H., Alitalo, K., and Vuorio, E., Enhanced expression of TGF-beta and c-*fos* mRNAs in the growth plates of developing human lung bones, *Development,* 102, 461, 1988.

586. De Togni, P., Niman, H., Raymond, V., Sawchenko, P., and Verma, I.M., Detection of *fos* protein during osteogenesis by monoclonal antibodies, *Mol. Cell. Biol.,* 8, 2251, 1988.

587. Gubits, R.M., Hazelton, J.L., and Simantov, R., Variations in c-fos gene expression during rat brain development, *Mol. Brain Res.,* 3, 197, 1988.

588. Dragunow, M., Peterson, M.R., and Robertson, H.A., Presence of c-fos-like immunoreactivity in the adult brain, *Eur. J. Pharmacol.,* 135, 113, 1987.

589. Dragunow, M. and Robertson, H.A., Localization and induction of c-fos protein-like immunoreactive material in the nuclei of adult mammalian neurons, *Brain Res.,* 440, 252, 1988.

590. Sagar, S.M., Sharp, F.R., and Curran, T., Expression of c-*fos* protein in brain: metabolic mapping at the cellular level, *Science,* 240, 1328, 1988.

591. Holt, J.T., Gopal, T.V., Moulton, A.D., and Nienhuis, A.W., Inducible production of c-fos antisense RNA inhibits 3T3 cell proliferation, *Proc. Natl. Acad. Sci. U.S.A.,* 83, 4794, 1986.

592. Nishikura, K. and Murray, J.M., Antisense RNA of proto-oncogene c-*fos* blocks renewed growth of quiescent 3T3 cells, *Proc. Natl. Acad. Sci. U.S.A.,* 7, 639, 1987.

593. Riabowol, K.T., Vosatka, R.J., Ziff, E.B., Lamb, N.J., and Feramisco, J.R., Microinjection of *fos*-specific antibodies blocks DNA synthesis in fibroblast cells, *Mol. Cell. Biol.,* 8, 167, 1988.

594. Curran, T., van Beveren, C., Ling, N., and Verma, I.M., Viral and cellular *fos* proteins are complexed with a 39,000-dalton cellular protein, *Mol. Cell. Biol.,* 5, 167, 1985.

595. Bohmann, D., Bos, T.J., Admon, A., Nishimura, T., Vogt, P.K., and Tjian, R., Human proto-oncogene c-*jun* encodes a DNA binding protein with structural and functional properties of transcriptional factor AP-1, *Science,* 238, 1386, 1987.

596. Angel, P., Allegretto, E.A., Okino, S.T., Hattori, K., Boyle, W.J., Hunter, T., and Karin, M., Oncogene *jun* encodes a sequence-specific *trans*-activator similar to AP-1, *Nature,* 332, 166, 1988.

597. Bos, T.J., Bohmann, D., Tsuchie, H., Tjian, R., and Vogt, P.K., v-*jun* encodes a nuclear protein with enhancer binding properties of AP-1, *Cell,* 52, 705, 1988.

598. Vogt, P.K. and Tjian, R., *jun*: a transcriptional regulator turned oncogene, *Oncogene,* 3, 3, 1988.

599. Sambucetti, L.C. and Curran, T., The Fos protein complex is associated with DNA in isolated nuclei and binds to DNA cellulose, *Science,* 234, 1417, 1986.

600. Barka, T., Gubits, R.M., and van der Noen, H.M., β-Adrenergic stimulation of c-*fos* gene expression in the mouse submandibular gland, *Mol. Cell. Biol.,* 6, 2984, 1986.

601. Lech, K., Anderson, K., and Brent, R., DNA-bound fos proteins activate transcription in yeast, *Cell,* 52, 179, 1988.

602. Mavilio, F., Testa, U., Sposi, N.M., Petrini, M., Pelosi, E., Bordignon, C., Amadori, S., Mandelli, F., and Peschle, C., Selective expression of *fos* proto-oncogene in human acute myelomonocytic and monocytic leukemias: a molecular marker of terminal differentiation, *Blood,* 69, 160, 1987.

603. Müller, R. and Wagner, E.F., Differentiation of F9 teratocarcinoma stem cells after transfer of c-*fos* proto-oncogenes, *Nature,* 311, 438, 1984.

604. Rüther, U., Wagner, E.F., and Müller, R., Analysis of the differentiation-promoting potential of inducible c-*fos* genes introduced into embryonal carcinoma cells, *EMBO J.,* 4, 1775, 1985.

605. Leibovitch, M.-P., Leibovitch, S.A., Hillion, J., Guillier, M., Schmitz, A., and Harel, J., Possible role of c-*fos*, c-N-*ras*, and c-*mos* proto-oncogenes in muscular development, *Exp. Cell Res.,* 170, 80, 1987.

606. Moore, J.P., Todd, J.A., Hesketh, T.R., and Metcalfe, J.C., c-*fos* and c-*myc* gene activation, ionic signals, and DNA synthesis in thymocytes, *J. Biol. Chem.,* 261, 8158, 1986.

607. Pompidou, A., Corral, M., Michel, P., Defer, N., Kruh, J., and Curran, T., The effects of phorbol ester and Ca ionophore on c-fos and c-myc expression and on DNA synthesis in human lymphocytes are not directly related, *Biochem. Biophys. Res. Commun.,* 148, 435, 1987.

608. Monroe, J.G., Up-regulation of c-*fos* expression is a component of the mIg signal transduction mechanism but is not indicative of competence for proliferation, *J. Immunol.,* 140, 1454, 1988.

609. Klinman, D.M., Mushinski, J.F., Honda, M., Ishigatsubo, Y., Mountz, J.D., Raveche, E.S., and Steinberg, A.D., Oncogene expression in autoimmune and normal peripheral blood mononuclear cells, *J. Exp. Med.,* 163, 1292, 1986.

610. Bravo, R., Burckhardt, J., Curran, T., and Müller, R., Expression of c-*fos* in NIH3T3 cells is very low but inducible throughout the cell cycle, *EMBO J.,* 5, 695, 1986.

611. Gutierrez, C., Guo, Z.-S., Farrell-Towt, J., Ju, G., and DePamphilis, M.L., c-*myc* protein and DNA replication: separation of c-*myc* antibodies from an inhibitor of DNA synthesis, *Mol. Cell. Biol.,* 7, 4594, 1987.

612. Reed, J.C., Alpers, J.D., Scherle, P.A., Hoover, R.G., Nowell, P.C., and Prystowsky, M.B., Proto-oncogene expression in cloned T lymphocytes: mitogens and growth factors induce different patterns of expression, *Oncogene,* 1, 223, 1987.

613. Curran, T. and Morgan, J.I., Superinduction of c-*fos* by nerve growth factor in the presence of peripherally active benzodiazepines, *Science,* 229, 1265, 1985.

614. Kruijer, W., Schubert, D., and Verma, I.M., Induction of the proto-oncogene *fos* by nerve growth factor, *Proc. Natl. Acad. Sci. U.S.A.,* 82, 7330, 1985.

615. Greenberg, M.E., Greene, L.A., and Ziff, E.B., Nerve growth factor and epidermal growth factor induce rapid transient changes in proto-oncogene transcription in PC12 cells, *J. Biol. Chem.,* 260, 14101, 1985.

616. Guerrero, I., Pellicer, A., and Burstein, D.E., Dissociation of c-fos from ODC expression and neuronal differentiation in PC12 subline stable transfected with an inducible N-ras oncogene, *Biochem. Biophys. Res. Commun.,* 150, 1185, 1988.

617. Curran, T. and Morgan, J.I., Barium modulates c-*fos* expression and post-translational modification, *Proc. Natl. Acad. Sci. U.S.A.,* 83, 8521, 1986.

618. Gonda, T.J. and Metcalf, D., Expression of *myb, myc,* and *fos* proto-oncogenes during differentiation of a murine myeloid leukaemia, *Nature,* 310, 249, 1984.

619. Müller, R., Curran, T., Müller, D., and Guilbert, L., Induction of c-*fos* during myelomonocytic differentiation and macrophage proliferation, *Nature,* 314, 546, 1985.

620. Barzilay, J., Kushtai, G., Plaksin, D., Feldman, M., and Eisenbach, L., Expression of major histocompatibility class I genes in differentiating leukemic cells is temporally related to activation of c-*fos* proto-oncogene, *Leukemia,* 1, 198, 1987.

621. Conscience, J.-F., Verrier, B., and Martin, G., Interleukin-3-dependent expression of the c-*myc* and c-*fos* proto-oncogenes in hemopoietic cells, *EMBO J.,* 5, 317, 1986.

622. Ruppert, C. and Wille, W., Proto-oncogene c-*fos* is highly induced by disruption of neonatal but not of mature brain tissue, *Mol. Brain Res.,* 2, 51, 1987.

623. Verrier, B., Müller, D., Bravo, R., and Müller, R., Wounding a fibroblast monolayer results in the rapid induction of the c-*fos* proto-oncogene, *EMBO J.,* 5, 913, 1986.

624. Wichelhaus, O., Olek, K., Wappenschmidt, C., and Wagener, C., Rapid expression of c-fos specific messenger RNA after wounding of a BALB/c-3T3 fibroblast monolayer, *J. Clin. Chem. Clin. Biochem.,* 25, 419, 1987.

625. Barka, T., Gubits, R.M., and van der Noen, H., Accumulation of c-*fos* mRNA in slices of mouse submandibular gland incubated *in vitro, Oncogene,* 1, 297, 1987.

626. Morgan, J.J., Cohen, D.R., Hempstead, J.L., and Curran, T., Mapping patterns of c-*fos* expression in the central nervous system after seizure, *Science,* 237, 192, 1987.

627. Hunt, S.P., Pini, A., and Evan, G., Induction of c-*fos*-like protein in spinal cord neurons following sensory stimulation, *Nature,* 328, 632, 1987.

628. Dragunow, M., and Robertson, H.A., Kindling stimulation induces c-*fos* protein(s) in granule cells of the rat dentate gyrus, *Nature,* 329, 441, 1987.

629. Dragunow, M. and Robertson, H.A., Generalized seizures induce c-*fos* protein(s) in mammalian neurons, *Neurosci. Lett.,* 82, 157, 1987.

630. Mellon, P., Pawson, A., Bister, K., Martin, M.S., and Duesberg, P.H., Specific RNA sequences and gene products of MC29 avian acute leukemia virus, *Proc. Natl. Acad. Sci. U.S.A.,* 75, 5874, 1978.

631. Kan, N.C., Flordellis, C.S., Garon, C.F., Duesberg, P.H., and Papas, T.S., Avian carcinoma virus MH2 contains a transformation-specific sequence, *mht*, and shares the *myc* sequence with MC29, CMII, and OK10 viruses, *Proc. Natl. Acad. Sci. U.S.A.,* 80, 6566, 1983.

632. Hayflick, J., Seeburg, P.H., Ohlsson, R., Pfeifer-Ohlsson, S., Watson, D., Papas, T., and Duesberg, P.H., Nucleotide sequence of two overlapping *myc*-related genes in avian carcinoma virus OK10 and their relation to the *myc* genes of other viruses and the cell, *Proc. Natl. Acad. Sci. U.S.A.,* 82, 2718, 1985.

633. Patchinsky, T., Walter, G., and Bister, K., Immunological analysis of v-*myc* gene products using antibodies against a *myc*-specific synthetic peptide, *Virology,* 136, 348, 1984.

634. Bunte, T., Donner, P., Pfaff, E., Reis, B., Greiser-Wilke, I., Schaller, H., and Moelling, K., Inhibition of DNA binding of purified p55$^{\text{v-myc}}$ *in vitro* by antibodies against bacterially expressed *myc* protein and a synthetic peptide, *EMBO J.,* 3, 1919, 1984.

635. Bader, J.P. and Ray, D.A., MC29 virus-coded protein occurs as monomers and dimers in transformed cells, *J. Virol.,* 53, 509, 1985.

636. Ramsay, G., Hayman, M.J., and Bister, K., Phosphorylation of specific sites in the *gag-myc* polyproteins encoded by MC29-type viruses correlates with their transforming ability, *EMBO J.,* 1, 1111, 1982.

637. Neiman, P., Wolf, C., Enrietto, P.J., and Cooper, G.M., A retroviral *myc* gene induces preneoplastic transformation of lymphocytes in a bursal transplantation assay, *Proc. Natl. Acad. Sci. U.S.A.,* 82, 222, 1985.

638. Bister, K., Trachmann, C., Jansen, H.W., Schroeer, B., and Patchinsky, T., Structure of mutant and wild-type MC29 v-*myc* alleles and biochemical properties of their protein products, *Oncogene,* 1, 97, 1987.

639. Kelly, K. and Siebenlist, U., The role of c-myc in the proliferation of normal and neoplastic cells, *J. Clin. Immunol.,* 5, 65, 1985.

640. Kelly, K. and Siebenlist, U., The regulation and expression of c-*myc* in normal and malignant cells, *Annu. Rev. Immunol.,* 4, 317, 1986.

641. Cole, M.D., The *myc* oncogene: its role in transformation and differentiation, *Annu. Rev. Genet.,* 20, 361, 1986.

642. DePinho, R.A., Hatton, K., Ferrier, P., Zimmerman, K., Legouy, E., Tesfaye, A., Collum, R., Yancopoulos, G., Nisen, P., and Alt, F., *myc* family genes: a dispersed multi-gene family, *Ann. Clin. Res.,* 18, 284, 1986.

643. Alitalo, K., Koskinen, P., Mäkelä, T.P., Saksela, K., Sistonen, L., and Winqvist, R., *myc* oncogenes: activation and amplification, *Biochim. Biophys. Acta,* 907, 1, 1987.

644. Ingvarsson, S., Asker, C., Axelson, H., Klein, G., and Sümegi, J., Structure and expression of B-*myc,* a new member of the *myc* gene family, *Mol. Cell. Biol.,* 8, 3168, 1988.

645. Neel, B.G., Jhanwar, S.C., Chaganti, R.S.K., and Hayward, W.S., Two human c-*onc* genes are located on the long arm of chromosome 8, *Proc. Natl. Acad. Sci. U.S.A.,* 79, 7842, 1982.

646. Colby, W.W., Chen, E.Y., Smith, D.M., and Levinson, A.D., Identification and nucleotide sequence of a human locus homologous to the v-*myc* oncogene of avian myelocytomatosis virus MC29, *Nature,* 301, 722, 1983.

647. Watt, R., Stanton, L.W., Marcu, K.B., Gallo, R.C., Croce, C.M., and Rovera, G., Nucleotide sequence of cloned cDNA of human c-*myc* oncogene, *Nature,* 303, 725, 1983.

648. Battey, J., Moulding, C., Taub, R., Murphy, W., Stewart, T., Potter, H., Lenoir, G., and Leder, P., The human c-*myc* oncogene: structural consequences of translocation into the IgH locus in Burkitt lymphoma, *Cell,* 34, 779, 1983.

649. Hann, S.R., King, M.W., Bentley, D.L., Anderson, C.W., and Eisenman, R.N., A non-AUG translational initiation in c-*myc* exon 1 generates an N-terminally distinct protein whose synthesis is disrupted in Burkitt's lymphomas, *Cell,* 52, 185, 1988.

650. Hamlyn, P. and Rabbitts, T., Translocation joins c-*myc* and immunoglobulin alpha 1 genes in a Burkitt lymphoma revealing a third exon in the c-*myc* oncogene, *Nature,* 304, 135, 1983.

651. Watt, R., Nishikura, K., Sorrentino, J., ar-Rushdi, A., Croce, C.M., and Rovera, G., The structure and nucleotide sequence of the 5′ end of the human c-*myc* oncogene, *Proc. Natl. Acad. Sci. U.S.A.,* 80, 6307, 1983.

652. ar-Rushdi, A., Nishikura, K., Erikson, J., Watt, R., Rovera, G., and Croce, C.M., Differential expression of the translocated and the untranslocated c-*myc* oncogene in Burkitt lymphoma, *Science,* 222, 390, 1983.

653. Nishikura, K., Activation of cryptic promoters of human c-*myc* genes in microinjected *Xenopus laevis* oocytes, *J. Mol. Biol.,* 193, 497, 1987.

654. Bentley, D.L. and Groudine, M., Novel promoter upstream of the human c-*myc* gene and regulation of c-*myc* expression in B-cell lymphomas, *Mol. Cell. Biol.,* 6, 3481, 1986.

655. Nishikura, K., Sequences involved in accurate and efficient transcription of human c-*myc* genes microinjected into frog oocytes, *Mol. Cell. Biol.,* 6, 4093, 1986.

656. Remmers, E.F., Yang, J.-Q., and Marcu, K.B., A negative transcriptional control element located upstream of the murine c-*myc* gene, *EMBO J.,* 5, 899, 1986.

657. Kakkis, E. and Calame, K., A plasmacytoma-specific factor binds the c-*myc* promoter region, *Proc. Natl. Acad. Sci. U.S.A.,* 84, 7031, 1987.

658. Lipp, M., Schilling, R., Wiest, S., Laux, G., and Bornkamm, G.W., Target sequences for *cis*-acting regulation within the dual promoter of the human c-*myc* gene, *Mol. Cell. Biol.,* 7, 1393, 1987.

659. Polack, A., Eick, D., Koch, E., and Bornkamm, G.W., Truncation does not abrogate transcriptional downregulation of the c-*myc* gene by sodium butyrate in Burkitt's lymphoma cells, *EMBO J.*, 6, 2959, 1987.

660. Riou, J.F., Vilarem, M.J., Larsen, C.J., and Riou, G., Characterization of the topoisomerase II-induced cleavage sites in the c-*myc* proto-oncogene: *in vitro* stimulation by the antitumoral intercalating drug mAMSA, *Biochem. Pharmacol.*, 35, 4409, 1986.

661. Riou, J.-F., Multon, E., Vilarem, M.-J., Larsen, C.-J., and Riou, G., *In vivo* stimulation by antitumor drugs of the topoisomerase II induced cleavage sites in c-*myc* protooncogene, *Biochem. Biophys. Res. Commun.*, 137, 154, 1986.

662. Nottenburg, C. and Varmus, H.E., Features of the chicken c-*myc* gene that influence the structure of c-*myc* RNA in normal cells and bursal lymphomas, *Mol. Cell. Biol.*, 6, 2800, 1986.

663. Lobanenkov, V.V., Nicolas, R.H., Plumb, M.A., Wright, C.A., and Goodwing, G.H., Sequence-specific DNA-binding proteins which interact with (G+C)-rich sequences flanking the chicken c-*myc* gene, *Eur. J. Biochem.*, 159, 181, 1986.

664. Heinke, C., Andersen, L., Hagan, S., and Guise, K.S., Tissue specific methylation of c-myc in adult chickens, *Biochem. Biophys. Res. Commun.*, 149, 313, 1987.

665. Kindy, M.S., McCormack, J.E., Buckler, A.J., Levine, R.A., and Sonenshein, G.E., Independent regulation of transcription of the two strands of the c-*myc* gene, *Mol. Cell. Biol.*, 7, 2857, 1987.

666. Dean, M., Kent, R.B., and Sonenshein, G.E., Transcriptional activation of immunoglobulin alpha heavy-chain genes by translocation of the c-*myc* oncogene, *Nature*, 305, 443, 1983.

667. Levine, R.A., McCormack, J.E., Buckler, A., and Sonenshein, G.E., Transcriptional and posttranscriptional control of c-*myc* gene expression in WEHI 231 cells, *Mol. Cell. Biol.*, 6, 4112, 1986.

668. Brewer, G. and Ross, J., Poly(A) shortening and degradation of the 3′ A+U-rich sequences of human c-*myc* mRNA in a cell-free system, *Mol. Cell. Biol.*, 8, 1697, 1988.

669. Stanton, L.W. and Bishop, J.M., Alternative processing of RNA transcribed from *NMYC*, *Mol. Cell. Biol.*, 7, 4266, 1987.

670. Sejersen, T., Rahm, M., Szabo, G., Ingvarsson, S., and Sümegi, J., Similarities and differences in the regulation of N-*myc* genes in murine embryonal carcinoma cells, *Exp. Cell Res.*, 172, 304, 1987.

671. Amy, C.M. and Bartholomew, J.C., Regulation of N-*myc* transcript stability in human neuroblastoma and retinoblastoma cells, *Cancer Res.*, 47, 6310, 1987.

672. Corral, M., Paris, B., Guguen-Guillozo, C., Corcos, D., Kruh, J., and Defer, N., Increased expression of the N-*myc* gene during normal and neoplastic rat liver growth, *Exp. Cell Res.*, 174, 107, 1988.

673. DePinho, R.A., Hatton, K.S., Tefaye, A., Yancopoulos, G.D., and Alt, F.W., The human *myc* gene family: structure and activity of L-*myc* and an L-*myc* pseudogene, *Genes Dev.*, 1, 1311, 1987.

674. Saksela, K., Expression of the L-*myc* gene is under positive control by short-lived proteins, *Oncogene*, 1, 291, 1987.

675. DeGreve, J., Battey, J., Fedorko, J., Birrer, M., Evan, G., Kaye, F., Sausville, E., and Minna, J., The human L-*myc* gene encodes multiple nuclear phosphoproteins from alternatively processed mRNAs, *Mol. Cell. Biol.*, 8, 4381, 1988.

676. Beimling, P., Benter, T., Sander, T., and Moelling, K., Isolation and characterization of the human cellular *myc* gene product, *Biochemistry*, 24, 6349, 1985.

677. Miyamoto, C., Chizzonite, R., Crowl, R., Rupprecht, K., Kramer, R., Schaber, M., Kumar, G., Poonian, M., and Ju, G., Molecular cloning and regulated expression of the human c-*myc* gene in *Escherichia coli* and *Saccharomyces cerevisiae*: comparison of the protein sequences, *Proc. Natl. Acad. Sci. U.S.A.*, 82, 7232, 1985.

678. Nishikura, K., Goldflam, A., and Vuocolo, G.A., Accurate and efficient transcription of human c-*myc* genes injected into *Xenopus laevis* oocytes, *Mol. Cell. Biol.*, 5, 1434, 1985.

679. Morgan, J.H., Papas, T.S., and Parsons, J.T., Isolation of antibodies specific for avian viral and cellular *myc* proteins, *J. Natl. Cancer Inst.*, 75, 937, 1985.

680. Morgan, J.H. and Parsons, J.T., Characterization of c-*myc* proteins from avian bursal lymphoma cell lines, *Virology*, 150, 178, 1986.

681. Evan, G.I., Lewis, G.K., Ramsay, G., and Bishop, J.M., Isolation of monoclonal antibodies specific for the human c-*myc* proto-oncogene product, *Mol. Cell. Biol.*, 5, 3610, 1985.

682. Ferré, F., Martin, P., Begue, A., Ghysdael, J., Saule, S., and Stéhelin, D., Préparation et caractérisation d'antisera spécifiques dirigés contre différents domains polypeptidiques codés par l'oncogène c-*myc* humain pour étudier l'expression de ce gène introduit dans des cellules de caille ou de rat, *C.R. Acad. Sci. Paris*, 303, 633, 1986.

683. Chan, S.Y.T., Evan, G.I., Ritson, A., Watson, J., Wraight, P., and Sikora, K., Localisation of lung cancer by a radiolabelled monoclonal antibody against the c-*myc* oncogene product, *Br. J. Cancer*, 54, 761, 1986.

684. Giallongo, A., Feo, S., Showe, L.C., and Croce, C.M., Isolation and partial characterization of a 48-kDa protein which is induced in normal lymphocytes upon mitogenic stimulation, *Biochem. Biophys. Res. Commun.*, 134, 1238, 1986.

685. Iwanaga, T., Fujita, T., Tsuchihashi, T., Yamaguchi, K., Abe, K., and Yanaihara, N., Immonocytochemical detection of the c-*myc* oncogene product in human fetuses, *Biomed. Res.*, 7, 161, 1986.

686. Gazin, C., Rigolet, M., Briand, J.P., Van Regenmortel, M.H.V., and Galibert, F., Immunochemical detection of proteins related to the human c-*myc* exon 1, *EMBO J.,* 5, 2241, 1986.

687. Eladari, M.E., Syed, S.H., Guilhot, S., d'Auriol, L., and Galibert, F., On the high conservation of the human c-*myc* first exon, *Biochem. Biophys. Res. Commun.,* 140, 313, 1986.

688. Butnick, N.Z., Miyamoto, C., Chizzonite, R., Cullen, B.R., Ju, G., and Skalka, A.M., Regulation of the human c-*myc* gene: 5' noncoding sequences do not affect translation, *Mol. Cell. Biol.,* 5, 3009, 1985.

689. Ferré, F., Martin, P., Lagrou, C., Raes, M.-B., Ghysdael, J., Saule, S., and Stéhelin, D., The human c-*myc* exon 1 product: preparation of antisera and analysis of its expression, *Oncogene,* 1, 387, 1987.

690. Slamon, D.J., Boone, T.C., Seeger, R.C., Keith, D.T., Chazin, V., Lee, H.C., and Souza, L.M., Identification and characterization of the protein encoded by the human N-*myc* oncogene, *Science,* 232, 768, 1988.

691. Kohl, N.E., Legouy, E., DePinho, R.A., Nisen, P.D., Smith, R.K., Gee, C.E., and Alt, F.W., Human N-*myc* is closely related in organization and nucleotide sequence to c-*myc,* *Nature,* 319, 73, 1986.

692. Stanton, L.W., Schwab, M., and Bishop, J.M., Nucleotide sequence of the human N-*myc* gene, *Proc. Natl. Acad. Sci. U.S.A.,* 83, 1772, 1986.

693. Ramsay, G., Stanton, L., Schwab, M., and Bishop, J.M., Human proto-oncogene N-*myc* encodes nuclear proteins that bind DNA, *Mol. Cell. Biol.,* 6, 4450, 1986.

694. Donner, P., Greiser-Wilke, I., and Moelling, K., Nuclear localization and DNA binding of the transforming gene product of avian myelocytomatosis virus, *Nature,* 296, 262, 1982.

695. Abrams, H.D., Rohrschneider, L.R., and Eisenman, R.N., Nuclear location of the putative transforming protein of avian myelocytomatosis virus, *Cell,* 29, 427, 1982.

696. Persson, H. and Leder, P., Nuclear localization and DNA binding properties of a protein expressed by human c-*myc* oncogene, *Science,* 225, 718, 1984.

697. Dang, C.V. and Lee, W.M.F., Identification of the human c-*myc* protein nuclear translocation signal, *Mol. Cell. Biol.,* 8, 4048, 1988.

698. Dang, C.V., McGuire, M., Buckmire, M., and Lee, W.M.F., Involvement of the "leucine zipper" region in the oligomerization and transforming activity of human c-myc protein, *Nature,* 337, 664, 1989.

699. Lüscher, B., Kuenzel, E.A., Krebs, E.G., and Eisenman, R.N., Myc proteins are phosphorylated by casein kinase II, *EMBO J.,* 8, 111, 1989.

700. Persson, H., Gray, H.E., Godeau, F., Braunhut, S., and Bellvè, A.R., Multiple growth-associated nuclear proteins immunoprecipitated by antisera raised against human c-*myc* peptide antigens, *Mol. Cell. Biol.,* 6, 942, 1986.

701. Hann, S.R. and Eisenman, R.N., Proteins encoded by the human c-*myc* oncogene: differential expression in neoplastic cells, *Mol. Cell. Biol.,* 4, 2486, 1984.

702. Ramsay, G., Evan, G.I., and Bishop, J.M., The protein encoded by the human proto-oncogene c-*myc,* *Proc. Natl. Acad. Sci. U.S.A.,* 81, 7742, 1984.

703. Eisenman, R.N., Tachibana, C.Y., Abrams, H.D., and Hann, S.R., v-*myc* and c-*myc*-encoded proteins are associated with the nuclear matrix, *Mol. Cell. Biol.,* 5, 114, 1985.

704. Evan, G.I. and Hancock, D.C., Studies on the interaction of the human c-*myc* protein with cell nuclei: p62^{c-myc} as a member of a discrete subset of nuclear proteins, *Cell,* 43, 253, 1985.

705. Van Straaten, J.P. and Rabbitts, T.H., The c-*myc* protein is associated with the nuclear matrix through specific metal interaction, *Oncogene Res.,* 1, 221, 1987.

706. Spector, D.L., Watt, R.A., and Sullivan, N.F., The v-*myc* and c-*myc* oncogene proteins colocalize *in situ* with small nuclear ribonucleoprotein particles, *Oncogene,* 1, 5, 1987.

707. Watt, R.A., Shatzman, A.R., and Rosenberg, M., Expression and characterization of the human c-*myc* DNA-binding protein, *Mol. Cell. Biol.,* 5, 448, 1985.

708. Bader, J.P., Hausman, F.A., and Ray, D.A., Intranuclear degradation of the transformation-inducing protein encoded by avian MC29 virus, *J. Biol. Chem.,* 261, 8303, 1986.

709. Winqvist, R., Saksela, K., and Alitalo, K., The *myc* proteins are not associated with chromatin in mitotic cells, *EMBO J.,* 3, 2947, 1984.

710. King, M.W., Roberts, J.M., and Eisenman, R.N., Expression of the c-*myc* proto-oncogene during development of *Xenopus laevis,* *Mol. Cell. Biol.,* 6, 4499, 1986.

711. Suzuki, T., Yanaihara, C., Hirota, M., Iwafuchi, M., Inoue, T., Mochizuki, T., Iguchi, K., Abe, K., and Yanaihara, N., Immunohistochemical demonstration of c-*myc* gene product in tumors induced in nude mice by human hepatoblastoma: a study with antiserum to a related synthetic peptide, *Biomed. Res.,* 7, 365, 1986.

712. Ferrari, S., Calabretta, B., Battini, R., Cosenza, S.C., Owen, T.A., Soprano, K.J., and Baserga, R., Expression of c-*myc* and induction of DNA synthesis by platelet-poor plasma in human diploid fibroblasts, *Exp. Cell Res.,* 174, 25, 1988.

713. Buckler, A.J., Rothstein, T.L., and Sonenshein, G.E., Two-step stimulation of B lymphocytes to enter DNA synthesis: synergy between anti-immunoglobulin antibody and cytochalasin on expression of c-*myc* and a G_1-specific gene, *Mol. Cell. Biol.,* 8, 1371, 1988.

714. Kaczmarek, L., Hyland, J.K., Watt, R., Rosenberg, M., and Baserga, R., Microinjected c-*myc* as a competence factor, *Science,* 228, 1313, 1985.

715. Studzinski, G.P., Brelvi, Z.S., Feldman, S.C., and Watt, R.A., Participation of c-*myc* protein in DNA synthesis of human cells, *Science,* 234, 467, 1986.

716. Heikkila, R., Schwab, G., Wickstrom, E., Loke, S.L., Pluznik, D.H., Watt, R., and Neckers, L.M., A c-*myc* antisense oligodeoxynucleotide inhibits entry into S phase but not progress from G_0 to G_1, *Nature,* 328, 445, 1987.

717. Zimmerman, K.A., Yancopoulos, G.D., Collum, R.G., Smith, R.K., Kohl, N.E., Denis, K.A., Nau, M.M., Witte, O.N., Toran-Allerand, D., Gee, C.E., Minna, J.D., and Alt, F.W., Differential expression of *myc* family genes during murine development, *Nature,* 319, 780, 1986.

718. Grady, E.F., Schwab, M., and Rosenau, W., Expression of N-*myc* and c-*src* during the development of fetal human brain, *Cancer Res.,* 47, 2931, 1987.

719. Schweinfest, C.W., Fujiwara, S., Lau, L.F., and Papas, T.S., c-*myc* can induce expression of G_0/G_1 transition genes, *Mol. Cell. Biol.,* 8, 3080, 1988.

720. Prendergast, G.C. and Cole, M.D., Posttranslational regulation of cellular gene expression by the c-*myc* oncogene, *Mol. Cell. Biol.,* 9, 124, 1989.

721. Van Beneden, R.J., Watson, D.K., Chen, T.T., Lautenberger, J.A., and Papas, T.S., Cellular *myc* (c-*myc*) in fish (rainbow trout): its relationship to other vertebrate *myc* genes and to the transforming genes of the MC29 family of viruses, *Proc. Natl. Acad. Sci. U.S.A.,* 83, 3698, 1986.

722. Madhavan, K., Bilodeau-Wentworth, D., and Wadsworth, S.C., Family of developmentally regulated, maternally expressed *Drosophila* RNA species detected by a v-*myc* probe, *Mol. Cell. Biol.,* 5, 7, 1985.

723. Voellmy, R., The heat shock genes: a family of highly conserved genes with a superbly complex expression pattern, *BioEssays,* 1, 213, 1984.

724. Bienz, M., Transient and developmental activation of heat-shock genes, *Trends Genet.,* 10, 157, 1985.

725. Craig, E.A., The heat shock response, *Crit. Rev. Biochem.,* 18, 239, 1985.

726. Kingston, R.E., Baldwin, A.S., and Sharp, P.A., Regulation of heat shock protein 70 gene expression by c-*myc*, *Nature,* 312, 280, 1984.

727. Aujame, L. and Morgan, C., Nonexpression of a major heat shock gene in mouse plasmacytoma MPC-11, *Mol. Cell. Biol.,* 5, 1780, 1985.

728. Ben-Mahrez, K., Perbal, B., Kryceve-Martinerie, C., Thierry, D., and Kohiyama, M., A protein of *Halobacterium halobium* immunologically related to the v-*myc* gene product, *FEBS Lett.,* 227, 56, 1988.

729. Ben-Mahrez, K., Sougakoff, W., Nakayama, M., and Kohiyama, M., Stimulation of an alpha like DNA polymerase by v-*myc* related protein of *Halobacterium halobium*, *Arch. Microbiol.,* 149, 175, 1988.

730. Crabbe, M.J.C., Partial sequence homology of human *myc* oncogene protein to β and γ crystallins, *FEBS Lett.,* 181, 157, 1985.

731. den Dunnen, J.T., Moormann, R.J.M., and Schoenmakers, J.G.G., Rat lens β-crystallins are internally duplicated and homologous to γ-crystallins, *Biochim. Biophys. Acta,* 824, 295, 1985.

732. Meakin, S.O., Breitman, M.L., and Tsui, L.-C., Structural and evolutionary relationships among five members of the human γ-crystallin gene family, *Mol. Cell. Biol.,* 5, 1408, 1985.

733. Villares, R. and Cabrera, C.V., The *achaete-scute* gene complex of *D. melanogaster:* conserved domains in a subset of genes required for neurogenesis and their homology to *myc*, *Cell,* 50, 415, 1987.

734. Cabrera, C.V., Martinez-Arias, A., and Bate, M., The expression of three members of the *achaete-scute* gene complex correlates with neuroblast segregation in *Drosophila*, *Cell,* 50, 425, 1987.

735. Bienz, B., Zakut-Houri, R., Givol, D., and Oren, M., Analysis of the gene coding for the murine cellular tumour antigen p53, *EMBO J.,* 3, 2179, 1984.

736. Rechsteiner, M., Do myc, fos, and E1A function as protein phosphatase inhibitors?, *Biochem. Biophys. Res. Commun.,* 143, 194, 1987.

737. Dean, M., Levine, R.A., Ran, W., Kindy, W., Sonenshein, G.E., and Campisi, J., Regulation of c-*myc* transcription and mRNA abundance by serum growth factors and cell contact, *J. Biol. Chem.,* 261, 9161, 1986.

738. Reed, J.C., Alpers, J.D., and Nowell, P.C., Expression of c-*myc* proto-oncogene in normal human lymphocytes: regulation by transcriptional and posttranscriptional mechanisms, *J. Clin. Invest.,* 80, 101, 1987.

739. Nepveu, A., Levine, R.A., Campisi, J., Greenberg, M.E., Ziff, E.B., and Marcu, K.B., Alternative modes of c-*myc* regulation in growth factor-stimulated and differentiating cells, *Oncogene,* 1, 243, 1987.

740. Blanchard, J.-M., Piechaczyk, M., Dani, C., Chambard, J.-C., Franchi, A., Pouyssegur, J., and Jeanteur, P., c-*myc* gene is transcribed at high rate in G_0-arrested fibroblasts and is post-transcriptionally regulated in response to growth factors, *Nature,* 317, 443, 1985.

741. Fahrlander, P.D., Piechaczyk, M., and Marcu, K.B., Chromatin structure of the murine c-*myc* locus: implications for the regulation of normal and chromosomally translocated genes, *EMBO J.,* 4, 3195, 1985.

742. Chung, J., Sinn, E., Reed, R.R., and Leder, P., Trans-acting elements modulate expression of the human c-*myc* gene in Burkitt lymphoma cells, *Proc. Natl. Acad. Sci. U.S.A.,* 83, 7918, 1986.

743. Boles, T.C. and Hogan, M.E., DNA structure equilibria in the human c-*myc* gene, *Biochemistry,* 26, 367, 1987.

744. Eick, D., Berger, R., Polack, A., and Bornkamm, G.W., Transcription of c-*myc* in human mononuclear cells is regulated by an elongation block, *Oncogene,* 2, 61, 1987.

745. Dani, C., Blanchard, J.M., Piechaczyc, M., El Sabouty, S., Marty, L., and Jeanteur, P., Extreme instability of myc mRNA in normal and transformed human cells, *Proc. Natl. Acad. Sci. U.S.A.,* 81, 7046, 1984.

746. Taylor, M.V., Gusse, M., Evan, G.I., Dathan, N., and Mechali, M., *Xenopus myc* proto-oncogene during development: expression as a stable maternal mRNA uncoupled from cell division, *EMBO J.,* 5, 3563, 1986.

747. Kindy, M.S. and Sonenshein, G.E., Regulation of oncogene expression in cultured aortic smooth muscle cells: post-transcriptional control of c-*myc* mRNA, *J. Biol. Chem.,* 261, 12865, 1986.

748. Swartwout, S.G., Preisler, H., Guan, W., and Kinniburgh, A., Relatively stable population of c-*myc* RNA that lacks poly(A), *Mol. Cell. Biol.,* 7, 2052, 1987.

749. Thompson, C.B., Challoner, P.B., Neiman, P.E., and Groudine, M., Levels of c-*myc* oncogene mRNA are invariant throughout the cell cycle, *Nature,* 314, 363, 1985.

750. Hann, S.R., Thompson, C.B., and Eisenman, R.N., c-*myc* oncogene protein synthesis is independent of the cell cycle in human and avian cells, *Nature,* 314, 366, 1985.

751. Rabbitts, P.H., Watson, J.V., Lamond, A., Forster, A., Stinson, M.A., Evan, G., Fischer, W., Atherton, E., Sheppard, R., and Rabbitts, T.H., Metabolism of c-*myc* gene products: c-*myc* mRNA and protein expression in the cell cycle, *EMBO J.,* 4, 2009, 1985.

752. Eisenman, R.N. and Hann, S.R., Proteins expressed by the c-*myc* oncogene in lymphomas of human and avian origin, *Proc. R. Soc. London,* B226, 73, 1985.

753. Snow, E.C., Fetherston, J.D., and Zimmer, S., Induction of the c-*myc* protooncogene after antigen binding to hapten-specific B cells, *J. Exp. Med.,* 164, 944, 1986.

754. Corcos, D., Vaulont, S., Denis, N., Lyonnet, S., Simon, M.-P., Kitzis, A., Kahn, A., and Kruh, J., Expression of c-*myc* is under dietary control in rat liver, *Oncogene Res.,* 1, 193, 1987.

755. Horikawa, S., Sakata, K., Hatanaka, M., and Tsukada, K., Expression of c-*myc* oncogene in rat liver by a dietary manipulation, *Biochem. Biophys. Res. Commun.,* 140, 574, 1986.

756. Nakamura, K.D., Turturro, A., and Hart, R.W., Elevated c-myc expression in progeria fibroblasts, *Biochem. Biophys. Res. Commun.,* 155, 996, 1988.

757. Dean, R., Kim, S.S., and Delgado, D., Expression of c-myc oncogene in human fibroblasts during *in vitro* senescence, *Biochem. Biophys. Res. Commun.,* 135, 105, 1986.

758. Tavassoli, M. and Shall, S., Transcription of the c-*myc* oncogene is altered in spontaneously immortalized rodent fibroblasts, *Oncogene,* 2, 337, 1988.

759. Ono, T., Tawa, R., Shinya, K., Hirose, S., and Okada, S., Methylation of the c-myc gene changes during aging process of mice, *Biochem. Biophys. Res. Commun.,* 139, 1299, 1986.

760. Matocha, M.F., Cosgrove, J.W., Atack, J.R., and Rapoport, S.I., Selective elevation of c-myc transcript levels in the liver of the aging Fischer-344 rat, *Biochem. Biophys. Res. Commun.,* 147, 1, 1987.

761. Ruppert, C., Goldowitz, D., and Wille, W., Proto-oncogene c-*myc* is expressed in cerebellar neurons at different developmental stages, *EMBO J.,* 5, 1897, 1986.

762. Phillips, N.E. and Parker, D.C., Fc-γ receptor effects on induction of c-*myc* mRNA expression in mouse B lymphocytes by anti-immunoglobulin, *Mol. Immunol.,* 24, 1199, 1987.

763. Billings, P.C., Shuin, T., Lillehaug, J., Miurs, T., Roy-Burman, P., and Landolph, J.R., Enhanced expression and state of the c-*myc* oncogene in chemically and X-ray-transformed C3H/10T1/2 mouse embryo cells, *Cancer Res.,* 47, 3643, 1987.

764. Schneider, M.D., Payne, P.A., Ueno, K., Perryman, M.B., and Roberts, R., Dissociated expression of c-*myc* and a *fos*-related competence gene during cardiac myogenesis, *Mol. Cell. Biol.,* 6, 4140, 1986.

765. Starksen, N.F., Simpson, P.C., Bishopric, N., Coughlin, S.R., Lee, W.M.F., Escobedo, J.A., and Williams, L.T., Cardiac myocyte hypertrophy is associated with c-*myc* protooncogene expression, *Proc. Natl. Acad. Sci. U.S.A.,* 83, 8348, 1986.

766. Mulvagh, S.L., Michael, L.H., Perryman, M.B., Roberts, R., and Schneider, M.D., A hemodynamic load in vivo induces cardiac expression of the cellular oncogene, c-*myc, Biochem. Biophys. Res. Commun.,* 147, 627, 1987.

767. Pfeifer-Ohlsson, S., Goustin, A.S., Rydnert, J., Wahlstrom, T., Bjersing, L., Stehelin, D., and Ohlsson, R., Spatial and temporal pattern of cellular *myc* oncogene expression in developing human placenta: implications for embryonic cell proliferation, *Cell,* 38, 585, 1984.

768. Maruo, T. and Mochizuki, M., Immunohistochemical localization of epidermal growth factor receptor and myc oncogene product in human placenta: implication for trophoblast proliferation and differentiation, *Am. J. Obstet. Gynecol.,* 156, 721, 1987.

769. Grausz, J.D., Fradelizi, D., Dautry, F., Monier, R., and Lehn, P., Modulation of c-fos and c-myc mRNA levels in normal human lymphocytes by calcium ionophore A23187 and phorbol ester, *Eur. J. Immunol.,* 16, 1217, 1986.

770. Smeland, E.B., Beiske, K., Ek, B., Watt, R., Pfeiffer-Ohlsson, S., Blomhoff, H.K., Godal, T., and Ohlsson, R., Regulation of c-*myc* transcription and protein expression during activation of normal human B cells, *Exp. Cell Res.,* 172, 101, 1987.

771. Lomo, J., Holte, H., de Lange Davies, C., Ruud, E., Laukas, M., Smeland, E.B., Godal, T., and Blomhoff, H.K., Downregulation of c-*myc* RNA is not a prerequisite for reduced cell proliferation, but is associated with G₁ arrest in B-lymphoid cell lines, *Exp. Cell Res.,* 172, 84, 1987.

772. Bains, M.A., Hoy, T.G., Baines, P., and Jacobs, A., Nuclear c-myc protein, maturation, and cell-cycle status on human haematopoietic cells, *Br. J. Haematol.*, 67, 293, 1987.

773. Sejersen, T., Björklund, H., Sümegi, J., and Ringertz, N.R., N-myc and c-src genes are differentially regulated in PCC7 embryonal carcinoma cells undergoing neuronal differentiation, *J. Cell. Physiol.*, 127, 274, 1986.

774. Chang, J.D., Billings, P.C., and Kennedy, A.R., c-myc expression is reduced in antipain-treated proliferating C3H 10T1/2 cells, *Biochem. Biophys. Res. Commun.*, 133, 830, 1985.

775. Filmus, J. and Buick, R.N., Relationship of c-*myc* expression to differentiation and proliferation of HL-60 cells, *Cancer Res.*, 45, 822, 1985.

776. Schofield, P.N., Engstrom, W., Lee, A.J., Biddle, C., and Graham, C.F., Expression of c-*myc* during differentiation of the human teratocarcinoma cell line Tera-2, *J. Cell Sci.*, 88, 57, 1987.

777. Mechti, N., Piechaczyk, M., Blanchard, J.-M., Marty, L., Bonnieu, A., Jeanteur, P., and Lebleu, B., Transcriptional and post-transcriptional regulation of c-myc expression during the differentiation of murine erythroleukemia Friend cells, *Nucleic Acids Res.*, 14, 9653, 1986.

778. Dmitrovsky, E., Kuehl, W.M., Hollis, G.F., Kirsch, I.R., Bender, T.P., and Segal, S., Expression of a transfected human c-*myc* oncogene inhibits differentiation of a mouse erythroleukaemia cell line, *Nature*, 322, 748, 1986.

779. Prochownik, E.V. and Kukowska, J., Deregulated expression of c-*myc* by murine erythroleukaemia cells prevents differentiation, *Nature*, 322, 848, 1986.

780. Nath, P., Getzenberg, R., Beebe, D., Pallansch, L., and Zelenka, P., c-*myc* mRNA is elevated as differentiating lens cells withdraw from the cell cycle, *Exp. Cell Res.*, 169, 215, 1987.

781. Hirayu, H., Dere, W.H., and Rapoport, B., Initiation of normal thyroid cells in primary culture is associated with enhanced c-myc messenger ribonucleic acid levels, *Endocrinology*, 120, 924, 1987.

782. Sejersen, T., Sümegi, J., and Ringertz, N.R., Density-dependent arrest of DNA replication is accompanied by decreased levels of c-myc mRNA in myogenic but not in differentiation defective myoblasts, *J. Cell. Physiol.*, 125, 465, 1985.

783. Denis, N., Blanc, S., Leibovitch, M.P., Nicolaiew, N., Dautry, F., Raymondjean, M., Kruh, J., and Kitzis, A., c-*myc* oncogene expression inhibits the initiation of myogenic differentiation, *Exp. Cell Res.*, 172, 212, 1987.

784. Endo, T. and Nadal-Ginard, B., Transcriptional and posttranscriptional contol of c-*myc* during myogenesis: its mRNA remains inducible in differentiated cells and does not suppress the differentiated phenotype, *Mol. Cell. Biol.*, 6, 1412, 1986.

785. Spizz, G., Hu, J.-S., and Olson, E.N., Inhibition of myogenic differentiation by fibroblast growth factor or type beta transforming growth factor does not require persistent c-*myc* expression, *Dev. Biol.*, 123, 500, 1987.

786. Watanabe, T., Sherman, M., Shafman, T., Iwata, T., and Kufe, D., Effects of ornithine decarboxylase inhibition on c-myc expression during murine erythroleukemia cell proliferation and differentiation, *J. Cell. Physiol.*, 127, 480, 1986.

787. Lee, J., Mehta, K., Blick, M.B., Gutterman, J.U., and Lopez-Berestein, G., Expression of c-*fos*, c-*myb*, and c-*myc* in human monocytes: correlation with monocytic differentiation, *Blood*, 69, 1542, 1987.

788. Reitsma, P.H., Rothberg, P.G., Astrin, S.M., Trial, J., Bar-Shavit, Z., Hall, A., Teitelbaum, S.L., and Kahn, A.J., Regulation of *myc* gene expression in HL-60 leukaemia cells by a vitamin D metabolite, *Nature*, 306, 492, 1983.

789. Simpson, R.U., Hsu, T., Begley, D.A., Mitchell, B.S., and Alizadeh, B.N., Transcriptional regulation of c-myc protooncogene by 1,25-dihydroxyvitamin D_3 in HL-60 promyelocytic leukemia cells, *J. Biol. Chem.*, 262, 4104, 1987.

790. Brelvi, Z.S. and Studzinski, G.P., Inhibition of DNA synthesis by an inducer of differentiation of leukemic cells, 1-α,25 dihydroxy vitamin D_3, precedes down regulation of the c-myc gene, *J. Cell. Physiol.*, 128, 171, 1986.

791. Thompson, N.L., Mead, J.E., Braun, L., Goyette, M., Shank, P.R., and Fausto, N., Sequential protooncogene expression during rat liver regeneration, *Cancer Res.*, 46, 3111, 1986.

792. Le Gros, J., De Feyter, R., and Ralph, R.K., Cyclic AMP and c-myc gene expression in PY815 mouse mastocytoma cells, *FEBS Lett.*, 186, 13, 1985.

793. Kubota, Y., Shuin, T., Yao, M., Inoue, H., and Yoshioka, T., The enhanced ^{32}P labeling of CDP-diacylglycerol in c-*myc* gene expressed human kidney cancer cells, *FEBS Lett.*, 212, 159, 1987.

794. Coughlin, S.R., Lee, W.M.F., Williams, P.W., Giels, G.M., and Williams, L.T., c-*myc* gene expression is stimulated by agents that activate protein kinase C and does not account for the mitogenic effect of PDGF, *Cell*, 43, 243, 1985.

795. Friedrich, B., Gullberg, M., and Lundgren, E., Uncoupling of c-*myc* mRNA expression from G1 events in human T lymphocytes, *Anticancer Res.*, 8, 23, 1988.

796. Bravo, R., Burckhardt, J., Curran, T., and Müller, R., Stimulation and inhibition of growth by EGF in different A431 cell clones is accompanied by the rapid induction of c-*fos* and c-*myc* proto-oncogenes, *EMBO J.*, 4, 1193, 1985.

797. Griep, A.E. and Westphal, H., Antisense *Myc* sequences induce differentiation of F9 cells, *Proc. Natl. Acad. Sci. U.S.A.*, 85, 6806, 1988.

798. Moscovici, M.G. and Moscovici, C., AMV-induced transformation of hematopoietic cells: growth patterns of producers and nonproducers, in *In Vivo and In Vitro Erytropoiesis: The Friend System,* Rossi, G.B., Ed., Elsevier-North Holland, Amsterdam, 1980, 503.

799. Moscovici, M.G., Klempnauer, K.-H., Symonds, G., Bishop, J.M., and Moscovici, C., Transformation-defective mutant of avian myeloblastosis virus that is temperature sensitive for production of transforming protein p45^{v-myb}, *Mol. Cell. Biol.,* 5, 3301, 1985.

800. Soret, J., Kryceve-Martinerie, C., Crochet, J., and Perbal, B., Transformation of Brown Leghorn chicken embryo fibroblasts by avian myeloblastosis virus proviral DNA, *J. Virol.,* 55, 193, 1985.

801. Lipsick, J.S., Ibanez, C.E., and Baluda, M.A., Expression of molecular clones of v-*myb* in avian and mammalian cells independently of transformation, *J. Virol.,* 59, 267, 1986.

802. Silva, R.F. and Moscovici, C., Spontaneous regression of leukemia in chickens infected with avian myeloblastosis virus, *Proc. Soc. Exp. Biol. Med.,* 143, 604, 1973.

803. Gonda, T.J., Sheiness, D.K., Fanshier, L., Bishop, J.M., Moscovici, C., and Moscovici, M.G., The genome and the intracellular RNAs of avian myeloblastosis virus, *Cell,* 23, 279, 1981.

804. Crochet, J., Soret, J., and Perbal, B., A cryptic promoter in the *myb* oncogene of avian myeloblastosis virus, *Virology,* 150, 252, 1986.

805. Bister, K., Nunn, M., Moscovici, C., Perbal, B., Baluda, M.A., and Duesberg, P.H., Acute leukemia viruses E26 and avian myeloblastosis virus have related transformation-specific RNA sequences but different genetic structures, gene products, and oncogenic properties, *Proc. Natl. Acad. Sci. U.S.A.,* 79, 3677, 1982.

806. Leprince, D., Gegonne, A., Coll, J., de Taisne, C., Schneeberg, A., Lagrou, C., and Stehelin, D., A putative second cell-derived oncogene of the avian leukaemia retrovirus E26, *Nature,* 306, 395, 1983.

807. Nunn, M.F., Seeburg, P.H., Moscovici, C., and Duesberg, P.H., Tripartite structure of the avian erythroblastosis virus E26 transforming gene, *Nature,* 306, 391, 1983.

808. Nunn, M., Weiher, H., Bullock, P., and Duesberg, P., Avian erythroblastosis virus E26: nucleotide sequence of the tripartite *onc* gene and of the LTR, and analysis of the cellular prototype of the viral *ets* sequence, *Virology,* 139, 330, 1984.

809. Evan, G.I., Lewis, G.K., and Bishop, J.M., Isolation of monoclonal antibodies specific for products of avian oncogene *myb*, *Mol. Cell. Biol.,* 4, 2843, 1984.

810. Moelling, K., Pfaff, E., Beug, H., Beimling, P., Bunte, T., Schaller, H.E., and Graf, T., DNA-binding activity is associated with purified *myb* proteins from AMV and E26 viruses and is temperature-sensitive for E26 *ts* mutants, *Cell,* 40, 983, 1985.

811. Boyle, W.J., Lampert, M.A., Li, A.C., and Baluda, M.A., Nuclear compartmentalization of the v-*myb* oncogene product, *Mol. Cell. Biol.,* 5, 3017, 1985.

812. Boyle, W.J. and Baluda, M.A., Subnuclear associations of the v-*myb* oncogene product and actin are dependent on ionic strength during nuclear isolation, *Mol. Cell. Biol.,* 7, 3345, 1987.

813. Lipsick, J.S., v-*myb* does not prevent the expression of c-*myb* in avian erythroblastosis, *J. Virol.,* 61, 3284, 1987.

814. Roussel, M., Saule, S., Lagrou, C., Rommens, C., Beug, H., Graf, T., and Stehelin, D., Three types of viral oncogene of cellular origin for hematopoietic cell transformation, *Nature,* 286, 452, 1979.

815. Souza, L.M., Stromer, J.N., Hilyard, R.L., Komaromy, M.C., and Baluda, M.A., Cellular sequences are present in the presumptive avian myeloblastosis virus genome, *Proc. Natl. Acad. Sci. U.S.A.,* 77, 5177, 1980.

816. Bergmann, D.G., Souza, L.M., and Baluda, M.A., Vertebrate DNAs contain nucleotide sequences related to the transforming gene of avian myeloblastosis virus, *J. Virol.,* 40, 450, 1981.

817. Katzen, A.L., Kornberg, T.B., and Bishop, J.M., Isolation of the proto-oncogene c-*myb* from *D. melanogaster,* *Cell,* 41, 449, 1985.

818. Perbal, B. and Kohiyama, M., Existence de séquences homologues de l'oncogéne *V-MYB* dans le génome des archaebactéries, *C.R. Acad. Sci. Paris,* 300, 177, 1985.

819. Nomura, N., Takahashi, M., Matsui, M., Ishii, S., Date, T., Sasamoto, S., and Ishizaki, R., Isolation of human cDNA clones of *myb*-related genes, A-*myb* and B-*myb*, *Nucleic Acids Res.,* 16, 11075, 1988.

820. Klempnauer, K.-H., Ramsay, G., Bishop, J.M., Moscovici, G.M., Moscovici, C., McGrath, J.P., and Levinson, A.D., The product of the retroviral transforming gene v-*myb* is a truncated version of the protein encoded by the cellular oncogene c-*myb*, *Cell,* 33, 345, 1983.

821. Rosson, D. and Reddy, E.P., Nucleotide sequence of chicken c-*myb* complementary DNA and implications for *myb* oncogene activation, *Nature,* 319, 604, 1986.

822. Gerondakis, S. and Bishop, J.M., Structure of the protein encoded by the chicken proto-oncogene c-*myb*, *Mol. Cell. Biol.,* 6, 3677, 1986.

823. Klempnauer, K.-H., Gonda, T.J., and Bishop, J.M., Nucleotide sequence of the retroviral leukemia gene v-*myb* and its cellular progenitor c-*myb*: the architecture of a transduced oncogene, *Cell,* 31, 453, 1982.

824. Kryceve-Martinerie, C., Soret, J., Crochet, J., Baluda, M., and Perbal, B., Expression of a truncated v-*myb* product in transformed chicken embryo fibroblasts, *FEBS Lett.,* 214, 81, 1987.

825. Klempnauer, K.-H., Symonds, G., Evan, G.I., and Bishop, J.M., Subcellular localization of proteins encoded by the oncogenes of avian erythroblastosis virus and avian leukemia virus E26 and by the chicken c-*myb* gene, *Cell,* 37, 537, 1984.

826. Boyle, W.J., Lampert, M.A., Lipsick, J.S., and Baluda, M.A., Avian myeloblastosis virus and E26 virus oncogene products are nuclear proteins, *Proc. Natl. Acad. Sci. U.S.A.,* 81, 4265, 1984.

827. Klempnauer, K.-H. and Sippel, A.E., Subnuclear localization of proteins encoded by the oncogene v-*myb* and its cellular homolog c-*myb*, *Mol. Cell. Biol.,* 6, 62, 1986.

828. Bender, T.P. and Kuehl, W.M., Murine *myb* protooncogene mRNA: cDNA sequence and evidence for 5′ heterogeneity, *Proc. Natl. Acad. Sci. U.S.A.,* 83, 3204, 1986.

829. Klempnauer, K.-H., Bonifer, C., and Sippel, A.E., Identification and characterization of the protein encoded by the human c-*myb* proto-oncogene, *EMBO J.,* 5, 1903, 1986.

830. Slamon, D.J., Boone, T.C., Murdock, D.C., Keith, D.E., Press, M.F., Larson, R.A., and Souza, L.M., Studies of the human c-*myb* gene and its product in human acute leukemias, *Science,* 233, 347, 1986.

831. Ishikura, H., Honma, Y., Honma, C., Hozumi, M., Black, J.D., Kieber-Emmons, T., and Bloch, A., Inhibition of messenger RNA transcriptional activity in ML-1 human myeloblastic leukemia cell nuclei by antiserum to a c-*myb*-specific peptide, *Cancer Res.,* 47, 1052, 1987.

832. Bading, H., Gerdes, J., Schwarting, R., Stein, H., and Moelling, K., Nuclear and cytoplasmic distribution of cellular *myb* protein in human haematopoietic cells evidenced by monoclinal antibody, *Oncogene,* 3, 257, 1988.

833. Bender, T.P., Thompson, C.B., and Kuehl, W.M., Differential expression of c-*myb* mRNA in murine B lymphomas by a block to transcription elongation, *Science,* 237, 1473, 1987.

834. Watson, R.J., A transcriptional arrest mechanism involved in controlling constitutive levels of mouse c-*myb* mRNA, *Oncogene,* 2, 267, 1988.

835. Thompson, C.B., Challoner, P.B., Neiman, P.E., and Groudine, M., Expression of the c-*myb* proto-oncogene during cellular proliferation, *Nature,* 319, 374, 1986.

836. Gewirtz, A.M. and Calabretta, B., A c-*myb* antisense oligodeoxynucleotide inhibits normal human hematopoieses *in vitro, Science,* 242, 1303, 1988.

837. Lipsick, J.S. and Boyle, W.J., c-*myb* protein expression is a late event during T-lymphocyte activation, *Mol. Cell. Biol.,* 7, 3358, 1987.

838. Kirsch, I.R., Bertness, V., Silver, J., and Hollis, G.F., Regulated expression of the c-*myb* and c-*myc* oncogenes during erythroid differentiation, *J. Cell. Biochem.,* 32, 11, 1986.

839. Watson, R.J., Dyson, P.J., and McMahon, J., Multiple c-*myb* transcript cap sites are variously utilized in cells of mouse haemopoietic origin, *EMBO J.,* 6, 1643, 1987.

840. Kastan, M.B., Slamon, D.J., and Civin, C.I., Expression of protooncogene c-*myb* in normal human hematopoietic cells, *Blood,* 73, 1444, 1989.

841. Sheiness, D. and Gardinier, M., Expression of a proto-oncogene (proto-*myb*) in hemopoietic tissues of mice, *Mol. Cell. Biol.,* 4, 1206, 1984.

842. Ferrari, S., Torelli, U., Selleri, L., Donelli, A., Venturelli, D., Narni, F., Moretti, L., and Torelli, G., Study of the levels of expression of two oncogenes, c-myc and c-myb, in acute and chronic leukemias of both lymphoid and myeloid lineage, *Leukemia Res.,* 9, 833, 1985.

843. Stern, J.B. and Smith, K.A., Interleukin-2 induction of T-cell G_1 progression and c-*myb* expression, *Science,* 233, 203, 1986.

844. Duprey, S.P. and Boettiger, D., Developmental regulation of c-*myb* in normal myeloid progenitor cells, *Proc. Natl. Acad. Sci. U.S.A.,* 82, 6937, 1985.

845. Yokota, S., Yuan, D., Katagiri, T., Eisenberg, R.A., Cohen, P.L., and Ting, J.P.-Y., The expression and regulation of c-*myb* transcription in B6/*lpr* Lyt-2⁻, L3T4⁻ T lymphocytes, *J. Immunol.,* 139, 2810, 1987.

846. Craig, R.W. and Bloch, A., Early decline in c-*myb* oncogene expression in the differentiation of human myeloblastic leukemia (ML-1) cells induced with 12-*O*-tetradecanoylphorbol-13-acetate, *Cancer Res.,* 44, 442, 1984.

847. Simonds, G., Klempnauer, K.-H., Evan, G.I., and Bishop, J.M., Induced differentiation of avian myeloblastosis virus-transformed myeloblasts: phenotypic alteration without altered expression of the viral oncogene, *Mol. Cell. Biol.,* 4, 2587, 1984.

848. Gozes, I., Nakai, H., Byers, M., Avidor, R., Weinstein, Y., Shani, Y., and Shows, T.B., Sequential expression in the nervous system of c-*MYB* and *VIP* genes, located in human chromosomal region 6q24, *Somat. Cell Mol. Genet.,* 13, 305, 1987.

849. Moloney, J.B., A virus-induced rhabdomyosarcoma of mice, *Natl. Cancer Inst. Monogr.,* 22, 139, 1966.

850. Aaronson, S.A. and Rowe, W.P., Nonproducer clones of murine sarcoma virus-transformed BALB/3Ts cells, *Virology,* 42, 9, 1970.

851. Frankel, A.E. and Fischinger, P.J., Nucleotide sequence in mouse DNA and RNA specific for Moloney sarcoma virus, *Proc. Natl. Acad. Sci. U.S.A.,* 73, 3705, 1976.

852. Cremer, K., Reddy, E.P., and Aaronson, S.A., Translational products of Moloney murine sarcoma virus RNA: identification of proteins encoded by the murine sarcoma virus *src* gene, *J. Virol.,* 38, 704, 1981.

853. Papkoff, J., Lai, M.H.-T., Hunter, T., and Verma, I.M., Analysis of transforming gene products from Moloney sarcoma virus, *Cell,* 27, 109, 1981.

854. Stanker, L.H., Horn, J.P., Gallick, G.E., Kloetzer, W.S., Murphy, E.C., Jr., Blair, D.G., and Arlinghaus, R.B., *gag-mos* polyproteins encoded by variants of the Moloney strain of mouse sarcoma virus, *Virology,* 126, 336, 1983.

855. Gallick, G.E., Sparrow, J.T., Singh, B., Maxwell, S.A., Stanker, L.H., and Arlinghaus, R.B., Recognition of *mos*-related proteins with an antiserum to a peptide of the v-*mos* gene product, *J. Gen. Virol.,* 66, 945, 1985.

856. Bold, R.J. and Donoghue, D.J., Biologically active mutants with deletions in the v-*mos* oncogene assayed with retroviral vectors, *Mol. Cell. Biol.,* 5, 3131, 1985.

857. Papkoff, J., Nigg, E.A., and Hunter, T., The transforming protein of Moloney murine sarcoma virus is a soluble cytoplasmic protein, *Cell,* 33, 161, 1983.

858. Papkoff, J., Verma, I.M., and Hunter, T., Detection of a transforming gene product in cells transformed by Moloney murine sarcoma virus, *Cell,* 29, 417, 1982.

859. Kloetzer, W.S., Maxwell, S.A., and Arlinghaus, R.B., Further characterization of the P85$^{gag\text{-}mos}$-associated protein kinase activity, *Virology,* 138, 143, 1984.

860. Gallick, G.E., Hamelin, R., Maxwell, S., Duyka, D., and Arlinghaus, R.B., The *gag-mos* hybrid protein of ts110 Moloney murine sarcoma virus: variation of gene expression with temperature, *Virology,* 139, 366, 1984.

861. Maxwell, S.A. and Arlinghaus, R.B., Serine kinase activity associated with Moloney murine sarcoma virus-124-encoded p37^{mos}, *Virology,* 143, 321, 1985.

862. Maxwell, S.A. and Arlinghaus, R.B., Use of site-specific antipeptide antibodies to perturb the serine kinase catalytic activity of p37^{mos}, *J. Virol.,* 55, 874, 1985.

863. Cizdziel, P.E., Nash, M.A., Blair, D.G., and Murphy, E.C., Jr., Molecular basis underlying phenotypic revertants of Moloney murine sarcoma virus MuSV*ts*110, *J. Virol.,* 57, 310, 1986.

864. Schmidt, M., Oskarsson, M.K., Dunn, J.K., Blair, D.G., Hughes, S., Propst, F., and Vande Woude, G.F., Chicken homolog of the *mos* proto-oncogene, *Mol. Cell. Biol.,* 8, 923, 1988.

865. Watson, R., Oskarsson, M., and Vande Woude, G.F., Human sequence homologous to the transforming gene (*mos*) of Moloney murine sarcoma virus, *Proc. Natl. Acad. Sci. U.S.A.,* 79, 4078, 1982.

866. Singh, B., Wittenberg, C., Reed, S.I., and Arlinghaus, R.B., Moloney murine sarcoma virus encoded p37^{mos} expressed in yeast has protein kinase activity, *Virology,* 152, 506, 1986.

867. Seth, A. and Vande Woude, G.F., Nucleotide sequence and biochemical activities of the Moloney murine sarcoma virus strain HT-1 *mos* gene, *J. Virol.,* 56, 144, 1985.

868. Singh, B., Hannink, M., Donoghue, D.J., and Arlinghaus, R.B., p37^{mos}-associated serine/threonine protein kinase activity correlates with the cellular transformation function of v-*mos*, *J. Virol.,* 60, 1148, 1986.

869. Singh, B., Wittenberg, C., Hannink, M., Reed, S.I., Donoghue, D.J., and Arlinghaus, R.B., The histidine-221 to tyrosine substitution in v-*mos* abolishes its biological function and its protein kinase activity, *Virology,* 164, 114, 1988.

870. Lai, C.-N., Gallick, G.E., Maxwell, S.A., Brinkley, B.R., and Becker, F.F., Potassium inhibition of transforming protein P85$^{gag\text{-}mos}$ and reversal of the transformed phenotype in 6m2 cells, *J. Cell. Physiol.,* 134, 445, 1988.

871. Seth, A., Priel, E., and Vande Woude, G.F., Nucleoside triphosphate-dependent DNA-binding properties of *mos* protein, *Proc. Natl. Acad. Sci. U.S.A.,* 84, 3560, 1987.

872. Barker, W.C. and Dayhoff, M.O., Viral *src* gene products are related to the catalytic chain of mammalian cAMP-dependent protein kinase, *Proc. Natl. Acad. Sci. U.S.A.,* 79, 2836, 1982.

873. Kamps, M.P., Taylor, S.S., and Sefton, B.M., Direct evidence that oncogenic tyrosine kinases and cyclic AMP-dependent protein kinase have homologous ATP-binding sites, *Nature,* 310, 589, 1984.

874. Hannink, M. and Donoghue, D.J., Lysine residue 121 in the proposed ATP-binding site of the v-*mos* protein is required for transformation, *Proc. Natl. Acad. Sci. U.S.A.,* 82, 7894, 1985.

875. Baldwin, G.S., Epidermal growth factor precursor is related to the translation product of the Moloney sarcoma virus oncogene *mos*, *Proc. Natl. Acad. Sci. U.S.A.,* 82, 1921, 1985.

876. Singh, B., Goldman, R., Hutton, L., Herzog, N.K., and Arlinghaus, R.B., The P55 protein affected by v-*mos* expression is vimentin, *J. Virol.,* 61, 3625, 1987.

877. Gattoni, S., Kirschmeier, P., Weinstein, I.B., Escobedo, J., and Dina, D., Cellular Moloney sarcoma (c-mos) sequences are hypermethylated and transcriptionally silent in normal and transformed rodent cells, *Mol. Cell. Biol.,* 2, 42, 1982.

878. Wood, T.G., McGeady, M.L., Baroudy, B.M., Blair, D.G., and Vande Woude, G.F., Mouse c-*mos* oncogene activation is prevented by upstream sequences, *Proc. Natl. Acad. Sci. U.S.A.,* 81, 7817, 1984.

879. Gojobori, T. and Yokoyama, S., Rates of evolution of the retroviral oncogene of Moloney murine sarcoma virus and of its cellular homologues, *Proc. Natl. Acad. Sci. U.S.A.,* 82, 4198, 1985.

880. van der Hoorn, F.A., Müller, V., and Pizer, L.I., Sequences upstream of c-*mos*(rat) that block RNA accumulation in mouse cells do not inhibit *in vitro* transcription, *Mol. Cell. Biol.,* 5, 406, 1985.

881. McGeady, M.L., Wood, T.G., Maizel, J.V., and Vande Woude, G.F., Sequences upstream from the mouse c-*mos* oncogene may function as a transcription termination signal, DNA, 5, 289, 1986.

882. van der Hoorn, F.A., c-*mos* upstream sequence exhibits species-specific enhancer activity and binds murine-specific nuclear proteins, *J. Mol. Biol.,* 193, 255, 1987.

883. Paules, R.S., Propst, F., Dunn, K.J., Blair, D.G., Kaul, K., Palmer, A.E., and Vande Woude, G.F., Primate c-*mos* proto-oncogene structure and expression: transcription inititaion both upstream and within the gene in a tissue-specific manner, *Oncogene*, 3, 59, 1988.

884. Propst, F. and Vande Woude, G.F., Expression of c-*mos* proto-oncogene transcripts in mouse tissues, *Nature*, 315, 516, 1985.

885. Goldman, D.S., Kiessling, A.A., Millette, C.F., and Cooper, G.M., Expression of c-*mos* RNA in germ cells of male and female mice, *Proc. Natl. Acad. Sci. U.S.A.*, 84, 4509, 1987.

886. Keshet, E., Rosenberg, M.P., Mercer, J.A., Propst, F., Vande Woude, G.F., Jenkins, N.A., and Copeland, N.G., Developmental regulation of ovarian-specific *Mos* expression, *Oncogene*, 2, 235, 1988.

887. Sagata, N., Oskarsson, M., Copeland, T., Brumbaugh, J., and Vande Woude, G.F., Function of c-*mos* proto-oncogene product in meiotic maturation in *Xenopus* oocytes, *Nature*, 335, 519, 1988.

888. Propst, F., Rosenberg, M.P., Iyer, A., Kaul, K., and Vande Woude, G.F., c-*mos* proto-oncogene RNA transcripts in mouse tissues: structural features, developmental regulation, and localization in specific cell types, *Mol. Cell. Biol.*, 7, 1629, 1987.

889. Horowitz, M., Luria, S., Rechavi, G., and Givol, D., Mechanism of activation of the mouse c-*mos* oncogene by the LTR of an intracisternal A-particle gene, *EMBO J.*, 3, 2937, 1984.

890. Blair, D.G., Oskarsson, M.K., Seth, A., Dunn, K.J., Dean, M., Zweig, M., Tainsky, M.A., and Vande Woude, G.F., Analysis of the transforming potential of the human homolog of *mos*, *Cell*, 46, 785, 1986.

891. Khillan, J.S., Oskarsson, M.K., Propst, F., Kuwabara, T., Vande Woude, G.F., and Westphal, H., Defects in lens fiber differentiation are linked to c-*mos* overexpression in transgenic mice, *Genes Dev.*, 1, 1327, 1987.

892. Ogiso, Y., Matsumoto, M., Morita, T., Nishino, H., Iwashima, A., and Matsuchiro, A., Expression of c-*mos* proto-oncogene in undifferentiated teratocarcinoma cells, *Biochem. Biophys. Res. Commun.*, 140, 477, 1986.

893. Papkoff, J. and Ringold, G.M., Use of the mouse mammary tumor virus long terminal repeat to promote steroid-inducible expression of v-*mos*, *J. Virol.*, 52, 420, 1984.

894. van der Hoorn, F.A. and Müller, V., Differential transformation of C3H10T1/2 cells by v-*mos*: sequential expression of transformation parameters, *Mol. Cell. Biol.*, 5, 2204, 1985.

895. Sergiescu, D., Gerfaux, J., Joret, A.-M., and Chany, C., Persistent expression of v-*mos* oncogene in transformed cells that revert to nonmalignancy after prolonged treatment with interferon, *Proc. Natl. Acad. Sci. U.S.A.*, 83, 5764, 1986.

896. Seliger, B., Kruppa, G., and Pfizenmaier, K., Murine gamma interferon inhibits v-*mos*-induced fibroblast transformation via down regulation of retroviral gene expression, *J. Virol.*, 61, 2567, 1987.

897. Seliger, B., Kollek, R., Stocking, C., Franz, T., and Ostertag, W., Viral transfer, transcription, and rescue of a selectable myeloproliferative sarcoma virus in embryonal cell lines: expression of the *mos* oncogene, *Mol. Cell. Biol.*, 6, 286, 1986.

898. Schmidt, A., Setoyama, C., and de Crombrugghe, B., Regulation of a collagen gene promoter by the product of viral *mos* oncogene, *Nature*, 314, 286, 1985.

899. Chan, J.C., Keck, M.E., and Li, W., Monoclonal antibody detection of transformation associated protein (TAP) in ts110 Moloney murine sarcoma virus transformed 6M2 cells that are different from the mos gene product, *Biochem. Biophys. Res. Commun.*, 134, 1223, 1986.

900. Donner, L., Fedele, L.A., Garon, C.F., Anderson, S.J., and Sherr, C.J., McDonough feline sarcoma virus: characterization of the molecularly cloned provirus and its feline oncogene (v-*fms*), *J. Virol.*, 41, 489, 1982.

901. Heisterkamp, N., Groffen, N.J., and Stephenson, J.R., Isolation of v-*fms* and its human cellular homolog, *Proc. Natl. Acad. Sci. U.S.A.*, 80, 383, 1983.

902. Heisterkamp, N., Groffen, J., and Stephenson, J.R., Isolation of v-*fms* and its human cellular homolog, *Virology*, 126, 248, 1983.

903. Rettenmier, C.W., Jackowski, S., Rock, C.O., Roussel, M.F., and Sherr, C.J., Transformation by the v-*fms* oncogene product: an analog of the CSF-1 receptor, *J. Cell. Biochem.*, 33, 109, 1987.

904. Manger, R., Najita, L., Nichols, E.J., Hakomori, S., and Rohrschneider, L., Cell surface expression of the McDonough strain of feline sarcoma virus *fms* gene product (gp^{fms}), *Cell*, 39, 327, 1984.

905. Wheeler, E.F., Roussel, M.F., Hampe, A., Walker, M.H., Fried, V.A., Look, A.T., Rettenmier, C.W., and Sherr, C.J., The amino-terminal domain of the v-*fms* oncogene product includes a functional signal peptide that directs synthesis of a transforming glycoprotein in the absence of feline leukemia virus *gag* sequences, *J. Virol.*, 59, 224, 1986.

906. Roussel, M.F., Rettenmier, C.W., Look, A.T., and Sherr, C.J., Cell surface expression of v-*fms*-coded glycoproteins is required for transformation, *Mol. Cell. Biol.*, 4, 1999, 1984.

907. Tamura, T., Simon, E., Niemann, H., Snoek, G.T., and Bauer, H., gp140^{v-fms} molecules expressed at the surface of cells transformed by the McDonough strain of feline sarcoma virus are phosphorylated in tyrosine and serine, *Mol. Cell. Biol.*, 6, 4745, 1986.

908. Wheeler, E.F., Askew, D., May, S., Ihle, J.N., and Sherr, C.J., The v-*fms* oncogene induces factor-independent growth and transformation of the interleukin-3-dependent myeloid cell line FDC-P1, *Mol. Cell. Biol.*, 7, 1673, 1987.

909. Sherr, C.J., Fibroblast and hematopoietic cell transformation by the *fms* oncogene (CSF-1 receptor), *J. Cell. Physiol.,* Suppl. 5, 83, 1987.

910. Lyman, S.D. and Rohrschneider, L.R., Analysis of functional domains of the v-*fms*-encoded protein of Susan McDonough strain feline sarcoma virus by linker insertion mutagenesis, *Mol. Cell. Biol.,* 7, 3287, 1987.

911. Majumder, S., Brown, K., Qiu, F.-H., and Besmer, P., c-*kit,* a transmembrane kinase: identification in tissues and characterization, *Mol. Cell. Biol.,* 8, 4896, 1988.

912. Rettenmier, C.W., Roussel, M.F., Quinn, C.O., Kitchingman, G.R., Look, A.T., and Sherr, C.J., Transmembrane orientation of glycoproteins encoded by the v-*fms* oncogene, *Cell,* 40, 971, 1985.

913. Nichols, E.J., Manger, R., Hakomori, S., Herscovics, A., and Rohrschneider, L.R., Transformation by the v-*fms* oncogene product: product of glycosylational processing and cell surface expression, *Mol. Cell. Biol.,* 5, 3467, 1985.

914. Nichols, E.J., Manger, R., Hakomori, S., and Rohrschneider, L.R., Transformation by the oncogene v-*fms*: the effects of castanospermine on transformation-related parameters, *Exp. Cell Res.,* 173, 486, 1987.

915. Browning, P.J., Bunn, H.F., Cline, A., Shuman, M., and Nienhuis, A.W., "Replacement" of COOH-terminal truncation of v-*fms* with c-*fms* sequences markedly reduces transformation potential, *Proc. Natl. Acad. Sci. U.S.A.,* 83, 7800, 1986.

916. Roussel, M.F., Downing, J.R., Rettenmier, C.W., and Sherr, C.J., A point mutation in the extracellular domain of the human CSF-1 receptor (c-*fms* proto-oncogene product) activates its transforming potential, *Cell,* 55, 979, 1988.

917. Sherr, C.J., Rettenmier, C.W., Sacca, R., Roussel, M.F., Look, A.T., and Stanley, E.R., The c-*fms* proto-oncogene product is related to the receptor for the mononuclear phagocyte growth factor, CSF-1, *Cell,* 41, 665, 1985.

918. Sherr, C.J., The *fms* oncogene, *Biochim. Biophys. Acta,* 948, 225, 1988.

919. Groffen, J., Heisterkamp, N., Spurr, N., Dana, S., Wasmuth, J.J., and Stephenson, J.R., Chromosomal localization of the human c-*fms* oncogene, *Nucleic Acids Res.,* 11, 6331, 1983.

920. Bartram, C.R., Böhlke, J.V., Adolph, S., Hameister, H., Ganser, A., Anger, B., Heisterkamp, N., and Groffen, J., Deletion of c-*fms* sequences in the 5q- syndrome, *Leukemia,* 1, 146, 1987.

921. Woolford, J., Rothwell, V., and Rohrschneider, L., Characterization of the human c-*fms* gene product and its expression in cells of the monocyte-macrophage lineage, *Mol. Cell. Biol.,* 5, 3458, 1985.

922. Coussens, L., Van Beveren, C., Smith, D., Chen, E., Mitchell, R.L., Isacke, C.M., Verma, I.M., and Ullrich, A., Structural alteration of viral homologue of receptor proto-oncogene *fms* at carboxyl terminus, *Nature,* 320, 277, 1986.

923. Furman, W.L., Rettenmier, C.W., Chen, J.H., Roussel, M.F., Quinn, C.O., and Sherr, C.J., Antibodies to distal carboxyl terminal epitopes in the v-*fms*-coded glycoprotein do not cross-react with the c-*fms* gene product, *Virology,* 152, 432, 1986.

924. Rettenmier, C.W., Chen, C.H., Roussel, M.F., and Sherr, C.J., The product of the c-*fms* proto-oncogene: a glycoprotein with associated tyrosine kinase activity, *Science,* 228, 320, 1985.

925. Rothwell, V.M. and Rohrschneider, L.R., Murine c-*fms* cDNA: cloning, sequence analysis and retroviral expression, *Oncogene Res.,* 1, 311, 1987.

926. Müller, R., Slamon, D.J., Adamson, E.D., Tremblay, J.M., Müller, D., Cline, M.J., and Verma, I.M., Transcription of c-*onc* gene c-*ras*^{Ki} and c-*fms* during mouse development, *Mol. Cell. Biol.,* 3, 1062, 1983.

927. Rettenmier, C.W., Sacca, R., Furman, W.L., Roussel, M.F., Holt, J.T., Nienhuis, A.W., Stanley, E.R., and Sherr, C.J., Expression of the human c-*fms* proto-oncogene product (colony-stimulating factor-1 receptor) on peripheral blood mononuclear cells and choriocarcinoma cell lines, *J. Clin. Invest.,* 77, 1740, 1986.

928. Wakamiya, N., Horiguchi, J., and Kufe, D., Detection of c-*fms* and CSF-1 RNA by *in situ* hybridization, *Leukemia,* 1, 518, 1987.

929. Rapp, U.R., Goldsborough, M.D., Mark, G.E., Bonner, T.I., Groffen, J., Reynolds, F.H., Jr., and Stephenson, J.R., Structure and biological activity of v-*raf*, a unique oncogene transduced by a retrovirus, *Proc. Natl. Acad. Sci. U.S.A.,* 80, 4218, 1983.

930. Coll, J., Righi, M., de Taisne, C., Dissous, C., Gegonne, A., and Stehelin, D., Molecular cloning of the avian acute transforming retrovirus MH2 reveals a novel cell-derived sequence (v-*mil*) in addition to the *myc* oncogene, *EMBO J.,* 2, 2189, 1983.

931. Kan, N.C., Flordellis, C.S., Mark, G.E., Duesberg, P.H., and Papas, T.S., A common *onc* gene sequence transduced by avian carcinoma virus MH2 and by murine sarcoma virus 3611, *Science,* 223, 813, 1984.

932. Flordellis, C.S., Kan, N.C., Lautenberger, J.A., Samuel, K.P., Garon, C.F., and Papas, T.S., Analysis of the cellular proto-oncogene *mht/raf*: relationship to the 5' sequences of v-*mht* in avian carcinoma virus MH2 and v-*raf* in murine sarcoma virus 3611, *Virology,* 141, 267, 1985.

933. Graf, T., von Weizsaecker, F., Grieser, S., Coll, J., Stehelin, D., Patschinsky, T., Bister, K., Bechade, C., Calothy, G., and Leutz, A., v-*mil* induces autocrine growth and enhanced tumorigenicity in v-*myc*-transformed avian macrophages, *Cell,* 45, 357, 1986.

934. Palmieri, S. and Vogel, M.L., Fibroblast transformation parameters induced by the avian v-*mil* oncogene, *J. Virol.,* 61, 1717, 1987.

935. Bechade, C., Calothy, G., Pessac, B., Martin, P., Coll, J., Denhez, F., Saule, S., Ghysdael, J., and Stéhelin, D., Induction of proliferation or transformation of neuroretina cells by the *mil* and *myc* viral oncogenes, *Nature, 316*, 559, 1985.

936. Béchade, C., Dambrine, G., David-Pfeuty, T., Esnault, E., and Calothy, G., Transformed and tumorigenic phenotypes induced by avian retroviruses containing the v-*mil* oncogene, *J. Virol., 62*, 1211, 1988.

937. Denhez, F., Heimann, B., d'Auriol, L., Graf, T., Coquillaud, M., Coll, J., Galibert, F., Moelling, K., Stehelin, D., and Ghysdael, J., Replacement of lys 622 in the ATP binding domain of P100$^{gag\text{-}mil}$ abolishes the *in vitro* autophosphorylation of the protein and the biological properties of the v-*mil* oncogene of MH2 virus, *EMBO J., 7*, 541, 1988.

938. Dozier, C., Denhez, F., Coll, J., Amouyel, P., Quatannens, B., Begue, A., Stehelin, D., and Saule, S., Induction of proliferation of neuroretina cells by long terminal repeat activation of the carboxy-terminal part of c-*mil*, *Mol. Cell. Biol., 7*, 1995, 1987.

939. Rapp, U.R., Reynolds, F.H., Jr., and Stephenson, J.R., New mammalian transforming retrovirus: demonstration of a polyprotein gene product, *J. Virol., 45*, 914, 1983.

940. Schultz, A.M., Copeland, T., Oroszlan, S., and Rapp, U.R., Identification and characterization of c-*raf* phosphoproteins in transformed murine cells, *Oncogene, 2*, 187, 1988.

941. Kolch, W., Schultz, A.M., Oppermann, H., and Rapp, U.R., Preparation of *raf*-oncogene-specific antiserum with *raf* protein produced in *E. coli, Biochim. Biophys. Acta, 949*, 233, 1988.

942. Patschinsky, T., Schroeer, B., and Bister, K., Protein product of proto-oncogene c-*mil, Mol. Cell. Biol., 6*, 739, 1986.

943. Bonner, T.I., Oppermann, H., Seeburg, P., Kerby, S.B., Gunnell, M.A., Young, A.C., and Rapp, U.R., The complete coding sequence of the human *raf* oncogene and the corresponding structure of the c-*raf*-1 gene, *Nucleic Acids Res., 14*, 1009, 1986.

944. Huebner, K., ar-Rushdi, A., Griffin, C.A., Isobe, M., Kozak, C., Emanuel, B.S., Nagarajan, L., Cleveland, J.L., Bonner, T.I., Goldsborough, M.D., Croce, C.M., and Rapp, U., Actively transcribed genes in the *raf* oncogene group, located on the X chromosome in mouse and human, *Proc. Natl. Acad. Sci. U.S.A., 83*, 3934, 1986.

945. Huleihel, M., Goldsborough, M., Cleveland, J., Gunnell, M., Bonner, T., and Rapp, U.R., Characterization of murine A-*raf*, a new oncogene related to the v-*raf* oncogene, *Mol. Cell. Biol., 6*, 2655, 1986.

946. Ikawa, S., Fukui, M., Ueyama, Y., Tamakoi, N., Yamamoto, T., and Toyoshima, K., B-*raf*, a new member of the *raf* family, is activated by DNA rearrangement, *Mol. Cell. Biol., 8*, 2651, 1988.

947. Mark, G.E., MacIntyre, R.J., Digan, M.E., Ambrosio, L., and Perrimon, N., *Drosophila melanogaster* homologs of the *raf* oncogene, *Mol. Cell. Biol., 7*, 2134, 1987.

948. Koenen, M., Sippel, A.E., Trachmann, C., and Bister, K., Primary structure of the chicken c-*mil* protein: identification of domains shared with or absent from the retroviral v-*mil* protein, *Oncogene, 2*, 179, 1988.

949. Dozier, C., Denhez, F., Henry, C., Coll, J., Begue, A., Quatannens, B., Saule, S., and Stehelin, D., Alternative splicing of RNAs transcribed from the chicken c-*mil* gene, *Mol. Cell. Biol., 8*, 1835, 1988.

950. Ishikawa, F., Takaku, F., Nagao, M., and Sugimura, T., Cysteine-rich regions conserved in amino-terminal halves of *raf* gene family products and protein kinase C, *Jpn. J. Cancer Res., 77*, 1183, 1986.

951. Ishikawa, F., Takaku, F., Nagao, M., and Sugimura, T., The complete primary structure of the rat A-*raf* cDNA coding region: conservation of the putative regulatory regions present in rat c-*raf, Oncogene Res., 1*, 243, 1987.

952. Bonner, T., O'Brien, S.J., Nash, W.G., Rapp, U.R., Morton, C.C., and Leder, P., The human homologues of *raf* (*mil*) oncogene are located on human chromosomes 3 and 4, *Science, 223*, 71, 1984.

953. Bonner, T.I., Kerby, S.B., Sutrave, P., Gunnell, M.A., Mark, G., and Rapp, U.R., Structure and biological activity of human homologs of the *raf/mil* oncogene, *Mol. Cell. Biol., 5*, 1400, 1985.

954. Kolch, W., Bonner, T.I., and Rapp, U.R., Expression of human c-raf-1 oncogene proteins in *E. coli, Biochem. Biophys. Res. Commun., 152*, 1045, 1988.

955. Beck, T.W., Huleihel, M., Gunnell, M., Bonner, T.I., and Rapp, U.R., The complete coding sequence of the human A-*raf*-1 oncogene and transforming activity of a human A-*raf* carrying retrovirus, *Nucleic Acids Res., 15*, 595, 1987.

956. Sariban, E., Mitchell, T., and Kufe, D., Expression of the c-*raf* proto-oncogene in human hematopoietic cells and cell lines, *Blood, 69*, 1437, 1987.

957. Ishikawa, F., Takaku, F., Nagao, M., and Sugimura, T., Rat c-*raf* oncogene activation by a rearrangement that produces a fused protein, *Mol. Cell. Biol., 7*, 1226, 1987.

958. Theilen, G.H., Zeigel, R.F., and Twiehaus, M.J., Biological studies with RE virus (strain T) that induces reticuloendotheliosis in turkeys, chickens, and Japanese quails, *J. Natl. Cancer Inst., 37*, 731, 1966.

959. Moore, B.E. and Bose, H.R., Jr., Transformation of avian lymphoid cells by reticuloendotheliosis virus, *Mutat. Res., 195*, 79, 1988.

960. Franklin, R.B., Maldonado, R.L., and Bose, H.R., Jr., Isolation and characterization of reticuloendotheliosis virus transformed bone marrow cells, *Intervirology, 3*, 342, 1974.

961. Beug, H., Müller, H., Grieser, S., Doederlein, G., and Graf, T., Hematopoietic cells transformed *in vitro* by REV-T avian reticuloendotheliosis virus express characteristics of very immature cells, *Virology, 115*, 295, 1981.

962. Chen, L., Lim, M.Y., Bose, H., Jr., and Bishop, J.M., Rearrangements of chicken immunoglobulin genes in lymphoid cells transformed by the avian retroviral oncogene v-*rel*, *Proc. Natl. Acad. Sci. U.S.A.*, 85, 549, 1988.

963. Garson, K. and Kang, C.Y., Identification of the v-rel protein in REV-T transformed chicken bone marrow cells and expression in COS1 cells, *Biochem. Biophys. Res. Commun.*, 134, 716, 1986.

964. Simek, S.L., Stephens, R.M., and Rice, N.R., Localization of the v-*rel* protein in reticuloendotheliosis virus strain T-transformed lymphoid cells, *J. Virol.*, 59, 120, 1986.

965. Gilmore, T.D. and Temin, H.M., Different localization of the product of the v-*rel* oncogene in chicken fibroblasts and spleen cells correlates with transformation by REV-T, *Cell*, 44, 791, 1986.

966. Gilmore, T.D. and Temin, H.M., v-*rel* oncoproteins in the nucleus and in the cytoplasm transform chicken spleen cells, *J. Virol.*, 62, 703, 1988.

967. Tung, H.Y.L., Bargmann, W.J., Lim, M.Y., and Bose, H.R., Jr., The v-*rel* oncogene product is complexed to a 40-kDa phosphoprotein in transformed lymphoid cells, *Proc. Natl. Acad. Sci. U.S.A.*, 85, 2479, 1988.

968. Moore, B.E. and Bose, H.R., Jr., Expression of the v-*rel* oncogene in reticuloendotheliosis virus-transformed fibroblasts, *Virology*, 162, 377, 1988.

969. Chen, I.S.Y. and Temin, H.M., Substitution of 5' helper virus sequences into non-*rel* portion of reticuloendotheliosis virus strain T suppresses transformation of chicken spleen cells, *Cell*, 31, 111, 1982.

970. Chen, I.S.Y., Wilhelmsen, K.C., and Temin, H.M., Structure and expression of c-*rel*, the cellular homolog to the oncogene of reticuloendotheliosis virus strain T, *J. Virol.*, 45, 104, 1983.

971. Wilhelmsen, K.C., Eggleton, K., and Temin, H.M., Nucleic acid sequences of the oncogene v-*rel* in reticuloendotheliosis virus strain T and its cellular homolog, the proto-oncogene c-*rel*, *J. Virol.*, 52, 172, 1984.

972. Sylla, B.S. and Temin, H.M., Activation of oncogenicity of the c-*rel* proto-oncogene, *Mol. Cell. Biol.*, 6, 4709, 1986.

973. Herzog, N.K., Bargmann, W.J., and Bose, H.R., Jr., Oncogene expression in reticuloendotheliosis virus-transformed lymphoid cell lines and avian tissues, *J. Virol.*, 57, 371, 1986.

974. Brownell, E., Ruscetti, F.W., Smith, R.G., and Rice, N.R., Detection of *rel*-related RNA and protein in human lymphoid cells, *Oncogene*, 3, 93, 1988.

975. Gélinas, C. and Temin, H.M., The v-*rel* oncogene encodes a cell-specific transcriptional activator of certain promoters, *Oncogene*, 3, 349, 1988.

976. Brownell, E., Fell, H.P., Tucker, P.W., Geurts van Kessel, A.H.M., Hagemeijer, A., and Rice, N.R., Regional localization of the human c-*rel* locus using translocation chromosome analysis, *Oncogene*, 2, 527, 1988.

977. Balduzzi, P.C., Notter, M.F.D., Morgan, H.R., and Shibuya, M., Some biological properties of two new avian sarcoma viruses, *J. Virol.*, 40, 268, 1981.

978. Neckameyer, W.S. and Wang, L.-H., Molecular cloning and characterization of avian sarcoma virus UR2 and comparison of its transforming sequence with those of other avian sarcoma viruses, *J. Virol.*, 50, 914, 1984.

979. Neckameyer, W.S., Shibuya, M., Hsu, M.-T., and Wang, L.-H., Proto-oncogene c-*ros* codes for a molecule with structural features common to those of growth factor receptors and displays tissue-specific and developmentally regulated expression, *Mol. Cell. Biol.*, 6, 1478, 1986.

980. Das, K.S., Christensen, J.R., and Balduzzi, P.C., Transfection and recombination with molecularly cloned derivatives of avian sarcoma virus UR2, *Virology*, 154, 415, 1986.

981. Garber, E.A., Hanafusa, T., and Hanafusa, H., Membrane association of the transforming protein of avian sarcoma virus UR2 and mutants temperature sensitive for cellular transformation and protein kinase activity, *J. Virol.*, 56, 790, 1985.

982. Balduzzi, P.C., Chovav, M., Christensen, J.R., and Macara, I.G., Specific inhibition of tyrosine kinase activity by an antibody to the v-*ros* oncogene product, *J. Virol.*, 60, 765, 1986.

983. Ellis, L., Morgan, D.O., Jong, S.-M., Wahg, L.-H., Roth, R.A., and Rutter, W.J., Heterologous transmembrane signalling by a human insulin receptor-v-ros hybrid in Chinese hamster ovary cells, *Proc. Natl. Acad. Sci. U.S.A.*, 84, 5101, 1987.

984. Wang, L.-H., Lin, B., Jong, S.-M.J., Dixon, D., Ellis, L., Roth, R.A., and Rutter, W.J., Activation of transforming potential of the human insulin receptor gene, *Proc. Natl. Acad. Sci. U.S.A.*, 84, 5725, 1987.

985. Podell, S.B. and Sefton, B.M., Chicken proto-oncogene c-*ros* cDNA clones: identification of a c-*ros* RNA transcript and deduction of the amino acid sequence of the carboxyl terminus of the c-*ros* product, *Oncogene*, 2, 9, 1987.

986. Matsushime, H., Wang, L.-H., and Shibuya, M., Human c-*ros*-1 gene homologous to the v-*ros* sequence of UR2 sarcoma virus encodes for a transmembrane receptorlike molecule, *Mol. Cell. Biol.*, 6, 3000, 1986.

987. Birchmeier, C., Birnbaum, D., Waitches, G., Fasano, O., and Wigler, M., Characterization of an activated human *ros* gene, *Mol. Cell. Biol.*, 6, 3109, 1986.

988. Satoh, H., Yoshida, M.C., Matsushime, H., Shibuya, M., and Sasaki, M., Regional localization of the human c-*ros*-1 on 6q22 and *flt* on 13q12, *Jpn. J. Cancer Res.*, 78, 772, 1987.

989. Matsushime, H., Yoshida, M.C., Sasaki, M., and Shibuya, M., A possible new member of tyrosine kinase family, human *frt* sequence, is highly conserved in vertebrates and located on human chromosome 13, *Jpn. J. Cancer Res.*, 78, 655, 1987.

990.   Nagarajan, L., Louie, E., Tsujimoto, Y., Balduzzi, P.C., Huebner, K., and Croce, C.M., The human c-*ros* gene (*ROS*) is located at chromosome region 6q16-6q22, *Proc. Natl. Acad. Sci. U.S.A.,* 83, 6568, 1986.

991.   Wallbank, A.M., Sperling, F.G., Hubben, K., and Stubbs, E.L., Isolation of a tumor virus from a chicken submitted to a poultry diagnostic laboratory: Esh sarcoma virus, *Nature,* 209, 1265, 1966.

992.   Itohara, S., Hirata, K., Inoue, M., Hatsuoka, M., and Sato, A., Isolation of a sarcoma virus from a spontaneous chicken tumor, *Jpn. J. Cancer Res.,* 69, 825, 1978.

993.   Kawai, S., Yoshida, M., Segawa, K., Sugiyama, H., Ishizaki, R., and Toyoshima, K., Characterization of Y73, an avian sarcoma virus: a unique transforming gene and its product, a phosphopolyprotein with protein kinase activity, *Proc. Natl. Acad. Sci. U.S.A.,* 77, 6199, 1980.

994.   Ghysdael, J., Neil, J.C., Wallbank, A.M., and Vogt, P.K., Esh avian sarcoma virus codes for a *gag*-linked transformation specific protein with an associated protein kinase activity, *Virology,* 111, 386, 1981.

995.   Kitamura, N., Kitamura, A., Toyoshima, K., Hirayama, Y., and Yoshida, M., Avian sarcoma virus Y73 genome sequence and structural similarity of its transforming gene product to that of Rous sarcoma virus, *Nature,* 297, 205, 1982.

996.   Sukegawa, J., Semba, K., Yamanashi, Y., Nishizawa, M., Miyajima, N., Yamamoto, T., and Toyoshima, K., Characterization of cDNA clones for the human c-*yes* gene, *Mol. Cell. Biol.,* 7, 41, 1987.

997.   Shibuya, M., Hanafusa, H., and Balduzzi, P.C., Cellular sequences related to three new *onc*-genes of avian sarcoma virus (*fps, yes,* and *ros*) and their expression in normal and transformed cells, *J. Virol.,* 42, 143, 1982.

998.   Sudol, M. and Hanafusa, H., Cellular proteins homologous to the viral *yes* gene product, *Mol. Cell. Biol.,* 6, 2839, 1986.

999.   Gentry, L.E. and Rohrschneider, L.R., Common features of the *yes* and *src* gene products define by peptide-specific antibodies, *J. Virol.,* 51, 539, 1984.

1000.   d'Auriol, L., Mattei, M.-G., Andre, C., and Galibert, F., Localization of the human c-*kit* protooncogene on the q11-q12 region of chromosome 4, *Hum. Genet.,* 78, 374, 1988.

1001.   Stahl, M.L., Ferenz, C.R., Kelleher, K.L., Kriz, R.W., and Knopf, J.L., Sequence similarity of phospholipase C with the non-catalytic region of src, *Nature,* 332, 269, 1988.

1002.   Mayer, B.J., Hamaguchi, M., and Hanafusa, H., A novel viral oncogene with structural similarity to phospholipase C, *Nature,* 332, 272, 1988.

1003.   Leprince, D., Gegonne, A., Coll, J., de Taisne, C., Schneeberger, A., Lagrou, C., and Stehelin, D., A putative second cell-derived oncogene of the avian leukaemia retrovirus E26, *Nature,* 306, 395, 1983.

1004.   Gegonne, A., Leprince, D., Duterque-Coquillaud, M., Vandenbunder, B., Flourens, A., Ghysdael, J., Debuire, B., and Stehelin, D., Multiple domains of the chicken cellular sequences homologous to the v-*ets* oncogene of the E26 retrovirus, *Mol. Cell. Biol.,* 7, 806, 1987.

1005.   Bister, K., Nunn, M., Moscovici, C., Perbal, B., Baluda, M.A., and Duesberg, P.H., Acute leukemia viruses E26 and avian myeloblastosis virus have related transformation-specific RNA sequences but different genetic structures, gene products, and oncogenic properties, *Proc. Natl. Acad. Sci. U.S.A.,* 79, 3677, 1982.

1006.   Watson, D.K., McWilliams, M.J., and Papas, T.S., Molecular organization of the chicken *ets* locus, *Virology,* 164, 99, 1988.

1007.   Ghysdael, J., Gegonne, A., Pognonec, P., Dernis, D., Leprince, D., and Stehelin, D., Identification and preferential expression in thymic and bursal lymphocytes of a c-*ets* oncogene-encoded M$_r$ 54,000 cytoplasmic protein, *Proc. Natl. Acad. Sci. U.S.A.,* 83, 1714, 1986.

1008.   Ghysdael, J., Gegonne, A., Pognonec, P., Boulukos, K., Leprince, D., Dernis, D., Lagrou, C., and Stehelin, D., Identification in chicken macrophages of a set of proteins related to, but distinct from, the chicken cellular c-*ets*-encoded protein p54$^{c\text{-}ets}$, *EMBO J.,* 5, 2251, 1986.

1009.   Boulukos, K.E., Pognonec, P., Begue, A., Galibert, F., Gesquière, J.C., Stéhelin, D., and Ghysdael, J., Identification in chickens of an evolutionarily conserved cellular *ets*-2 gene (c-*ets*-2) encoding nuclear proteins related to the products of the c-*ets* proto-oncogene, *EMBO J.,* 7, 697, 1988.

1010.   Watson, D.K., McWilliams, M.J., Lapis, P., Lautenberger, J.A., Schweinfest, C.W., and Papas, T.S., Mammalian *ets*-1 and *ets*-2 genes encode conserved proteins, *Proc. Natl. Acad. Sci. U.S.A.,* 85, 7862, 1988.

1011.   Watson, D.K., McWilliams-Smith, M.J., Nunn, M.F., Duesberg, P.H., O'Brien, S.J., and Papas, T.S., The *ets* sequence from the transforming gene of avian erythroblastosis virus, E26, has unique domains on human chromosomes 11 and 21: both loci are transcriptionally active, *Proc. Natl. Acad. Sci. U.S.A.,* 82, 7294, 1985.

1012.   Fujiwara, S., Fisher, R.J., Seth, A., Bhat, N.K., Showalter, S.D., Zweig, M., and Papas, T.S., Characterization and localization of the products of the human homologs of the v-*ets* oncogene, *Oncogene,* 2, 99, 1988.

1013.   Watson, D.K., Sacchi, N., McWilliams-Smith, M.J., O'Brien, S.J., and Papas, T.S., The avian and mammalian *ets* genes: molecular characterization, chromosome mapping, and implication in human leukemia, *Anticancer Res.,* 6, 631, 1986.

1014.   Pognonec, P., Boulukos, K.E., Gesquière, J.C., Stéhelin, D., and Ghysdael, J., Mitogenic stimulation of thymocytes results in calcium-dependent phosphorylation of c-*ets*-1 proteins, *EMBO J.,* 7, 977, 1988.

1015.   Ferguson, J., Ho, J.-Y., Peterson, T.A., and Reed, S.I., Nucleotide sequence of the yeast cell division cycle start genes *CDC28, CDC36, CDC37,* and *CDC39,* and a structural analysis of the predicted products, *Nucleic Acids Res.,* 14, 6681, 1986.

1016. Fong, H.K.W., Hurley, J.B., Hopkins, R.S., Miake-Lye, R., Johnson, M.S., Doolittle, R.F., and Simon, M.I., Repetitive segmental structure of the transducin beta subunit: homology with the *CDC4* gene and identification of related mRNAs, *Proc. Natl. Acad. Sci. U.S.A.,* 83, 2162, 1986.

1017. Lörincz, A.T. and Reed, S.I., Primary structure homology between the product of yeast cell division control gene *CDC28* and vertebrate oncogenes, *Nature,* 307, 183, 1984.

1018. Reed, S.I., Hadwiger, J.A., and Lörincz, A.T., Protein kinase activity associated with the product of the yeast cell division cycle gene *CDC28, Proc. Natl. Acad. Sci. U.S.A.,* 82, 4055, 1985.

1019. Patterson, M., Sclafani, R.A., Fangman, W.L., and Rosamond, J., Molecular characterization of cell cycle gene *CDC7* from *Saccharomyces cerevisiae,* Mol. Cell. Biol., 6, 1590, 1986.

1020. Chen, J.H., The proto-oncogene c-*ets* is preferentially expressed in lymphoid cells, *Mol. Cell. Biol.,* 5, 2993, 1985.

1021. Bhat, N.K., Fisher, R.J., Fujiwara, S., Ascione, R., and Papas, T.S., Temporal and tissue-specific expression of mouse *ets* genes, *Proc. Natl. Acad. Sci. U.S.A.,* 84, 3161, 1987.

1022. Amouyel, P., Gégonne, A., Delacourte, A., Défossez, and Stéhelin, D., Expression of ETS proto-oncogenes in astrocytes in human cortex, *Brain Res.,* 447, 149, 1988.

1023. Rao, V.N., Papas, T.S., and Reddy, E.S.P., *erg,* a human *ets*-related gene on chromosome 21: alternative splicing, polyadenylation, and translation, *Science,* 237, 635, 1987.

1024. Maki, Y., Bos, T.J., Davis, C., Starbuck, M., and Vogt, P.K., Avian sarcoma virus 17 carries the *jun* oncogene, *Proc. Natl. Acad. Sci. U.S.A.,* 84, 2848, 1987.

1025. Vogt, P.K., Bos, T.J., and Doolittle, R.F., Homology between the DNA-binding domain of the GCN4 regulatory protein of yeast and the carboxyl-terminal region of a protein coded for by the oncogene *jun, Proc. Natl. Acad. Sci. U.S.A.,* 84, 3316, 1987.

1026. Struhl, K., The DNA-binding domains of the jun oncoprotein and the yeast GCN4 transcriptional activator proteins are functionally homologous, *Cell,* 50, 841, 1987.

1027. Haluska, F.G., Huebner, K., Isobe, M., Nishimura, T., Croce, C.M., and Vogt, P.K., Localization of the human *JUN* protooncogene to chromosome region 1p31-32, *Proc. Natl. Acad. Sci. U.S.A.,* 85, 2215, 1988.

1028. Cooper, C.S., Park, M., Blair, D.G., Tainsky, M.A., Huebner, K., Croce, C.M., and Vande Woude, G.F., Molecular cloning of a new transforming gene from a chemically transformed human cell line, *Nature,* 311, 29, 1984.

1029. Park, M., Testa, J.R., Blair, D.G., Parsa, N.Z., and Vande Woude, G.F., Two rearranged *MET* alleles in MNNG-HOS cells reveal the orientation of *MET* on chromosome 7 to other markers tightly linked to the cystic fibrosis locus, *Proc. Natl. Acad. Sci. U.S.A.,* 85, 2667, 1988.

1030. Tempest, P.R., Cooper, C.S., and Major, G.N., The activated human *met* gene encodes a protein tyrosine kinase, *FEBS Lett.,* 209, 357, 1986.

1031. Gonzatti-Haces, M., Seth, A., Park, M., Copeland, T., Oroszlan, S., and Vande Woude, G.F., Characterization of the *TRP-MET* oncogene p65 and the *MET* proto-oncogene p140 protein-tyrosine kinases, *Proc. Natl. Acad. Sci. U.S.A.,* 85, 21, 1988.

1032. Chan, A.M.-L., King, H.W.S., Tempest, P.R., Deakin, E.A., Cooper, C.S., and Brookes, P., Primary structure of the *met* protein tyrosine kinase domain, *Oncogene,* 1, 229, 1987.

1033. Park, M., Dean, M., Cooper, C.S., Schmidt, M., O'Brien, S.J., Blair, D.G., and Vande Woude, G.F., Mechanism of *met* oncogene activation, *Cell,* 45, 895, 1986.

1034. Tempest, P.R., Reeves, B.R., Spurr, N.K., Rance, A.J., Chan, A.M.-L., and Brookes, P., Activation of the *met* oncogene in the human MNNG-HOS cell line involves a chromosomal rearrangement, *Carcinogenesis,* 7, 2051, 1986.

1035. Dean, M., Park, M., and Vande Woude, G.F., Characterization of the rearranged *trp-met* oncogene breakpoint, *Mol. Cell. Biol.,* 7, 921, 1987.

1036. Cooper, C.S., Tempest, P.R., Beckman, M.P., Heldin, C.-H., and Brookes, P., Amplification and overexpression of the *met* gene in spontaneously transformed NIH3T3 fibroblasts, *EMBO J.,* 5, 12623, 1986.

1037. Yoshida, M.C., Satoh, H., Sasaki, M., Semba, K., Yamamoto, T., and Toyoshima, K., Regional localization of a novel *yes*-related proto-oncogene, *syn,* on human chromosome 6 at band q21, *Jpn. J. Cancer Res.,* 77, 1059, 1986.

1038. Kawakami, T., Pennington, C.Y., and Robbins, K.C., Isolation and oncogenic potential of a novel human *src*-like gene, *Mol. Cell. Biol.,* 6, 4195, 1986.

1039. Kypta, R.M., Hemming, A., and Courtneidge, S.A., Identification and characterization of p59^{fyn} (a *src*-like protein tyrosine kinase) in normal and polyoma virus transformed cells, *EMBO J.,* 7, 3837, 1988.

1040. Marth, J.D., Peet, R., Krebs, E.G., and Perlmutter, R.M., A lymphocyte-specific protein-tyrosine kinase gene is rearranged and overexpressed in the murine T cell lymphoma LSTRA, *Cell,* 43, 393, 1985.

1041. Voronova, A.F. and Sefton, B.M., Expression of a new tyrosine protein kinase is stimulated by retrovirus promoter insertion, *Nature,* 319, 682, 1986.

1042. Marth, J.D., Disteche, C., Pravtcheva, D., Ruddle, F., Krebs, E.G., and Perlmutter, R.M., Localization of a lymphocyte-specific protein tyrosine kinase gene (*lck*) at a site of frequent chromosomal abnormalities in human lymphomas, *Proc. Natl. Acad. Sci. U.S.A.,* 83, 7400, 1986.

1043. Voronova, A.R., Buss, J.E., Patschinsky, T., Hunter, T., and Sefton, B.M., Characterization of the protein apparently responsible for the elevated tyrosine protein kinase activity in LSTRA cells, *Mol. Cell. Biol.,* 4, 2705, 1984.

1044. Trevillyan, J.M., Lin, Y., Chen, S.J., Phillips, C.A., Canna, C., and Linna, T.J., Human T lymphocytes express a protein-tyrosine kinase homologous to p56^LSTRA, *Biochim. Biophys. Acta,* 888, 286, 1986.

1045. Trevillyan, J.M., Canna, C., Maley, D., Linna, T.J., and Phillips, C.A., Identification of the human T-lymphocyte protein-tyrosine kinase by peptide-specific antibodies, *Biochem. Biophys. Res. Commun.,* 140, 392, 1986.

1046. Boulet, I., Fagard, R., and Fischer, S., Correlation between phosphorylation and kinase activity of a tyrosine protein kinase: p56 *lck, Biochem. Biophys. Res. Commun.,* 149, 56, 1987.

1047. Koga, Y., Kimura, N., Minowada, J., and Mak, T.W., Expression of the human T-cell-specific tyrosine kinase YT16 (*lck*) message in leukemic T-cell lines, *Cancer Res.,* 48, 856, 1988.

1048. Marth, J.D., Lewis, D.B., Wilson, C.B., Gearn, M.E., Krebs, E.G., and Perlmutter, R.M., Regulation of pp56^lck during T-cell activation: functional implications for the *src*-like protein tyrosine kinases, *EMBO J.,* 6, 2727, 1987.

1049. Veillette, A., Foss, F.M., Sausville, E.A., Bolen, J.B., and Rosen, N., Expression of the *lck* tyrosine kinase gene in human colon carcinoma and other non-lymphoid human tumor cell lines, *Oncogene Res.,* 1, 357, 1987.

1050. Marth, J.D., Overell, R.W., Meier, K.E., Krebs, E.G., and Perlmutter, R.M., Translational activation of the *lck* proto-oncogene, *Nature,* 332, 171, 1988.

1051. Marth, J.D., Cooper, J.A., King, C.S., Ziegler, S.F., Tinker, D.A., Overell, R.W., Krebs, E.G., and Perlmutter, R.M., Neoplastic transformation induced by an activated lymphocyte-specific protein tyrosine kinase (pp56^lck), *Mol. Cell. Biol.,* 8, 540, 1988.

1052. Garvin, A.M., Pawar, S., Marth, J.D., and Perlmutter, R.M., Structure of the murine *lck* gene and its rearrangement in a murine lymphoma cell line, *Mol. Cell. Biol.,* 8, 3058, 1988.

1053. Quintrell, N., Lebo, R., Varmus, H., Bishop, J.M., Pettenati, M.J., Le Beau, M.M., Diaz, M.O., and Rowley, J.D., Identification of a human gene (*HCK*) that encodes a protein-tyrosine kinase and is expressed in hemopoietic cells, *Mol. Cell. Biol.,* 7, 2267, 1987.

1054. Ziegler, S.F., Marth, J.D., Lewis, D.B., and Perlmutter, R.M., Novel protein-tyrosine kinase gene (*hck*) preferentially expressed in cells of hematopoietic origin, *Mol. Cell. Biol.,* 7, 2276, 1987.

1055. Holtzman, D.A., Cook, W.D., and Dunn, A.R., Isolation and sequence of a cDNA corresponding to a *src*-related gene expressed in murine hemopoietic cells, *Proc. Natl. Acad. Sci. U.S.A.,* 84, 8325, 1987.

1056. Yamanashi, Y., Fukushige, S.-I., Semba, K., Sukegawa, J., Miyajima, N., Matsubara, K.-I., Yamamoto, T., and Toyoshima, K., The *yes*-related cellular gene *lyn* encodes a possible tyrosine kinase similar to p56^lck, *Mol. Cell. Biol.,* 7, 237, 1987.

1057. Strebhardt, K., Mullins, J.I., Bruck, C., and Rübsamen-Waigmann, H., Additional member of the protein-tyrosine kinase family: the *src*- and *lck*-related protooncogene c-*tkl, Proc. Natl. Acad. Sci. U.S.A.,* 84, 8778, 1987.

1058. Sakamoto, H., Mori, M., Taira, M., Yoshida, T., Matsukawa, S., Shimizu, K., Sekiguchi, M., Terada, M., and Sugimura, T., Transforming gene from human stomach cancers and a noncancerous portion of stomach mucosa, *Proc. Natl. Acad. Sci. U.S.A.,* 83, 3997, 1986.

1059. Taira, M., Yoshida, T., Miyagawa, K., Sakamoto, H., Terada, M., and Sugimura, T., cDNA sequence of human transforming gene *hst* and identification of the coding sequence required for transforming activity, *Proc. Natl. Acad. Sci. U.S.A.,* 84, 2980, 1987.

1060. Delli Bovi, P. and Basilico, C., Isolation of a rearranged human transforming gene following transfection of Kaposi sarcoma DNA, *Proc. Natl. Acad. Sci. U.S.A.,* 84, 5660, 1987.

1061. Delli Bovi, P., Curatola, A.M., Kern, F.G., Greco, A., Ittmann, M., and Basilico, C., An oncogene isolated by transfection of Kaposi's sarcoma DNA encodes a growth factor that is a member of the FGF family, *Cell,* 50, 729, 1987.

1062. Mester, J., Wagenaar, E., Sluyser, M., and Nusse, R., Activation of *int*-1 and *int*-2 mammary oncogenes in hormone-dependent and -independent mammary tumors of GR mice, *J. Virol.,* 61, 1073, 1987.

1063. Dickson, C. and Peters, G., Potential oncogene product related to growth factors, *Nature,* 326, 833, 1987.

1064. Jaye, M., Lyall, R.M., Mudd, R., Schlessinger, J., and Sarver, N., Expression of acidic fibroblast growth factor cDNA confers growth advantage and tumorigenesis to Swiss 3T3 cells, *EMBO J.,* 7, 963, 1988.

1065. Yuasa, Y. and Sudo, K., Transforming genes in human hepatomas detected by a tumorigenicity assay, *Jpn. J. Cancer Res.,* 78, 1036, 1987.

1066. Adelaide, J., Mattei, M.-G., Marics, I., Raybaud, F., Planche, J., De Lapeyriere, O., and Birnbaum, D., Chromosomal localization of the *hst* oncogene and its co-amplification with the *int*.2 oncogene in a human melanoma, *Oncogene,* 2, 423, 1988.

1067. Inoue, C., Shiga, K., Takasawa, S., Kitagawa, M., Yamamoto, H., and Okamoto, H., Evolutionary conservation of the insulinoma gene *rig* and its possible function, *Proc. Natl. Acad. Sci. U.S.A.,* 84, 6659, 1987.

1068. Eva, A. and Aaronson, S.A., Isolation of a new human oncogene from a diffuse B-cell lymphoma, *Nature,* 316, 273, 1985.

1069. Eva, A., Vecchio, G., Diamond, M., Tronick, S.R., Ron, D., Cooper, G.M., and Aaronson, S.A., Independently activated *dbl* oncogenes exhibit similar yet distinct structural alterations, *Oncogene,* 1, 355, 1987.

1070. Eva, A., Vecchio, G., Rao, C.D., Tronick, S.R., and Aaronson, S.A., The predicted *DBL* oncogene product defines a distinct class of transforming proteins, *Proc. Natl. Acad. Sci. U.S.A.,* 85, 2061, 1988.

1071. Srivastave, S.K., Wheelock, R.H.P., Aaronson, S.A., and Eva, A., Identification of the protein encoded by the human diffuse B-cell lymphoma (*dbl*) oncogene, *Proc. Natl. Acad. Sci. U.S.A.,* 85, 8868, 1986.

1072. Tsujimoto, Y., Finger, L.R., Yunis, J., Nowell, P.C., and Croce, C.M., Cloning of the chromosome breakpoint of neoplastic B cells with the t(14;18) chromosome translocation, *Science,* 226, 1097, 1984.

1073. Tsujimoto, Y. and Croce, C.M., Analysis of the structure, transcripts, and protein products of *bcl-2,* the gene involved in human follicular lymphoma, *Proc. Natl. Acad. Sci. U.S.A.,* 83, 5214, 1986.

1074. Tsujimoto, Y., Ikegaki, N., and Croce, C.M., Characterization of the protein product of *bcl-2,* the gene involved in human follicular lymphoma, *Oncogene,* 2, 3, 1987.

1075. Reed, J.C., Tsujimoto, Y., Alpers, J.D., Croce, C.M., and Nowell, P.C., Regulation of *bcl-2* proto-oncogene expression during normal human lymphocyte proliferation, *Science,* 236, 1295, 1987.

1076. Gurfinkel, N., Unger, T., Givol, D., and Mushinski, J.F., Expression of the *bcl-2* gene in mouse B lymphocytic cell lines is differentiation stage specific, *Eur. J. Immunol.,* 17, 567, 1987.

1077. Lane, M.-A., Sainten, A., and Cooper, G.M., Stage-specific transforming genes of human and mouse B- and T-lymphocyte neoplasms, *Cell,* 28, 873, 1982.

1078. Diamond, A., Cooper, G.M., Ritz, J., and Lane, M.-A., Identification and molecular cloning of the human *Blym* transforming gene activated in Burkitt's lymphomas, *Nature,* 305, 112, 1983.

1079. Lane, M.-A., Sainten, A., Doherty, K.M., and Cooper, G.M., Isolation and characterization of a stage-specific transforming gene, *Tlym-I,* from T-cell lymphomas, *Proc. Nat. Acad. Sci. U.S.A.,* 81, 2227, 1984.

1080. Devine, J.M., Diamond, A., Lane, M.-A., and Cooper, G.M., Characterization of the Blym-1 transforming genes of chicken and human B-cell lymphomas, *J. Cell Physiol.,* Suppl. 3, 193, 1984.

1081. Neiman, P., The *BLYM* oncogenes, *Adv. Cancer Res.,* 45, 107, 1985.

1082. Goubin, G., Goldman, D.S., Luce, J., Neiman, P.E., and Cooper, G.M., Molecular cloning and nucleotide sequence of a transforming gene detected by transfection of chicken B-cell lymphoma DNA, *Nature,* 302, 114, 1983.

1083. Diamond, A., Devine, J.M., and Cooper, G.M., Nucleotide sequence of a human *Blym* transforming gene activated in a Burkitt's lymphoma, *Science,* 225, 516, 1984.

1084. Rogers, J., Relationship of *Blym* genes to repeated sequences, *Nature,* 320, 579, 1986.

1085. Devine, J.M., Mechanism of activation of *HuBlym-*1 gene unresolved, *Nature,* 321, 437, 1986.

1086. Wolf, D., Harris, N., and Rotter, V., Reconstitution of p53 expression in a nonproducer Ab-MuLV-transformed cell line by transfection of a functional p53 gene, *Cell,* 38, 119, 1984.

1087. Eliyahu, D., Raz, A., Gruss, P., Givol, D., and Oren, M., Participation of p53 cellular tumour antigen in transformation of normal embryonic cells, *Nature,* 312, 646, 1984.

1088. Jenkins, J.R., Rudge, K., and Currie, G.A., Cellular immortalization by a cDNA clone encoding the transformation-associated phosphoprotein p53, *Nature,* 312, 651, 1984.

1089. Rotter, V. and Wolff, D., Biological and molecular analysis of p53 cellular-encode tumor antigen, *Adv. Cancer Res.,* 43, 113, 1985.

1090. Oren, M., The p53 cellular tumor antigen: gene structure, expression and protein properties, *Biochim. Biophys. Acta,* 823, 67, 1985.

1091. Crawford, L., Human p53 and human tumours, *BioEssays,* 3, 117, 1985.

1092. Zakut-Houri, R., Oren, M., Bienz, B., Lavie, V., Hazum, S., and Givol, D., A single gene and a pseudogene for the cellular tumor antigen p53, *Nature,* 306, 594, 1983.

1093. Rotter, V., Wolf, D., Pravtcheva, D., and Ruddle, F.H., Chromosomal assignment of the murine gene encoding the transformation-related protein p53, *Mol. Cell. Biol.,* 4, 383, 1984.

1094. Jenkins, J.R., Rudge, K., Redmond, S., and Wade-Evans, A., Cloning and expression analysis of full length mouse cDNA sequences encoding the transformation associated protein p53, *Nucleic Acids Res.,* 12, 5609, 1984.

1095. Pinhasi, O. and Oren, M., Expression of the mouse p53 cellular tumor antigen in monkey cells, *Mol. Cell. Biol.,* 4, 2180, 1984.

1096. Bienz-Tadmor, B., Zakut-Houri, R., Libresco, S., Givol, D., and Oren, M., The 5' region of the p53 gene: evolutionary conservation and evidence for a negative regulatory element, *EMBO J.,* 4, 3209, 1985.

1097. Matlashewski, G., Lamb, P., Pim, D., Peacock, J., Crawford, L., and Benchimol, S., Isolation and characterization of a human p53 cDNA clone: expression of the human p53 gene, *EMBO J.,* 3, 3257, 1984.

1098. Wade-Evans, A. and Jenkins, J.R., Precise epitope mapping of the murine transformation-associated protein, p53, *EMBO J.,* 4, 699, 1985.

1099. Zakut-Houri, R., Bienz-Tadmor, B., Givol, D., and Oren, M., Human p53 cellular tumor antigen: cDNA sequence and expression in COS cells, *EMBO J.,* 4, 1251, 1985.

1100. Harlow, E., Williamson, N.M., Ralston, R., Helfman, D.M., and Adams, T.E., Molecular cloning and *in vitro* expression of a cDNA clone for human cellular tumor antigen p53, *Mol. Cell. Biol.,* 5, 1601, 1985.

1101. Isobe, M., Emanuel, B.S., Givol, D., Oren, M., and Croce, C.M., Localization of gene for human p53 tumour antigen to band 17p13, *Nature,* 320, 84, 1986.

1102. Lamb, P. and Crawford, L., Characterization of the human p53 gene, *Mol. Cell. Biol.,* 6, 1379, 1986.

1103. Soussi, T., Caron de Fromentel, C., Méchali, M., May, P., and Kress, M., Cloning and characterization of a cDNA from *Xenopus laevis* coding for a protein homologous to human and murine p53, *Oncogene,* 1, 71, 1987.

1104. Samad, A., Anderson, C.W., and Carroll, R.B., Mapping of phosphomonoester and apparent phosphodiester bonds of the oncogene product p53 from simian virus 40-transformed 3T3 cells, *Proc. Natl. Acad. Sci. U.S.A.,* 83, 897, 1986.

1105. Meek, D.W. and Eckhart, W., Phosphorylation of p53 in normal and simian virus 40-transformed NIH 3T3 cells, *Mol. Cell. Biol.,* 8, 461, 1988.

1106. Banks, L., Matlashewski, G., and Crawford, L., Isolation of human-p53-specific monoclonal antibodies and their use in the studies of human p53 expression, *Eur. J. Biochem.,* 159, 529, 1986.

1107. Yewdell, J.W., Gannon, J.V., and Lane, D.P., Monoclonal antibody analysis of p53 expression in normal and transformed cells, *J. Virol.,* 59, 444, 1986.

1108. Milner, J. and Sheldon, M., A new anti-p53 monoclonal antibody, previously reported to be directed against the large T antigen of simian virus-40, *Oncogene,* 1, 453, 1987.

1109. Milner, J., Different forms of p53 detected by monoclonal antibodies in non-dividing and dividing lymphocytes, *Nature,* 310, 143, 1984.

1110. Milner, J. and Cook, A., The cellular tumour antigen p53: evidence for transformation-related immunological variants of p53, *Virology,* 154, 21, 1986.

1111. Harris, N., Brill, E., Shohat, O., Prokocimer, M., Wolf, D., Arai, N., and Rotter, V., Molecular basis for heterogeneity of the human p53 protein, *Mol. Cell. Biol.,* 6, 4650, 1986.

1112. Stürzbecher, H.-W., Chumakov, P., Welch, W.J., and Jenkins, J.R., Mutant p53 proteins bind hsp 72/73 cellular heat shock-related proteins in SV40-transformed monkey cells, *Oncogene,* 1, 201, 1987.

1113. Kaczmarek, L., Oren, L., and Baserga, R., Co-operation between the p53 protein tumor antigen and platelet-poor plasma in the induction of cellular DNA synthesis, *Exp. Cell Res.,* 162, 268, 1986.

1114. Mercer, W.E. and Baserga, R., Expression of the p53 protein during the cell cycle of human peripheral blood lymphocytes, *Exp. Cell Res.,* 160, 31, 1985.

1115. Reich, N.C. and Levine, A.J., Growth regulation of a cellular tumour antigen, p53, in nontransformed cells, *Nature,* 308, 199, 1984.

1116. Mercer, W.E., Nelson, D., DeLeo, A.B., Old, L.J., and Baserga, R., Microinjection of monoclonal antibody to protein p53 inhibits serum-induced DNA synthesis in 3T3 cells, *Proc. Natl. Acad. Sci. U.S.A.,* 79, 6309, 1982.

1117. Coulier, F., Imbert, J., Albert, J., Jeunet, E., Lawrence, J.-J., Crawford, L., and Birg, F., Permanent expression of p53 in FR 3T3 rat cells but cell cycle-dependent association with large-T antigen in simian virus 40 transformants, *EMBO J.,* 4, 3413, 1985.

1118. Darzynkiewicz, A., Staiano-Coico, L., Kunicka, J.E., DeLeo, A.B., and Old, L.J., p53 content in relation to cell growth and proliferation in murine L1210 leukemia and normal lymphocytes, *Leukemia Res.,* 1383, 1986.

1119. Shohat, O., Greenberg, M., Reisman, D., Oren, M., and Rotter, V., Inhibition of cell growth mediated by plasmids encoding p53 anti-sense, *Oncogene,* 1, 277, 1987.

1120. Steinmeyer, K. and Deppert, W., DNA binding properties of murine p53, *Oncogene,* 3, 501, 1988.

1121. Baker, S.J., Fearon, E.R., Nigro, J.M., Hamilton, S.R., Preisinger, A.C., Jessup, J.M., van Tuinen, P., Ledbetter, D.H., Barker, D.F., Nakamura, Y., White, R., and Vogelstein, B., Chromosome 17 deletions and p53 gene mutations in colorectal carcinomas, *Science,* 244, 217, 1989.

1122. Jackson, T.R., Blair, L.A.C., Marshall, J., Goedert, M., and Hanley, M.R., The *mas* oncogene encodes an angiotensin receptor, *Nature,* 335, 437, 1988.

Chapter 8

THE ROUS SARCOMA VIRUS ONCOGENE AND ITS PROTOONCOGENE COUNTERPART

I. INTRODUCTION

Rous sarcoma virus (RSV) is an avian sarcoma virus (ASV) that was first isolated in 1911.[1] RSV and its oncogene, v-*src*, as well as the cellular counterpart of this oncogene, c-*src*, and the respective products of these oncogenes, the proteins pp60^{v-src} and pp60^{c-src}, are historically important and have been subjected to extensive studies by many investigators. In addition to RSV, the ASV family is composed of acute retroviruses transducing oncogenes closely related to v-*src*, including the oncogenes v-*fps*, v-*yes*, and v-*ros*.[2] A recently identified ASV, the acute retrovirus ASV-17, transduces the oncogene v-*jun*.[3] Transduction of oncogenes by ASVs requires the occurrence of at least two recombinational events between cellular and viral DNA.[4]

II. THE ROUS SARCOMA VIRUS

Cells from many animal species can be infected *in vitro* with RSV. The virus induces phenotypic transformation of chicken embryo fibroblasts (CEFs) within less than 24 h after infection *in vitro*. Numerous alterations are observed in the RSV-infected cultured fibroblasts, including changes in morphology, growth, and metabolism.[5-7] RSV-transformed CEFs generally exhibit a rounded morphology but some mutants induce the appearance of CEFs with elongated spindled shape characteristics.[8] Human diploid fibroblasts are susceptible to infection by RSV, which results in their morphological transformation and the production of small numbers of virus particles that are infectious in bioassay.[9,10] The complete proviral sequence was shown to be integrated in the human cells and comparable amounts of pp60^{v-src} are produced by avian and human cells infected with RSV. Human cell lines infected with RSV can induce progressive tumors in nude mice.

Not all cells infected with RSV express viral-specific functions. Normal early chicken embryonic cells from the pregastrulation stage can be infected at high efficiency with RSV but, in spite of this and the fact that RSV DNA is integrated into the host cell genome, the levels of viral mRNA produced by the infected cell are very low and are not sufficient to generate competent viral particles.[11] The chicken embryo can regulate the susceptibility of tissues to RSV infection and/or expression and modulates the spread of the virus through tissues that may or may not be transformation competent.[12] In general, RSV infection and expression are compatible with differentiation and expression of differentiated characteristics *in ovo*. It is thus apparent that not all cells are susceptible to the effects of RSV infection.

RSV and other ASVs are not involved in the transmission of malignant diseases under natural conditions, but can cause visible fibrosarcomas (Rous sarcomas) a few days after injection into young chicks. Rous sarcoma is a recruitment tumor in which growth is primarily due to the spread of infectious progeny viral particles to adjacent cells which then become part of an enlarging tumor mass.[13] Inoculation of RSV into the wing web of a chicken will often induce a tumor within 1 week, but usually the initial growth is followed by tumor regression due to an immune response directed against viral and/or tumor antigens.[14,15] Regressing RSV-induced chicken sarcomas produce little or no infectious progeny virus.[16] The tumor cells which are found during Rous sarcoma regression apparently survive specific antitumor immune responses of the host because of their inability to express relevant antigens at their surface. The specific pp60^{v-src} kinase activity was found to be reduced by about 75% in the cells from regressing Rous sarcomas.[17] Direct injection of phorbol ester (PMA) into growing RSV-induced chicken sarcomas results in accelerated tumor regression which is associated with inhibition of both the pp60[c-src] kinase and DNA synthesis.[18]

ASV inoculation in mammals may result in tumor induction. All neonatal and adult F344 rats inoculated with the B77 isolate of ASV developed brain tumors (astrocytomas).[19] Marmosets of the genus *Sanguinus* injected with RSV can develop sarcomas.[20] In contrast to nontransplantable sarcomas induced by RSV of chicken origin, RSV rescued from the virus-free marmosets sarcomas induces tumors that are transplantable to young but not to adult marmosets. Several transplantable RSV-induced tumors were established, propagated in culture, and partially characterized in this experimental study. The transplanted tumors enlarged rapidly, metastasized to several organs, and killed the recipients 29 to 59 d after inoculation.

A recombinant murine retrovirus, termed MRSV, carrying the v-src oncogene has been constructed, thus facilitating the study of v-src action in mammalian cell systems.[21] MRSV lacks a functional *env* gene resulting from the fact that the v-src gene was inserted at this site but is able to infect, transform, and replicate in cells from a variety of species in the presence of appropriate helper virus. Injection of MRSV into mice results in the appearance of an erythroproliferative disease, and MRSV is able to transform erythroid progenitor cells *in vitro*.[22]

A. STRUCTURE OF RSV

The core of RSV consists of a single-stranded diploid RNA genome composed of two identical 35S RNA molecules associated in a 70S complex. A cloverleaf model for the structure of RSV 35S RNA has been proposed.[23] Many strains of RSV and other avian sarcoma viruses have been described, depending on differences in the recombinational events occurring between viral and cellular sequences during the integration and isolation processes. The Schmidt-Ruppin and Prague strains of RSV are nondefective in replication, the genome being complete in these strains, whereas other RSV strains are replication defective, lacking the genome segments coding for virus structural components. The genome of nondefective RSV strains contains three viral genes (*gag*, *pol*, and *env*) plus the v-src oncogene, which is derived from c-src protoonco-gene sequences contained in normal, noninfected chicken cells.[4] The original RSV was, as other RSV strains, replication defective.[24] The RSV genome is associated with a basic protein and reverse transcriptase which is surrounded by a protein capsid.[7] In addition to products encoded by the virus genome, purified virions of the Schmidt-Ruppin strain of RSV contain some enzymatic and nonenzymatic components which may be of cellular origin and are incorporated into the viral particle.[25] Such components are probably picked up from the cytoplasm during assembly of the virions. They include nucleotides and nucleotide kinase, phosphatase, hexokinase, and lactate dehydrogenase activities.

Both reverse transcriptase and endonuclease activities are associated with RSV virions.[26-28] After virus infection, the RNA is transcribed by reverse transcriptase into a single-stranded DNA copy (cDNA), which is then converted by host DNA polymerase into a double-stranded DNA copy of the virus, the RSV provirus, the latter being integrated into the cellular DNA. Division of RSV-infected chicken embryo fibroblast is required for the initiation, but not for the maintenance, of transcription of virus RNA.[29] Integration of ASVs can occur at multiple sites within the mammalian genome.[30] RSV-transformed Chinese hamster fibroblasts may contain several copies of the RSV provirus, which are generated by amplification of the proviral sequences and are distributed among different nonhomologous chromosomes.[31] Duplications of variable segments of proviral RSV DNA have been detected in RSV-transformed rat cells, suggesting that upstream rearrangements may influence provirus expression which is usually low in mammalian cells.[32]

The complete sequence of the v-src gene has been determined and, more recently, the complete sequence of the RSV genome (Prague C strain) has also been determined, the genome being composed of 9312 nucleotides.[33,34] Sequence variations of the RSV genome are frequently found, which indicates that the genome supports a very high incidence of spontaneous mutations in the course of replication, thus explaining the genetic diversity observed in avian retroviruses.[35] An RSV mutant (*SE*21Q1b) has been used to demonstrate that the retroviral particle contains all that is necessary for stable gene transfer from an mRNA molecule into a quail cell line.[36]

B. TRANSCRIPTION AND TRANSLATION OF THE RSV GENOME

Apparently, the RSV genome is transcribed into a single RNA species which serves as the precursor for four different RSV mRNAs: *gag* mRNA, *gag-pol* mRNA, *env* mRNA, and *src* mRNA, the latter having most *gag*, *pol*, and *env* sequences removed by splicing. The v-*src* message is apparently polycistronic, producing two polypeptides, a very small (nine-amino acid) peptide that is initiated at the *gag* AUG codon and the 60,000-dDa pp60$^{v\text{-}src}$ protein that is initiated at the *src* AUG codon.[37]

At least three species of RSV mRNA (38S, 28S, and 21S mRNAs) have been identified in the cytoplasm of RSV-infected cells The 21S mRNA corresponds to the transcription of the 3' end of the viral genome, where the *src* gene is located. The 21S polyadenylated mRNA of RSV has been translated in cell-free systems and the protein product of the v-*src* gene, pp60$^{v\text{-}src}$, has been identified by immunoprecipitation with antisera obtained from rabbits bearing RSV-induced tumors and by partial digestion with proteases followed by separation on polyacrylamide gels. In addition, the 21S mRNA from RSV has been purified from total cellular RNA by molecular hybridization with virus-specific cDNA, and the purified RNA has been translated in a cell-free system to obtain the pp60$^{v\text{-}src}$ protein.[38] Ribosomes may bind to two or more AUG codons at the 5' end of RSV RNA and translation *in vitro* of RSV virion RNA results in the synthesis of at least two polypeptides.[39] The efficiency of RSV *env* gene expression from an SV40 vector appears to depend on differences in the efficiency with which the *env*-specific transcripts are translated according to the use of AUG codons present in the vector and intrinsic properties of the *env* gene.[40]

Fluctuations in the transcriptional activity of RSV proviruses are observed in RSV-infected cells and can occur either spontaneously or under the influence of different exogenous factors. In certain cells, e.g., in the preneoplastic cell line 10W transfected with RSV DNA, no expression of RSV RNA is observed in spite of the presence of multiple copies of the RSV genome.[41] However, tumorigenic sublines of these cells which exhibit amplification of the v-*src* gene sequences associated with the presence of DM chromosomes may express v-*src* RNA and may form tumors in nude mice. The reason for the lack of RSV transcription in RSV-transfected 10W cells is unknown but it is clear that RSV genomes are not expressed in all infected cells. The inefficient expression of RSV genomes in different types of cells can be attributed, at least in part, to the site of integration. Cellular sequences near the integration site can regulate provirus expression in *cis*. Moreover, there are fluctuations in proviral expression according to the predominant physiologic conditions and position-dependent fluctuations in proviral repression may be mediated by *trans*-acting factors.[42] It is thus evident that complex cellular factors are critically involved in the regulation of RSV provirus expression.

RSV encodes a transcriptional activator that increases transient expression of the RSV LTR as well as from adventitious host cell promoters.[43] Genomic duplications located at the 5' side of the integrated RSV provirus may have an important regulatory role on the provirus transcriptional activity.[44] The duplications may either attenuate a negative effect of flanking elements at the host chromosome integration site or augment the positive regulation of conventional provirus expression or both. DNA rearrangements 5' to the RSV provirions are common in transformed rat cells, but not seen in infected but untransformed cells.[45] These rearrangements seem to occur near the time of virus integration and would determine the fate of the virus-infected cells. In any case, transformation of mammalian cells by RSV is a relatively rare event and the provirus remains transcriptionally silent in the majority of infected cells.[46] Other control mechanisms of RSV transcription are exerted by differences in methylation of

CCGG sequences located mainly at the 3' half of the provirus, close to the *src* gene, and not at the 5' end of the provirus where transcription is initiated.[47]

The transcriptional activity of integrated RSV genomes may depend, at least in part, on enhancers contained within the LTR. In turn, the activity of these enhancers may be controlled by specific proteins of either viral or cellular origin. Two protein factors, termed EF-I and EF-II, extracted from avian cell nuclei, can recognize particular nucleotide sequences contained in different enhancer elements from RSV LTR.[48] EF-I and EF-II can asymmetrically protect 25- to 30-nucleotide regions on alternate DNA strands of the RSV LTR enhancer. The protected nucleotides have only weak homologies with several consensus sequence motifs known to be essential for the activity of other enhancers.

Other elements that may influence RSV provirus expression are sequences from the *gag-pol* region of the provirus.[44] A *cis*-acting element contained within the *gag* gene of RSV may act as a transcriptional enhancer in the regulation of RSV expression.[49] The synthesis of RNA from the integrated RSV provirus may be studied by using constructed point mutations of the 3' end of the RSV *pol* gene.[50] The *pol* gene of RSV is positioned downstream of the *gag* gene in a different, briefly overlapping reading frame; nevertheless, the primary translation product of *pol* is a *gag-pol* fusion protein which is produced by an interesting, novel mechanism of ribosomal frameshifting.[51] The analysis of different cloned variants of the Prague strain of RSV showed that the different relative levels of the pp60^{src} product found in RSV-infected cells may be due to differences in splicing of the transcripts containing v-*src*-specific sequences.[52]

Some RSV isolates with reduced tumorigenic properties may have alterations at the amino-terminal sequences of the oncogene product. For example, the protein of the rASV157 isolate consists at the amino terminus of 30 amino acids of the *env* signal peptide attached to serine-6 of the *src* sequence, and the protein of the rASV1702 isolate consists at the same region of 45 amino acids of the *env* signal peptide attached to alanine-76 of the *src* sequence.[53] The *in vivo* tumorigenicity of rASV157 and rASV1702 isolates is greatly reduced; they induce benign, noninvasive tumors that regress rapidly. In contrast to RSV isolates nondefective in transformation, the *src* proteins rASV157 and rASV1702 are not myristylated and have an altered subcellular localization. Amino-terminal deletion mutants of the RSV glycoprotein do not block signal peptide cleavage but can block intracellular transport of the protein.[54]

III. THE C-*SRC* PROTOONCOGENE

In chicken cells the c-*src* protooncogene is composed of 12 exons.[55] Exon 1 codes for a 5' untranslated region of mRNA. The entire sequences of the chicken c-*src* coding regions were determined. The chicken c-*src* gene has been cloned in chimeric plasmid and retroviral vectors and the cloned gene are able to direct the synthesis of high amounts of c-*src* mRNA and protein upon its transfection into rat, mouse or monkey cell lines.[56-58] The v-*src* and c-*src* genes have also been expressed in the yeast *Saccharomyces cerevisiae*.[59] While the posttranslational modification and enzymatic activities of pp60^{v-src} produced in yeast are indistinguishable from those of pp60^{v-src} produced in RSV-infected cells, the avian c-*src* protein produced in yeast is different from that produced in CEF cells with regard to both its *in vivo* state of phosphorylation and its *in vitro* kinase activity.

It was proposed that the human genome contains two c-*src* protooncogenes, one in chromosome 1p34-p36 (locus c-*src*-2) and the other in chromosome 20q12-q13 (locus c-*src*-1).[60,61] Both human c-*src* loci are expressed and the isolation and structural mapping of of the duplicated human c-*src* genes was reported.[62-64] However, all the available data, including chromosome localization and nucleotide sequence analysis, indicate that the c-*src*-2 gene is identical to the c-*fgr* protooncogene.[65] The following discussion is thus limited to the classic c-*src* gene.

In contrast to the coding regions of the chicken c-*src* gene, which spans a distance of 6 kb, the human c-*src* gene is much more larger and contains 11 coding exons spanning a distance of 19.5 kb. The nucleotide sequences of the human c-*src* gene exhibit 89% homology with the chicken c-*src* gene, which corresponds to 98% amino acid homology between the products of the human and chicken pp60^{c-src} products in the same region. These facts reflect strong functional constraints on the evolution of the pp60^{c-src} molecule region associated with tyrosine-specific protein kinase activity. In contrast, the region of human c-*src* coding for the amino-terminal one third of pp60^{c-src} exhibits considerably less homology to chicken c-*src* and RSV v-*src*.[64] Sequence analysis of the one-third 5′ coding region of the human c-*src* gene revealed that the region of the protein encoded by the second exon of the gene contains sequences specific for the *src* proteins from different species.[66] These sequences could be involved in the recognition of a *src*-specific substrate or receptor. A molecularly cloned human c-*src* gene has been expressed by using a replication-competent retroviral vector cloned from RSV.[67]

A. EXPRESSION OF THE C-*SRC* PROTOONCOGENE IN NORMAL CELLS AND TISSUES

The c-*src* gene is expressed in a diversity of normal metazoan cells and tissues, ranging from human and other mammals down to sponges.[68-72] Studies with antisense RNA (anti-mRNA) complementary to pp60^{c-src} mRNA lead to the suggestion that perhaps all metazoan cells may require some low level of pp60^{c-src} synthesis to remain viable.[73] A differential expression of the c-*src* gene has been observed in normal *Drosophila* and chicken cells and tissues, with age-dependent changes occurring in some tissues.[74-76] In the adult *Drosophila*, the majority of c-*src* transcripts are contained in the ovaries, especially in oocytes and nurse cells.[75,77] Transcripts of the *Drosophila* c-*src* gene are expressed predominantly during embryogenesis of the insect, in imaginal discs of third-instar larvae.

Tyrosine-specific protein kinase activity can be detected in normal human sera and blood cells, especially lymphocytes and polymorphonuclear cells, by an antiserum specific to pp60^{src}.[78] Activation of pp60^{c-src} kinase may be a normal physiological event associated with differentiation of myeloid cells.[79] High levels of pp60^{c-src}-specific protein-tyrosine kinase are expressed in human and rabbit platelets, which indicates that expression of this activity is not limited to proliferating cells.[80] Whereas the major tyrosine-protein kinase present in human platelets is apparently identical to pp60^{c-src}, or a degradation product of pp60^{src}, the endogenous phosphorylation of the anion channel band 3 in human erythrocyte membranes is not due to pp60^{c-src} activity but is associated with the activity of an unidentified enzyme.[81]

1. Expression of c-*src* in Neural Tissues

High levels of c-*src* expression are found in the central nervous system of vertebrates, where they are also subjected to developmental regulation.[74,82-85] In contrast to the protooncogene N-*myc*, which is expressed predominantly in undifferentiated human neural cells, expression of the c-*src* protooncogene increases in the primordial gray matter of human fetal brain and the ganglion cell layer of the retina with increasing fetal development.[86] pp60^{c-src} is specifically expressed at high levels in neurons and astrocytes but the structure of the protooncogene product in these cells is qualitatively different in two aspects: (1) the pp60^{c-src} protein from neurons exhibits a 6- to 12-times higher tyrosine-specific protein kinase activity than the protein from astrocytes and (2) the pp60^{c-src} protein from neurons contains a structural alteration within the amino-terminal domain of the molecule.[87] The latter alteration results in altered electrophoretic mobility of the protein and is not produced by posttranslational modification, but is probably generated by an alteration in the processing of c-*src* mRNA expressed in neurons.[88] In addition, the neuronal pp60^{c-src} protein contains a unique serine phosphorylation site within the amino-terminal part of the molecule.

Analysis of a c-*src* cDNA clone isolated from a mouse brain cDNA library revealed that it encodes a pp60^{c-src} protein that differs from chicken or human pp60^{c-src} in having an insert of six extra amino acids within the amino-terminal 16 kDa of the molecule.[89] S1 protection analysis confirmed that brain c-*src* mRNA contains a 18-nucleotide insertion at the position corresponding to the six extra amino acids. These differences are not species but organ specific. The evidence further indicated that brain-specific c-*src* mRNA may be originated by cell-specific differences in splicing of c-*src* mRNA. The specifically altered form of pp60^{c-src} present in the mouse brain is developmentally regulated,[90] which indicates its physiological importance. This molecular form of pp60^{c-src} is specific to the central nervous tissue and is not expressed at significant amounts in peripheral nervous system tissues.[91] The functional role of pp60^{c-src} in the central nervous system and other animal tissues is unknown. However, there is histochemical and experimental evidence in favor of a role of pp60^{c-src} in the differentiation of nervous tissue.[84,92] The pp60^{c-src} protein is a normal product of sensory neurons.[93]

Accumulation of pp60^{c-src} is developmentally regulated at the transcriptional level in tissues such as the embryonic neural retina.[94] The amount of c-*src* mRNA gradually increases during development of the neural retina in chicken embryos, reaching a peak by days 11 to 13 of embryonic life and decreasing thereafter to a level which persists also in adult retina. High levels of pp60^{c-src} expression have been detected in the membranes of chromaffin granules (secretory vesicles) from adrenal medullary chromaffin tissue, which suggests that the pp60^{c-src} kinase may function in the regulation of neurotransmitter release.[95]

2. Molecular Forms of pp60^{c-src}

In addition to the altered molecular form of the pp60^{c-src} protein present in neuronal cells, other normal or transformed cells may also contain variant molecular forms of the protein. Normal human fibroblasts and A431 human epidermoid carcinoma cells contain two forms of the normal protein product of c-*src*, differing in their molecular weights and phosphorylation sites.[96] More recently, different molecular forms of pp60^{v-src} and pp60^{c-src} have been detected.[97-99] Human tumors of neuroectodermal origin contain a molecular form of pp60^{c-src} with elevated level of specific kinase activity.[100] The tyrosine-specific protein kinase activity of pp60^{c-src} obtained from human colon cancer tissue specimens and tumor-derived cell lines is consistently elevated over the activity of pp60^{c-src} molecules isolated from normal human colon mucosa tissues and cultures of normal colonic mucosa cells.[101,102] Quantitative and qualitative changes of the pp60^{c-src} kinase occur during retinoic acid-induced differentiation of an embryonal carcinoma cell line into neuron-like cells.[103] An increased activity of the pp60^{c-src} kinase (4- to 11-fold), without concomitant increase in the protein, was observed in tumor derived SHE cell lines derived from *in vitro* induction of neoplastic transformation by chemical carcinogens.[104] No structural changes of the protein or alterations in the phosphorylation of tyrosine-527 or tyrosine-416, two sites involved in the regulation of the pp60^{c-src} kinase, were detected in these cells. The mechanism of activation remained uncharacterized but they could involve *trans*-acting factors present in the tumor cells. The possible role of elevated pp60^{c-src}-associated protein kinase activity in tumorigenic processes is unknown.

3. Expression of the c-*src* Gene in Skeletal Muscle

In skeletal muscle of the chicken, expression of the c-*src* gene was found to be different from that of other tissues, including cardiac and smooth muscles.[105] Whereas all other chicken tissues, as well as the embryonic chicken skeletal muscle, are characterized by the expression of a single c-*src* mRNA of 4.0 kb, shortly before hatching this transcript is replaced in the skeletal muscle by a smaller-sized (2.8 to 3.3 kb) class of c-*src* mRNAs, which persist into adulthood. These smaller c-*src* mRNAs are probably generated by alternative splicing and code for proteins which lack most of the kinase domain. The function of these skeletal muscle-specific c-*src*-related proteins is unknown.

B. PHILOGENY OF THE *SRC* PROTOONCOGENE

The protein product of the viral *src* oncogene, pp60^{v-src}, was initially considered as a marker for RSV infection.[106] However, it was found that nucleotide sequences related to the v-*src* oncogene and a protein similar to pp60$^{v\text{-}src}$, termed pp60$^{c\text{-}src}$, are present in uninfected animal cells.[107-112] Apparently, the c-*src* protooncogene exists in all metazoan species, including mammals, birds, fishes, insects, and sponges.[68,113-117] Two divergent c-*src* genes are expressed in *Xenopus laevis* and three loci related to the *src* oncogene are contained in the genome of *Drosophila*.[118,119] The third c-*src Drosophila* gene has been sequenced and it was found that the gene shares significant structural homology to other genes of vertebrate and *Drosophila* c-*src* family.[75] The third c-*src* gene of *Drosophila* is located at position 28C in the polytene chromosome map of the insect and contains an ORF capable of encoding a 66-kDa protein which is apparently expressed predominantly during embryogenesis as well as in the ovaries of the adult female insect. Another *Drosophila* c-*src* protooncogene was also sequenced and its differential expression in the tissues of the insect was determined.[76]

There is evidence for maternal inheritance of RNA transcripts from the three *Drosophila src*-related genes.[75] RNA transcripts from each of the *Drosophila* c-*src* genes are present in preblastoderm embryos, indicating that they are of maternal origin. As embryogenesis proceeds, the levels of these RNAs decline. The preblastoderm c-*src* RNAs of *Drosophila* contain polyadenylic acid and are present on polyribosomes, suggesting that they are functional mRNAs. It is thus clear that pp60$^{c\text{-}src}$ must be involved in some essential cellular function(s) during embryogenesis as well as in later stages of development.

Phosphotyrosine has been identified in yeast (*Saccharomyces cerevisiae*) proteins and tyrosine-specific protein kinase activity is associated with the plasma membrane of yeast cells.[120,121] Protein kinases with homology to the products of members of the *src* gene family may be involved in the initiation of the cell cycle in yeast.[122] Tyrosine kinase activity may exist even in bacteria. Phosphotyrosine and tyrosine kinase activity have been detected, for example, in the photosynthetic bacterium *Rhodospirillum rubrum* growing under photoautotrophic conditions.[123] Tyrosine-specific protein kinases and phosphotyrosine-containing proteins have also been detected in plants (peanut plantlets).[124] Thus, it seems that tyrosine-specific protein kinases and phosphotyrosine-containing proteins are universally present in living organisms.

In general, pp60$^{c\text{-}src}$ expression appears to be more related to cellular differentiation processes than to cellular proliferation.[125] However, the precise role of pp60$^{c\text{-}src}$ in processes of cell proliferation and cell differentiation is unknown. Whereas expression of c-*src* increases by 300 to 500% when PCC7 embryonal carcinoma cells are induced to differentiate into nerve-like cells, no c-*src* gene transcripts are detectable in either proliferating or differentiated F9 embryonal carcinoma cells.[126]

1. The *src* Oncogene Family

The c-*src* gene is member of a superfamily of evolutionary related genes and some of the products of this family are characterized by possessing tyrosine-specific protein kinase activity. This family includes, in addition to c-*src*, the protooncogenes c-*abl*, c-*yes*, c-*fps*, c-*fes*, c-*raf/mil/mht*, c-*erb*-B, c-*ros*, and c-*mos*.[127-129] Probably, these protooncogenes derive from a common ancestral gene, from which c-*mos* would represent the oldest known derivative, the next sequences being c-*raf* and c-*erb*-B.[130] The protein products of c-*mos*, c-*raf*, and c-*erb*-B do not possess tyrosine kinase activity, which would had been acquired later in evolution by the other members of the family, including the protein product of c-*src*.

2. pp60^{src} and the Catalytic Subunit of cAMP-Dependent Protein Kinase

Residues 259-485 of pp60^{src} have 22% sequence identity with residues 33 to 258 of the catalytic subunit of cAMP-dependent protein kinase, an enzyme that has specificity for serine phosphorylation.[131] The ATP analogue *p*-fluorosulfonylbenzoyl 5′-adenosine (FSBA) inactivates the tyrosine-specific protein kinase activity of pp60^{src} by reacting with lysine at position 295.[132] Neither arginine nor histidine can carry out the function of lysine-295 in the ATP-binding site of pp60^{src}.[133] When aligned for maximum sequence identity, lysine-295 of pp60^{src} and the lysine in the catalytic subunit of the kinase, which also reacts with FSBA, are superimposed precisely. This functional homology is strong evidence that the protein kinases, irrespective of amino acid substrate specificity, comprise a single divergent gene family.[132]

IV. THE PROTEIN PRODUCT OF THE V-*SRC* ONCOGENE AND ITS ASSOCIATED KINASE ACTIVITY

The protein product of the v-*src* oncogene is a 60-kDa phosphoprotein kinase composed of 526 amino acids.[134] The RSV *src* protein has been purified over 2400-fold by affinity chromatography techniques.[135,136] pp60[v-*src*] with functional activity has been obtained by cloning the v-*src* gene in molecular vectors, followed by introduction of the vectors into bacteria or mouse cells.[137-139] The latter (immature murine lymphoid cells) become transformed and express high amounts of pp60[v-*src*] after transfection with a recombinant retrovirus (MRSV) containing the v-*src* gene. Rat cells are also transformed upon transfection with chimeric plasmids containing a cloned v-*src* gene, whereas the same cells are not transformed when the chimeric plasmid contains a c-*src* gene cloned from the chicken genome.[140] The location of v-*src* in a retrovirus vector would determine whether the viral product is toxic or transforming.[141] Inserting the v-*src* gene near the 5' end of a viral vector genome (a modified spleen necrosis virus (SNV) vector) results in a vector with an acute toxic effect on cultured chicken and dog cells, whereas insertion of the oncogene near the 3' end of the viral vector (i.e., in a similar location as in ASV) results in less toxic and more marked transforming effects. Recombinant M-MuLV carrying the v-*src* gene induce transformation *in vitro* and pathological changes *in vivo*.[142]

The purified pp60[v-*src*] protein obtained from bacterial recombinants can be used as an antigen for injection into rabbits and production of a highly specific cross-reactive serum that recognizes the v-*src* protein from many different strains of RSV.[143,144] Antibodies to pp60[src] can also be obtained by using as antigens synthetic oligopeptides corresponding to specific regions of the primary structure of pp60[v-*src*].[145,146] Monoclonal antibodies have been produced by hybridoma techniques against the oncogene product of RSV and some of these antibodies cross-react with pp60[c-*src*] from chicken, rodent, or human origin.[147-149]

The purified protein product of the v-*src* oncogene possesses cAMP-independent protein kinase activity.[150,151] This kinase has specificity for phosphorylation of tyrosine residues on different protein substrates.[152,153] Phosphorylation of cellular proteins on tyrosine residues seems to be relatively infrequent. In normal chicken embryo fibroblasts only about 0.03% of the acid-stable phosphorylated amino acids in protein are phosphotyrosines, this level being increased six- to tenfold after transformation by RSV. The tyrosine-specific protein kinase activity of pp60[v-*src*] can be specifically inhibited *in vivo* by the isoflavone compound genistein, which does not affect the activity of serine and threonine kinases.[154] A monoclonal antibody, R2D2, can inhibit the specific kinase activity of the pp60[v-*src*] protein as well as the specific activity of the products of two other members of the v-*src* family, pp70[gag-fgr] and pp90[gag-yes].[155] Binding sites in both the amino-terminal 110 amino acid residues and the carboxy-terminal 240 residues of pp60[v-*src*] have been identified for the R2D2 antibody. These results indicate that at least a part of the epitope recognized by R2D2 resides within the carboxy-terminal region of the pp60[v-*src*] protein which is essentially required for protein kinase activity.

A. PHOSPHORYLATION OF THE *SRC* PROTEIN

The pp60[v-*src*] protein contains several phosphorylation sites. One major phosphorylation site is a serine residue situated in the amino-terminal portion of the molecule and the other site is a tyrosine residue in the carboxy-terminal portion.[153,156-158]

1. Phosphorylation of pp60[src] on Serine and Threonine

Some regions of the pp60[src] molecule are structurally related to the catalytic chain of mammalian cAMP-dependent protein kinase,[131] and cAMP may increase the phosphorylation of pp60$^{v\text{-}src}$ on serine, which enhances the associated kinase activity in intact cells.[159] The major site of serine phosphorylation in both the v-*src*- and c-*src*-encoded proteins is serine-17, which is the target of cAMP-dependent protein kinase.[111,156] An elevated expression of v-*src* coincides with a marked decrease of type-I cAMP-dependent protein kinase activity in baby hamster kidney (BHK) cells.[160]

The growth factor PDGF and the phorbol ester TPA induce quiescent, serum-deprived chicken embryo cells to enter the cell cycle and this phenomenon is accompanied by a two- to fourfold increase in serine phosphorylation of pp60$^{c\text{-}src}$.[161] The phosphorylation occurs very soon after the initial stimulation to growth by either PDGF or TPA and is localized to the amino-terminal end of the pp60$^{c\text{-}src}$ molecule, a region which has an essential role for transformation, not necessarily dependent on tyrosine phosphorylation. The enzyme responsible for phosphorylation of pp60$^{c\text{-}src}$ on serine has not been identified but one possible candidate is protein kinase C. Phosphorylation on the amino-terminal part of the pp60^{src} molecule, at serine-12, may depend on protein kinase C activity.[162] TPA activates protein kinase C, and induces phosphorylation of pp60^{src} exclusively on the serine-12 residue.[163,164] Stimulation of T lymphocytes or the Jurkat T-cell line with soluble antibodies to the CD3/T-cell receptor complex results in activation and translocation of protein kinase C and phosphorylation of pp60$^{c\text{-}src}$ on serine-12.[165] The biological significance of phosphorylation of pp60$^{v\text{-}src}$ on serine-12 is not understood, since it is apparently not reflected in a change in the kinetic properties of the pp60$^{v\text{-}src}$ kinase.[166]

The pp60$^{c\text{-}src}$ protein of mouse fibroblasts (modified NIH/3T3 cells) may undergo a cell cycle-specific modification which consists in threonine and, possibly, serine phosphorylation within its 16-kDa amino-terminal region during mitosis.[167] At the same time, serine-17, the site of cAMP-dependent phosphorylation, appears to be dephosphorylated during mitosis. While the amount of pp60$^{c\text{-}src}$ is not significantly altered during the cell cycle, the specific kinase activity of modified pp60$^{c\text{-}src}$ is enhanced during mitosis. This activation is independent of phosphorylation on either tyrosine-416 or tyrosine-527. These results suggest that pp60$^{c\text{-}src}$ may be involved in the regulation of mitotic events.

2. Phosphorylation of pp60^{src} on Tyrosine

The viral protein, pp60$^{v\text{-}src}$, is phosphorylated both *in vivo* and *in vitro* predominantly at tyrosine-416.[168] In contrast, only a trace amount of phosphorylation of the cellular protein, pp60$^{c\text{-}src}$, at tyrosine-416 is observed *in vivo*.[169] The major site of pp60$^{c\text{-}src}$ tyrosine phosphorylation is located on one or more of the three tyrosine residues located on the carboxy-terminal portion of the molecule, at positions 511, 519, and 527.[170,171] Tyrosines 519 and 527 are situated in the carboxy-terminal 19-amino acid segment of the cellular protein that is deleted and replaced by an unrelated sequence the viral protein. Tyrosine-511 is in the region common to both the cellular and the viral protein and is situated four residues from the junction where the sequences of pp60$^{c\text{-}src}$ and pp60$^{v\text{-}src}$ diverge.[170]

Since tyrosine-527 is not present in pp60$^{v\text{-}src}$ it has been suggested that the increase in transforming ability and kinase activity that occurred in the genesis of pp60$^{v\text{-}src}$ may have resulted from the loss of this site that would be involved in negative regulation of the protein function.[171] Phosphorylation of tyrosine-527 may be important for maintaining the lower kinase activity of pp60$^{c\text{-}src}$, as compared to the higher kinase activity of pp60$^{v\text{-}src}$. Dephosphorylation of pp6060$^{c\text{-}src}$ by phosphatase treatment *in vitro* causes a 10- to 20-fold increase in pp60$^{c\text{-}src}$ protein-tyrosine kinase activity and a similar increase is obtained by the binding of specific antibody to the region of pp60$^{c\text{-}src}$ which contains phosphotyrosine-527.[172] The avian pp60$^{c\text{-}src}$ produced in genetically manipulated yeast is underphosphorylated at tyrosine-527 and this is accompanied by a significant increase in its tyrosine-specific protein kinase activity.[59,173] Artificial replacement of phenylalanine for tyrosine at position 527 strongly activates pp60$^{c\text{-}src}$ transforming and kinase activities, whereas the additional introduction of a similar replacement at position 416 suppresses these activities.[174] Tyr-Phe mutation of normal pp60$^{c\text{-}src}$ eliminates its partial transforming activity in particular experimental systems. Unfortunately, almost nothing is known about the molecular mechanisms involved in the regulation of pp60$^{c\text{-}src}$ kinase activity within normal or transformed cells. Studies with site-directed mutagenesis in which the ATP-binding site of pp60$^{c\text{-}src}$ is destroyed, and its kinase activity is abolished, strongly suggest that phosphorylation of tyrosine-527 in the pp60$^{c\text{-}src}$ protein depends not on autophosphorylation but on the action of another tyrosine kinase present in normal chicken cells.[175]

Protein pp60$^{c\text{-}src}$ associated with the polyoma virus middle-T antigen contains a phosphorylation site on a tyrosine residue located within the carboxy-terminal portion of the molecule.[176] This phosphorylation site is absent in pp60$^{c\text{-}src}$ molecules which are not associated with polyoma virus middle-T antigen. The biological meaning of these qualitative differences is not understood.

3. Biological Significance of pp60^{src}-Induced Phosphorylation

The specific kinase activity of pp60$^{v\text{-}src}$ can be inhibited by means of a synthetic decapeptide homologous to the amino acid sequence located around the tyrosine phosphorylation site of the enzyme.[177] Moreover, antibodies generated against two synthetic peptides corresponding to two defined regions of pp60$^{v\text{-}src}$ interact specifically with the EGF receptor protein.[178] In particular, the cytoplasmic (carboxy-terminal) portion of the EGF receptor, which contains the tyrosine and autophosphorylation domains of the molecule, is antigenically related to pp60$^{v\text{-}src}$.

Viral factors in addition to those related to the specific kinase activity of pp60$^{v\text{-}src}$ are probably necessary for expression of the growth control properties associated with the viral protein product.[179] In cells infected with temperature-conditional RSV mutants, pp60$^{v\text{-}src}$ kinase activity shows no consistent correlation with several parameters of cell transformation.[180,181] Thus, it is important to identify the primary cellular targets of pp60$^{v\text{-}src}$ kinase activity for understanding the mechanisms of transformation associated with this oncogene product.

Different physical and immunologic species of pp60$^{v\text{-}src}$ can be identified in RSV-transformed cells but their functional significance is not understood. Fractions of pp60$^{v\text{-}src}$ obtained from RSV-transformed cells by immunoprecipitation with a specific monoclonal antibody differ in their phosphoaminoacid profile but these fractions do not show differences in their tyrosyl kinase specific activities.[182] Thus, yet to be defined modifications of the v-src protein may be involved in its functional regulation.

4. Alteration of pp60$^{c\text{-}src}$ Phosphorylation by Viral Oncogene Products

Quail, chicken, and rat cells infected with the AEV (which transduces both the v-erb-A and v-erb-B oncogenes) exhibit a marked reduction in the specific activity of the endogenous pp60$^{c\text{-}src}$ kinase as well as an hypophosphorylation of this kinase on serine and threonine residues.[183] A similar reduction of the pp60$^{c\text{-}src}$ kinase is observed when cells are transformed by other acute retroviruses whose oncogene products are characterized by tyrosine-specific protein kinase activity, e.g., v-fms, v-yes, and v-fgr. The mechanisms by which the inhibition of pp60$^{c\text{-}src}$ activity occurs in these cells is unknown, but the observed hypophosphorylation of pp60$^{c\text{-}src}$ in AEV-infected cells suggests a role for both serine and tyrosine phosphatases.

V. CELLULAR MECHANISMS OF ACTION OF PP60^{src}

In spite of extensive experimental studies, the cellular mechanisms of action of pp60^{src} (of either viral or cellular origin) are little understood.[184-187] However, as a general rule, there is a strong correlation between the biological effects of the *src* protein products and their respective tyrosine-specific kinase activities. This correlation may be studied with the aid of specific inhibitors of these type of activity such as the isoflavone compound genistein.[154]

Many cellular components are modified by the kinase action of pp60^{src} and it seems likely that this oncogene product acts on more than one primary cellular target,[187-189] although it is difficult to discard the possibility of a single primary target followed by some type of "cascade phenomenon". The specific cellular alterations produced by pp60^{v-src} may be explained on the basis that the cellular proteins modified by infection of mouse or rat cells by RSV are different from those modified by the action of other oncogenes of the *src* family, like *fps*, *fes*, and *abl*.[190]

A. EFFECTS OF PP60^{src} ON THE PLASMA MEMBRANE

After synthesis, pp60^{src} forms a complex with two proteins in the cytoplasmic compartment of the cell, and the kinase is thereafter attached to some component of the plasma membrane.[191] The pp60^{src} protein of either viral or cellular origin is associated with the inner face of the plasma membrane,[192-195] although it was also found to be associated with the external aspect of the membrane.[196]

1. Association of pp60^{src} with the Cell Membrane

Protein pp60^{src} is anchored to the plasma membrane by some portion of its amino-terminal domain, whereas the kinase activity is carried by the carboxy-terminal half of the molecule.[197] Myristic acid, a rare 14-carbon saturated fatty acid, is attached to glycine at the amino terminal region of pp60^{src} of either viral or cellular origin immediately after synthesis and is present in both soluble and membrane bound forms of the protein.[198-201] Changes in the amino-terminal sequence of pp60^{v-src} decrease both the membrane association of the protein and its tumorigenic action,[202] and the first ten amino acids within this region are required for pp60^{src} myristoylation, from which depends pp60^{src} membrane association and pp60^{src}-induced transformation.[198,203,204] RSV point mutants in which the amino-terminal glycine residue of pp60^{v-src} is changed to an alanine or a glutamic acid residue fail to become myristylated and are not able to transform cells.[205] The mutant pp60^{v-src} proteins are as active as the wild-type oncogene protein but exhibit a lack of association with cell membranes, remaining at a cytosolic location. These results lend support to the hypothesis that membrane association is critically required for the transforming potential of pp60^{v-src} and that the elevation of cellular phosphotyrosine content produced by the tyrosine-specific protein kinase activity of the oncogenic product is, by itself, insufficient for cellular transformation. However, the specific kinase activity is required for transformation. Changes produced by site-directed mutagenesis techniques in a restricted region of the carboxy-terminal region of the protein lead to a decrease in the specific kinase activity and also result in a concomitant loss of the transforming potential of the mutant virus.[206,207]

2. pp60^{src}-Induced Modification of Cell Surface Proteins

The infection of susceptible cells with RSV results in an array of functional changes occurring at the level of plasma membrane, including alterations in the hexose and amino acid transport and an increase in thymidine transport.[208] The biochemical changes responsible for the functional alterations observed in the plasma membrane of RSV-infected cells are not well understood but they may be related to the synthesis, degradation, or specific structural modification of particular cell surface proteins. RSV-transformed chicken cells are characterized by a highly efficient glucose transport system, which is due not to increased synthesis or phosphorylation of the transporter protein but to a decrease in the transporter protein degradation rate.[209] In contrast, glucose starvation increases the rate of glucose transport into the cells by affecting the biosynthesis of the specific transport protein.

Phosphorylation of cell surface proteins is associated with RSV-induced transformation of chick embryo fibroblasts.[210,211] Different plasma membrane components are apparently phosphorylated on tyrosine residues by the action of pp60^{src} but they are not well characterized. The band 3 protein, which is one of the major integral membrane glycoproteins of the human erythrocytes (and probably also of other cell types), is phosphorylated on tyrosine residues by the purified pp60^{v-src} kinase by the purified pp60^{v-src} kinase as well as by the purified EGF receptor kinase.[212] Other membrane proteins may be specifically dephosphorylated as a result of pp60^{src} activity.[213] The phenomenon of dephosphorylation observed in RSV-transformed cells could be produced as a consequence of secondary effects related in some manner to the primary action of pp60^{src}.

RSV-induced transformation of BHK cells is associated with alteration in complex-type N-linked oligosaccharides expressed on the cell surface.[214] In particular, RSV-transformed BHK cells express more relative amounts of asparagine-linked oligosaccharides containing the sequence N-acetylglucosamine-β^{1,6}mannose-α^{1,6}mannose than do parental BHK cells. However, this modification is apparently not characteristic of RSV-transformed cells since it is also present in polyoma virus-transformed BHK cells.[214]

3. Cell Surface Antigens in RSV-Transformed Cells

A tumor-specific cell surface antigen, not related to the pp60^{v-src} protein, is expressed in RSV-transformed mouse and rat cells, but not in cells infected with retroviruses transducing other oncogenes of the *src* family.[190] Two antigens of the human MHC system, HLA-A2 and HLA-B7, are phosphorylated *in vitro* by pp60^{v-src}.[215] The phosphorylation occurs at a tyrosine residue encoded in a highly conserved exon of the antigen intracellular domain.

4. Fibronectin and Adhesion Plaques in RSV-Transformed Cells

Fibronectin is a major extracellular adhesive protein and its local degradation is believed to play an important role in the migration of cells through the extracellular matrix during tumor invasion. Fibronectin is lost from the cell surface of cells after transformation with RSV and newly expressed pp60^{v-src} is localized at the cytoplasmic surface of the cell membrane, corresponding to the cell contact sites where the degradation of extracellular fibronectin occurs.[216] Some ASV isolates encode pp60^{v-src} size-variant proteins with alterations in the amino-terminal membrane binding domain and these proteins behave as peripheral membrane proteins, being localized in adhesion plaques and regions of cell-to-cell contact.[217] Adhesion plaques and fibronectin expression in the cellular matrix may be interconnected phenomena and could be related to the maintenance of a transformed morphology.[7] The predominant cellular shape caused by infection with wild-type RSV is highly rounded and refractile but a number of RSV mutants have been isolated that induce a very elongated spindle shape called fusiform. In fusiform mutant-infected cells, pp60^{v-src} is made in amounts equivalent to those in wild-type RSV-infected cells and the oncogene product has full tyrosine-specific protein kinase activity. Furthermore, fusiform mutant-infected cells grow in soft agar and are tumorigenic. This suggests that one domain of the v-*src* gene controls oncogenic transformation and another, independent domain influences the transformed cell shape. It has been shown that, whereas cells transformed with wild-type RSV contain pp60^{v-src} in adhesion plaques and lack fibronectin in the extracellular matrix, all fusiform mutant-transformed cells lack significant location of pp60^{v-src} in the adhesion plaques but express an abundant extracellular matrix of fibronectin.[7]

An adhesion-plaque protein complex, the fibronectin receptor, was identified as a substrate for phosphorylation induced in CEF cells by RSV and other acute transforming retroviruses whose products possess tyrosine-specific protein kinase activity.[218] Three fibronectin receptor protein components of 160, 140, and 120 kDa are expressed on the surface of both normal and transformed cells and two of these proteins (those of 140 and 120 kDa) are selectively phosphorylated in the RSV-transformed cells but not in the normal cells. The three proteins comprising the avian fibronectin receptor presumably span the plasma membrane, with the extracellular domain binding to fibronectin and laminin and the intracellular domain forming attachments to the cytoskeleton through talin.[218] Thus, the fibronectin receptor functions both as a receptor for extracellular matrix proteins and as a link with cytoskeletal elements and may represent an important substrate for the morphological alterations observed in RSV-transformed cells. A concomitant loss of fibronectin and the 140-kDa fibronectin receptor are observed in

CEF cells after RSV-induced transformation.[219] However, both normal and RSV-transformed cells contain enzymes capable of degrading fibronectin and other components of the extracellular matrix, and fibronectin degrading activities are apparently similar in normal and transformed cells.[220]

B. EFFECTS OF PP60^{src} ON THE CYTOPLASM

Several cytoplasmic proteins are phosphorylated on tyrosine residues, as well as on serine and threonine residues, as a primary or secondary result of pp60^{src} action.[221] However, the relative importance of these proteins in RSV-induced neoplastic transformation is little understood.

1. The p36 Protein

A possible primary target of pp60^{src} is a 36,000-Da protein (36K or p36 protein). A cDNA clone complementary to sequences for the p36 protein has been constructed.[222] Using the cDNA probe for p36 it has been determined that the size of p36 mRNA is 1100 nucleotides and that the levels of p36 mRNA are approximately the same in all adult chicken tissues examined but are significantly higher in cultured chicken cells. A method for calcium-dependent isolation of p36 has been proposed and the fractionation of the phosphorylated p36 species has been reported.[223] In the absence of Ca^{2+} chelators, three cellular proteins copurify with p36 extracted from a cytosolic or membrane fraction of CEF cells.[224]

Protein p36 is phosphorylated *in vitro* by pp60^{v-src} and is also phosphorylated in avian and mammalian cells after RSV infection.[211,225-228] The pp60^{src} protein kinase is intimately associated with the plasma membrane and p36 is localized mainly on the inner, cytoplasmic face of the plasma membrane.[229,230] Moreover, the p36 protein substrate of pp60^{v-src} is myristylated in a transformation-sensitive manner.[231]

Protein p36 has domains related to Ca^{2+} and lipid binding.[232] This protein belongs to the Ca^{2+}-dependent membrane-binding protein family and shows structural homology to a 67-kDa protein isolated from the bovine aorta.[233] Phosphorylation of p36 on tyrosine residues is enhanced by Ca^{2+} and it is possible that p36, like protein kinase C, is a Ca^{2+}-activated, phospholipid-dependent protein.[234] Protein p36 is phosphorylated *in vitro* and *in vivo* on serine and threonine residues by protein kinase C in a Ca^{2+}- and phospholipid-dependent process.[235] p36 is phosphorylated on tyrosine-23 by tyrosine-specific kinases, including the pp60^{c-src} kinase, and on serine-25 by protein kinase C.[236] Modulation of p36 phosphorylation on serine and tyrosine induced by growth factors has been studied in human cells using two anti-p36 monoclonal antibodies.[237]

Protein p36 is found in cytoplasmic (85%) and nuclear (15%) cellular fractions, and in both fractions it is associated with small ribonucleoprotein particles.[238] The function of such p36-RNP complexes is unknown. Protein p36 is expressed only in certain rodent tissues (fibroblasts, epithelial cells, cardiac muscle cells, macrophages, testicular interstitial cells) and is absent in other tissues (smooth muscle cells, erythrocytes, lymphocytes, nerve cells).[239] Phosphorylation of p36 is significantly reduced in full revertant cell clones originated from RSV-transformed cells.[240] However, phosphorylation of p36 is not an exclusive property of RSV or other acute retroviruses since it also occurs in cells treated with growth factors such as EGF and PDGF.[241-244]

The precise function of the p36 protein, also called calpactin I,[245] has not been characterized. Expression of p36 is developmentally regulated in the avian embryonic limb and it has been suggested that p36 may have a structural or mechanical function.[246] Protein p36 exhibits structural homology to lipocortin.[247] Recent evidence indicates that p36 and a related protein, p35, are identical to lipocortins II and I, respectively.[248,249] Lipocortins are phosphoproteins with an inhibiting effect on the activity of phospholipase A$_2$, an enzyme involved in the generation of leukotrienes and prostaglandins from phospholipid metabolite precursors. In any case, the role of p36 in neoplastic transformation has not been elucidated.

2. Proteins pp50 and pp90

Two cytoplasmic phosphoproteins of 50 kDa (pp50) and 90 kDa (pp90) interact with pp60^{src} but their respective functions are not understood.[250,251] Both pp50 and pp90 proteins display stable noncovalent interaction with *gag-onc* fusion proteins of different FeSV isolates.[252] The pp90 phosphoprotein is an abundant cytoplasmic protein present in normal cells and is associated with steroid hormone receptors.[253,254] Protein pp90 is apparently identical to the chicken and mouse heat-shock protein HSP90.[255] Circumstantial evidence supports a transport or membrane-directing function for a complex between pp60^{src}, pp50, and pp90.[256] Protein pp90/HSP90 is an actin-binding protein that can cross-link actin filaments.[257] The interaction of pp90/HSP90 and F-actin is inhibited by calmodulin.[258] Protein pp90/HSP90 forms a highly stable complex with the protein products of the oncogenes v-*src*, v-*fps*, v-*yes*, v-*fes*, and v-*fgr*, which are members of the tyrosine-protein kinase family of oncogenes. Protein pp90/HSP90 also form stable complexes with steroid hormone receptors.[254,259,260] The results suggest a modulatory action of pp90/HSP90 on both the oncogene protein products and the steroid hormone receptors. They also suggest that the transforming action of some oncogene protein products may be exerted, at least in part, through their interaction with particular HSPs, which would involve an alteration of actin components of the cytoskeleton.

3. Higher Molecular Weight Proteins

Other protein substrates for pp60^{src} kinase may have higher molecular weight. Approximately 30% of phosphotyrosine-containing protein molecules present in RSV-transformed cells have sizes greater than 100 kDa.[261] A protein of 120 kDa containing phosphotyrosine is coimmunoprecipitated with pp60^{v-src} in RSV-transformed mammalian cells.[262] Phosphotyrosine-containing proteins of 230 and 130 kDa are prominent in RSV-transformed cells, but other proteins of lower molecular weight are also immunoprecipitated in the same cells by antibodies specific for phosphotyrosine.[263]

4. Cytoskeletal Components

Cytoskeletal proteins are important substrates for tyrosine-specific protein kinases *in vitro* and probably also *in vivo*. Cytoskeletal association of pp60^{v-src} has been ascertained by different methods, including electronmicroscopic techniques and immunoferritin labeling.[264] In RSV-transformed NRK cells, pp60^{v-src} was found to be localized on different components of the cytoskeleton, including actin microfilaments present in adhesion plaques, adherent junctions between cells, and microfilament bundles. Association of pp60^{v-src} with cytoskeletal components may be relevant to its transforming potential. While more than 70% of this viral product has been found to be associated with detergent-insoluble cytoskeletal proteins in RSV-transformed cells, nontransforming proteins, including pp60^{c-src}, are found mainly in the fraction solubilized by the detergent extraction.[265,266] This difference in the affinities of the v-*src* and c-*src* protein products for cytoskeletal proteins may explain, at least in part, the lack of ability of pp60^{c-src} to transform cells.

The microfilament and microtubule protein substrates of the pp60^{v-src} kinase are different from those of the EGF and insulin receptor kinases.[267] A well-identified target, phosphorylated on tyrosine residues by the action of pp60^{src}, is vinculin,[268,269] a 130-kDa cytoskeletal protein involved in the anchorage of microfilaments to the plasma membrane. Additional phosphorylation of tyrosine residues in vinculin does not occur upon transformation by ASVs containing oncogenes other than v-*src*, like v-*fps*, v-*ros*, and v-*fes*.[270] The functional significance of phosphorylation of vinculin on tyrosine remains unknown. Addition of fibronectin to the medium of RSV-transformed CEFs restores morphology similar to that of untransformed cells, but this reversion is not accompanied by a decrease in tyrosine-specific phosphorylation of vinculin.[271] Studies with a *ts* mutant of RSV (*ts* LA32), which displays no detectable defect in tyrosine-specific kinase activity but cannot transform cells at the restrictive temperature, clearly show that the presence of an active pp60[v-src] tyrosine-specific kinase and phosphorylation of vinculin on tyrosine are not sufficient to perturb cell morphology in a characteristic transformation-associated manner.[272] These results suggest that phosphorylation of tyrosine residues on vinculin is not a key determinant in the rounded morphology characteristic of RSV-transformed CEFs.

Other modification found in vinculin is the covalently attachment of fatty acid.[273] Palmitic acid, or a derivative of it, is linked to vinculin and a reduction of this binding accompanies transformation of CEFs by RSV and correlates with a change in cell morphology. The mechanism involved in pp60[v-src]-induced acylation of vinculin is unknown but this modification could provide a mechanism to alter the organization of vinculin within the cells and thereby may play a regulatory role in anchoring or stabilizing microfilament bundles at the plasma membrane.[273] However, the possible role of vinculin modification in the expression of a morphologically transformed phenotype remains to be determined.

Another protein present in the focal adhesions where stress fibers are attached to the membrane is talin, a 215-kDa protein. Talin might mediate interactions between the cytoskeleton and the extracellular matrix. In RSV-transformed CEFs, talin exhibits a significant increase (about threefold) in its phosphotyrosine content and a marked intracellular redistribution of talin is observed in these cells.[274] However, only 3% of the talin molecules contain phosphotyrosine residues in RSV-transformed CEFs. Tyrosine phosphorylation of talin, like that of vinculin, is insufficient to induce any of the known parameters of transformation and does not correlate with any transformed morphology.[275] Other proteins associated with the stress fibers of normal CEFs, e.g., filamin, α-actinin, and myosin, do not show increased phosphorylation on tyrosine after RSV-induced transformation.

The major cytoskeletal component of both normal and transformed cells is the contractile protein actin. This protein is present both as monomeric globular (G) actin and as large macromolecular assemblies which include long polymers of filamentous (F) actin, some appearing as single filaments and others as thicker filament bundles.[276] The larger actin complexes also contain several actin-associated proteins and there is evidence that two mammalian heat shock proteins, HSP90 and HSP100, are actin-binding proteins.[257] RSV-induced transformation of Rat-1 fibroblasts is associated with depolymerization of cytosolic actin and increased proportion of actin polymers in the cytoskeleton cores.[276] The shifts observed in the cytosolic actin monomer/polymer equilibrium state could play a significant role in some of the morphological features of RSV-induced transformation, including alteration in cell shape towards a more "rounded up" morphology and also in the decreased adhesiveness of cells. A marked reduction of binding sites for cytochalasins (fungal alkaloid metabolites that have potent activity on actin-related cytoskeletal and motile functions) is found on actin filaments of RSV-transformed CEF cells.[277] Moreover, extracts of the transformed cells have a significant higher level of endogenous cytochalasin-like activity that extracts of nontransformed cells.

Studies have been performed using purified native microfilament- and microtubule-related proteins as substrates for the purified pp60[v-src] kinase *in vitro*.[267] Among the filament proteins, the purified *src* kinase preferentially phosphorylates the α subunit of fodrin on tyrosine residues and this phosphorylation is not inhibited by F-actin. Among microtubule proteins, the *src* kinase favors the phosphorylation of tubulin as compared to protein MAP2. The peptide mapping of MAP2 phosphorylated by the *src* kinase is different from that of the insulin and EGF receptor kinases, which show marked similarities.

5. Ribosomal Protein S6

The S6 ribosomal protein kinase is also phosphorylated by the action of pp60[v-src].[278] This phosphorylation occurs not on tyrosine but on serine residues and a similar modification is induced by a variety of tumor viruses as well as by serum or phorbol ester.[279-282] Apparently, all of these agents stimulate S6 phosphorylation by acting through some common pathway(s).

Exposure of quiescent mouse fibroblasts to different mitogenic stimuli indicate that a common kinase, termed mitogen-activated S6 kinase, is involved in the response generated by all the various factors.[283] The same S6 kinase could mediate the pp60[src]-induced phosphorylation of the ribosomal protein S6. Similar S6 kinase activity is found in insulin-treated 3T3-L1 cells and RSV-transformed chick embryo fibroblasts.[284] Microinjection of pp60[v-src] into *Xenopus* oocytes increases phosphorylation of protein S6 and other proteins and accelerates the rate of progesterone-induced meiotic maturation.[285,286]

6. Protein Phosphatase 1

Protein phosphatase 1 is one of four major protein phosphatases involved in cellular regulation. The function of this enzyme is best understood in skeletal muscle where it participates in the control of glycogen metabolism. However, protein phosphatase 1 is active towards other phosphorylated proteins involved in the regulation of such diverse cellular processes as glycolysis, gluconeogenesis, fatty acid synthesis, cholesterol synthesis, protein synthesis, muscle contraction, aromatic amino acid breakdown, and neurotransmission. Phosphorylation of the enzyme on tyrosine *in vitro* by the pp60[v-src] kinase is accompanied by a loss of the enzyme activity.[287] Phosphorylation of phosphatase 1 by pp60[v-src] decreases its activity towards phosphorylase kinase and glycogen synthase as well as towards phosphorylase a.[288] The pp60[v-src] phosphorylation sites are in a region of protein phosphatase 1 which influences substrate binding and which may be near the active site of the enzyme.

7. Glycolytic Enzymes

Protein pp60[v-src] phosphorylates in cultured cells three glycolytic enzymes (enolase, phosphoglycerate mutase, and lactate dehydrogenase).[289] These enzymes catalyze three out of the last four steps of glycolysis and their modification may contribute to the high rate of aerobic glycolysis observed in transformed cells, evident from the rapid glucose uptake and lactate production observed in cells transformed by different agents, including RSV.

The rate of glycolysis is increased in RSV-transformed cells, as it is in many other types of transformed cells. This change correlates with increased activity of the enzyme 6-phosphofructo-2-kinase (PFK-2) which results in a threefold increase in the concentration of fructose 2,6-bisphosphate.[290] The PFK-2/fructose 2,6-bisphosphate system is involved in the control of glycolysis by mitogens and tumor promoters (phorbol esters).

8. Calmodulin and Caldesmon

In RSV-transformed cultured fibroblasts the normal, ordered pattern of actin-containing stress fibers is altered and is replaced by a diffuse network of actin-containing matrix. By use of the indirect immunofluorescence technique, it has been found that in these cells the calmodulin- and F-actin-binding protein caldesmon is decreased and that its intracellular distribution is changed to a diffuse and blurred appearance, which is very much the same of the antiactin pattern observed in the transformed state.[291] Phosphorylation of calmodulin at tyrosine residues is observed in RSV-transformed cells.[135] In an *in vitro* system, tyrosine phosphorylation of calmodulin by pp60[v-src] is inhibited by Ca^{2+} and the structure of calmodulin-Ca^{2+} complex may be altered by tyrosine phosphorylation.[292] These changes of caldesmon and calmodulin in transformed cells may correlate with the loss of Ca^{2+} regulation which is associated with malignant transformation.

9. Glutamic Acid Decarboxylase

In neuronal cells (quail embryo neuroretina cultures), pp60[v-src] can selectively stimulate the activity of the enzyme glutamic acid decarboxylase (GAD), which is responsible for the synthesis of the neurotransmitter γ-aminobutyric acid (GABA).[293] GAD activity is also stimulated in the same cells by retroviruses carrying the v-*mil* oncogene. The possible physiological significance of these observations is unclear but this is an example of a differentiated cellular function activated by pp60$^{v\text{-}src}$. In both chick neural retina and cerebellum, expression of the c-*src* protooncogene occurs in developing neurons at the onset of differentiation, at a stage when cell proliferation ceases.[82,84]

C. EFFECTS OF PP60^{src} ON THE NUCLEUS

Profound changes in genome expression occur in RSV-infected cells. Moreover, rearrangements of viral and cellular DNA are often associated with RSV expression in these cells.[32] There is evidence that RSV encodes a transcriptional activator that may influence the expression of cellular genes and that pp60^{src} produces selective changes in genomic functions, activating the transcription of particular gene subsets.[43,294]

1. Cellular Genes Activated for the pp60^{src}-Induced Mitogenic Response

The putative genes responding to pp60^{src} are almost unknown. It may be true that the activation of only a few cellular genes is sufficient for the mitogenic action of pp60^{src}. While serum stimulation of serum-deprived NRK cells results in the synthesis of over 100 cellular proteins during G_1 transit, pp60$^{v\text{-}src}$ action do not produce an increase in total protein synthesis and only six proteins (18.5 to 44 kDa) are clearly increased when the quiescent cells are stimulated to transit G_1 by pp60$^{v\text{-}src}$ action.[295] The appearance of the six proteins and the subsequent initiation of DNA replication may have resulted from pp60$^{v\text{-}src}$ stimulating only a small number of cellular genes because both the protein changes and DNA replication are completely suppressed by the transcription inhibitor actinomycin D. Transcription of the c-*myc* protooncogene may be strongly activated by RSV infection in both rat fibroblasts and chick embryo cells.[296]

By studying RSV mutants it has been concluded that the expression of the mitogenic action of pp60$^{v\text{-}src}$ does not account per se for cell tumorigenicity and that tumor formation is compatible with low levels of pp60$^{v\text{-}src}$ protein kinase activity.[297] In fact, some experimental results suggest that an RSV-induced transformed phenotype can occur independently of cell division after infection.[298]

Apparently, pp60^{src} induces activation of genes that may lead to DNA replication and mitosis without help from external growth factors.[299,300] Autocrine growth is induced by *src*-related oncogenes in chicken myeloid cells transformed by avian acute retroviruses containing the v-*myb* or v-*myc* oncogenes.[301] Such cells would be rendered capable of producing a growth factor that stimulates their proliferation in an autocrine fashion. These phenomena may depend on specific phosphorylation processes that are stimulated by the kinase activity associated with these oncogene products and pp60$^{c\text{-}src}$ itself is a substrate for phosphorylation when cells are stimulated to enter the cell cycle.

2. Mechanisms of pp60^{src}-Induced Gene Regulation

The mechanisms responsible for pp60^{src}-induced genomic changes are unknown. A possible mechanism is alteration of DNA topoisomerases, which are enzymes involved in controlling the topological state of DNA, including DNA supercoiling and relaxation.[302,303] Such changes are importantly involved in the regulation of DNA functions (transcription and translation). All topological interconversions of DNA are associated with the transient breakage and rejoining of DNA strands. It is thus most interesting that pp60^{src} is able to interact with and nick supercoiled double-stranded DNA in an ATP-dependent manner.[304] Incubation of *Escherichia coli* or calf thymus type-I topoisomerases with pp60$^{v\text{-}src}$ or a tyrosine-specific protein kinase purified from normal rat liver results in a tenfold loss of topoisomerase activity.[305]

3. Induction of DNA Replication

In particular types of cells, RSV infection or transfection of a v-*src* oncogene may result in stimulation of DNA replication and mitosis. For example, introduction by electroporation of a v-*src* oncogene linked to the rat insulin II promoter into β-cells from fetal rat pancreatic islets resulted in stimulation of ^{3}H-thymidine incorporation into the cell DNA.[306] The effect observed with v-*src* transfection in fetal islet cells was more pronounced than any effect previously reported on extrinsically induced β-cell replication. Similar, but less pronounced results were obtained by transfection of a combination of c-*myc* and mutant c-H-*ras* genes. The c-*myc* protooncogene alone was ineffective in this system.

VI. MECHANISMS OF V-*SRC*-INDUCED TRANSFORMATION

In spite of numerous studies the mechanisms responsible for the phenotypic transformation of cells induced by the v-*src* oncogene product remain unknown. However, some clues to the solution of this complex problem have been obtained by the results of experiments performed in the last few years.

A. SUSCEPTIBILITY TO V-*SRC*-INDUCED TRANSFORMATION

Specific types of cells are either susceptible or resistant to the transforming action of the v-*src* oncogene product. Fibroblasts are most susceptible to RSV-induced transformation but other types of cells have been transformed with RSV infection. However, unlike fibroblasts, other cells can be irreversibly committed to differentiate and die after RSV infection. Chicken erythroid cells can be transformed by RSV but the transformation appears to be very unstable.[307,308] The expression of v-*src* in avian macrophages fails to elicit a transformed cell phenotype.[309] The physiological conditions of the particular cell are also important for determining susceptibility or resistance to transformation. Very young (4-d-old) chicken embryos can support RSV infection in the absence of neoplasia.[310] Apparently, chickens that are undergoing active morphogenesis can modulate the use of RSV sequences by chick cells. In general, chicken embryos *in ovo* are resistant to the tumorigenic action of RSV in spite of the expression of high levels of pp60^{v-src}-associated tyrosine kinase activity but the ability to display a transformed phenotype is rapidly acquired when the infected cells are placed in culture.[311] Transformation of diploid Syrian hamster embryo (SHE) cells by transfection with RSV DNA occurs with a low frequency and only after a long latency period (more than 14 weeks).[312] In contrast, transfection of different preneoplastic cell lines with RSV DNA results in the efficient induction of tumor formation with a short latency period (3 to 4 weeks) after injection into nude mice.

Madin-Darby canine kidney (MDCK) cells were derived from renal tubular epithelium and retain the morphogenetic determinants required to form polarized multicellular epithelial structures *in vitro*. Low levels of expression of pp60^{v-src} in MDCK cells elicits plasticity in these multicellular structures and perturbs lateral membrane contacts and the formation of the zonula adherens between cells.[313] However, pp60^{v-src} expression in MDCK cells is not associated with a mitogenic effect or neoplastic transformation. These results indicate that pp60^{v-src} may display, in particular cellular systems, physiological effects which are dissociable from neoplastic transformation.

The construction of recombinant murine leukemia virus containing the v-*src* oncogene has facilitated the study of this oncogene in mammalian cells.[314] After infection of long-term marrow cultures from mice with the molecular recombinant virus, it is observed that the v-*src* gene produces a dramatic increase in the stem cell compartment and the committed progenitor cell compartment, and a decrease in mature granulocytes, but, unlike its effects in other systems, no evidence for neoplastic transformation is apparent.[315] Thus, specific types of cellular responses, which depend on host factors, are of critical importance for the appearance, or lack of appearance, of a transformed phenotype in cells where the v-*src* oncogene is expressed. Interferon can inhibit the expression of the transformed phenotype in RSV-transformed rat cells by selectively reducing the synthesis of pp60^{v-src}.[316]

B. DIFFERENCES IN THE TRANSFORMING ABILITIES OF V-*SRC* AND C-*SRC* PRODUCTS

The viral oncogene product, pp60$^{v\text{-}src}$, is much more efficient in inducing experimental cell transformation than its normal cellular counterpart, pp60$^{c\text{-}src}$, but the mechanisms responsible for this difference are not understood. In contrast to the cloned v-*src* oncogene, an intact human c-*src* protooncogene carried by a molecular vector is unable to induce neoplastic transformation in the focus-forming assay.[67] However, cotransfection of the c-*src* gene and genes coding for nuclear proteins such as v-*myc*, c-*myc*, adenovirus E1A, and polyoma virus large T antigen results in induction of anchorage-independent growth and focus formation in the NIH/3T3 assay system.[317] Quantitative and/or qualitative differences between the viral and cellular oncogene proteins could explain the observed differences in v-*src* and c-*src* transforming ability.

1. Quantitative Differences in the Levels of Expression of c-*src* and v-*src*

A simple dosage phenomenon could be responsible for the observed differences between the transforming capabilities of c-*src* and v-*src* gene products. The level of pp60$^{c\text{-}src}$ present in normal cells is much lower than the level of pp60$^{v\text{-}src}$ present in RSV-infected cells.[318] By placing the v-*src* oncogene under the control of a regulatable promoter such as MMTV LTR and manipulating glucocorticoid concentrations, it has been shown that there is a distinct threshold dose for v-*src*-induced cellular transformation.[319]

The c-*src* gene is expressed in most cell types of vertebrate species but only about one to four c-*src* mRNA copies are present in a typical cultured or tissue cell.[320] The highest normal levels of pp60$^{c\text{-}src}$ are found in the neural tissues, especially in the brain and the retina.[82,321] Intracellular levels of the *src* product that are 10- to 100-times higher than the normal levels are found after RSV infection, which could explain the emergence of a transformed phenotype. High-level expression of c-*src* sequences from molecular vectors containing an SV40 or retroviral promoter does not result in transformation of cultured chicken fibroblasts or mammalian fibroblastic cell lines.[56,67,322,323] However, a slight transformation capacity of c-*src* has been observed in some experimental systems. Overexpression of pp60$^{c\text{-}src}$ by means of plasmids containing M-MuSV LTRs and chicken c-*src* genes induces focus formation in NIH/3T3 cells, but only at about 1% the frequency of focus formation induced by a similar expression plasmid carrying the v-*src* oncogene.[324] A fully transformed phenotype is not induced by the expression vector carrying, not v-*src*, but the c-*src* protooncogene. A constructed recombinant murine retrovirus which efficiently transduces pp60$^{c\text{-}src}$ into NIH/3T3 cells is unable to induce cell transformation in spite of the fact that the levels of functional pp60$^{c\text{-}src}$ protein kinase within the cells are increased 3- to 15-fold above the endogenous murine levels in control lines.[58]

Increased levels of pp60$^{c\text{-}src}$-dependent tyrosyl kinase activity have been found in human neuroblastomas, and the alteration is associated with amino-terminal tyrosine phosphorylation of the c-*src* gene product.[325] Very high levels of pp60$^{c\text{-}src}$-specific kinase activity, comparable to the levels observed in RSV-transformed cells, have been detected in human and rabbit normal blood platelets.[80] Since platelets are anuclear cells, it is clear that high levels of tyrosine protein kinase activity do not necessarily correlate with cell proliferation, but may be involved in other cellular functions, possibly including the transduction of extracellular signals at the level of the cell membrane. A similar function may be postulated for the presence of high levels of pp60$^{c\text{-}src}$ kinase in the central nervous system.

2. Qualitative Differences between c-*src* and v-*src*

There are two important structural differences between the protein products of v-*src* and c-*src* genes: (1) the 19 carboxy-terminal amino acids of pp60$^{c\text{-}src}$ are replaced by a new set of 12 amino acids in pp60$^{v\text{-}src}$ and (2) the two products show several differences in amino acid sequences. Comparison of the amino acid sequences of the v-*src*- and c-*src*-encoded proteins reveals amino acid changes throughout the protein sequences: about 7 for the Schmidt-Ruppin strain of RSV and 17 for the Prague strain of RSV. The structure of the carboxy-terminal region of the v-*src* product is most important for the transforming capability of the protein, probably by affecting substrate specificity.[326] There is, however, much controversy about how structural differences may account for the marked differences in the oncogenic potential of the v-*src* and c-*src* proteins.[327]

The functional properties of the protein products of v-*src* and c-*src* are similar but subtle differences may exist.[56] In particular, the kinase activity with specificity for tyrosine residues is about tenfold higher in the pp60^{v-src} protein than in the pp60^{c-src} protein, and this difference may account, at least in part, for the transforming ability of the viral oncogene product.[322,328] Overproduced pp60^{c-src} is only capable of inducing low-level phosphorylation of cellular proteins, which may account for its inability to transform cells.[169] The expression of relatively low numbers of pp60^{v-src} molecules per cell can increase tyrosine phosphorylation to high levels but, in contrast, a tripling of pp60^{c-src} content does not significantly increase phosphotyrosine content of total cell proteins nor lead to phosphorylation of known pp60^{v-src} substrates.[329]

The direct injection into chickens of genomic cloned DNA carrying the v-*src* gene is sufficient to determine the induction of sarcomas *in vivo* and the cells from the tumors induced by these procedure acquire v-*src* sequences in their genomes and express high levels of v-*src* messages.[330] On the other hand, RSV variants that carry the c-*src* gene instead of the v-*src* gene are not able to induce transformation in chicken embryo fibroblasts.[322] Plasmids carrying the c-*src* gene are not able to induce focus formation in NIH/3T3 cells in spite of the presence of high levels of the c-*onc* protein product, whereas plasmids carrying the v-*src* gene, either alone or associated with c-*src*, are very efficient for the induction of oncogenic transformation in the same cells.[323] The infection of long-term murine bone marrow cultures with a recombinant murine amphotropic virus carrying the v-*src* oncogene results in an alteration of the normal differentiation program of the stem cells.[331] Thus, qualitative differences between v-*src* and c-*src* may be responsible for the different oncogenic potential of their respective protein products.

Differences have been observed in the peptide mapping and phosphotyrosine site of the v-*src* and c-*src* protein products.[168,332] Differences are also observed by inhibition of the kinase activity of these products with a specific dinucleotide.[333] Oncogenic activation of the c-*src* gene may result from only an alteration affecting the carboxyl terminus of the pp60^{src} protein and enhanced expression by LTRs.[334] Single amino acid substitutions at different sites can activate the transforming potential of pp60^{c-src}.[335] A single point mutation at nucleotide 1321 of the c-*src* gene, resulting in conversion of amino acid 441 of pp60^{c-src} from isoleucine to phenylalanyne, is sufficient to activate the transforming capability of the protein. Mutation at codon 378 of the c-*src* gene, which results in substitution of glutamic acid for glycine, also results in activation of the transforming potential. Both substitutions reside in the tyrosine kinase domain of pp60^{c-src} and may contribute to a conformational change of the protein that activates its kinase activity.[335] However, high level of expression of the altered protein is necessary for cellular transformation, which indicates that both qualitative and quantitative changes are responsible for differences in the transforming capability of v-*src* and c-*src*.

C. STUDY OF RSV MUTANTS

Among many different classes of RSV mutants that have been described, the study of transformation-defective (*td*) and temperature-sensitive (*ts*) mutants have yielded interesting results.

1. Proliferation-Defective Mutants

Analysis of v-*src* deletion mutants has revealed that the amino-terminal one third of pp60^{v-src}, including the membrane-binding domain and the site of myristylation, are essential for cell transformation but not for the induction of cell proliferation.[336] These findings suggest that the target(s) required for the mitogenic response to *src* proteins could be a cytoplasmic substrate, whereas those required for morphological transformation and anchorage independence could be membrane proteins.

2. Transformation-Defective RSV Deletion Mutants

Transformation-defective (*td*) RSV deletion mutants are frequently generated as spontaneous segregants from nondefective RSV.[337] In such mutants the viruses have deleted part or all of the v-*src* oncogene coding sequences.[338,339] Although the mechanisms of generation of RSV *td* deletion mutants are not clear, retention of a short stretch of the 3′ v-*src* coding sequence is necessary and sufficient for the generation of recovered RSVs by recombination with the c-*src* protooncogene in the host cell.[340]

The study of *td* RSV deletion mutants can contribute to define the regions of the RSV genome which are essentially involved in the induction of neoplastic transformation. Particular regions from the amino-terminal part of the pp60[v-*src*] protein are essential for the induction of transformation. However, the occurrence of recombinational events between the virus mutants and homologous cellular sequences makes difficult the characterization of the transformation-related sequences.[340,341] RSVs generated by recombination between *td* genomes and c-*src* sequences can transduce not only the coding sequences (exons) of the c-*src* gene but also various lengths of c-*src* intervening sequences (introns), especially internal intron 1 sequences.[342] Thus, some recombination junctions can be formed by splicings involving cryptic donor and acceptor sites in the *td* RSV genome and c-*src* sequences. The results suggest that such recombinational events occur at the DNA level.

The spontaneous variant of RSV, *dl*PA105, carries a deletion in the amino-terminal portion of the v-*src* oncogene coding sequence, which results in the production of a truncated pp60[v-*src*] protein of 45 kDa, termed p45[v-*src*], which lacks amino acid residues 33 to 126.[343,344] Protein p45[v-*src*] contains both phosphoserine and phosphotyrosine, is myristylated, and possesses tyrosine kinase activity indistinguishable from that of wild-type pp60[v-*src*]. Quail neuroretina cells infected with the mutant RSV became morphologically transformed and formed colonies in soft agar. In contrast, the *dl*PA105 mutant virus induced only limited morphological alterations in quail fibroblasts and was defective in promoting anchorage-independent growth of these cells. Synthesis and tyrosine kinase activity of the mutant p45[v-*src*] protein were similar in both cell types. These data indicate that the portion of the v-*src* protein deleted in p45[v-*src*] is dispensable for the mitogenic and tumorigenic properties of wild-type pp60[v-*src*], whereas it is required for *in vitro* transformation of fibroblasts. The ability of *dl*PA105 to induce different transformation phenotypes in quail fibroblasts and quail neuroretina cells is a property unique to this RSV mutant and provides evidence for the existence of cell-type-specific responses to v-*src* proteins. Such differential responses may be due to the interaction of v-*src* with different, cell-specific substrates in different types of cells.

3. Temperature-Sensitive RSV Mutants

The study of temperature-sensitive (*ts*) RSV mutants is also interesting for the characterization of molecular phenomena associated with RSV-induced neoplastic transformation. The important role of pp60[v-*src*] in the proliferation of cells transformed by RSV is documented by the fact that cells transformed with *ts* mutants of the viral oncogene product are temperature-sensitive for *in vivo* growth.[345] In general, the genetic and biochemical analysis of *ts* mutants of v-*src* genes indicate that the function of the specific kinase domain of the protein is essential for the stimulation of cell proliferation, morphological alteration, and anchorage independence.[346-348]

Two mutations in the putative tyrosine kinase domain are essential for the *ts* phenotype of an RSV mutant (tsNY68) and elimination of one of the two essential mutations of tsNY68 is sufficient to restore the wild-type phenotype.[349] However, the studies with transformation-defective *ts* RSV mutants suggest that there is no simple relationship between pp60$^{v\text{-}src}$, pp60$^{v\text{-}src}$-associated kinase activity, and transformation, supporting the idea of multifunctionality of the *v-src* gene protein product.[350] Different pp60$^{v\text{-}src}$ proteins of particular types of RSV *ts* mutants may be perturbed not only in the kinase activity but may be altered in their intracellular localization and processing.[351] Two *ts* mutations of RSV were due to distinct but close single amino acid changes near the carboxyl terminus of the *v-src* oncogene product, but back mutations to wild type could result from second mutations at either nearby or distant sites.[352]

The study of *ts* mutants of RSV indicates the existence of structural and functional pp60$^{v\text{-}src}$ domains that are required for transformation of chick embryo fibroblasts but do not grossly affect tyrosine-protein kinase activity.[353] Other *ts* mutants of RSV have amino acid changes at the carboxy-terminal domain of the protein molecule involved in kinase activity, including a change at position 461.[354] However, chimeric *src* protein containing only the Met-461 mutation is indistinguishable from the wild-type protein and a second carboxy-terminal mutation is required for full temperature sensitivity *in vivo*. No significant change in the secondary structure of the protein is associated with Met-461 mutation alone, but pp60^{src} proteins carrying additional mutations at the carboxyl terminus have an altered secondary structure and exhibit stable binding to cellular proteins p50 and p90.[354]

A close correlation exists between *ts* expression of the pp60$^{v\text{-}src}$ product and the characteristics of cellular compartments and fluxes for calcium.[355] Since calcium is importantly involved in the control mechanisms of cell proliferation, the results obtained with *ts* mutants suggest that RSV could alter these mechanisms by producing a redistribution of calcium between different cellular compartments. The study of RSV *ts* mutants also demonstrates that pp60$^{v\text{-}src}$ can stimulate cells to enter mitosis without help from external serum growth factors and is, therefore, a complete mitogen.[300]

4. Fusiform Mutants

Chicken embryo fibroblasts infected with wild-type RSV develop a characteristic rounded transformed cell morphology. In contrast, some RSV mutants, termed fusiform or *morf*^{f} mutants, exhibit an elongated spindle shape.[8] Although the molecular mechanisms responsible for the morphological characteristics of *morf*^{f} RSV mutants have not been clarified, the available evidence indicates that a region within the terminal one-third coding region of the *v-src* gene contributes to a structural domain of the pp60$^{v\text{-}src}$ protein that is important for controlling some morphological parameters of transformation in cells infected with RSV.[356]

5. Constructed RSV Mutants

Studies with local mutagenesis of RSV strongly suggest that the two major sites of phosphorylation of pp60$^{v\text{-}src}$ (serine at position 17 and tyrosine at position 416) are dispensable for kinase activity and transformation of chicken embryo fibroblasts.[357] However, an RSV mutant (RSV-SF1) in which tyrosine at position 416 is replaced by phenylalanine results in a marked reduction of the oncogenic potential of the viral protein product when tested in mouse cells.[358] RSV-SF1 pp60$^{v\text{-}src}$ has several properties in common with pp60$^{v\text{-}src}$ of wild-type viral origin, including tyrosine-specific kinase activity and interaction with different cellular proteins, but it is tumorigenic only if tested in immunodeficient (mt$^+$/mt$^+$) mice. These results suggest that tyrosine kinase activity may not be fully responsible for pp60$^{v\text{-}src}$-induced tumorigenesis, and that evasion of the host immune response is a necessary step in tumorigenesis induced by the *v-src* oncogene.[358]

In another mutant, RSV-SF2, lysine 295 is replaced by methionine at the ATP-binding site of pp60$^{v\text{-}src}$.[359] SF2 pp60$^{v\text{-}src}$ has a half-life similar to that of wild-type pp60$^{v\text{-}src}$ and is localized in the membranous fraction of the cells but rat cells expressing the modified protein remain morphologically untransformed and are not tumorigenic. SF2 pp60$^{v\text{-}src}$ isolated from these cells lacks kinase activity.

Replacement of the carboxyl region of pp60^{c-src} with that of pp60^{v-src} results in activation of pp60^{c-src} transforming activity in NIH/3T3 cells, whereas replacement of the carboxy-terminal region of pp60^{v-src} with that of pp60^{c-src} reduces pp60^{v-src} transforming activity.[326] In contrast, replacement of the carboxy-terminal region of pp60^{v-src} with a randomly selected sequence does not affect transforming activity. These results indicate that the v-*src* modifications which are most important for transformation are those in the carboxy-terminal region of the molecule and that the specific c-*src* carboxy-terminal region is required for suppression of transformation potential.

Constructed mutants containing alterations of the carboxyl terminus of pp60^{v-src} have a deleterious effect on both cell transformation and protein kinase activity, which suggests that the carboxy-terminal portion of pp60^{v-src} is involved in maintaining the overall tertiary structure of the enzymatically active v-*src* protein.[360] The region of pp60^{c-src} from residue 515 to the carboxyl terminus, comprising 19 amino acids, is replaced by an unrelated sequence of 12 residues in pp60^{v-src}. This region includes a phosphorylation site at tyrosine-527, and the absence of this site, which could exert a negative regulatory function, may be responsible for the acquisition of transforming potential in the viral product.[171] Leucine-516 is highly conserved among the protein tyrosine kinases and its replacement abrogates the transforming ability of pp60^{v-src}.[361]

Tyrosine-527 is a major element of the carboxy-terminal part of the pp60^{c-src} molecule responsible for regulating the activity of pp60^{c-src} *in vivo*.[362] Whereas the major site of tyrosine phosphorylation in pp60^{v-src} is tyrosine-416, the major site of *in vivo* phosphorylation of pp60^{c-src} is the carboxy-terminal residue, tyrosine-527. A good but not perfect correlation exists between lack of phosphorylation at tyrosine-527 and increased phosphorylation on tyrosine-416, and between elevated phosphorylation on tyrosine-416 and enhanced kinase activity. Studies with *in vitro* phosphatase treatment indicate that dephosphorylation of tyrosine-527 results in activation of the pp60^{c-src}-associated kinase activity.[172] Studies with site-directed mutagenesis indicate that carboxy-terminal alteration which either remove or replace tyrosine-527 serve to activate the c-*src* protein, resulting in increased *in vivo* tyrosine protein kinase activity and capability for inducing cellular transformation.[363]

Constructed chimeric molecules involving specific amino acid changes in the amino-terminal region of the c-*src* protein indicate that some of these changes are sufficient to convert pp60^{c-src} into a transforming protein.[328] In particular, the change from threonine to isoleucine at position 338 or the replacement of a fragment of pp60^{c-src} containing glycine-63, arginine-95, and threonine-96 with a corresponding fragment of pp60^{v-src} containing asparagine-63, triptophane-95, and isoleucine-96 converts pp60^{c-src} into a transforming protein by the criteria of focus formation, anchorage-independent growth, and tumor formation in newborn chickens. These mutations are associated with an elevation in the specific kinase activity of the pp60^{c-src} protein, which supports the idea that this activity is essential for the transforming ability of the protein.

Results obtained with constructed deletion mutants of RSV suggest that a short sequence of the amino-terminal region of pp60^{v-src} (amino acids 2 to 15) is required for myristylation, membrane association, and cell transformation.[198,203,204,364] These mutants have little alteration in tyrosine kinase activity and the results obtained with them suggest the following sequence of events: (1) a critical amino acid sequence in the amino terminal region of pp60^{v-src} is required for fatty acid attachment (myristoylation in an amide linkage, probably to glycine at position 2, which blocks the N terminus of the protein), (2) myristoylation is required for membrane association of pp60^{v-src}, and (3) association of pp60^{v-src} with the cell membrane is required for the expression of its ability to induce malignant transformation. An amino-terminal peptide from pp60^{v-src} can direct myristoylation and plasma membrane localization when fused to heterologous proteins.[365] RSV mutants with different tyrosine kinase activities have also been used to study the relationships between vinculin phosphorylation, pp60^{v-src} location, and adhesion plaque integrity.[272]

D. TYROSINE PHOSPHORYLATION

There is strong evidence that phosphorylation on tyrosine residues in particular cellular proteins is essential for the induction of transformation by RSV.[366] However, in rat cell lines transformed with relatively low amounts of pp60^{v-src} no increase in phosphorylation was detected in a major cellular protein target for v-*src*-induced tyrosine phosphorylation.[319]

Inhibition of the pp60^{v-src}-associated protein kinase may result in reversion of RSV-transformed cells to a normal phenotype.[362] Benzenoid ansamycin antibiotics (herbimycin, macbecin, and geldanamycin) reduce the intracellular phosphorylation of pp60^{src} at the permissive temperature in NRK cells infected with a *ts* mutant of RSV, and this effect in accompanied by a morphological reversion from the transformed to the normal phenotype.[368,369] Herbimycin is effective in inducing reversion of the transformed phenotype in cells transformed by oncogenes encoding tyrosine kinases (v-*src*, v-*yes*, v-*ros*, v-*abl*, and v-*erb*-B), but not other oncogenes (v-*raf*, v-*ras*, and v-*myc*).[370] Removal of the antibiotics allow the cells to revert to the transformed morphology. Apparently, benzenoid ansamycins have no direct effect on *src* kinase but destroy its intracellular environment, which results in an irreversible alteration of pp60^{src} and loss of its catalytic activity. However, the mechanism of pp60^{src} kinase inactivation in the antibiotic-treated cells has not been elucidated. Another agent, oxanosine, inhibits the growth of *ts* RSV mutants at the permissive temperature by mechanisms which are apparently independent of the pp60^{v-src}-associated kinase activity.[371]

The possible role of the endogenous protein, pp60^{c-src}, in experimental and spontaneous neoplastic transformation is not understood. The action of potent tumor promoters such as phorbol myristate acetate (PMA) is apparently independent from the protein kinase encoded by the c-*src* protooncogene.[372,373] Proteins with tyrosine kinase activity and antigenically related to pp60^{src} (and, more particularly, to the carboxy-terminal sequence of pp60^{src}) are present in human lymphoblastoid cell of either malignant origin (Raji cell line) or normal origin (Priess cell line).[70] The level of pp60^{c-src} kinase activity in human neuroblastoma cells is increased 20- to 40-fold over that found in either glioblastomas or normal human fibroblasts but is not significantly different from normal brain tissue.[325] The tyrosine-specific kinase activity of pp60^{c-src} from human colon cancer tissue specimens and tumor-derived cell lines is consistently elevated over the activity of pp60^{c-src} molecules isolated from normal human colon mucosa tissues and cultures of normal colonic mucosa cells.[101] This elevation is not related to an increased amount of the pp60^{c-src} protein in the tumor cells but is due to some alteration in the posttranslational modification of the protein which results in enhancement of the specific kinase activity.[102] Tyrosine-specific kinases are present in normal cells and are responsible for the phosphorylation of a number of proteins. The possible relationship between these kinase activities and pp60^{c-src} is largely unknown.

E. HORMONES AND GROWTH FACTORS OR THEIR CELLULAR RECEPTORS

The cellular mechanisms of action of many hormones and growth factors are intimately associated with biochemical processes involving protein phosphorylation. There are some interesting relationships between these phosphorylation processes and those related to pp60^{src} kinase activity.

1. Insulin Receptor

The purified insulin receptors present in cultured IM-9 human lymphocytes are immunoprecipitated by antibodies to pp60^{src} and this precipitation is competitively inhibited by purified pp60^{v-src}.[374] In contrast, the product of v-*raf* does not inhibit precipitation of the insulin receptor. Since the cellular insulin receptor possesses tyrosine kinase activity,[375] the latter results suggest the existence of structural and functional homologies between pp60^{src} and the insulin receptor. It is unlikely that pp60^{v-src} represents a truncated form of the insulin receptor because three other antibodies to pp60^{v-src}, including a monoclonal antibody, were unable to induce precipitation of the receptor. Most probably, there is a similarity between certain epitopes of both proteins.[376] The human insulin receptor is structurally related to the tyrosine-specific kinase family of oncogenes.[377]

The solubilized insulin receptor is phosphorylated and activated by the pp60[v-src] kinase.[378,379] However, exogenous proteins like angiotensin and calmodulin are also phosphorylated in vitro by the kinase activity of pp60[v-src],[135,380] and the biological significance of this phosphorylation is not understood.

2. Epidermal Growth Factor Receptor

Antibodies generated against two synthetic peptides corresponding to two defined regions of pp60[src] interact specifically with the EGF receptor kinase.[178] The results from these studies suggest that at least two domains within the cytoplasmic portion of the EGF receptor are antigenically related to two domains of the pp60[src] molecule. One domain is the major phosphotyrosine site on pp60[src] and the second domain is either part of the kinase domain of pp60[src] or can somehow modulate its activity.[178] A similar antigenic and structural homology exists between the cytoplasmic portion of the EGF receptor, the *erb*-B oncogene, and other members of the *src* oncogene family, including the oncogenes *fes, mos, yes, fps,* and *abl*.[381]

RSV-induced transformation of mouse and rat fibroblasts is associated with a marked reduction in the level of expression of EGF receptors on the cell surface.[382] The role of this change in RSV-induced transformation is not clear but it is not specific of the v-*src* oncogene since transformation induced by other oncogenes or non-oncogene factors may be associated with similar changes in the EGF receptor levels. Moreover, NR6 cells, which lack EGF receptors, are also transformed by RSV infection, which indicates that the presence of functional EGF receptors is not obligatory for transformation induced by the v-*src* oncogene.[382] Murine fibroblasts overexpressing chicken pp60[c-src] show a two- to fivefold enhanced incorporation of ^{3}H-thymidine into DNA in response to EGF relative to that of the parent line.[383] The pp60[c-src] protein may interact with the mitogenic transduction pathway of EGF in some event distal to EGF binding.

3. Platelet-Derived Growth Factor

The growth factor PDGF or the phorbol ester TPA induce quiescent, serum-deprived chicken embryo cells to enter the cell cycle and this phenomenon is accompanied by a two- to fourfold increase in serine phosphorylation of pp60[c-src].[161] The phosphorylation occurs very soon after the initial stimulation to growth by either PDGF or TPA and is localized to the amino-terminal end of the pp60[c-src] molecule, a region with an essential role for transformation, not necessarily dependent of tyrosine phosphorylation. The enzyme responsible for phosphorylation of pp60[c-src] on serine has not been identified but one possible candidate is protein kinase C. In addition to serine phosphorylation, PDGF also induces rapid phosphorylation of tyrosine residues located on the amino-terminal portion of pp60[c-src] and this is accompanied by both increased kinase activity of pp60[c-src] and increased phosphorylation of the p36 protein substrate *in vivo*.[384] These results are compatible with the hypothesis that pp60[c-src] may play a role in the mitogenic response to PDGF.

4. Abrogation of Growth Factor Requirement

Expression of a v-*src* oncogene may result in abrogation of the requirement for specific growth factors in some, but not all, types of cells. The murine cell lines CTLL-2 and FD.C/1 are dependent for growth on the interleukins IL-2 and IL-3, respectively. Expression of a retroviral vector carrying the v-*src* oncogene in CTLL-2 cells results in abrogation of the requirement for exogenous supply of IL-2, but expression of the same vector in FD.C/1 cells does not abrogate their requirement for exogenous supply of IL-3.[385] Moreover, only a small fraction of CTLL-2 cells expressing v-*src* become IL-3 independent, suggesting that expression of the oncogene is insufficient by itself for the induction of growth factor abrogation and that secondary progression factors are required for this abrogation. In any case, this abrogation is not associated with an endogenous production of IL-3.

F. TYROSINE SULFATION

A general sulfation of tyrosine residues on proteins has been observed in both normal and transformed cells.[386,387] Tyrosine sulfation is apparently a widespread protein modification. In a human hepatoma cell line (HepG2), 7 of 15 proteins are sulfated on tyrosine and 3 of them (fibrinogen, α-fetoprotein, and fibronectin) contain tyrosine-O-sulfate.[388]

In contrast with the increase in phosphotyrosine induced by pp60^{v-src}, a sometimes rather drastic reduction in tyrosine-O-sulfated proteins parallels infection of rat embryo fibroblasts (cell line 3Y1) with either RSV or FSV.[389] The decrease in tyrosine-O-sulfate occurring in cells infected with these acute transforming retroviruses is apparently due to increased secretion of compounds containing tyrosine-O-sulfate, possibly including a loss of fibronectin from the cell membrane coincident with malignant transformation.[389,390] The tyrosine sulfation site in fibronectin secreted by 3Y1 cells is located in the carboxy-terminal fibrin-binding region of the molecule.[391] The relationship between tyrosine phosphorylation and tyrosine sulfation of proteins, if any, remains to be identified.

G. ACTIVATION OF PROTEIN KINASE C

It has been suggested that the transforming ability of pp60^{v-src} would depend not on its tyrosine kinase activity but on its ability to activate protein kinase C through the phosphoinositide metabolic pathway, which is an important transductional intracellular system.[392-396] pp60^{v-src} would be capable of phosphorylating phosphatidylinositol to form both mono- and diphosphorylated derivatives, and 1,2-diacylglycerol would be phosphorylated to form phosphatidic acid.[397] If this is true, pp60^{v-src} would be involved in both the generation and removal of 1,2-diacylglycerol, a catabolite that activates protein kinase C. High levels of protein kinase C activity have been found in NIH/3T3 cells transformed by transfection with a plasmid carrying the v-src oncogene.[398] The product of the acute retrovirus UR2 is the protein p60^{v-ros}, which also possesses tyrosine protein kinase activity. The v-ros oncogene is a member of the src oncogene family and it has also been suggested that its transforming activity may be associated with an ability to phosphorylate phosphatidylinositol and generate 1,2-diacylglycerol, thus activating protein kinase C.[399]

However, the results obtained in other studies clearly demonstrate that the phosphorylation of phosphatidylinositol metabolites is catalyzed by proteins that are different from tyrosine protein kinases.[400] In the electric ray *Narke japonica* a tyrosine-specific protein kinase from the acetylcholine receptor-rich membranes of the electroplax is related to pp60^{v-src} kinase and a phosphatidylinositol kinase activity is associated with this enzyme, but these enzymes are different and the tyrosine-specific protein kinase has no intrinsic phosphatidylinositol kinase activity.[401] These results cast serious doubt on the validity of interpretations about a presumed direct phosphorylation of phosphatidylinositol derivatives by oncogene proteins possessing tyrosine protein kinase activity, including pp60^{src} and p68^{ros}. Moreover, phosphatidylkinase activity in chicken embryo fibroblasts is not immunoprecipitated by an antibody that recognizes pp60^{c-src}, and overproduction of pp60^{c-src} do not increase the phosphatidylinositol kinase level in the cells.[402] These results demonstrate that phosphatidylinositol kinase activity is not encoded by the v-src and c-src genes. Most probably, the activation of protein kinase C in v-src-transformed cells proceeds by indirect mechanisms which depend on the primary tyrosine-specific activity of the oncogene product.

H. INTERCELLULAR COMMUNICATION

The pp60^{c-src} protein may be involved in junctional cell-to-cell communication. The pp60$^{v\text{-}src}$ oncogene product or an overexpressed pp60$^{c\text{-}src}$ protooncogene product may delay this communication. The formation of gap junctions between cultured chicken lens epithelial cells is inhibited by pp60$^{v\text{-}src}$.[403] Overexpression of the c-*src* gene in NIH/3T3 cells transfected with constructed vectors causes reduction of cell-to-cell transmission of molecules in the 400- to 700-Da range.[404] This down regulation of gap junctional communication correlates with the level of tyrosine protein kinase activity of the c-*src* gene product. The down regulation is enhanced by point mutation at tyrosine-527, a site whose phosphorylation results in inhibition of p60$^{c\text{-}src}$-associated tyrosine protein kinase activity. Substitution of the v-*src* carboxy-terminal coding region has a similar effect. Mutation of tyrosine-416 (a site phosphorylated upon tyrosine-527 mutation) suppresses the down regulation of cell communication caused by tyrosine-527 mutation and gene overexpression.

Intercellular communication, as measured by ^{3}H-uridine nucleotide transfer, is reduced in NIH/3T3 cells transformed by transfection with a plasmid carrying the v-*src* oncogene, as compared to parental untransformed cells.[398] A similar effect is produced by treatment with the tumor promoter PMA. Hypothetically, an inhibition of the transfer, via gap junctions, of important regulatory molecules from normal cells to cells expressing an oncogene may provide an explanation for the altered behavior of transformed cells. However, no direct proof exists in favor of the general validity of this hypothesis.

Studies performed in MDCK cells maintained in culture suggest that pp60$^{c\text{-}src}$ may be involved in regulating the shape of highly differentiated epithelial cells without changes in cell proliferation.[405] A natural function of pp60$^{c\text{-}src}$ may be to confer on differentiated cells and multicellular structures the ability to undergo changes in shape, which would allow the plasticity necessary for the occurrence of dynamic changes in spatial organization.

I. GLUCOSE TRANSPORT

An accelerated rate of glucose transport is one of the most important characteristics of neoplastic transformation. A marked increase in the rate of glucose uptake is observed in REF cells transfected with a v-*src* oncogene.[406] A similar increase is observed in cells transfected with a mutant EJ c-*ras* gene as well as in cells exposed to phorbol ester (TPA), but not in cells transfected with an activated c-*myc* gene. The increased glucose transport rate is paralleled by a marked increase in the amount of glucose transporter mRNA and protein.

J. ION FLUXES AND INTRACELLULAR CALCIUM REGULATION

Changes in ion fluxes across the cell membrane may have an important role in the expression of a transformed phenotype induced by pp60$^{v\text{-}src}$ and other oncogene products. Intracellular concentrations of Na$^+$ in chick embryo cells transformed with the Schmidt-Ruppin strain of RSV are higher than in uninfected cells or in cells transformed with the Bryan strain of the same virus.[407] On the other hand, there is a correlation between higher intracellular K$^+$ level and the expression of transformation parameters by chick cells infected with the Bryan strain of RSV. Moreover, uninfected chick embryo cells incubated in medium containing an elevated concentration of K$^+$ (an increase from 5 to 30 mM) exhibit several, but not all, of the transformation parameters expressed by chicken embryo cells infected with the Bryan strain of RSV.[407] Unlike growth factors, pp60$^{v\text{-}src}$ can induce, either directly or indirectly, a major change in membrane permeability to monovalent cations, with permanent depolarization of the plasma membrane.[408] These results suggest that monovalent ions may act as mediators of the biochemical events associated with RSV-induced transformation.

Changes in the intracellular distribution or concentration of calcium may also be relevant to the expression of a transformed phenotype induced by RSV. The calmodulin-binding protein caldesmon is decreased in RSV-transformed cells and its pattern of intracellular distribution is altered in these cells.[291] Phosphorylation of tyrosine residues of the intracellular Ca^{2+}-binding protein calmodulin is observed in RSV-transformed cells.[135] In an *in vitro* system, tyrosine phosphorylation of calmodulin by pp60^{v-src} kinase is inhibited by Ca^{2+}, and there is evidence that the structure of the Ca^{2+}-calmodulin complex may be altered by tyrosine phosphorylation. In contrast, serine and threonine phosphorylation of calmodulin occurs in both normal and RSV-transformed cells.

K. EXPRESSION OF HOST CELL SURFACE ANTIGENS

Tumor surface antigens (TSAs) expressed in RSV-transformed cells may be encoded not by the virus but by the host cell. Rat sarcomas induced by the Schmidt-Ruppin strain of RSV express a 60,000-mol wt TSA which is distinct from all the tested viral products.[82] This TSA is, at least in part, a host protein and, moreover, its expression appears to be restricted by cell type. The biological significance of this TSA is unknown. Cytotoxic T lymphocytes may display specific responses against multiple antigenic sites present in RSV-induced tumor cells.[409]

HLA class I antigen and β_2-microglobulin expression is reduced in RSV-transformed human fibroblasts.[410] This reduction is associated with decreased amounts of HLA class I transcripts but no rearrangement or hypermethylation of the HLA class I genes was detected. Reduction in MHC antigen expression is observed in other types of transformed cells and may contribute to tumor progression *in vivo*.

L. ABROGATION OF IDF45 ACTIVITY

Density-dependent inhibition of 3T3 fibroblast growth would depend on the release of a 45-kDa protein, termed IDF45, which is capable of decreasing DNA synthesis in CEF cells and inhibits CEF growth in a reversible manner.[411] Studies with Ny68 virus (a mutant of RSV with *ts* properties for the expression of transformation) suggest that pp60^{v-src} may induce loss of sensitivity to IDF45, which would explain why RSV-transformed cells escape to the mechanisms controlling density-dependent inhibition of growth and would continue to proliferate up until depletion of the culture medium.[412]

M. PROTOONCOGENE EXPRESSION

The possible role of protooncogene expression in RSV-induced transformation is little understood. Infection of either rat fibroblasts (3Y1 cell line) or chick embryo fibroblasts with the Schmidt-Ruppin strain of RSV results in a marked (30- to 100-fold) increase in the amount of c-*myc* transcripts.[296] The mechanisms responsible for this increase are unknown. Determination of the levels of expression of 19 protooncogenes in RSV-infected or RSV-transformed CEF cells showed a marked increase in the transcriptional activity of c-*fgr* and a slight increase in c-*fos* and c-*myc*, compared with uninfected CEF cells.[413] However, the observed alterations in protooncogene expression were apparently caused by the viral infection itself and were not due to the process of neoplastic transformation.

N. DESTABILIZATION OF THE HOST CELL GENOME

The continued presence of an integrated v-*src* oncogene may not be required for the expression of a transformed phenotype in RSV-infected cells.[414,415] The evidence suggests that the v-*src* product may produce, at least in some cellular systems, a kind of permanent damage that can be transmitted to the successive cell generations, which become independent on the presence of the v-*src* oncogene for expressing a transformed phenotype. Although the exact mechanism of this type of "hit-and-run" phenomenon is unknown, it may be hypothesized that it is associated with a destabilization of the host cell genome induced by the v-*src* oncogene.

O. EFFECT OF PHORBOL ESTERS ON ASV-INDUCED TRANSFORMATION

Injection of phorbol ester (PMA) directly into ASV-induced tumors results in increased expression of viral antigens at the cell surface and increased production of progeny virus in comparison to untreated cells. Unexpectedly, however, the PMA-treated tumors show regression and express diminished levels of the kinase activity associated with the pp60$^{v\text{-}src}$ oncogene product.[416] The molecular mechanisms involved in these opposite effects of phorbol ester are unknown.

P. REVERSION OF RSV-INDUCED TRANSFORMATION

As discussed previously, in some cellular systems the continued presence of the v-*src* product is required for the expression of a transformed phenotype, and inactivation of the cellular effects of this product with compounds such as benzoquinoid ansamycin antibiotics (herbamycin, macbecin, or geldanamycin) may result in reversion to morphological normalcy.[367-370] This reversion is not permanent, since removal of the antibiotics results in the reappearance of the transformed phenotype. Treatment of RSV-transformed cells with retinoic acid may also result in reversion of the transformed phenotype.[417] The molecular mechanisms of these reversions are unknown.

VII. CONCLUSION

An array of biochemical, functional, and morphological changes occurs in RSV-transformed cells but, in spite of many important studies on this topic, the primary mechanisms involved in the transforming action of the v-*src* oncogene are little understood. The ensemble of the available evidence supports the concept that the oncogenic activity of the v-*src* protein product critically depends on its higher tyrosine-specific kinase activity as compared to the activity of its cellular counterpart, the c-*src* kinase. However, the primary cellular targets whose alteration results in the expression of a transformed phenotype in RSV-infected cells have not been defined. Human cells are generally resistant to RSV-induced neoplastic transformation. The v-*src* oncogene can convert rat embryo fibroblasts to a fully transformed and tumorigenic phenotype but has no demonstrable effect on diploid human fibroblasts.[418]

The normal functions of the c-*src* protooncogene product remain largely unknown, and no definite proof exists about a possible oncogenic action of this product under natural conditions. The exact role of the c-*src* protein in the processes of cell differentiation and cell proliferation is unknown. In vertebrates, the highest concentrations of pp60$^{c\text{-}src}$ kinase are found in nonproliferating, fully differentiated cells like platelets and neurons. Almost nothing is known about the mechanisms involved in the regulation of pp60$^{c\text{-}src}$ kinase activity within normal or transformed cells.

REFERENCES

1. Rous, P., A sarcoma of the fowl transmissible by an agent separable from the tumor cells, *J. Exp. Med.*, 13, 397, 1911.
2. Wang, L.-H. and Hanafusa, H., Avian sarcoma viruses, *Virus Res.*, 9, 159, 1988.
3. Maki, Y., Bos, T.J., Davis, C., Starbuck, M., and Vogt, P.K., Avian sarcoma virus 17 carries the *jun* oncogene, *Proc. Natl. Acad. Sci. U.S.A.*, 84, 2848, 1987.
4. Wang, L.-H., The mechanism of transduction of proto-oncogene c-*src* by avian retroviruses, *Mutat. Res.*, 186, 135, 1987.
5. Hanafusa, H., Cell transformation by RNA tumor viruses, in *Comprehensive Virology*, Vol. 10, Fraenkel-Conrat, H. and Wagner, R., Eds., Plenum Press, New York, 1977, 401.
6. Rohrschneider, L. and Reynolds, S., Regulation of cellular morphology by the Rous sarcoma virus *src* gene: analysis of fusiform mutants, *Mol. Cell. Biol.*, 5, 3097, 1985.
7. Svoboda, J., Rous sarcoma virus, *Intervirology*, 26, 1, 1986.
8. Temin, H.M., The control of cellular morphology in embryonic cells infected with Rous sarcoma virus, *Virology*, 10, 182, 1960.

9. Transformation de fibroblastes diploides humains avec production virale après infection par des rétrovirus aviaires, *C.R. Acad. Sci. Paris,* 297, 17, 1983.

10. Rabotti, G., Teutsch, B., Mariller, M., Pavloff, N., Mongiat, F., Auger, J., and Semmel, M., Integration and expression of provirus in human cells transformed by avian sarcoma virus, *J. Natl. Cancer Inst.,* 78, 817, 1987.

11. Mitrani, E., Coffin, J., Boedtker, H., and Doty, P., Rous sarcoma virus is integrated but not expressed in chicken early embryonic cells, *Proc. Natl. Acad. Sci. U.S.A.,* 84, 2781, 1987.

12. Howlett, A.R., Cullen, B., Hertle, M., and Bissell, M.J., Tissue tropism and temporal expression of Rous sarcoma virus in embryonic avian limb *in ovo, Oncogene Res.,* 1, 255, 1987.

13. Ponten, J., The *in vivo* growth mechanism of avian Rous sarcoma, *Natl. Cancer Inst. Monogr.,* 17, 131, 1964.

14. Freire, P.M. and Duran-Reynals, F., Growth and regression of the Rous sarcoma as a function of the age of the host, *Cancer Res.,* 13, 386, 1953.

15. Wainberg, M.A., Yu, M., Schwartz-Luft, E., and Israel, E., Cellular and humoral antitumor immune responsiveness in chickens bearing tumors induced by avian sarcoma virus, *Int. J. Cancer,* 19, 680, 1977.

16. Wainberg, M.A., Israel, E., and Yu, M., Immune selection of tumor cell variants in chicken bearing tumors induced by avian sarcoma viruses, *Cancer Res.,* 42, 1669, 1982.

17. Poulin, L., Grise-Miron, L., Spira, B., and Wainberg, M.A., Altered pp60[src] kinase activity in regressing tumors induced by Rous sarcoma virus, *Cancer Lett.,* 36, 99, 1987.

18. Poulin, L., Skalski, V., and Wainberg, M.A., Effect of phorbol ester on growth of tumors induced by Rous sarcoma virus on pp60[src] kinase activity in these tumors, *Cancer Res.,* 47, 3637, 1987.

19. Copeland D.D. and Bigner, D.D., Influence of age at inoculation on avian oncornavirus-induced brain tumor incidence, tumor morphology, and postinoculation survival in F344 rats, *Cancer Res.,* 37, 1657, 1777.

20. Marczynska B. and Massey, R.J., Transplantable primate tumors induced by Rous sarcoma virus. I. Induction of tumors transplantable into young marmosets, *J. Natl. Cancer Inst.,* 77, 537, 1986.

21. Anderson, S.M. and Scolnick, E.M., Construction and isolation of a transforming murine retrovirus containing the *src* gene of Rous sarcoma virus, *J. Virol.,* 46, 594, 1983.

22. Anderson, S.M., Klinken, S.P., and Hankins, W.D., A murine recombinant retrovirus containing the *src* oncogene transforms erythroid precursor cells *in vitro, Mol. Cell. Biol.,* 5, 3369, 1985.

23. Darlix, J.-L., Schwager, M., Spahr, P.-F., and Bromley, P.A., Analysis of the secondary and tertiary structures of Rous sarcoma virus RNA, *Nucleic Acids Res.,* 8, 3335, 1980.

24. Dutta, A., Wang, L.-H., Hanafusa, T., and Hanafusa, H., Partial nucleotide sequence of Rous sarcoma virus-29 provides evidence that the original Rous sarcoma virus was replication defective, *J. Virol.,* 55, 728, 1985.

25. Mizutani, S. and Temin, H.M., Enzymes and nucleotides in virions of Rous sarcoma virus, *J. Virol.,* 8, 409, 1971.

26. Temin, H.M. and Mizutani, S., RNA-dependent DNA polymerase in virions of Rous sarcoma virus, *Nature,* 226, 1211, 1970.

27. Mizutani, S., Boettiger, D., and Temin, H.M., A DNA-dependent DNA polymerase and a DNA endonuclease in virions of Rous sarcoma virus, *Nature,* 228, 424, 1970.

28. Coffin, J.M. and Temin, H.M., Ribonuclease-sensitive deoxyribonucleic acid polymerase activity in uninfected rat cells and rat cells infected with Rous sarcoma virus, *J. Virol.,* 8, 630, 1971.

29. Humphries, E.H. and Temin, H.M., Requirement for cell division for initiation of transcription of Rous sarcoma virus RNA, *J. Virol.,* 14, 531, 1974.

30. Collins, C.J., Boettiger, D., Green, T.L., Burgess, M.B., Devlin, B.H., and Parsons, J.T., Arrangement of integrated avian sarcoma virus DNA sequences within the cellular genomes of transformed and revertant mammalian cells, *J. Virol.,* 33, 760, 1980.

31. Hillova, J., Hill, M., Mariage-Samson, R., and Belehradek, J., Jr., RSV provirus with same flanking sequences is found on different size classes of Chinese hamster chromosomes, *Intervirology,* 23, 29, 1985.

32. Gillespie, D.A.F., Hart, K.A., and Wyke, J.A., Rearrangements of viral and cellular DNA are often associated with expression of Rous sarcoma virus in rat cells, *Cell,* 41, 279, 1985.

33. Takeya, T., Feldman, R.A., and Hanafusa, H., DNA sequence of the viral and cellular *src* gene of chickens. I. Complete nucleotide sequence of an *Eco*RI fragment of recovered avian sarcoma virus which codes for gp37 and pp60[src], *J. Virol.,* 44, 1, 1982.

34. Schwartz, D.E., Tizard, R., and Gilbert, W., Nucleotide sequence of Rous sarcoma virus, *Cell,* 32, 853, 1983.

35. Darlix, J.-L. and Spahr, P.-F., High spontaneous mutation rate of Rous sarcoma virus demonstrated by direct sequencing of the RNA genome, *Nucleic Acids Res.,* 11, 5953, 1983.

36. Linial, M., Creation of a processed pseudogene by retroviral infection, *Cell,* 49, 93, 1987.

37. Hughes, S., Mellstrom, K., Kosik, E., Tamanoi, F., and Brugge, J., Mutation of a termination codon affects *src* initiation, *Mol. Cell. Biol.,* 4, 1738, 1984.

38. Weiss, S.R., Varmus, H.E., and Bishop, J.M., Cell-free translation of purified avian sarcoma virus *src* mRNA, *Virology,* 110, 476, 1981.

39. Petersen, R.B. and Hackett, P.B., Characterization of ribosome binding on Rous sarcoma virus RNA *in vitro, J. Virol.,* 56, 683, 1985.

40. Perez, L., Wills, J.W., and Hunter, E., Expression of the Rous sarcoma virus *env* gene from a simian virus 40 late-region replacement vector: effects of upstream initiation codons, *J. Virol.,* 61, 1276, 1987.

41. Gilmer, T.M., Lamb, P.W., Oshimura, M., and Barrett, J.C., Correlation of v-*src* gene amplification with the tumorigenic phenotype in a Syrian hamster embryo cell line, *Cancer Res.,* 47, 4663, 1987.

42. Akroyd, J., Fincham, V.J., Green, A.R., Levantis, P., Searle, S., and Wyke, J.A., Transcription of Rous sarcoma proviruses in rat cells is determined by chromosomal position effects that fluctuate and can operate over long distances, *Oncogene,* 1, 347, 1987.

43. Broome, S. and Gilbert, W., Rous sarcoma virus encodes a transcriptional activator, *Cell,* 40, 537, 1985.

44. Levantis, P., Gillespie, D.A.F., Hart, K., Bissell, M.J., and Wyke, J.A., Control of expression of an integrated Rous sarcoma provirus in rat cells: role of 5′ genomic duplications reveals unexpected patterns of gene transcription and its regulation, *J. Virol.,* 57, 907, 1986.

45. Green, A.R., Searle, S., Gillespie, D.A.F., Bissell, M., and Wyke, J.A., Expression of integrated Rous sarcoma viruses: DNA rearrangements 5′ to the provirus are common in transformed rat cells but not seen in infected but untransformed cells, *EMBO J.,* 5, 707, 1986.

46. Boettiger, D., Virogenic nontransformed cells isolated following infection of normal rat kidney cells with B77 strain of Rous sarcoma virus, *Cell,* 3, 71, 1977.

47. Searle, S., Gillespie, D.A.F., Chiswell, D.J., and Wyke, J.A., Analysis of variations in proviral cytosine methylation that accompany transformation and morphological reversion in a line of Rous sarcoma virus-infected Rat-1 cells, *Nucleic Acids Res.,* 12, 5193, 1984.

48. Sealey, L. and Chalkey, R., At least two nuclear proteins bind specifically to the Rous sarcoma virus long terminal repeat enhancer, *Mol. Cell. Biol.,* 7, 787, 1987.

49. Stoltzfus, C.M., Chang, L.-J., Cripe, T.P., and Turek, L.P., Efficient transformation by Prague A Rous sarcoma virus plasmid DNA requires the presence of *cis*-acting regions within the *gag* gene, *J. Virol.,* 61, 3401, 1987.

50. Hippenmeyer, P.J. and Grandgenett, D.P., Mutants of the Rous sarcoma virus reverse transcriptase gene are nondefective in early replication events, *J. Biol. Chem.,* 260, 8520, 1985.

51. Jacks, T. and Varmus, H.E., Expression of the Rous sarcoma virus *pol* gene by ribosomal frameshifting, *Science,* 230, 1237, 1985.

52. Stoltzfus, C.M., Lorenzen, S.K., and Berberich, S.L., Noncoding region between the *env* and *src* genes of Rous sarcoma virus influences splicing efficiency at the *src* gene 3′ splice site, *J. Virol.,* 61, 177, 1987.

53. Garber, E.A. and Hanafusa, H., NH_2-terminal sequences of two src proteins that cause aberrant transformation, *Proc. Natl. Acad. Sci. U.S.A.,* 84, 80, 1987.

54. Hardwick, J.M., Shaw, K.E.S., Wills, J.W., and Hunter, E., Amino-terminal deletion mutants of the Rous sarcoma virus glycoprotein do not block signal peptide cleavage but can block intracellular transport, *J. Cell Biol.,* 103, 829, 1986.

55. Takeya, T. and Hanafusa, H., Structure and sequence of the cellular gene homologous to the RSV *src* gene and the mechanism for generating the transforming virus, *Cell,* 32, 881, 1983.

56. Parker, R.C., Varmus, H.E., and Bishop, J.M., Expression of v-*src* and chicken c-*src* in rat cells demonstrates qualitative differences between pp60$^{v\text{-}src}$ and pp60$^{c\text{-}src}$, *Cell,* 37, 131, 1984.

57. Gilmer, T.M., Expression of the chicken c-*src* gene in COS cells, *Mol. Cell. Biol.,* 4, 846, 1984.

58. Piwnica-Worms, H., Kaplan, D.R., Whitman, M., and Roberts, T.M., Retrovirus shuttle vector for study of kinase activities of pp60$^{c\text{-}src}$ synthesized *in vitro* and overproduced *in vivo*, *Mol. Cell. Biol.,* 6, 2033, 1986.

59. Kornbluth, S., Jove, R., and Hanafusa, H., Characterization of avian and viral p60^{src} proteins expressed in yeast, *Proc. Natl. Acad. Sci. U.S.A.,* 84, 4455, 1987.

60. Le Beau, M.M., Westbrook, C.A., Diaz, M.O., and Rowley, J.D., Evidence for two distinct c-*src* loci on human chromosomes 1 and 20, *Nature,* 312, 70, 1984.

61. Sakaguchi, A.Y., Mohandas, T., and Naylor, S.L., A human c-*src* gene resides on the proximal long arme of chromosome 20 (cen—q131), *Cancer Genet. Cytogenet.,* 18, 123, 1985.

62. Gibbs, C.P., Tanaka, A., Anderson, S.K., Radul, J., Baar, J., Ridgway, A., Kung, H.-J., and Fujita, D.J., Isolation and structural mapping of a human c-*src* gene homologous to the transforming gene (v-*src*) of Rous sarcoma virus, *J. Virol.,* 53, 19, 1985.

63. Parker, R.C., Mardon, G., Lebo, R.V., Varmus, H.E., and Bishop, J.M., Isolation of duplicated human c-*src* genes located on chromosomes 1 and 20, *Mol. Cell. Biol.,* 5, 831, 1985.

64. Anderson, S.K., Gibbs, C.P., Tanaka, A., Kung, H.-J., and Fujita, D.J., Human cellular *src* gene: nucleotide sequence and derived amino acid sequence of the region coding for the carboxy-terminal two-thirds of pp60$^{c\text{-}src}$, *Mol. Cell. Biol.,* 5, 1122, 1985.

65. Nishizawa, M., Semba, K., Yoshida, M.C., Yamamoto, T., Sasaki, M., and Toyoshima, K., Structure, expression, and chromosomal location of the human c-*fgr* gene, *Mol. Cell. Biol.,* 6, 511, 1986.

66. Tanaka, A., Gibbs, C.P., Arthur, R.R., Anderson, S.K., Kung, H.-J., and Fujita, D.J., DNA sequence encoding the amino-terminal region of the human c-*src* protein: implications of the sequence divergence among *src*-type kinase oncogenes, *Mol. Cell. Biol.,* 7, 1978, 1987.

67. Tanaka, A. and Fujita, D.J., Expression of a molecularly cloned human c-*src* oncogene by using a replication-competent retroviral vector, *Mol. Cell. Biol.,* 6, 3900, 1986.

68. Schartl, M. and Barnekow, A., The expression in eukaryotes of a tyrosine kinase which is reactive with pp60^{v-src} antibodies, *Differentiation,* 23, 109, 1982.
69. Jacobs, C. and Rubsamen, H., Expression of pp60^{c-src} protein kinase in adult and fetal human tissue: high activities in some sarcomas and mammary carcinomas, *Cancer Res.,* 43, 1696, 1983.
70. Pavloff, N., Biquard, J.-M., Hanania, N., and Semmel, M., Isolation of proteins with kinase activity and related to pp60 src from human cells, *Biochem. Biophys. Res. Commun.,* 121, 779, 1984.
71. Barnekow, A. and Schartl, M., Cellular *src* gene product detected in the freshwater sponge *Spongilla lacustris*, *Mol. Cell. Biol.,* 4, 1179, 1984.
72. Sorge, J.P., Sorge, L.K., and Maness, P.F., pp60^{c-src} is expressed in human fetal and adult brain, *Am. J. Pathol.,* 119, 151, 1985.
73. Amini, S., DeSeau, V., Reddy, S., Shalloway, D., and Bolen, J.B., Regulation of pp60^{c-src} synthesis by inducible RNA complementary to c-*src* mRNA in polyomavirus-transformed rat cells, *Mol. Cell Biol.,* 6, 2305, 1986.
74. Barnekow, A. and Bauer, H., The differential expression of the cellular *src*-gene product pp60^{src} and its phosphokinase activity in normal chicken cells and tissues, *Biochim. Biophys. Acta,* 792, 94, 1984.
75. Wadsworth, S.C., Madhavan, K., and Bilodeau-Wentworth, D., Maternal inheritance of transcripts from three *Drosophila src*-related genes, *Nucleic Acids Res.,* 13, 2153, 1985.
76. Simon, M.A., Drees, B., Kornberg, T., and Bishop, J.M., The nucleotide sequence and the tissue-specific expression of Drosophila c-*src*, *Cell,* 42, 841, 1985.
77. Gregory, R.J., Kammermeyer, K.L., Vincent, W.S., III, and Wadsworth, S.G., Primary sequence and developmental expression of a novel *Drosophila melanogaster src* gene, *Mol. Cell. Biol.,* 7, 2119, 1987.
78. Haas, A., Heller, I., and Presek, P., Detection of a tyrosine kinase in human sera and blood cells by pp60^{src} antiserum, *Biochem. Biophys. Res. Commun.,* 135, 426, 1986.
79. Gee, C.E., Griffin, J., Sastre, L., Miller, L.J., Springer, T.A., Piwnica-Worms, H., and Roberts, T.M., Differentiation of myeloid cells is accompanied by increased levels of pp60^{c-src} protein and kinase activity, *Proc. Natl. Acad. Sci. U.S.A.,* 83, 5131, 1986.
80. Golden, A., Nemeth, S.P., and Brugge, J.S., Blood platelets express high levels of the pp60^{c-src}-specific tyrosine kinase activity, *Proc. Natl. Acad. Sci. U.S.A.,* 83, 852, 1986.
81. Varshney, G.C., Henry, J., Kahn, A., and Phan-Dinh-Tuy, F., Tyrosine kinases in normal human blood cells: platelet but not erythrocyte band 3 tyrosine kinase is p60^{c-src}, *FEBS Lett.,* 205, 97, 1986.
82. Sorge, L.K., Levy, B.T., and Maness, P.F., pp60^{c-src} is developmentally regulated in the neural retina, *Cell,* 36, 249, 1984.
83. Levy, B.T., Sorge, L.K., Meymandi, A., and Maness, P.F., pp60^{c-src} kinase is in chick and human embryonic tissues, *Dev. Biol.,* 104, 9, 1984.
84. Fults, D.W., Towle, A.C., Lauder, J.M., and Maness, P.F., pp60^{c-src} in the developing cerebellum, *Mol. Cell. Biol.,* 5, 27, 1985.
85. Neer, E.J. and Lok, J.M., Partial purification and characterization of a pp60^{v-src}-related tyrosine kinase from bovine brain, *Proc. Natl. Acad. Sci. U.S.A.,* 82, 6025, 1985.
86. Grady, E.F., Schwab, M., and Rosenau, W., Expression of N-*myc* and c-*src* during the development of fetal human brain, *Cancer Res.,* 47, 2931, 1987.
87. Brugge, J.S., Cotton, P.C., Queral, A.E., Barrett, J.N., Nonner, D., and Keane, R.W., Neurones express high levels of a structurally modified, activated form of pp60^{c-src}, *Nature,* 316, 554, 1985.
88. Brugge, J., Cotton, P., Lustig, A., Yonemoto, W., Lipsich, L., Coussens, P., Barrett, J.N., Nonner, D., and Keane, R.W., Characterization of the altered form of the c-*src* gene product in neuronal cells, *Genes Dev.,* 1, 287, 1987.
89. Martinez, R., Mathey-Prevot, B., Bernards, A., and Baltimore, D., Neuronal pp60^{c-src} contains a six-amino acid insertion relative to its non-neuronal counterpart, *Science,* 237, 411, 1987.
90. Wiestler, O.D. and Walter, G., Developmental expression of two forms of pp60^{c-src} in mouse brain, Mol. Cell. Biol., 8, 502, 1988.
91. Le Beau, J.M., Wiestler, O.D., and Walter, G., An altered form of pp60^{c-src} is expressed primarily in the central nervous system, *Mol. Cell. Biol.,* 7, 4115, 1987.
92. Alema, S., Casalbore, P., Agostini, E., and Tato, F., Differentiation of PC12 phaeochromocytoma cells induced by v-*src* oncogene, *Nature,* 316, 557, 1985.
93. Maness, P.F., pp60^{c-src} encoded by the proto-oncogene c-*src* is a product of sensory neurons, *J. Neurosci. Res.,* 16, 127, 1986.
94. Vardimon, L., Fox, L.E., and Moscona, A.A., Accumulation of c-*src* mRNA is developmentally regulated in embryonic neural retina, *Mol. Cell. Biol.,* 6, 4109, 1986.
95. Parsons, S.J. and Creutz, C.E., p60^{c-src} activity detected in the chromaffin granule membrane, *Biochem. Biophys. Res. Commun.,* 134, 736, 1986.
96. Shealy, D.J. and Erikson, R.L., Human cells contain two forms of pp60^{c-src}, *Nature,* 293, 666, 1981.
97. Collett, M.S., Belzer, S.K., and Purchio, A.F., Structurally and fucntionally modified forms of pp60^{v-src} in Rous sarcoma virus-transformed cell lysates, *Mol. Cell. Biol.,* 4, 1213, 1984.

98. Collett, M.S., Belzer, S.K., and Kamp, L.E., Enzymatic characteristics of pp60^{v-src} isolated from vanadium-treated transformed cells, *J. Cell. Biochem.,* 26, 95, 1984.

99. Resh, M.D. and Erikson, R.L., Highly specific antibody to Rous sarcoma virus *src* gene product recognizes a novel population of pp60^{v-src} and pp60^{c-src} molecules, *J. Cell Biol.,* 100, 409, 1985.

100. Rosen, N., Bolen, J.B., Schwartz, A.M., Cohen, P., DeSeau, V., and Israel, M.A., Analysis of pp60^{c-src} protein kinase activity in human tumor cell lines and tissues, *J. Biol. Chem.,* 261, 13754, 1986.

101. Bolen, J.B., Veillette, A., Schwartz, A.M., DeSeau, V., and Rosen, N., Activation of pp60^{c-src} protein kinase activity in human colon carcinoma, *Proc. Natl. Acad. Sci. U.S.A.,* 84, 2251, 1987.

102. Bolen, J.B., Veillette, A., Schwartz, A.M., DeSeau, V., and Rosen, N., Analysis of pp60^{c-src} in human colon carcinoma and normal human colon mucosal cells, *Oncogene Res.,* 1, 149, 1987.

103. Lynch, S.A., Brugge, J.S., and Levine, J.M., Induction of altered c-*src* product during neural differentiation of embryonal carcinoma cells, *Science,* 234, 873, 1986.

104. Kanner, S.B., Parsons, S.J., Parsons, J., and Gilmer, T.M., Activation of pp60^{c-src} tyrosine kinase specific activity in tumor-derived Syrian hamster embryo cells, *Oncogene,* 2, 327, 1988.

105. Wang, L.-H., Iijima, S., Dorai, T., and Lin, B., Regulation of the expression of proto-oncogene c-*src* by alternative RNA splicing in chicken skeletal muscle, *Oncogene Res.,* 1, 43, 1987.

106. Brugge, J.S. and Erikson, R.L., Identification of a transformation-specific antigen induced by an avian sarcoma virus, *Nature,* 269, 346, 1977.

107. Stehelin, D., Varmus, H.E., Bishop, J.M., and Vogt, P.K., DNA related to the transforming gene(s) of avian sarcoma viruses is present in normal avian DNA, *Nature,* 260, 170, 1976.

108. Spector, D.H., Varmus, H.E., and Bishop, J.M., Nucleotide sequences related to the transforming gene of avian sarcoma virus are present in the DNA of uninfected vertebrates, *Proc. Natl. Acad. Sci. U.S.A.,* 75, 4100, 1978.

109. Collett, M.S., Brugge, J.S., and Erikson, R.L., Characterization of a normal avian cell protein related to the avian sarcoma virus transforming gene product, *Cell,* 15, 1363, 1978.

110. Oppermann, H., Levinson, A.D., Varmus, H.E., Levinton, L., and Bishop, J.M., Uninfected vertebrate cells contain a protein that is closely related to the product of the avian sarcoma virus transforming gene (*src*), *Proc. Natl. Acad. Sci. U.S.A.,* 76, 1804, 1979.

111. Collett, M.S., Erikson, E., Purchio, A.F., Brugge, J.S., and Erikson, R.L., A normal cell protein similar in structure and function to the avian sarcoma virus transforming gene product, *Proc. Natl. Acad. Sci. U.S.A.,* 76, 3159, 1979.

112. Sefton, B.M., Hunter, T., and Beemon, K., Relationship of polypeptide products of the transforming gene of Rous sarcoma virus and the homologous gene of vertebrates, *Proc. Natl. Acad. Sci. U.S.A.,* 77, 2959, 1980.

113. Barnekow, A., Schartl, M., Anders, F., and Bauer, H., Identification of a fish protein associated with a kinase activity related to the Rous sarcoma virus transforming protein, *Cancer Res.,* 42, 2429, 1982.

114. Shilo, B. and Weinberg, R.A., DNA sequences homologous to vertebrate oncogenes are conserved in *Drosophila melanogaster*, *Proc. Nat. Acad. Sci. U.S.A.,* 78, 6789, 1981.

115. Lev, Z., Leibovitz, N., Segev, O., and Shilo, B.-Z., Expression of the *src* and *abl* cellular oncogenes during development of *Drosophila melanogaster*, *Mol. Cell. Biol.,* 4, 982, 1984.

116. Gessler, M. and Barnekow, A., Differential expression of the cellular oncogenes c-*src* and c-*yes* in embryonal and adult chicken tissues, *Biosci. Rep.,* 4, 757, 1984.

117. Barnekow, A. and Schartl, M., Cellular *src* gene product detected in the freshwater sponge *Spongilla lacustris*, *Mol. Cell. Biol.,* 4, 1179, 1984.

118. Simon, M.A., Kornberg, T.B., and Bishop, J.M., Three loci related to the *src* oncogene and tyrosine-specific protein kinase activity in *Drosophila*, *Nature,* 302, 837, 1983.

119. Steele, R.E., Two divergent cellular *src* genes are expressed in *Xenopus laevis*, *Nucleic Acids Res.,* 13, 1747, 1985.

120. Castellanos, R.M.P. and Mazón, M.J., Identification of phosphotyrosine in yeast proteins and of a protein tyrosine kinase associated with the plasma membrane, *J. Biol. Chem.,* 260, 8240, 1985.

121. Schieven, G., Thorner, J., and Martin, G.S., Protein-tyrosine kinase activity in *Saccharomyces cerevisiae*, *Science,* 231, 390, 1986.

122. Dahl, C., Biemann, H.-P., and Dahl, J., A protein kinase antigenically related to pp60^{v-src} possibly involved in yeast cell cycle control: positive *in vivo* regulation by sterol, *Proc. Natl. Acad. Sci. U.S.A.,* 84, 4012, 1987.

123. Vallejos, R.H., Holuigue, L., Lucero, H.A., and Torruella, M., Evidence of tyrosine kinase activity in the photosynthetic bacterium *Rhodospirillum rubrum*, *Biochem. Biophys. Res. Commun.,* 126, 685, 1985.

124. Torruella, M., Casano, L.M., and Vallejos, R.H., Evidence of the activity of tyrosine kinase(s) and of the presence of phosphotyrosine proteins in pea plantlets, *J. Biol. Chem.,* 261, 6651, 1986.

125. Schartl, M. and Barnekow, A., Differential expression of the cellular src gene during vertebrate development, *Dev. Biol.,* 105, 415, 1984.

126. Sejersen, T., Björklund, H., Sümegi, J., and Ringertz, N.R., N-myc and c-src genes are differentially regulated in PCC7 embryonal carcinoma cells undergoing neuronal differentiation, *J. Cell. Physiol.,* 127, 274, 1986.

127. Hoffman-Falk, H., Einat, P., Shilo, B.-Z., and Hoffmann, F.M., Drosophila melanogaster DNA clones homologous to vertebrate oncogenes: evidence for a common ancestor to the *src* and *abl* cellular genes, *Cell,* 32, 589, 1983.

128. Hoffmann, F.M., Fresco, L.D., Hoffman-Falk, H., and Shilo, B.-Z., Nucleotide sequences of the Drosophila *src* and *abl* homologs: conservation and variability in the *src* family of oncogenes, *Cell,* 35, 393, 1983.

129. Shilo, B.-Z., Evolution of cellular oncogenes, *Adv. Viral Oncol.,* 4, 29, 1984.

130. Mark, G.E. and Rapp, U.R., Primary structure of v-*raf*: relatedness to the *src* family of oncogenes, *Science,* 224, 285, 1984.

131. Barker, W.C. and Dayhoff, M.O., Viral *src* gene products are related to the catalytic chain of mammalian cAMP-dependent protein kinase, *Proc. Natl. Acad. Sci. U.S.A.,* 79, 2836, 1982.

132. Kamps, M.P., Taylor, S.S., and Sefton, B.M., Direct evidence that oncogenic tyrosine kinases and cyclic AMP-dependent protein kinase have homologous ATP-binding sites, *Nature,* 310, 589, 1984.

133. Kamps, M.P. and Sefton, B.M., Neither arginine nor histidine can carry out the function of lysine-295 in the ATP-binding site of pp60^{src}, *Mol. Cell. Biol.,* 6, 751, 1986.

134. Wyke, J.A. and Stoker, A.W., Genetic analysis of the form and function of the viral *src* oncogene product, *Biochim. Biophys. Acta,* 907, 47, 1987.

135. Fukami, Y. and Lipmann, F., Purification of the Rous sarcoma virus *src* kinase by casein-agarose and tyrosine-agarose affinity chromatography, *Proc. Natl. Acad. Sci. U.S.A.,* 82, 321, 1985.

136. Sugimoto, Y., Erikson, E., Graziani, Y., and Erikson, R.L., Inter- and intramolecular interactions of highly purified Rous sarcoma virus-transforming protein, pp60^{v-src}, *J. Biol. Chem.,* 260, 13838, 1985.

137. Gilmer, T.M. and Erikson, R.L., Rous sarcoma virus transforming protein p60^{src}, expressed in *E. coli,* functions as a protein kinase, *Nature,* 294, 771, 1981.

138. McGrath, J.P. and Levinson, A.D., Bacterial expression of an enzymatically active protein encoded by RSV *src* gene, *Nature,* 295, 423, 1982.

139. Pierce, J.H., Aaronson, S.A., and Anderson, S.M., Hematopoietic cell transformation by a murine recombinant retrovirus containing the *src* gene of Rous sarcoma virus, *Proc. Natl. Acad. Sci. U.S.A.,* 81, 2374, 1984.

140. Parker, R.C., Varmus, H.E., and Bishop, J.M., Expression of v-*src* and chicken c-*src* in rat cells demonstrates qualitative differences between pp60^{v-src} and pp60^{c-src}, *Cell,* 37, 131, 1984.

141. Tarpley, W.G. and Temin, H.M., The location of v-*src* in a retrovirus vector determines whether the virus is toxic or transforming, *Mol. Cell. Biol.,* 4, 2653, 1984.

142. Feuerman, N.H., Davis, B.R., Pattengale, P.K., and Fan, H., Generation of a recombinant Moloney murine leukemia virus carrying the v-*src* gene of avian sarcoma virus: transformation in vitro and pathogenesis *in vivo, J. Virol.,* 54, 804, 1985.

143. Gilmer, T.M. and Erikson, R.L., Development of anti-pp60^{src} serum with antigen produced in *Escherichia coli, J. Virol.,* 45, 462, 1983.

144. Development and characterization of antisera specific for amino- and carboxy-terminal regions of pp60^{src}, *J. Virol.,* 55, 242, 1985.

145. Tamura, T. and Bauer, H., Monoclonal antibody against the carboxy terminal peptide of pp60^{src} of Rous sarcoma virus reacts with native pp60^{src}, *EMBO J.,* 1, 1479, 1982.

146. Tamura, T., Bauer, H., Birr, C., and Pipkorn, R., Antibodies against synthetic peptides as a tool for functional analysis of the transforming protein pp60^{src}, *Cell,* 34, 587, 1983.

147. Tanaka, T. and Kurth, R., Monoclonal antibodies specific for the avian sarcoma virus transforming protein pp60^{src}, *Virology,* 133, 202, 1984.

148. Parsons, S.J., McCarley, D.J., Ely, C.M., Benjamin, D.C., and Parsons, J.T., Monoclonal antibodies to Rous sarcoma virus pp60^{src} react with enzymatically active cellular pp60^{src} of avian and mammalian origin, *J. Virol.,* 51, 272, 1984.

149. Parsons, S.J., McCarley, D.J., Raymond, V.W., and Parsons, J.T., Localization of conserved and nonconserved epitopes within the Rous sarcoma virus-encoded *src* protein, *J. Virol.,* 59, 755, 1986.

150. Collett, M.S. and Erikson, R.L., Protein kinase activity associated with the avian sarcoma virus *src* gene product, *Proc. Natl. Acad. Sci. U.S.A.,* 75, 2021, 1978.

151. Levinson, A.D., Oppermann, H., Levintow, L., Varmus, H.E., and Bishop, J.M., Evidence that the transforming gene of avian sarcoma virus encodes a protein kinase associated with a phosphoprotein, *Cell,* 15, 561, 1978.

152. Hunter, T. and Sefton, B.M., Transforming gene product of Rous sarcoma virus phosphorylates tyrosine, *Proc. Natl. Acad. Sci. U.S.A.,* 77, 1311, 1980.

153. Collett, M.S., Purchio, A.F., and Erikson, R.L., Avian sarcoma virus transforming protein, pp60^{src}, shows protein kinase activity specific for tyrosine, *Nature,* 285, 167, 1980.

154. Akiyama, T., Ishida, J., Nakagawa, S., Ogawara, H., Watanabe, S., Itoh, N., Shibuya, M., and Fukami, Y., Genistein, a specific inhibitor of tyrosine-specific protein kinase, *J. Biol. Chem.,* 262, 5592, 1987.

155. McCarley, D.J., Parsons, J.T., Benjamin, D.C., and Parsons, S.J., Inhibition of the tyrosine kinase activity of v-*src*, v-*fgr*, and v-*yes* gene products by a monoclonal antibody which binds both amino and carboxy peptide fragments of pp60^{v-src}, *J. Virol.,* 61, 1927, 1987.

156. Collett, M.S., Erikson, E., and Erikson, R.L., Structural analysis of the avian sarcoma virus transforming protein: sites of phosphorylation, *J. Virol.,* 29, 770, 1979.

157. Resh, M.D. and Erickson, R.L., Characterization of pp60^{src} phosphorylation in vitro in Rous sarcoma virus-transformed cell membranes, *Mol. Cell. Biol.,* 5, 916, 1985.

158. Patschinsky, T., Hunter, T., and Sefton, B.M., Phosphorylation of the transforming protein of Rous sarcoma virus: direct demonstration of phosphorylation of serine 17 and identification of an additional site of tyrosine phosphorylation in p60^{v-src} of Prague Rous sarcoma virus, *J. Virol.,* 59, 73, 1986.

159. Roth, C.W., Richert, N.D., Pastan, I., and Gottesman, M.M., Cyclic AMP treatment of Rous sarcoma virus-transformed Chinese hamster ovary cells increases phosphorylation of pp60^{src} and increases pp60^{src} kinase activity, *J. Biol. Chem.,* 258, 10768, 1983.

160. Clinton, G.M. and Roskoski, R., Jr., Tyrosyl and cyclic AMP-dependent protein kinase activities in BHK cells that express viral pp60^{src}, *Mol. Cell. Biol.,* 4, 973, 1984.

161. Tamura, T., Friis, R.R., and Bauer, H., pp60^{c-src} is a substrate for phosphorylation when cells are stimulated to enter cell cycle, *FEBS Lett.,* 177, 151, 1984.

162. Gould, K.L., Woodgett, J.R., Cooper, J.A., Buss, J.E., Shalloway, D., and Hunter, T., Protein kinase C phosphorylates pp60^{src} at a novel site, *Cell,* 42, 849, 1985.

163. Purchio, A.F., Shoyab, M., and Gentry, L.E., Site-specific increased phosphorylation of pp60^{v-src} after treatment of RSV-transformed cells with a tumor promoter, *Science,* 229, 1393, 1985.

164. Purchio, A.F., Gentry, L., and Shoyab, M., Phosphorylation of pp60^{v-src} by the TPA receptor kinase (protein kinase C), *Virology,* 150, 524, 1986.

165. Ledbetter, J.A., Gentry, L.E., June, C.H., Rabinovitch, P.S., and Purchio, A.F., Stimulation of T cells through the CD3/T-cell receptor complex: role of cytoplasmic calcium, protein kinase C translocation, and phosphorylation of pp60^{c-src} in the activation pathway, *Mol. Cell. Biol.,* 7, 650, 1987.

166. Gentry, L.E., Chaffin, K.E., Shoyab, M., and Purchio, A.F., Novel serine phosphorylation of pp60^{c-src} in intact cells after tumor promoter treatment, *Mol. Cell. Biol.,* 6, 735, 1986.

167. Chackalaparampil, I. and Shalloway, D., Altered phosphorylation and activation of pp60^{c-src} during fibroblast mitosis, *Cell,* 52, 801, 1988.

168. Smart, J.E., Oppermann, H., Czernilofsky, A.P., Purchio, A.F., Erikson, R.L., and Bishop, J.M., Characterization of sites for tyrosine phosphorylation in the transforming protein of Rous sarcoma virus (pp60^{v-src}) and its normal cellular homologue (pp60^{c-src}), *Proc. Natl. Acad. Sci. U.S.A.,* 78, 6013, 1981.

169. Iba, H., Cross, F.R., Garber, E.A., and Hanafusa, H., Low level of cellular protein phosphorylation in nontransforming overproduced p60^{c-src}, *Mol. Cell. Biol.,* 5, 1058, 1985.

170. Laudano, A.P. and Buchanan, J.M., Phosphorylation of tyrosine in the carboxyl-terminal tryptic peptide of pp60^{c-src}, *Proc. Natl. Acad. Sci. U.S.A.,* 83, 892, 1986.

171. Cooper, J.A., Gould, K.L., Cartwright, C.A., and Hunter, T., Tyr^{527} is phosphorylated in pp60^{c-src}: implications for regulation, *Science,* 231, 1431, 1986.

172. Cooper, J.A. and King, C.S., Dephosphorylation or antibody binding to the carboxy terminus stimulates pp60^{c-src}, *Mol. Cell. Biol.,* 6, 4467, 1986.

173. Cooper, J.A. and Runge, K., Avian pp60^{c-src} is more active when expressed in yeast than in vertebrate fibroblasts, *Oncogene Res.,* 1, 297, 1987.

174. Kmiecik, T.E. and Shalloway, D., Activation and suppression of pp60^{c-src} transforming ability by mutation of its primary sites of tyrosine phosphorylation, *Cell,* 49, 65, 1987.

175. Jove, R., Kornbluth, S., and Hanafusa, H., Enzymatically inactive p60^{c-src} mutant with altered ATP-binding site is fully phosphorylated in its carboxy-terminal regulatory region, *Cell,* 50, 937, 1987.

176. Yonemoto, W., Jarvis-Morar, M., Brugge, J.S., Bolen, J.B., and Israel, M.A., Tyrosine phosphorylation within the amino-terminal domain of pp60^{c-src} molecules associated with polyoma virus middle-sized tumor antigen, *Proc. Natl. Acad. Sci. U.S.A.,* 82, 4568, 1985.

177. Wong, T.W. and Goldberg, A.R., Synthetic peptide fragment of *src* gene product inhibits the *src* protein kinase and crossreacts immunologically with avian *onc* kinases and cellular phosphoproteins, *Proc. Natl. Acad. Sci. U.S.A.,* 78, 7412, 1981.

178. Lax, I., Bar-Eli, M., Yarden, Y., Liberman, T.A., and Schlessinger, J., Antibodies to two defined regions of the transforming protein pp60^{src} interact specifically with the epidermal growth factor receptor kinase system, *Proc. Natl. Acad. Sci. U.S.A.,* 81, 5911, 1984.

179. Parry, G., Bartholomew, J.C., and Bissell, M.J., Role of the *src* gene in growth regulation of Rous sarcoma virus-infected chicken embryo fibroblasts, *Nature,* 288, 720, 1980.

180. Weber, M.J., Rubsamen, H., and Friis, R.R., Lack of correlation between pp60^{src} kinase activity and transformation parameters in cells infected with temperature-conditional mutants of Rous sarcoma virus, *J. Gen. Virol.,* 52, 395, 1981.

181. Cooper, J., Nakamura, K.D., Hunter, T., and Weber, M.J., Phosphotyrosine-containing proteins and expression of transformation parameters in cells infected with partial transformation mutants of Rous sarcoma virus, *J. Virol.,* 46, 15, 1983.

182. Collett, M.S. and Belzer, S.K., Forms of pp60^{v-src} isolated from Rous sarcoma virus-transformed cells, *J. Virol.*, 61, 1593, 1987.

183. McCarley, D.J. and Parsons, S.J., Reduced tyrosine kinase specific activity is associated with hypo-phosphorylation of pp60^{c-src} in cells infected with avian erythroblastosis virus, *Proc. Natl. Acad. Sci. U.S.A.*, 84, 5793, 1987.

184. Erikson, R.L., Purchio, A.F., Erikson, E., Collett, M.S., and Brugge, J.S., Molecular events in cells transformed by Rous sarcoma virus, *J. Cell Biol.*, 87, 319, 1980.

185. Bauer, H., Barnekow, A., and Rose, G., The transforming protein of Rous sarcoma virus, pp60^{src}: growth and cell proliferation inducing properties, in *Hormones and Cell Regulation*, Dumont, J.E., Nunez, J., and Schultz, G., Eds., Elsevier, Amsterdam, 1982, 187.

186. Erikson, R.L., Towards a biochemical description of malignant transformation: identification and functional characteristics of the Rous sarcoma virus transforming gene product, *Cancer*, 53, 2041, 1984.

187. Weber, M.J. and Friis, R.R., Dissociation of transformation parameters using temperature-conditional mutants of Rous sarcoma virus, *Cell*, 16, 25, 1979.

188. Anderson, D.D., Beckmann, R.P., Harms, E.H., Nakamura, K., and Weber, M.J., Biological properties of "partial" transformation mutants of Rous sarcoma virus and characterization of their pp60^{src} kinase, *J. Virol.*, 37, 445, 1981.

189. Martinez, R., Nakamura, K.D., and Weber, M.J., Identification of phosphotyrosine-containing proteins in untransformed and Rous sarcoma virus-transformed chicken embryo fibroblasts, *Mol. Cell. Biol.*, 2, 653, 1982.

190. Kuzumaki, N., Yamagiwa, S., and Oikawa, T., No expression of a Rous sarcoma virus-induced tumor antigen in mammalian cells infected with retroviruses transducing other oncogenes of the *src* family, *J. Natl. Cancer Inst.*, 74, 889, 1985.

191. Courtneidge, S.A. and Bishop, J.M., Transit of pp60^{v-src} to the plasma membrane, *Proc. Natl. Acad. Sci. U.S.A.*, 79, 7117, 1982.

192. Courtneidge, S.A., Levinson, A.D., and Bishop, J.M., The protein encoded by the transforming gene of avian sarcoma virus (pp60^{src}) and a homologous protein in normal cells (pp60$^{proto-src}$) are associated with the plasma membrane, *Proc. Natl. Acad. Sci. U.S.A.*, 77, 3783, 1980.

193. Krueger, J.G., Wang, E., Garber, E.A., and Goldberg, A.R., Differences in intracellular location of pp60^{src} in rat and chicken cells transformed by Rous sarcoma virus, *Proc. Natl. Acad. Sci. U.S.A.*, 77, 4142, 1980.

194. Krzyzek, R.A., Mitchell, R.L., Lau, A.F., and Faras, A.J., Association of pp60^{src} protein kinase activity with plasma membrane of nonpermissive and permissive avian sarcoma virus-infected cells, *J. Virol.*, 36, 805, 1980.

195. Nigg, E.A., Sefton, B.M., Hunter, T., Walter, G., and Singer, S.J., Immunofluorescent localization of the transforming protein of Rous sarcoma virus with antibodies against a synthetic peptide, *Proc. Natl. Acad. Sci. U.S.A.*, 79, 5322, 1982.

196. Barnekow, A., Boschek, C.B., Ziemiecki, A., Friis, R.R., and Bauer, H., Demonstration of the Rous sarcoma virus pp60^{src} and its associated protein kinase on the surface of intact cells, in *Genes and Tumor Genes*, Winnacker, E. and Schoene, H.-H., Eds., Raven Press, New York, 1982, 65.

197. Levinson, A.D., Courtneidge, S.A., and Bishop, J.M., Structural and functional domains of the Rous sarcoma virus transforming protein (pp60^{src}), *Proc. Natl. Acad. Sci. U.S.A.*, 78, 1624, 1981.

198. Cross, F.R., Garber, E.A., Pellman, D., and Hanafusa, H., A short sequence in the p60^{src} N terminus is required for p60^{src} myristylation and membrane association and for cell transformation, *Mol. Cell. Biol.*, 4, 1834, 1984.

199. Buss, J.E., Kamps, M.P., and Sefton, B.M., Myristic acid is attached to the transforming protein of Rous sarcoma virus during or immediately after synthesis and is present in both soluble and membrane-bound forms of the protein, *Mol. Cell. Biol.*, 4, 2697, 1984.

200. Buss, J.E. and Sefton, B.M., Myristic acid, a rare fatty acid, is the lipid attached to the transforming protein of Rous sarcoma virus and its cellular homolog, *J. Virol.*, 53, 7, 1985.

201. Schultz, A.M., Henderson, L.E., Oroszlan, S., Garber, E.A., and Hanafusa, H., Amino terminal myristylation of the protein kinase p60src, a retroviral transforming protein, *Science*, 227, 427, 1985.

202. Krueger, J.G., Garber, E.A., Goldberg, A.R., and Hanafusa, H., Changes in amino-terminal sequences of pp60^{src} lead to decreased membrane association and decreased *in vivo* tumorigenicity, *Cell*, 28, 889, 1982.

203. Pellman, D., Garber, E.A., Cross, F.R., and Hanafusa, H., Fine structural mapping of a critical NH$_2$-terminal region of p60^{src}, *Proc. Natl. Acad. Sci. U.S.A.*, 82, 1623, 1985.

204. Kamps, M.P, Buss, J.E., and Sefton, B.M., Mutation of NH$_2$-terminal glycine of p60^{src} prevents both myristoylation and morphological transformation, *Proc. Natl. Acad. Sci. U.S.A.*, 82, 4625, 1985.

205. Buss, J.E., Kamps, M.P., Gould, K., and Sefton, B.M., The absence of myristic acid decreases membrane binding of p60^{src} but does not affect tyrosine protein kinase activity, *J. Virol.*, 58, 468, 1986.

206. Bryant, D. and Parsons, J.T., Site-directed point mutation in the *src* gene of Rous sarcoma virus results in an inactive *src* gene product, *J. Virol.*, 45, 1211, 1983.

207. Bryant, D.L. and Parsons, J.T., Amino acid alterations within a highly conserved region of the Rous sarcoma virus *src* gene product pp60^{src} inactivate tyrosine protein kinase activity, *Mol. Cell. Biol.*, 4, 862, 1984.

208. Uehara, Y., Hori, M., and Umezawa, H., Specific increase in thymidine transport at a permissive temperature in the rat kidney cells infected with *src^ts*-Rous sarcoma virus, *Biochem. Biophys. Res. Commun.,* 125, 129, 1984.

209. Shawyer, L.K., Olson, S.A., White, M.K., and Weber, M.J., Degradation and biosynthesis of the glucose transporter protein in chicken embryo fibroblasts transformed by the *src* oncogene, *Mol. Cell. Biol.,* 7, 2112, 1987.

210. Yee, S.-P. and Branton, P.E., External cell surface protein phosphorylation in normal and Rous sarcoma virus transformed chick embryo fibroblasts, *J. Cell. Physiol.,* 106, 149, 1981.

211. Dehazya, P. and Martin, G.S., pp60^src^-dependent protein phosphorylation in membranes from Rous sarcoma virus-transformed chicken embryo fibroblasts, *Virology,* 143, 407, 1985.

212. Shiba, T., Akiyama, T., Kadowaki, T., Fukami, Y., Tsuji, T., Osawa, T., Kasuga, M., and Takaku, F., Purified tyrosine kinases, the EGF receptor kinase and the src kinase, can catalyze the phosphorylation of the band 3 protein from human erythrocytes, *Biochem. Biophys. Res. Commun.,* 135, 720, 1986.

213. Witt, D.P. and Gordon, J.A., Specific dephosphorylation of membrane proteins in Rous sarcoma virus-transformed chick embryo fibroblasts, *Nature,* 287, 241, 1980.

214. Pierce, M. and Arango, J., Rous sarcoma virus-transformed baby hamster kidney cells express higher levels of asparagine-linked tri- and tetraantennary glycopeptides containning (GlcNAc-β(1,6)man-α(1,6)man) and poly-*N*-acetyllactosamine sequences than baby hamster kidney cells, *J. Biol. Chem.,* 261, 10772, 1986.

215. Guild, B.C., Erikson, R.L., and Strominger, J.L., HLA-A2 and HLA-B7 antigens are phosphorylated *in vitro* by Rous sarcoma virus kinase (pp60^v-src^) at a tyrosine residue encoded in a highly conserved exon of the intracellular domains, *Proc. Natl. Acad. Sci. U.S.A.,* 80, 2894, 1983.

216. Chen, W.-T., Chen, J.-M., Parsons, S.J., and Parsons, J.T., Local degradation of fibronectin at sites of expression of the transforming gene product pp60^src^, *Nature,* 316, 156, 1985.

217. Krueger, J.G., Garber, E.A., Chin, S.S.-M., Hanafusa, H., and Goldberg, A.R., Size-variant pp60^src^ proteins of recovered avian sarcoma viruses interact with adhesion plaques as peripheral membrane proteins: effects on cell transformation, *Mol. Cell. Biol.,* 4, 454, 1984.

218. Hirst, R., Horwitz, A., Buck, C., and Rohrschneider, L., Phosphorylation of the fibronectin receptor complex in cells transformed by oncogenes that encode tyrosine kinases, *Proc. Natl. Acad. Sci. U.S.A.,* 83, 6470, 1986.

219. Chen, W.-T., Wang, J., Hasegawa, T., Yamada, S.S., and Yamada, K.M., Regulation of fibronectin receptor distribution by transformation, exogenous fibronectin, and synthetic peptides, *J. Cell Biol.,* 103, 1649, 1986.

220. Chan, L.-M., Hatier, C., Parry, G., Werb, Z., and Bissell, M.J., Collagen-fibronectin interactions in normal and Rous sarcoma virus-transformed tendon cells: possible mechanisms for increased extracellular matrix turnover after transformation, *In Vitro Cell. Dev. Biol.,* 23, 308, 1987.

221. Cooper, J.A. and Hunter, T., Changes in protein phosphorylation in Rous sarcoma virus transformed chicken embryo cells, *Mol. Cell. Biol.,* 1, 165, 1981.

222. Tomasiewicz, H.G., Cook-Degan, R., and Chikaraishi, D.M., Isolation of a cDNA clone complementary to sequences for a 34-kilodalton protein which is a pp60^v-src^ substrate, *Mol. Cell. Biol.,* 4, 1935, 1984.

223. Soric, J. and Gordon, J.A., Calcium-dependent isolation of the 36-kilodalton substrate of pp60^src^-kinase. Fractionation of the phosphorylated and unphosphorylated species, *J. Biol. Chem.,* 261, 14490, 1986.

224. Simon, M., Arrigo, A.-P., and Spahr, P.-F., Association of three chicken proteins with the 34 kD target of Rous sarcoma virus tyrosine kinase, *Exp. Cell Res.,* 169, 419, 1987.

225. Radke, K. and Martin, G.S., Transformation by Rous sarcoma virus: effects of *src* gene expression on the synthesis and phosphorylation of cellular polypeptides, *Proc. Natl. Acad. Sci. U.S.A.,* 76, 5212, 1979.

226. Radke, K., Gilmore, T., and Martin, G.S., Transformation by Rous sarcoma virus: a cellular substrate for transformation-specific protein phosphorylation contains phosphotyrosine, *Cell,* 21, 821, 1980.

227. Erikson, E. and Erikson, R.L., Identification of a cellular protein substrate phosphorylated by the avian sarcoma virus-transforming gene product, *Cell,* 21, 829, 1980.

228. Erikson, E., Tomasiewicz, G., and Erikson, R.L., Biochemical characterization of a 34-kilodalton normal cellular substrate of pp60^v-src^ and an associated 6-kilodalton protein, *Mol. Cell. Biol.,* 4, 77, 1984.

229. Greenberg, M.E. and Edelman, G.M., The 34 kd pp60^src^ substrate is located at the inner face of the plasma membrane, *Cell,* 33, 767, 1983.

230. Lehto, V.-P., Virtanen, I., Paasivuo, R., Ralston, R., and Alitalo, K., The p36 substrate of tyrosine-specific protein kinsinc co-localizes with non-erythrocyte alpha-spectrin antigen, p230, in surface lamina of cultured fibroblasts, *EMBO J.,* 2, 1701, 1983.

231. Soric, J. and Gordon, J.A., The 36-kilodalton substrate of pp60^v-src^ is myristylated in a transformation-sensitive manner, *Science,* 230, 563, 1985.

232. Johnsson, N., Vandekerckhove, J., Van Damme, J., and Weber, K., Binding sites for calcium, lipid and p11 on p36, the substrate of retroviral tyrosine-specific protein kinases, *FEBS Lett.,* 198, 361, 1986.

233. Martin, F., Derancourt, J., Capony, J.-P., and Colote, S., Sequence homologies between p36, the substrate of pp60^src^ tyrosine kinase and a 67 kDa protein isolated from bovina aorta, *Biochem. Biophys. Res. Commun.,* 145, 961, 1987.

234. Glenney, J.R., Jr., Phosphorylation of p36 *in vitro* with pp60^{src}: regulation by Ca^{2+} and phospholipid, FEBS Lett., 192, 79, 1985.

235. Khanna, N.C., Tokuda, M., Chong, S.M., and Waisman, D.M., Phosphorylation of p36 in vitro by protein kinase C, *Biochem. Biophys. Res. Commun.*, 137, 397, 1986.

236. Gould, K.L., Woodgett, J.R., Isacke, C.M., and Hunter, T., The protein-tyrosine kinase substrate p36 is also a substrate for protein kinase C *in vitro* and *in vivo*, *Mol. Cell. Biol.*, 6, 2738, 1986.

237. Isacke, C.M., Trowbridge, I.S., and Hunter, T., Modulation of p36 phosphorylation in human cells: studies using anti-p36 antibodies, *Mol. Cell. Biol.*, 6, 2745, 1986.

238. Arrigo, A.-P., Darlix, J.-L., and Spahr, P.-F., A cellular protein phosphorylated by the avian sarcoma virus transforming gene product is associated with ribonucleoprotein particles, *EMBO J.*, 2, 309, 1983.

239. Gould, K.L., Cooper, J.A., and Hunter, T., The 46,000-dalton tyrosine protein kinase substrate is widespread, whereas the 36,000-dalton substrate is only expressed at high levels in certain rodent tissues, *J. Cell Biol.*, 98, 487, 1984.

240. Nawrocki, J.F., Lau, A.F., and Faras, A.J., Correlation between phosphorylation of a 34,000-molecular-weight protein, pp60^{src}-associated kinase activity, and tumorigenicity in transformed and revertant vole cells, *Mol. Cell. Biol.*, 4, 212, 1984.

241. Erikson, E., Cook, R., Miller, G.J., and Erikson, R.L., The same normal cell protein is phosphorylated after transformation by avian sarcoma viruses with unrelated transforming genes, *Mol. Cell. Biol.*, 1, 43, 1981.

242. Hunter, T. and Cooper, J.A., Epidermal growth factor induces rapid tyrosine phosphorylation of proteins in A431 human tumor cells, *Cell*, 24, 741, 1981.

243. Cooper, J.A., Bowen-Pope, D.F., Raines, E., Ross, R., and Hunter, T., Similar effects of platelet-derived growth factor and epidermal growth factor on the phosphorylation of tyrosine in cellular proteins, *Cell*, 31, 263, 1982.

244. Zendegui, J.G. and Carpenter, G., Substrates of the epidermal growth factor receptor-kinase, *Cell Biol. Int. Rep.*, 8, 619, 1984.

245. Glenney, J., Two related but distinct forms of the M$_r$ 36,000 tyrosine kinase substrate (calpactin) that interact with phospholipid and actin in a Ca^{2+}-dependent manner, *Proc. Natl. Acad. Sci. U.S.A.*, 83, 4258, 1986.

246. Carter, V.C., Howlett, A.R., Martin, G.S., and Bissell, M.J., The tyrosine phosphorylation substrate p36 is developmentally regulated in embryonic avian limb and is induced in cell culture, *J. Cell Biol.*, 103, 2017, 1986.

247. Weber, K. and Johnsson, N., Repeating sequence homologies in the p36 target protein of retroviral protein kinases and lipocortin, the p37 inhibitor of phospholipase A$_2$, *FEBS Lett.*, 203, 95, 1986.

248. Huang, K.-S., Wallner, B.P., Mattaliano, R.J., Tizard, R., Burne, C., Frey, A., Hession, C., McGray, P., Sinclair, L.K., Chow, E.P., Browning, J.L., Ramachandran, K.L., Tang, J., Smart, J.E., and Pepinsky, R.B., Two human 35 kd inhibitors of phospholipase A$_2$ are related to substrates of pp60^{v-src} and of the epidermal growth factor receptor/kinase, *Cell*, 46, 191, 1986.

249. Brugge, J.S., The p35/p36 substrates of protein-tyrosine kinases as inhibitors of phospholipase A$_2$, *Cell*, 46, 149, 1986.

250. Brugge, J.S., Erikson, E., and Erikson, R.L., The specific interaction of the Rous sarcoma virus transforming protein, pp60^{src}, with two cellular proteins, *Cell*, 25, 363, 1981.

251. Brugge, J.S. and Darrow, D., Rous sarcoma virus-induced phosphorylation of a 50,000-molecular weight cellular protein, *Nature*, 295, 250, 1982.

252. Ziemiecki, A., Characterization of the monomeric and complex-associated forms of the *gag-onc* fusion proteins of three isolates of feline sarcoma virus: phosphorylation, kinase activity, acylation, and kinetics of complex formation, *Virology*, 151, 265, 1986.

253. Catelli, M.G., Binart, N., Jung-Testas, I., Renoir, J.M., Baulieu, E.E., Feramisco, J.R., and Welch, W.J., The common 90-kd protein component of non-transformed "8S" steroid receptors is a heat-shock protein, *EMBO J.*, 4, 3131, 1985.

254. Ziemiecki, A., Catelli, M.-G., Joab, I., and Moncharmont, B., Association of the heat shock protein hsp90 with steroid hormone receptors and tyrosine kinase oncogene products, *Biochem. Biophys. Res. Commun.*, 138, 1298, 1986.

255. Schuh, S., Yonemoto, W., Brugge, J., Bauer, V.J., Riehl, R.M., Sullivan, W.P., and Toft, D.O., A 90,000-dalton binding protein common to both steroid receptors and the Rous sarcoma virus transforming protein, pp60^{v-src}, *J. Biol. Chem.*, 260, 14292, 1985.

256. Brugge, J.S., Interaction of the Rous sarcoma virus protein pp60^{src} with the cellular proteins pp50 and pp90, *Curr. Top. Microbiol. Immunol.*, 123, 1, 1986.

257. Koyasu, S., Nishida, E., Kadowaki, T., Matsuzaki, F., Iida, K., Harada, F., Kasuga, M., Sakai, H., and Yahara, I., Two mammalian heat shock proteins, HSP90 and HSP100, are actin-binding proteins, *Proc. Natl. Acad. Sci. U.S.A.*, 83, 8054, 1986.

258. Nishida, E., Koyasu, S., Sakai, H., and Yahar, I., Calmodulin-regulated binding of the 90-kDa heat shock protein to actin filaments, *J. Biol. Chem.*, 261, 16033, 1986.

259. Oppermann, H., Levinson, W., and Bishop, J.M., A cellular protein that associates with the transforming protein of Rous sarcoma virus is also a heat-shock protein, *Proc. Natl. Acad. Sci. U.S.A.*, 78, 1067, 1981.

260. Lipsich, L.A., Cutt, J.R., and Brugge, J.S., Association of transforming proteins of Rous, Fujinami and Y73 avian sarcoma viruses with the same two cellular proteins, *Mol. Cell. Biol.,* 2, 875, 1982.

261. Beemon, K., Ryden, T., and McNelly, E.A., Transformation by avian sarcoma viruses leads to phosphorylation of multiple cellular proteins on tyrosine residues, *J. Virol.,* 42, 742, 1982.

262. Lau, A.F., Phosphotyrosine-containing 120,000-dalton protein coimmunoprecipitated with pp60^{v-src} from Rous sarcoma virus-transformed mammalian cells, *Virology,* 151, 86, 1986.

263. Seki, J., Owada, M.K., Sakato, N., and Fujio, H., Direct identification of phosphotyrosine-containing proteins in some retrovirus-transformed cells by use of anti-phosphotyrosine antibody, *Cancer Res.,* 46, 907, 1986.

264. Henderson, D. and Rohrschneider, L., Cytoskeletal association of pp60^{src}, the transforming protein of the Rous sarcoma virus, *Exp. Cell Res.,* 168, 411, 1987.

265. Hamaguchi, M. and Hanafusa, H., Association of p60^{src} with Triton X-100-resistant cellular structure correlates with morphological transformation, *Proc. Natl. Acad. Sci. U.S.A.,* 84, 2312, 1987.

266. Loeb, D.M., Woolford, J., and Beemon, K., pp60^{c-src} has less affinity for the detergent-insoluble cellular matrix than do pp60^{v-src} and other viral protein-tyrosine kinases, *J. Virol.,* 61, 2420, 1987.

267. Akiyama, T., Kadowaki, T., Nishida, E., Kadooka, T., Ogawara, H., Fukami, Y., Sakai, H., Takaku, F., and Kasuga, M., Substrate specificities of tyrosine-specific protein kinases toward cytoskeletal proteins *in vitro,* *J. Biol. Chem.,* 261, 14797, 1986.

268. Sefton, B.M., Hunter, T., Ball, E., and Singer, S.J., Vinculin: a cytoskeletal target of the transforming protein of Rous sarcoma virus, *Cell,* 24, 165, 1981.

269. Rohrschneider, L. and Rosok, M.J., Transformation parameters and pp60^{src} localization in cells infected with partial transformation mutants of Rous sarcoma virus, *Mol. Cell. Biol.,* 3, 731, 1983.

270. Antler, A.M., Greenberg, M.E., Edelman, G.M., and Hanafusa, H., Increased phosphorylation of tyrosine in vinculin does not occur upon transformation by some avian sarcoma viruses, *Mol. Cell. Biol.,* 5, 263, 1985.

271. Kellie, S., Patel, B., Mitchell, A., Critchley, D.R., Wigglesworth, N.M., and Wyke, J.A., Comparison of the relative importance of tyrosine-specific vinculin phosphorylation and the loss of surface-associated fibronectin in the morphology of cells transformed by Rous sarcoma virus, *J. Cell Sci.,* 82, 129, 1986.

272. Kellie, S., Patel, B., Wigglesworth, N.M., Critchley, D.R., and Wyke, J.A., The use of Rous sarcoma virus transformation mutants with differing tyrosine kinase activities to study the relationships between vinculin phosphorylation, pp60^{v-src} location and adhesion plaque integrity, *Exp. Cell Res.,* 165, 216, 1986.

273. Burn, P. and Burger, M., The cytoskeletal protein vinculin contains transformation-sensitive, covalently bound lipid, *Science,* 235, 476, 1987.

274. Pasquale, E.B., Maher, P.A., and Singer, S.J., Talin is phosphorylated on tyrosine in chicken embryo fibroblasts transformed by Rous sarcoma virus, *Proc. Natl. Acad. Sci. U.S.A.,* 83, 5507, 1986.

275. DeClue, J.E. and Martin, G.S., Phosphorylation of talin at tyrosine in Rous sarcoma virus-transformed cells, *Mol. Cell. Biol.,* 7, 371, 1987.

276. Holme, T.C., Kellie, S., Wyke, J.A., and Crawford, N., Effect of transformation by Rous sarcoma virus on the character and distribution of actin in Rat-1 fibroblasts: a biochemical and microscopical study, *Br. J. Cancer,* 53, 465, 1986.

277. Magargal, W.W. and Lin, S., Transformation-dependent increase in endogenous cytochalasin-like activity in chicken embryo fibroblasts infected by Rous sarcoma virus, *Proc. Natl. Acad. Sci. U.S.A.,* 83, 8201, 1986.

278. Decker, S., Phosphorylation of ribosomal protein S6 in avian sarcoma virus-transformed chicken embryo fibroblasts, *Proc. Natl. Acad. Sci. U.S.A.,* 78, 4112, 1981.

279. Blenis, J. and Erikson, R.L., Phosphorylation of the ribosomal protein S6 is elevated in cells transformed by a variety of tumor viruses, *J. Virol.,* 50, 966, 1984.

280. Blenis, J., Spivack, J.G., and Erikson, R.L., Phorbol ester, serum, and Rous sarcoma virus transforming gene product induce similar phosphorylation of ribosomal protein S6, *Proc. Natl. Acad. Sci. U.S.A.,* 81, 6408, 1984.

281. Blenis, J. and Erickson, R.L., Regulation of a ribosomal protein S6 kinase activity by the Rous sarcoma virus transforming protein, serum, or phorbol ester, *Proc. Natl. Acad. Sci. U.S.A.,* 82, 7621, 1985.

282. Blenis, J. and Erikson, R.L., Stimulation of ribosomal protein S6 kinase activity by pp60^{v-src} or by serum: dissociation from phorbol ester-stimulated activity, *Proc. Natl. Acad. Sci. U.S.A.,* 83, 1733, 1986.

283. Pelech, S.L. and Krebs, E.G., Mitogen-activated S6 kinase is stimulated via protein kinase C-dependent and independent pathways in Swiss 3T3 cells, *J. Biol. Chem.,* 262, 11598, 1987.

284. Cobb, M.H., Burr, J.G., Linder, M.E., Gray, T.B., and Gregory, J.S., Similar ribosomal protein S6 kinase activity is found in insulin-treated 3T3-L1 cells and chick embryo fibroblasts transformed by Rous sarcoma virus, *Biochem. Biophys. Res. Commun.,* 137, 702, 1986.

285. Spivack, J.G., Erikson, R.L., and Maller, J.L., Microinjection of pp60^{v-src} into *Xenopus* oocytes increases phosphorylation of ribosomal protein S6 and accelerates the rate of progesterone-induced meiotic maturation, *Mol. Cell. Biol.,* 4, 1631, 1984.

286. Spivack, J.G. and Maller, J.L., Phosphorylation and protein synthetic events in *Xenopus laevis* oocytes microinjected with pp60^{v-src}, *Mol. Cell. Biol.,* 5, 3629, 1985.

287. Johansen, J.W. and Ingebritsen, T.S., Phosphorylation and inactivation of protein phosphatase 1 by pp60^{v-src}, *Proc. Natl. Acad. Sci. U.S.A.,* 83, 207, 1986.

288. Johansen, J.W. and Ingebritsen, T.S., Effects of phosphorylation of protein phosphatase 1 by pp60$^{v\text{-}src}$ on the interaction of the enzyme with substrates and inhibitor proteins, *Biochim. Biophys. Acta*, 928, 63, 1987.

289. Cooper, J.A., Reiss, N.A., Schwartz, R.J., and Hunter, T., Three glycolytic enzymes are phosphorylated at tyrosine in cells transformed by Rous sarcoma virus, *Nature*, 302, 218, 1983.

290. Bosca, L., Mojena, M., Ghysdael, J., Rousseau, G.G., and Hue, L., Expression of the v-*src* or v-*fps* oncogene increases fructose 2,6-bisphosphate in chick-embryo fibroblasts, *Biochem. J.*, 236, 595, 1986.

291. Owada, M.K., Hakura, A., Iida, K., Yahar, I., Sobue, K., and Kakiuchi, S., Occurrence of caldesmon (a calmodulin-binding protein) in cultured cells: comparison of normal and transformed cells, *Proc. Natl. Acad. Sci. U.S.A.*, 81, 3133, 1984.

292. Fukami, Y., Nakamura, T., Nakayama, A., and Kanehisa, T., Phosphorylation of tyrosine residues of calmodulin in Rous sarcoma virus-transformed cells, *Proc. Natl. Acad. Sci. U.S.A.*, 83, 4190, 1986.

293. Crisanti, P., Lorinet, A.M., Calothy, G., and Pessac, B., Glutamic acid decarboxylase activity is stimulated in quail retina neuronal cells transformed by Rous sarcoma virus and is regulated by pp60$^{v\text{-}src}$, *EMBO J.*, 4, 1467, 1985.

294. Groudine, M. and Weintraub, H., Activation of cellular genes by avian RNA tumor viruses, *Proc. Natl. Acad. Sci. U.S.A.*, 77, 5351, 1980.

295. Durkin, J.P. and Whitfield, J.F., The selective induction of a small number of proteins during G$_1$ transit results from the mitogenic action of pp60$^{v\text{-}src}$ in *ts*ASV-infected rat cells, *J. Cell. Physiol.*, 125, 51, 1985.

296. Kuchino, Y., Nemoto, K., Kawai, S., and Nishimura, S., Activation of c-*myc* gene transcription by Rous sarcoma virus infection, *Jpn. J. Cancer Res.*, 76, 75, 1985.

297. Poirier, F., Julien, P., Dezelee, P., Dambrine, G., Esnault, E., Benatre, A., and Calothy, G., Role of the mitogenic property and kinase activity of p60^{src} in tumor formation by Rous sarcoma virus, *J. Virol.*, 49, 325, 1984.

298. Bader, J.P., Virus-induced transformation without cell division, *Science*, 180, 1069, 1973.

299. Durkin, J.P. and Whitfield, J.F., Partial characterization of the mitogenic action of pp60$^{v\text{-}src}$, the oncogenic protein product of the *src* gene of avian sarcoma virus, *J. Cell. Physiol.*, 120, 135, 1984.

300. Durkin and Whitfield, J.F., The mitogenic activity of pp60$^{v\text{-}src}$, the oncogenic protein product of the *src* gene of avian sarcoma virus, is independent of external serum growth factors, *Biochem. Biophys. Res. Commun.*, 123, 411, 1984.

301. Adkins, B., Leutz, A., and Graf, T., Autocrine growth induced by *src*-related oncogenes in transformed chicken cells, *Cell*, 39, 439, 1984.

302. Gellert, M., DNA topoisomerases, *Annu. Rev. Biochem.*, 50, 879, 1981.

303. Wang, J.C., DNA topoisomerases, *Annu. Rev. Biochem.*, 54, 665, 1985.

304. Mroczkowski, B., Mosig, G., and Cohen, S., ATP-stimulated interaction between epidermal growth factor receptor and supercoiled DNA, *Nature*, 309, 270, 1984.

305. Tse-Dinh, Y.-C., Wong, T.W., and Goldberg, A.R., Virus- and cell-encoded tyrosine protein kinases inactivate DNA topoisomerases *in vitro*, *Nature*, 312, 785, 1984.

306. Welsh, M., Welsh, N., Nilsson, T., Arkhammar, P., Pepinsky, R.B., Steiner, D.F., and Berggren, P.-O., Stimulation of pancreatic islet beta-cell replication by oncogenes, *Proc. Natl. Acad. Sci. U.S.A.*, 85, 116, 1988.

307. Kahn, P., Adkins, B., Beug, H., and Graf, T., *src*- and *fps*-containing avian sarcoma viruses transform chicken erythroid cells, *Proc. Natl. Acad. Sci. U.S.A.*, 81, 7122, 1984.

308. Palmieri, S., Transformation of erythroid cells by Rous sarcoma virus (RSV), *Virology*, 140, 269, 1985.

309. Lipsich, L., Brugge, J.S., and Boettiger, D., Expression of the Rous sarcoma virus *src* gene in avian macrophages fails to elicit transformed cell phenotype, *Mol. Cell. Biol.*, 4, 1420, 1984.

310. Milford, J.J. and Duran-Reynals, F., Growth of a chicken sarcoma virus in the chick embryo in the absence of neoplasia, *Cancer Res.*, 3, 578, 1943.

311. Dolberg, D.S. and Bissell, M.J., Inability of Rous sarcoma virus to cause sarcomas in the avian embryo, *Nature*, 309, 552, 1984.

312. Gilmer, T.M., Annab, L.A., Oshimura, M., and Barrett, J.C., Neoplastic transformation of normal and carcinogen-induced preneoplastic Syrian hamster embryo cells by the v-*src* oncogene, *Mol. Cell. Biol.*, 5, 1707, 1985.

313. Warren, S.L. and Nelson, W.J., Nonmitogenic morphoregulatory action of pp60$^{v\text{-}src}$ on multicellular epithelial structures, *Mol. Cell. Biol.*, 7, 1326, 1987.

314. Anderson, S.M. and Scolnick, E.M., Construction and isolation of a transforming murine retrovirus containing the *src* gene of Rous sarcoma virus, *J. Virol.*, 46, 594, 1983.

315. Boettiger, D., Anderson, S., and Dexter, T.M., Effect of *src* infection on long-term marrow cultures: increased self-renewal of hemopoietic progenitor cells without leukemia, *Cell*, 36, 763, 1984.

316. Lin, S.L., Garber, E.A., Wang, E., Caliguiri, L.A., Schellekens, H., Goldberg, A.R., and Tamm, I., Reduced synthesis of pp60^{src} and expression of the transformation-related phenotype in interferon-treated Rous sarcoma virus transformed rat cells, *Mol. Cell. Biol.*, 3, 1656, 1983.

317. Shalloway, D., Johnson, P.J., Freed, E.O., Coulter, D., and Flood, W.A., Jr., Transformation of NIH 3T3 cells by cotransfection with c-*src* and nuclear oncogenes, *Mol. Cell. Biol.*, 7, 3582, 1987.

318. Karess, R.E., Hayward, W.S., and Hanafusa, H., Cellular information in the genome of recovered avian sarcoma virus directs the synthesis of transforming protein, *Proc. Natl. Acad. Sci. U.S.A.,* 76, 3154, 1979.

319. Jakobovits, E.B., Majors, J.E., and Varmus, H.E., Hormonal regulation of the Rous sarcoma virus *src* gene via a heterologous promoter defines a threshold dose for cellular transformation, *Cell,* 38, 757, 1984.

320. Shibuya, M., Hanafusa, H., and Balduzzi, P.C., Cellular sequences related to thre new *onc*-genes of avian sarcoma virus (*fps, yes,* and *ros*) and their expression in normal and transformed cells,*J. Virol.,* 42, 143, 1982.

321. Cotton, P.C. and Brugge, J.S., Neural tissues express high levels of the cellular *src* gene product pp60^{c-src}, *Mol. Cell. Biol.,* 3, 1157, 1983.

322. Iba, H., Takeya, T., Cross, F.R., Hanafusa, T., and Hanafusa, H., Rous sarcoma virus variants that carry the cellular *src* gene instead of the viral *src* gene cannot transform chicken embryo fibroblasts, *Proc. Natl. Acad. Sci. U.S.A.,* 81, 4424, 1984.

323. Shalloway, D., Coussens, P.M., and Yaciuk, P., Overexpression of the c-*src* protein does not induce transformation of NIH 3T3 cells, *Proc. Natl. Acad. Sci. U.S.A.,* 81, 7071, 1984.

324. Johnson, P.J., Coussens, P.M., Danko, A.V., and Shalloway, D., Overexpressed pp60^{c-src} can induce focus formation without complete transformation of NIH 3T3 cells, *Mol. Cell. Biol.,* 5, 1073, 1985.

325. Bolen, J.B., Rosen, N., and Israel, M.A., Increased pp60^{c-src} tyrosyl kinase activity in human neuroblastomas is associated with amino-terminal tyrosine phosphorylation of the *src* gene product, *Proc. Natl. Acad. Sci. U.S.A.,* 82, 7275, 1985.

326. Reddy, S., Yaciuk, P., Kmiecik, T.E., Coussens, P.M., and Shalloway, D., v-*src* mutations outside the carboxyl-coding region are not sufficient to fully activate transformation by pp60^{c-src} in NIH 3T3 cells, *Mol. Cell. Biol.,* 8, 704, 1988.

327. Ikawa, S., Hagino-Yamagishi, K., Kawai, S., Yamamoto, T., and Toyoshima, K., Activation of the cellular *src* gene by transducing retrovirus, *Mol. Cell. Biol.,* 6, 2420, 1986.

328. Kato, J.-Y., Takeya, T., Grandori, C., Iba, H., Levy, J.B., and Hanafusa, H., Amino acid substitutions sufficient to convert the nontransforming p60^{c-src} protein to a transforming protein, *Mol. Cell. Biol.,* 6, 4155, 1986.

329. Cooper, J.A., Hunter, T., and Shalloway, D., Protein-tyrosine kinase activity of pp60^{c-src} is restricted in intact cells, *Cancer Cells,* 3, 321, 1985.

330. Fung, Y.-K.T., Crittenden, L.B., Fadly, A.M., and Kung, H.-J., Tumor induction by direct injection of cloned v-*src* DNA into chickens, *Proc. Natl. Acad. Sci. U.S.A.,* 80, 353, 1983.

331. Boettiger, D. and Dexter, T.M., Altered stem cell (CFU-S) function following infection of hematopoietic cells with a virus carrying v-*src*, *Blood,* 67, 398, 1986.

332. Parker, R.C., Varmus, H.E., and Bishop, J.M., Cellular homologue (c-*src*) of the transforming gene of Rous sarcoma virus: isolation, mapping, and transcriptional analysis of c-*src* and flanking regions,*Proc. Natl. Acad. Sci. U.S.A.,* 78, 5842, 1981.

333. Barnekow, A., Effect of several nucleotides on the phosphorylating activities of the Rous-sarcoma-virus transforming protein pp60^{v-src} and its cellular homologue, pp60^{c-src}, *Biosci. Rep.,* 3, 153, 1983.

334. Ikawa, S., Yamamoto, T., and Toyoshima, K., Modification of carboxyl-terminal region is the cause of activation of the *src* gene in avian sarcoma virus S2, *Jpn. J. Cancer Res.,* 77, 611, 1986.

335. Levy, J.B., Iba, H., and Hanafusa, H., Activation of the transforming potential of p60^{c-src} by a single amino acid change, *Proc. Natl. Acad. Sci. U.S.A.,* 83, 4228, 1986.

336. Calothy, G., Laugier, D., Cross, F.R., Jove, R., Hanafusa, T., and Hanafusa, H., The membrane-binding domain and myristylation of p60^{v-src} are not essential for stimulation of cell proliferation, *J. Virol.,* 61, 1678, 1987.

337. Vogt, P.K., Spontaneous segregation of nontransforming viruses from cloned sarcoma viruses, *Virology,* 46, 939, 1971.

338. Kawai, S., Duesberg, P.H., and Hanafusa, H., Transformation-defective mutants of Rous sarcoma virus with *src* gene deletions of varying length, *J. Virol.,* 24, 910, 1977.

339. Lai, M.M.C., Hu, S.S.F., and Vogt, P.K., Occurrence of partial deletion and substitution of the *src* gene in the RNA genome of ASV, *Proc. Natl. Acad. Sci. U.S.A.,* 74, 4781, 1977.

340. Parvin, J.D. and Wang, L.-H., Mechanisms for the generation of *src*-deletion mutants and recovered sarcoma viruses: identification of viral sequences involved in *src* deletions and in recombination with c-*src* sequences, *Virology,* 138, 236, 1984.

341. Enrietto, P.J., Payne, L.N., and Wyke, J.A., Analysis of the pathogenicity of transformation defective partial deletion mutants of avian sarcoma virus: characterization of recovered viruses which encode novel *src* specific proteins, *Virology,* 127, 397, 1983.

342. Soong, M.-M., Iijima, S., and Wang, L.-H., Transduction of c-*src* coding and intron sequences by a transformation-defective deletion mutant of Rous sarcoma virus, *J. Virol.,* 59, 556, 1986.

343. Laugier, D., Marx, M., Barnier, J.V., Poirier, F., Genvrin, P., Dezélée, P., and Calothy, G., N-terminal deletion in the *src* gene of Rous sarcoma virus results in syntheis of a 45,000-M$_r$ protein with mitogenic activity,*J. Virol.,* 61, 2523, 1987.

344. Poirier, F., Laugier, D., Marx, M., Dambrine, G. Garber, E.A., Gevrin, P., David-Pfeuty, T., and Calothy, G., Rous sarcoma virus mutant *dl*PA105 induces different transformed phenotypes in quail embryonic fibroblasts and neuroretina cells, *J. Virol.,* 61, 2530, 1987.

345. Chambers, A.F. and Wilson, S., Cells transformed with a *ts* viral *src* mutant are temperature sensitive for in vivo growth, *Mol. Cell. Biol.,* 5, 728, 1985.

346. Jove, R., Mayer, B.J., Iba, H., Laugier, D., Poirier, F., Calothy, G., Hanafusa, T., and Hanafusa, H., Genetic analysis of p60^{v-src} domains involved in the induction of different cell transformation parameters, *J. Virol.,* 60, 840, 1986.

347. Jove, R., Garber, E.A., Iba, H., and Hanafusa, H., Biochemical properties of p60^{v-src} mutants that induce different cell transformation parameters, *J. Virol.,* 60, 849, 1986.

348. Mayer, B.J., Jove, R., Krane, J.F., Poirier, F., Calothy, G., and Hanafusa, H., Genetic lesions involved in temperature sensitivity of the *src* gene products of four Rous sarcoma virus mutants, *J. Virol.,* 60, 858, 1986.

349. Nishizawa, M., Mayer, B.J., Takeya, T., Yamamoto, T., Toyoshima, K., Hanafusa, H., and Kawai, S., Two independent mutations are required for temperature-sensitive cell transformation by a Rous sarcoma virus temperature-sensitive mutant, *J. Virol.,* 56, 743, 1985.

350. Rubsamen, H., Ziemicki, A., Friis, R.R., and Bauer, H., The expression of pp60^{src} and its associated protein kinase activity in cells infected with different transformation-defective temperature-sensitive mutants of Rous sarcoma virus, *Virology,* 102, 453, 1980.

351. Stoker, A.W., Kellie, S., and Wyke, J.A., Intracellular localization and processing of pp60^{v-src} proteins expressed by two distinct temperature-sensitive mutants of Rous sarcoma virus, *J. Virol.,* 58, 876, 1986.

352. Fincham, V.J. and Wyke, J.A., Localization of temperature-sensitive transformation mutations and back mutations in the Rous sarcoma virus *src* gene, *J. Virol.,* 58, 694, 1986.

353. Stoker, A.W., Enrietto, P.J., and Wyke, J.A., Functional domains of the pp60^{v-src} protein as revealed by analysis of temperature-sensitive Rous sarcoma virus mutants, *Mol. Cell. Biol.,* 4, 1508, 1984.

354. Garber, E.A., Mayer, B.J., Jove, R., and Hanafusa, H., Analysis of p60^{v-src} mutants carrying lesions involved in temperature sensitivity, *J. Virol.,* 61, 354, 1987.

355. Seuwen, K. and Adam, G., Calcium compartments and fluxes are affected by the *src* gene product of Rat-1 cells transformed by temperature-sensitive Rous sarcoma virus, *Biochem. Biophys. Res. Commun.,* 125, 337, 1984.

356. Anderson, S.K. and Fujita, D.J., Morph^f mutants of Rous sarcoma virus: nucleotide sequencing analysis suggests that a class of morph^f mutants was generated through splicing of a cryptic intron, *J. Virol.,* 61, 1893, 1987.

357. Cross, F.R. and Hanafusa, H., Local mutagenesis of Rous sarcoma virus: the major sites of tyrosine and serine phosphorylation of p60^{src} are dispensable for transformation, *Cell,* 34, 597, 1983.

358. Snyder, M.A. and Bishop, J.M., A mutation at the major phosphotyrosine in pp60^{v-src} alters oncogenic potential, *Virology,* 136, 375, 1984.

359. Snyder, M.A., Bishop, J.M., McGrath, J.P. and Levinson, A.D., A mutation at the ATP-binding site of pp60^{v-src} abolishes kinase activity, transformation, and tumorigenicity, *Mol. Cell. Biol.,* 5, 1772, 1985.

360. Wilkerson, V.W., Bryant, D.L., and Parsons, T.J., Rous sarcoma virus variants that encode *src* proteins with an altered carboxy terminus are defective for cellular transformation, *J. Virol.,* 55, 314, 1985.

361. Yaciuk, P. and Shalloway, D., Features of the pp60^{v-src} carboxyl terminus that are required for transformation, *Mol. Cell. Biol.,* 6, 2807, 1986.

362. Cheng, S.H., Piwnica-Worms, H., Harvey, R.W., Roberts, T.M., and Smith, A.E., The carboxy terminus of pp60^{c-src} is a regulatory domain and is involved in complex formation with the middle-T antigen of polyomavirus, *Mol. Cell. Biol.,* 8, 1736, 1988.

363. Reynolds, A.B., Vila, J., Lansing, T.J., Potts, W.M., Weber, M.J., and Parson, J.T., Activation of the oncogenic potential of the avian cellular *src* protein by specific structural alteration of the carboxy terminus, *EMBO J.,* 6, 2359, 1987.

364. Kamps, M.P., Buss, J.F., and Sefton, B.M., Rous sarcoma virus transforming protein lacking myristic acid phosphorylates know polypeptide substrates without inducing transformation, *Cell,* 45, 105, 1986.

365. Pellman, D., Garber, E.A., Cross, F.R., and Hanafusa, H., An N-terminal peptide from p60^{src} can direct myristylation and plasma membrane localization when fused to heterologous proteins, *Nature,* 314, 374, 1985.

366. Sefton, B.M., Hunter, T., Beemon, K., and Eckhart, W., Evidence that the phosphorylation of tyrosine is essential for cellular transformation by Rous sarcoma virus, *Cell,* 20, 807, 1980.

367. Uehara, Y., Hori, M., Takeuchi, T., and Umezawa, H., Screening of agents which convert "transformed morphology" of Rous sarcoma virus-infected rat kidney cells to "normal morphology": identification of an active agent as herbimycin and its inhibition of intracelullar *src* kinase, *Jpn. J. Cancer Res.,* 76, 672, 1985.

368. Uehara, Y., Hori, M., Takeuchi, T., and Umezawa, H., Phenotypic change from transformed to normal induced by benzoquinonoid ansamycins accompanies inactivation of p60^{src} in rat kidney cells infected with Rous sarcoma virus, *Mol. Cell. Biol.,* 6, 2198, 1986.

369. Murakami, Y., Mizuno, S., Hori, M., and Uehara, Y., Reversal of transformed phenotypes by herbimycin A in *src* oncogene expressed rat fibroblasts, *Cancer Res.,* 48, 1587, 1988.

370. Uehara, Y., Murakami, Y., Mizuno, S., and Kawai, S., Inhibition of transforming activity of tyrosine kinase oncogenes by herbimycin A, *Virology,* 164, 294, 1988.

371. Uehara, Y., Hasegawa, M., Hori, M., and Umezawa, H., Increased sensitivity to oxanosine, a novel nucleoside antibiotic, or rat kidney cells upon expression of the integrated viral *src* gene, *Cancer Res.,* 45, 5230, 1985.

372. Goldberg, A.R., Delclos, K.B., and Blumberg, P.M., Phorbol ester action is independent of viral and cellular *src* kinase levels, *Science*, 208, 191, 1980.

373. Pietropaolo, C., Laskin, J.D., and Weinstein, I.B., Effect of tumor promoters on *sarc* expression in normal and transformed chick embryo fibroblasts, *Cancer Res.*, 41, 1565, 1981.

374. Perrotti, N., Taylor, S.I., Richert, N.D., Rapp, U.R., Pastan, I.H., and Roth, J., Immunoprecipitation of insulin receptors from cultured human lymphocytes (IM-9 cells) by antibodies to pp60*src*, *Science*, 227, 761, 1985.

375. Kalia, M., Fujita-Yamaguchi, Y., Blithe, D.L., and Kahn, C.R., Tyrosine-specific protein kinase activity is associated with the purified insulin receptor,*Proc. Natl. Acad. Sci. U.S.A.*, 80, 2137, 1983.

376. Perrotti, N., Grunberger, G., Richert, N.D., and Taylor, S.I., Immunological similarity between the insulin receptor and the protein encoded by the *src* oncogene,*Endocrinology*, 118, 2349, 1986.

377. Ullrich, A., Bell, J.R., Chen, E.Y., Herrera, R., Petruzzelli, L.M., Dull, T.J., Gray, A., Coussens, L., Liao, Y.-C., Tsubokawa, M., Mason, A., Seeburg, P.H., Grunfield, C., Rosen, O.M., and Ramachandran, J., Human insulin receptor and its relationship to the tyrosine kinase family of oncogenes, *Nature*, 313, 756, 1985.

378. White, M.F., Werth, D.K., Pastan, I., and Kahn, C.R., Phosphorylation of the solubilized insulin receptor by the gene product of the Rous sarcoma virus, pp60*src*, *J. Cell. Biochem.*, 26, 169, 1984.

379. Yu, K.-T., Werth, D.K., Pastan, I.H., and Czech, M.P., *src* catalyzes the phosphorylation and activation of the insulin receptor kinase, *J. Biol. Chem.*, 260, 5838, 1985.

380. Wong, T.W. and Goldberg, A.R., Kinetics and mechanism of angiotensin phosphorylation by the transforming gene product of Rous sarcoma virus, *J. Biol. Chem.*, 259, 3127, 1984.

381. Privalsky, M.L. and Bishop, J.M., Subcellular localization of the v-*erb*-B protein, the product of a transforming gene of avian erythroblastosis virus, *Virology*, 135, 356, 1984.

382. Wasilenko, W.J., Shawver, L.K., and Weber, M.J., Down-modulation of EGF receptors in cells transformed by the *src* oncogene,*J. Cell. Physiol.*, 131, 450, 1987.

383. Luttrell, D.K., Luttrell, L.M., and Parsons, S.J., Augmented mitogenic responsiveness to epidermal growth factor in murine fibroblasts that overexpress pp60*c-src*, *Mol. Cell. Biol.*, 8, 497, 1988.

384. Ralston, R. and Bishop, J.M., The product of the protooncogene c-*src* is modified during the cellular response to platelet-derived growth factor, *Proc. Natl. Acad. Sci. U.S.A.*, 82, 7845, 1985.

385. Overell, R.W., Watson, J.D., Gallis, B., Weisser, K.E., Cosman, D., and Widmer, M.B., Nature and specificity of lymphokine independence induced by a selectable retroviral vector expressing v-*src*, *Mol. Cell. Biol.*, 7, 3394, 1987.

386. Huttner, W.B., Sulphation of tyrosine residues: a widespread modification of proteins, *Nature*, 299, 273, 1982.

387. Brand, S.J., Andersen, B.N., and Rehfeld, J.F., Complete tyrosine-*O*-sulphation of gastrin in neonatal rat pancreas, *Nature*, 309, 456, 1984.

388. Liu, M.-C., Yu, S., Sy, J., Redman, C.M., and Lipmann, F., Tyrosine sulfation of proteins from the human hepatoma cell line HepG2, *Proc. Natl. Acad. Sci. U.S.A.*, 82, 7160, 1985.

389. Liu, M.-C. and Lipmann, F., Decrease of tyrosine-*O*-sulfate-containing proteins found in rat fibroblasts infected with Rous sarcoma virus or Fujinami sarcoma virus, *Proc. Natl. Acad. Sci. U.S.A.*, 81, 3695, 1984.

390. Liu, M.-C. and Lipmann, F., Isolation of tyrosine-*O*-sulfate by Pronase hydrolysis from fibronectin secreted by Fujinami sarcoma virus-infected rat fibroblasts, *Proc. Natl. Acad. Sci. U.S.A.*, 82, 34, 1985.

391. Liu, M.-C. and Suiko, M., Tyrosine sulfation site is located in the C-terminal fibrin-binding domain in secreted fibronectin from rat embryo fibroblasts, lyne 3Y1, *Arch. Biochem. Biophys.*, 255, 162, 1987.

392. Berridge, M.J., Inositol triphosphate and diacylglycerol as second messengers, *Biochem. J.*, 220, 345, 1984.

393. Farese, R.V., Phospholipids as intermediates in hormone action, *Mol. Cell. Endocrinol.*, 35, 1, 1984.

394. Kuo, J.F., Schatzman, R.C., Turner, R.S., and Mazzei, G.J., Phospholipid-sensitive Ca^{2+}-dependent protein kinase: a major protein phosphorylation system, *Mol. Cell. Endocrinol.*, 35, 65, 1984.

395. Majerus, P.W., Neufeld, E.J., and Wilson, D.B., Production of phosphoinositide-derived messengers, *Cell*, 37, 701, 1984.

396. Berridge, M.J., Inositol lipids and cell proliferation, *Biochim. Biophys. Acta*, 907, 33, 1987.

397. Sugimoto, Y., Whitman, M., Cantley, L.C., and Erikson, R.L., Evidence that the Rous sarcoma virus transforming gene product phosphorylates phosphatidylinositol and diacylglycerol, *Proc. Natl. Acad. Sci. U.S.A.*, 81, 2117, 1984.

398. Chang, C.-C., Trosko, J.E., Kung, H.-J., Bombick, D., and Matsumura, F., Potential role of the *src* gene product in inhibition of gap-junctional communication in NIH-3T3 cells, *Proc. Natl. Acad. Sci. U.S.A.*, 82, 5360, 1985.

399. Macara, I.G., Marinetti, G.V., and Balduzzi, P.C., Transforming protein of avian sarcoma virus UR2 is associated with phosphatidylinositol kinase activity: possible role in tumorigenesis, *Proc. Natl. Acad. Sci. U.S.A.*, 81, 1984.

400. MacDonald, M.L., Kuenzel, E.A., Glomset, J.A., and Krebs, E.G., Evidence from two transformed cell lines that phosphorylation of peptide tyrosine and phosphatidylinositol are catalyzed by different proteins, *Proc. Natl. Acad. Sci. U.S.A.*, 82, 3993, 1985.

401. Fukami, Y., Owada, M.K., Sumi, M., and Hayashi, F., A p60*v-src*-related kinase in the acetylcholine receptor-rich membranes of *Narke japonica*: association and dissociation of phosphatidylinositol kinase activity, *Biochem. Biophys. Res. Commun.*, 139, 473, 1986.

402. Sugano, S. and Hanafusa, H., Phosphatidylinositol kinase activity in virus-transformed and nontransformed cells, *Mol. Cell. Biol.*, 5, 2399, 1985.

403. Menko, A.S. and Boettiger, D., Inhibition of chicken embryo lens differentiation and lens junction formation in culture by pp60^{v-src}, *Mol. Cell. Biol.*, 8, 1414, 1988.

404. Azarnia, R., Reddy, S., Kmiecik, T.E., Shalloway, D., and Loewenstein, W.R., The cellular *src* gene product regulates junctional cell-to-cell communication, *Science*, 239, 398, 1988.

405. Warren, S.L., Handel, L.M., and Nelson, W.J., Elevated expression of pp60^{c-src} alters a selective morphogenetic property of epithelial cells in vitro without a mitogenic effect, *Mol. Cell. Biol.*, 8, 632, 1988.

406. Flier, J.S., Mueckler, M.M., Usher, P., and Lodish, H.F., Elevated levels of glucose transport and transporter messenger RNA are induced by *ras* or *src* oncogenes, *Science*, 235, 1492, 1987.

407. Garry, R.F. and Bostick, D.A., Intracellular K$^+$ and the expression of transformation parameters by chick cells transformed with the Bryan strain of Rous sarcoma virus, *Virology*, 150, 439, 1986.

408. van der Valk, J., Verlaan, I., de Laat, S.W., and Molenaar, W.H., Expression of pp60^{v-src} alters the ionic permeability of the plasma membrane in rat cells, *J. Biol. Chem.*, 262, 2431, 1987.

409. Haraguchi, S., Kurakata, S., Fujii, T., Matsuo, T., and Yoshida, T.O., Recognition of Rous sarcoma virus-induced tumor antigens by cytotoxic T lymphocytes (CTL): studies on specificity of killing by CTL employing H-2 congenic and recombinant mouse tumor cells, *Cell. Immunol.*, 105, 340, 1987.

410. Gogusev, J., Teutsch, B., Morin, M.T., Mongiat, F., Haguenau, F., Suskind, F., and Rabotti, G.F., Inhibition of HLA class I antigen and mRNA expression induced by Rous sarcoma virus in transformed human fibroblasts, *Proc. Natl. Acad. Sci. U.S.A.*, 85, 203, 1988.

411. Blat, C., Chatelain, G., Dasauty, G., and Harel, L., Inhibitory diffusible factor IDF45, a G1 phase inhibitor, *FEBS Lett.*, 203, 175, 1986.

412. Blat, C., Villaudy, J., Rouillard, D., Golde, A., and Harel, L., Modulation by the src oncogene of the effect of inhibitory diffusible factor IDF45, *J. Cell. Physiol.*, 130, 416, 1987.

413. Bullacher, C. and Barnekow, A., Transcription of proto-oncogene in Rous sarcoma virus infected and transformed chicken embryo cells, *Arch. Virol.*, 100, 185, 1988.

414. Wyke, J.A., Stoker, A.W., Searle, S., Spooncer, E., Simmons, P., and Dexter, T.M., Perturbed hemopoiesis and the generation of multipotential cell clones in *src*-infected bone marrow cultures is an indirect or transient effect of the oncogene, *Mol. Cell. Biol.*, 6, 959, 1986.

415. Marczynska, B., Gilles, P.N., and Ogston, C.W., Instability of v-*src* sequences in nonhuman primate tumors cultured *in vitro*, *Virology*, 159, 154, 1987.

416. Wainberg, M.A., Skalski, V., and Poulin, L., Differential effects of phorbol ester on tumor cells induced by avian sarcoma virus, *Anticancer Res.*, 7, 81, 1987.

417. Chackalaparampil, I., Banerjee, D., Poirier, Y., and Mukerjee, B.B., Altered processing of a major secreted phosphoprotein correlates with tumorigenicity in Rous sarcoma virus-transformed mammalian cells, *J. Virol.*, 53, 841, 1985.

418. Hjelle, B., Liu, E., and Bishop, J.M., Oncogene v-*src* transforms and establishes embryonic rodent fibroblasts but not diploid human fibroblasts, *Proc. Natl. Acad. Sci. U.S.A.*, 85, 4355, 1988.

Chapter 9

PROTOONCOGENES AND CANCER

I. INTRODUCTION

Protooncogenes are normal components of the genome in probably all of the metazoan species. Their possible role in the origin and/or maintenance of malignant cell transformation is supported by the following experimental observations:

1. Infection of cultured normal cells by acute transforming retroviruses (which contain oncogenes of cellular origin) results in the appearance of a transformed phenotype.[1] However, cells transformed by an acute retrovirus such as A-MuLV may be able to differentiate without a decrease in the expressed amount or specific activity of the oncogene product.[2] Thus, expression of a viral oncogene product may be necessary to induce neoplastic transformation in cells infected by acute retroviruses, but it is in itself not sufficient for the maintenance of the transformed state.

2. Infection of animals with acute transforming retroviruses results in development of malignant tumors within weeks after inoculation of the virus.[1,3]

3. Transfection of DNA extracted from tumor cells to NIH/3T3 cells (which are nononcogenic cells of murine origin) results in the production of foci of transformed cells, whereas DNA transfection from normal cells does not induce such foci.[4,5]

4. Transfection to NIH/3T3 cells of DNA extracted from cells transformed by chemical carcinogens induces the appearance of foci of cells with transformed phenotype and, more importantly, the previous treatment of the DNA with different restriction enzymes suggests that the same transforming genes are transferred in all cases.[6]

5. Transfection to NIH/3T3 cells of DNA containing the c-*mos* protooncogene with a promoter LTR at position 5′ results in the efficient and rapid induction of a malignant phenotype.[7]

6. Transfection of cultured normal human bronchial epithelial cells (NHBE cells) with a plasmid carrying the v-H-*ras* oncogene results in the appearance of a transformed phenotype, including alterations in growth requirements and terminal differentiation, and appearance of tumorigenic properties.[8] Introduction by gene transfer of an activated N-*ras* gene derived from tumorigenic late-passage PA-1 human teratocarcinoma cells into nontumorigenic, early passage revertants of these cells induces their tumorigenic conversion.[9] However, transfection of normal quiescent human lymphocytes with v-H-*ras* and v-*myc* oncogenes is not sufficient for the induction of cell growth and immortalization.[10] In contrast to the susceptibility of some established rodent cell lines to transformation by c-*ras* gene containing activating point mutations, normal human cells (cultured mesothelial cells and fibroblasts) are resistant to neoplastic transformation induced by introduction of these genes and remain dependent on the exogenous supply of serum factors for their growth *in vitro*.[11] Plasmid-mediated transfection of the normal human c-*myc* gene is incapable of inducing neoplastic transformation and tumorigenic properties in primary rat embryo fibroblast (REF) cells.[12] Transfection of REF cells with several different oncogenes (activated v-*myc*, mutated EJ or T24 c-H-*ras*, plasmids encoding polyoma virus large T or middle T antigen) does not correlate with differences in invasive or metastatic capability.[13] Moreover, cells transformed by transfection with a mutated EJ c-H-*ras* gene exhibit a normal phenotype after fusion to normal hamster cells in spite of the continued expression of the altered protooncogene.[14]

7. Induction of tumors in mice by means of defined chemical carcinogens is associated with

activation of protooncogenes in the tumor cells, although a similar or identical activation is also observed in chemically induced benign skin papillomas.[15,16]

8. Injection of a cloned viral oncogene (v-*src*) to susceptible animals (chickens) results in the effective induction of malignant tumors (sarcomas) within weeks after injection.[17] However, chick embryos *in ovo* are resistant to the tumorigenic action of RSV, and RSV variants that carry the cellular *src* gene (c-*src*) instead of the viral *src* gene (v-*src*) cannot transform chicken embryo fibroblasts *in vitro*.[18-20] A constructed recombinant murine retrovirus which efficiently transduces the avian c-*src* gene into murine cells (NIH/3T3 cells) is unable to induce cell transformation in the recipient cells in spite of the fact that the levels of functional pp60^{src} protein within the cells are increased 3- to 15-fold above the endogenous murine levels in control cell lines.[21]

9. An activated v-H-*ras* oncogene from H-MuSV can replace chemical carcinogens and act as initiator of two-stage mouse skin carcinogenesis *in vivo*.[22] This experimental system requires a critical interaction between the v-H-*ras*-initiated cell and a tumor promoter phorbol ester.

10. Transfection of a mutant EJ c-H-*ras* gene into nontumorigenic LE/6 cell lines established from the livers of carcinogen-treated rats results in the generation of transformed cells capable of producing tumors at the site of subcutaneous inoculation in nude mice.[23] Transfection of the mouse mammary adenocarcinoma cell line SP1 (a tumorigenic but not metastasizing cell line) with a mutant T24 c-H-*ras* gene, but not a normal c-H-*ras* gene, results in the formation of lung metastases from a subcutaneous site where the transfected cells are implanted in syngeneic mice.[24] The EJ c-H-*ras* gene is capable of inducing a rapid conversion of first-passage rat embryo cells to a tumorigenic but not metastatic phenotype; cotransfection of a c-*myc* protooncogene with the EJ c-H-*ras* gene is necessary to produce the conversion of the rat embryo cells into cells possessing both tumorigenic and metastatic potential.[25]

11. NIH/3T3 cells transformed by a human protooncogene (c-H-*ras*-1) activated with retroviral LTR can be phenotypically reverted after treatment with mouse IFN.[26] However, mouse IFN does not induce reversion in NIH/3T3 cells transformed with a mutant (EJ/T24) c-*ras* oncogene.[27]

12. Injection of a specific monoclonal antibody into animals bearing tumors composed of NIH/3T3 cells transformed by the protooncogene c-*neu* may result in inhibition of tumor growth and prolonged survival of the animals.[28] However, in all of these experiments the treated animals eventually died from their tumors.

13. Systematic deletion of oncogene DNA sequences by experimental procedures indicates that within oncogenes there are regions specifically involved in their transforming ability.[29]

14. Induction of site-directed point mutation in a viral oncogene (the v-*src* gene) may abolish or markedly reduce its potential transforming properties.[29-32] Other mutation sites may be dispensable for transformation.[33] Moreover, clonal NIH/3T3 cell lines expressing multiple copies of the mutant protooncogene have a more transformed phenotype than cells expressing only the single copy c-*ras* gene.[34]

15. Specific point mutations at codons 12 and 61 of c-*ras* protooncogenes may be associated with marked enhancement in the transforming ability of these genes as tested in the DNA transfection assay with NIH/3T3 cells.[35]

16. Transfection of rat cells with molecular vectors expressing different levels of a mutant c-*ras* gene results in the graded appearance of morphologic and functional alterations characteristic of neoplastic transformation.[36,37] Reversion of these phenotypic changes occurs when the vectors are functionally manipulated to inhibit the production of the mutant c-*ras* product. On the other hand, even high levels of expression of the nonmutant c-*ras* product are ineffective in inducing transformation.

17. The human fibrosarcoma cell line HT1080 contains an activated N-*ras* gene (mutated at codon 61), and genetic variants of these cells expressing reduced levels of the p21^{N-ras} protein exhibit reversion of the transformed phenotype.[38] The revertants undergo reacquisition of the transformed phenotype after transfection of cloned activated c-*ras* genes.

18. Transgenic mice carrying a mutated c-H-*ras* gene cloned in a molecular vector which is specifically expressed in pancreatic acinar cells develop pancreas carcinomas.[39] A cloned normal c-H-*ras* gene or a normal c-*myc* gene does not produce tumors under the same experimental conditions. However, up to 80% of female transgenic mice specifically expressing in the mammary gland high levels of a c-*myc* transgene during late pregnancy and lactation develop mammary adenocarcinomas.[40] The tumors appear as early as 2 months after the onset of c-*myc* transgene expression, and their appearance is associated with deregulated milk protein gene expression and adquisition of hormone and growth factor-independent growth. A very low incidence of mammary tumors is observed in female mice expressing in the mammary gland an activated c-*ras* transgene,[41] which suggests that the oncogenic potential of different activated protooncogenes may show tissue specificity. The c-*myc* transgene expressed in these mice is not structurally normal but is altered by replacement of 5′ regulatory sequences and deletion of the first exon. The fact that only a fraction of the mammary gland cells expressing the deregulated c-*myc* transgene become neoplastically transformed indicates that other genetic and/or epigenetic alterations are required in order for malignant transformation to occur.

19. In certain experimental systems, e.g., in aflatoxin B$_1$-induced rat liver tumors, oncogenic activation of c-*ras* genes is generally detected.[42] However, in other systems, using different cell types and different carcinogens, c-*ras* activation is a late and infrequent event in the multistage processes associated with the neoplastic transformation of cells.[43-45] Protooncogenes other than c-*ras* or other genetic changes may be responsible for the initiation of transformation in experimental and spontaneous tumors.

The ensemble of the results mentioned above, as well as the results obtained in many other similar experiments, strongly support the concept that oncogenes, especially viral oncogenes, are genes with defined potential for the induction of cell transformation. Some structurally and/or functionally altered protooncogenes seem to have a similar potential. Numerous clinical and experimental studies give evidence in favor of the participation of altered protooncogenes, in conjunction with other cellular genes, in the origin and/or development of malignant diseases in human and other animal species.[43-63] The mechanisms by which viral oncogenes or altered protooncogenes may cause neoplastic transformation are not clear but one possibility is the disruption of the activity of the normal, wild-type gene by a kind of dominant negative effect.[64] Quantitative and/or qualitative changes could hypothetically be responsible for the oncogenic activation of protooncogene sequences. The basic types of mechanisms that could be associated with activation of protooncogenes in tumors include altered expression of protooncogenes at abnormal times or sites, amplification of protooncogene sequences, translocation and/or rearrangement of protooncogenes, and mutation or truncation of protooncogenes. Another possibility to be considered is the deletion of protooncogenes; however, a more important aspect would consist in the physical or functional loss of tumor suppressor genes (antioncogenes or emerogenes).

Direct proof that cellular oncogenes (protooncogenes) are causally related to spontaneous tumors occurring in humans and other animals is still lacking. The hypothesis that protooncogenes are latent equivalents to viral oncogenes, i.e., that they represent true cancer genes, has been challenged.[65] It has been hypothesized that the products of activated protooncogenes are not necessary for tumor initiation but may be responsible for tumor growth and development.[66] However, the role of protooncogenes in invasion and metastasization, which are the most important characteristics of malignant tumors, is still uncertain.[67,68] As may be concluded from the discussion contained in the remaining part of this chapter, the exact role of protooncogenes in the complex, multistage carcinogenic processes remains to be determined. However, there may be little doubt that protooncogenes are importantly involved in many carcinogenic processes.

II. ONCOGENICALLY ACTIVE PROTOONCOGENES IN TUMOR CELLS

Since protooncogenes are genes with apparent oncogenic potential, and since they are apparently present in all animal cells, including human cells, it is conceivable that some kind of activation of protooncogenes could be associated with the origin and/or growth of neoplastic cell populations. However, this association would not be a simple one because there are more than 30 different oncogenes and their respective levels of expression are frequently different in different animal tissues, and even in different stages of cellular differentiation. Thus, the assumed association between protooncogenes and neoplastic diseases must have some kind of specificity for both the protooncogene and the tumor.

The presence of active protooncogenes in some, but not all, human tumors became apparent through the positive results obtained already in the first experiments with transfection of DNA extracted from different human tumor cell lines.[69-71] In such experiments, as in many consecutive ones,[72] it was found that DNAs extracted from different types of human tumor cell lines contain a gene, or genes, capable of transforming NIH/3T3 cells. The donor cell lines studied by transfection assays were of varied origin, including carcinomas from different sites (urinary bladder, lung, colon, pancreas, mammary gland) as well as tumors of the nervous system and hematopoietic malignancies. The same gene, or closely related genes, are responsible for positive results, as may be deduced from digestion of donor DNA with restriction enzymes.

A. ACTIVATION OF C-*RAS* GENES

Oncogenic activation of c-*ras* genes, as demonstrated in the NIH/3T3 DNA transfection/transformation assay, has been detected in a diversity of human tumors as well as in tumors experimentally induced in animals by carcinogenic agents.

1. Activation of c-*ras* Genes in Human Tumors

Protooncogenes of the c-*ras* family (c-H-*ras*, c-K-*ras*, N-*ras*) have been found to be active in a number of human carcinoma cell lines and primary human tumor specimens of several sites, including colon, lung, gall bladder, urinary bladder, and pancreas carcinomas, as well as melanomas and rhabdomyosarcomas.[73-75] Members of the same protooncogene family were also found to be active in human hematopoietic neoplasms including cell lines or primary samples from different types of leukemias (AML, ALL, CML, and T-cell leukemias).[76-78] According to the results of several studies, there would be a correlation between the member of the c-*ras* family that is activated in the NIH/3T3 assay and the site of the tumor. The gene c-H-*ras* would be preferentially activated in urinary tract tumors, the gene c-K-*ras* in lung and colon carcinomas, and the gene N-*ras* in hematopoietic neoplasms. Activation of N-*ras* was detected in human sarcoma, rhabdomyosarcoma, neuroblastoma and myeloid leukemia cell lines.[79-86] The same protooncogene was found to be activated by a point mutation in 2 of 32 samples of fresh bone marrow cells obtained from patients with a diversity of leukemias.[87] One of the two positive cases had CML and the other ALL. Of this series of 32 patients, 2 additional cases gave positive results in the NIH/3T3 transfection assay but the active transforming genes were different from c-*ras* or B-*lym* and remained unidentified. Activated N-*ras* genes were also detected in three of six human tissues infiltrated by AML cells.[85]

Most primary human tumors are negative for the presence of active protooncogenes in DNA transfection assays with the NIH/3T3 system.[72] Using this assay, activated genes of the c-*ras* family have been detected in less than 20% of the total human tumors, including carcinomas of different sites, sarcomas, neuroblastomas, lymphomas, and leukemias. Activation of c-*ras* genes may not correlate with either tissue type or stage of differentiation of neoplasms.[88] In a clinical study, only 2 of 38 randomly selected specimens of primary human tumors of the urinary tract had activated c-H-*ras* genes, and the 2 positive patients had no special clinical or pathological features that could serve to distinguish them from the cases that were negative for protooncogene activation.[89,90] Of 13 tissue samples obtained directly from human melanomas, 1 contained an activated N-*ras* gene, corresponding to a mutation at codon 12; the other 12 melanomas were negative for activated c-*ras* genes.[91] One of eight samples from primary prostatic cancer contained an activated c-K-*ras* gene detected in the NIH/3T3 DNA transfection assay.[92] Only 1 of 18 human ovarian carcinomas or ovarian carcinoma cell lines yielded DNA active in transformation of NIH/3T3 cells, and the positive case, which corresponded to activation of N-*ras*, was probably associated with N-*ras* rearrangement during the transfection experiment and was not present in the original tumor cells.[93] No active c-*ras* genes were detected by the NIH/3T3 assay among 16 primary human mammary carcinomas and only one from five established human mammary carcinoma cell lines scored as positive in the NIH/3T3 DNA transfection assay.[94] In an independent study, only 1 of 10 human mammary tumor cell lines was scored as positive in the assay.[95] Consistently negative results were obtained with the same system by screening of normal cells from patients with high cancer risk syndromes.[96] Only 4 of 30 human melanoma cell lines yielded transforming c-*ras* genes in the NIH/3T3 assay and, interestingly, of 5 cell lines originating from separate metastases of a single patient, only 1 contained an active c-*ras* gene.[97] These results suggest that activation of c-*ras* genes is heterogeneous among neoplastic cell populations, even within a given tumor. However, some types of human tumors may be associated more frequently with activated c-*ras* genes. For example, four of six malignant tumors of the thyroid gland (one anaplastic tumor, one follicular moderately differentiated tumor, and two papillary tumors) were found to contain activated c-*ras* genes, while no such genes were detected in normal thyroid tissue, benign thyroid adenomas, or thyroid tissue from Graves' disease.[98] Somatic mutation of the c-*ras* genes at particular codons (codons 12 and 61) is usually responsible for their activation as assessed in the NIH/3T3 assay.

2. Activation of c-*ras* Genes in Experimental Carcinogenesis

Oncogenic activation of c-*ras* genes and other protooncogenes may occur as a consequence of experimental cancer induction with radiation and chemical mutagens and carcinogens. A rather high incidence of c-*ras* activation due to specific types of mutations has been found in some of these studies.[99-101] On the other hand, no protooncogene activation was detected in other experiments. For example, rat urothelial cell lines transformed with NMU did not contain activated protooncogenes, according to the focus assay in NIH/3T3 cells and a tumorigenic assay in nude mice.[102] The reason for such large differences is unknown but the results of several studies suggest a specificity of protooncogene activation related to both the cell type and the carcinogenic agent.

An activated c-*ras* gene was detected in an osteosarcoma cell line obtained from a bone tumor induced in mouse with ^{90}Sr.[103] An activated c-K-*ras* gene was detected by the NIH/3T3 transfection assay and by Southern blot analysis in 6 of 12 rat skin tumors induced by ionizing radiation.[104] The DNAs of 10 of 12 tumors also showed c-*myc* amplification (5- to 20-fold). Evidence for tissue specificity was observed in patterns of protooncogene activation, with each of the radiation-induced three clear cell carcinomas exhibiting activation of both c-*myc* and c-H-*ras* genes.[104] However, the expression of these two genes was not clearly increased in the tumors as compared with rat epidermis.

High molecular weight DNA from mouse skin carcinomas induced by sequential treatment of mouse skin with initiators and promoters may cause morphological transformation of NIH/3T3 cells, and the transforming properties are due to the transfer of an activated c-H-*ras* protooncogene.[15] The protooncogene c-K-*ras* was found to be active in two of four methyl-cholanthrene (MCA)-induced mouse fibrosarcomas.[105]

Examination of fibrosarcomas induced in rats by subcutaneous injection of the potent mutagenic agent 1,8-dinitropyrene by the DNA transfection assay indicated the presence of activated c-K-*ras* genes in 1 of 9 tumors examined; the other tumors could contain unidentified c-*onc* genes other than those from the c-*ras* family.[106] Of 11 fibrosarcomas induced in rats by 1,6-dinitropyrene, 2 were positive for transformation in the DNA transfection assay, but the DNA from one of the original tumors which gave positive results for activation of an N-*ras* gene did not give any transformants by several transfection assays, suggesting either selection of cells containing an activated N-*ras* gene in the tumor or activation of the protooncogene during cell manipulation or culture *in vitro*.[107] The results further suggest that activation of c-*ras* genes does not occur frequently in sarcomas induced in rats by dinitropyrene. DNAs from a nontumorigenic hamster epidermal cell line and from two neoplastic cell lines transformed by benzo(*a*)pyrene (BP) were not capable of transforming NIH/3T3 cells.[108] The same cells acquired tumorigenic properties in nude mice after transfection with a plasmid containing a mutated EJ c-H-*ras* gene.

Transfection analysis of DNAs from thymic lymphomas induced in RJF mice by percutaneous application of MCA revealed that 10 of the 12 tumors contained an activated c-K-*ras* gene.[109] DNA from 10 of 11 hepatocellular carcinomas induced in rats with intraperitoneal injection of aflatoxin B$_1$ contained transforming sequences, as detected in the DNA transfection assay.[110] However, only two of the liver tumor DNAs contained an activated c-*ras* gene (c-K-*ras*), and the alteration corresponded to an amplification of the gene sequences. Moreover, this alteration was not present in the original tumor tissue. In another study, only 1 of 18 hepatocellular carcinomas induced in rats by continuous administration of 3 different carcinogens contained an activated c-*ras* gene, which was identified as N-*ras*.[111] Only 14 of 33 mouse liver tumors and 1 of 28 rat liver tumors induced with *N*-nitrosodiethylamine were positive in the NIH/3T3 DNA transfection assay.[112] Genetic loci other than c-*ras* genes are probably involved in experimental hepatocarcinogenesis in mice and rats.

Chemically induced transformation of human cells is difficult to attain and has rarely been reported. DNA prepared from an MCA-transformed human 312H cell line induced foci upon transfection into NIH/3T3 cells, and analysis of the p21^{c-ras} product contained in these cells by immunoprecipitation and gel electrophoresis indicated that it contained a c-H-*ras* gene activated by mutation at the 61st codon.[113] On the other hand, DNA prepared from DMBA-transformed and DMSO-treated control 312H cell lines failed to induce foci.

Whenever possible, positive results obtained with the DNA transfection assay should be confirmed by studying DNA from the original tumor. DNA of 1 of 5 intestinal adenocarcinomas induced in rats with an organic compound that is present in broiled fish was positive in the NIH/3T3 transfection assay and contained a mutation (G-T transversion) in the 12th codon of N-*ras*.[114] However, this mutation was not present in the original tumor DNA, as tested with a specific oligonucleotide probe, thus indicating that it probably occurred during the transfection procedure.

An interesting aspect is the induction of transforming ability by treatment of cloned c-*ras* genes with ultimate carcinogens *in vitro*. Plasmids containing cloned human c-H-*ras* genes have been treated with ultimate carcinogens capable of forming DNA adducts, and the cloned protooncogenes were altered by the treatment by mutation at codons 12 or 61, thus acquiring transforming ability when tested in the NIH/3T3 assay.[115-117] Studies with DNA amplification *in vitro* using the polymerase chain reaction (PCR) method, followed by oligonucleotide probe hybridization analysis, should make more clear the role of protooncogene mutation in experimental carcinogenesis.

3. Host Cell Factors Involved in c-*ras* Activation

Activation of c-*ras* genes may be a late result of the growth of tumor cells under particular conditions, either *in vitro* or *in vivo*. For example, in one study an activated N-*ras* gene was detected in late but not early passage human PA1 teratocarcinoma cultured cells.[118] A similar situation occurs in the mouse, where active c-*ras* genes, which were detected in a minority of tumors (5/21), were present only in the metastatic variants of the tumors, which suggests a possible role of protooncogenes in the progression of certain tumors.[119] Studies *in vitro* suggest that cells that have accumulated genetic (karyotypic) alterations as a consequence of prolonged culture may be more susceptible to neoplastic transformation associated with mutational activation of c-*ras* gene.[120]

The genetic constitution of the host may be important for the activation or lack of activation of c-*ras* genes by carcinogenic agents. In some inbred mouse strains with genetic predisposition to cancer, the incidence of protooncogene activation in the tumors may be rather high. For example, male mice of the strain B6C31F exhibit a high incidence of hepatocellular adenoma and carcinoma, and 3/10 of the adenomas and 10/13 of the carcinomas examined scored positive in the DNA transfection/transformation assay.[121] In contrast, none (0/29) of a variety of spontaneous tumors from Fischer 344/N rats gave positive results in the same assay.

B. ACTIVE C-*LYM* GENES

By means of the NIH/3T3 transfection/transformation assay an active B-*lym*-1 gene was detected in the majority of neoplasms of intermediate stage B lymphocytes of chicken, mouse, and human origin, and an active T-*lym*-I gene was found in also a majority of mouse and human neoplasms of early and intermediate stage T lymphocytes.[88,122-125] Genes such as B-*lym*-1 and T-*lym*-I may have a normal function at specific stages of differentiation within discrete lymphoid cell lineages. The mechanisms of activation of *lym* genes have not been elucidated. Both the DNA sequences and the level of expression of B-*lym*-1 are apparently normal in Burkitt's lymphoma cells.[126] Mouse B-*lym*-1 gene is apparently a portion of LINES repetitive elements contained in the mouse genome and the human B-*lym*-1 gene is 50 to 60% homologous to the mouse sequence, although it shows no significant homology to human LINES elements.[127,128] The human B-*lym*-1 gene, however, contains an *Alu* sequence repeat. The functional role of *lym* genes in normal and transformed cells is unknown.

C. ACTIVE C-*RAF* GENE

A gene active for inducing foci in the NIH/3T3 assay was isolated from a primary stomach cancer and was identified as c-*raf*.[129] The active DNA sequence encompassed about 60 kbp but the mechanism of activation was not elucidated. DNA from the metastasized lymph node of the same patient, as well as DNA from similar tumors resected from other two patients, were negative in the same assay system. An active c-*raf*-1 gene was detected by the NIH/3T3 DNA transfection assay in the radiation-resistant human laryngeal carcinoma cell line SQ-20B, but the mechanism of activation was not elucidated and the original tumor tissue was not examined.[130] Activation of c-*raf*-1 genes detected in other human tumor cells, including neural, colonic, and laryngeal cancers, as well as in a chemically induced rat hepatocellular carcinoma, was found to occur during the DNA transfection procedure and the active genes were not present in the original tumor DNAs.[131-135]

D. ACTIVATION OF OTHER GENES IN TUMORS

The NIH/3T3 and other DNA transfection/transformation assays have been used to detect cellular genes with transforming capability that do not seem to have v-*onc* counterparts. In addition to c-*ras*, c-*lym,* and c-*raf*, other genes have occasionally been detected to be activated in different tumors or tumor cell lines. Such genes, frequently considered as protooncogenes, have been designated as *met*,[136] *dbl*,[137,138] and *ret*.[139] Activation of the *met* gene in the chemically transformed human cell line MNNG-HOS occurred not by mutation but by a chromosomal rearrangement that generated a chimeric gene which is transcribed to produce a hybrid mRNA.[140,141] The transforming sequence, termed *tpr-met*, resulted from a recombinational event.[142] The *dbl* gene codes for a 66-kDa protein (p66) which is phosphorylated on serine residues and lacks tyrosine kinase activity.[143,144] The mechanism of *dbl* activation is unknown.

Another putative protooncogene, termed *hst*, was detected with the same transfection assay in 3 of 58 DNA samples obtained from a total of 26 patients with stomach cancers.[145] The *hst* gene was active not only in the tumor samples from two patients but also in a noncancerous portion of the stomach from one of these two patients. None of the 58 samples of DNAs in this study of stomach cancer contained active c-*ras* genes, and the normal functional role and the mechanism of activation of *hst* were not characterized. One possible mechanism of *hst* oncogenic activation is rearrangement. In a series of stomach cancers, the *hst* gene was found to be rearranged in all transformants tested (5 out of 15 stomach cancers) but DNA samples from the original stomach cancer tissues contained only the non-rearranged *hst* gene.[146] Thus, the *hst* gene could be activated by rearrangement that occurred *in vitro* during transfection. Apparent oncogenic activation of the *hst* gene in a human hepatoma occurred during or after the DNA transfection procedure and was not present in the original DNA from tumor cells.[147] In an independent study, the DNAs from 2 of 12 human hepatocellular carcinomas tested in the NIH/3T3 assay were scored as positive and the transforming gene was identified as *hst*.[148] An oncogenically activated gene sequence detected with the NIH/3T3 transfection assay in DNA from human Kaposi's sarcoma is apparently identical to *hst*.[149] Interestingly, *hst* shows homology to the growth factor FGF.[150] The possible role of the *hst* gene in human tumorigenic processes is not understood but it has been found to be coamplified with the *int*-2 protooncogene in a human melanoma.[151]

A DNA sequence, termed *lca*, was detected in a primary human hepatocellular carcinoma using the NIH/3T3 transfection assay.[152] This sequence has a linkage to an *Alu* sequence and spans more than 10 kbp. It shows no significant homology with known oncogenes and is normally located on human chromosome 2. The *lca* gene was detected in another sample of human hepatocellular carcinoma from a survey of 12 specimens of this type of tumor.[152] The mechanism of *lca* activation is unknown. Molecular hybridization analyses using *lca* DNA as a probe did not demonstrate any difference between *lca* isolated from hepatocellular carcinoma and the respective DNA sequence contained in normal human placenta.

An active transforming gene, termed *trk*, detected in a human colon carcinoma, was generated not by mutation but by somatic recombination of a truncated tyrosine kinase receptor gene with the tropomyosin gene.[153,154] The truncated kinase sequences of the *trk* gene can also be activated by recombination with other genomic sequences.[155]

Unidentified genes with transforming ability in the NIH/3T3 assay were also detected in DNAs extracted from human solid, primary squamous cell carcinomas of the head and neck,[156] and from a human pancreatic adenocarcinoma cell line (HPAF).[157] Two human cell lines, one derived from an Ewing sarcoma and the other from a leiomyosarcoma, were positive in the DNA transfection assay but their transforming DNA sequences showed no homology to a diversity of cloned oncogene sequences.[131] Similar findings were obtained in spontaneous liver tumors occurring in B6C3F1 mice and in a human hepatoma cell line which contained the HBV DNA sequence.[158,159] Not being present in acute retroviruses, the criterion applied to designate these genes as protooncogenes is based on their transforming ability in the NIH/3T3 DNA transfection/transformation assay.

Activation of a particular DNA sequence, which is apparently distinct from the known oncogenes, has been detected in hamster and mouse cells transformed *in vitro* by X-irradiation.[160] DNA transfected from the irradiated cells produced transformed colonies upon transfection into mouse recipient cell lines (NIH/3T3 and C3H/10T1/2) and a rat cell line (Rat-2). The transfectants were capable of growing in soft agar and formed tumors after implantation in nude mice. Treatment of the DNAs with restriction endonucleases prior to transfection indicated that the same transforming gene was present in each of the transformed mouse or hamster cells.

E. ACTIVE PROTOONCOGENES IN NONCANCEROUS LESIONS

Genes displaying transforming activity in the NIH/3T3 DNA transfection assay may be present in lesions from nonmalignant (noncancerous) diseases. Transforming genes, apparently different from c-*ras* genes, have been detected, for example, in the DNA from human atherosclerotic plaques.[161] The transforming genes detected in these lesions have not been identified as yet, but they could have a role in the origin of atherosclerotic plaques, which have been considered as clonal lesions representing a kind of primary benign neoplasm.[162]

F. SUMMARY

Using the NIH/3T3 DNA transfection/transformation assay, oncogenic activation of proto-oncogenes, especially of c-*ras* genes, has been detected in a number of human tumor cell lines and, less frequently, in primary human tumors. A much higher frequency of c-*ras* activation is found in tumors induced in rodent species by either ionizing radiation or chemical carcinogens. The exact role of the protooncogene activation in tumor origin and/or development *in vivo* is not understood. Active protooncogenes may be present in noncancerous lesions such as human atherosclerotic plaques but their possible role in the origin or development of these lesions is uncertain.

III. ALTERED EXPRESSION OF PROTOONCOGENES IN TUMORS

The expression of protooncogenes in tumors may be appraised either by measuring their transcriptional activity in the tumor cells or by determining the specific protein products in the tumor tissue or body fluids. Due to the possibility of spurious cross-reactions with other cellular proteins, the results obtained with immunologic methods using either monoclonal or polyclonal antibodies should be confirmed, whenever possible, by studies performed at the nucleic acid level with molecular hybridization techniques.

A. EXPRESSION OF PROTOONCOGENES IN TUMOR CELL LINES

The transcriptional activity of one or more oncogenes could be altered in malignant cells as compared to their normal counterparts. The transcriptional activity of genes is frequently inferred from the levels of specific mRNA, but these levels depend not only on the actual rate of transcription but also on RNA processing or RNA stability. Moreover, increased levels of a particular type of mRNA in proliferating cells, including tumor cells, may not indicate overexpression of the respective gene, but may simply reflect the fraction of proliferating cells.[163] In any case, high levels of expression of protooncogenes, or other genes, in tumor cells, or in cells surrounding tumors, do not necessarily indicate that these genes are critically or causally involved in the tumorigenic processes.

Increased mRNA levels corresponding to transcription of c-*sis* and c-*myc* genes have been found in some cell lines derived from different human tumors.[164,165] Constitutive high levels of c-*myc* gene expression have been observed in the human hepatoma cell line HepG2.[166] High levels of c-*myc* transcripts were also detected in two of seven different human tumor cell lines examined; the two lines with elevated levels of c-*myc* mRNA corresponded to giant cell carcinoma of the lung (line C-Lu99) and a colon cancer (line C1).[167] No amplification or rearrangement involving the c-*myc* gene was detected in these two cell lines, and low levels of c-*myc* transcripts were present in three of the same seven cell lines. In another study, two of seven cell lines established from human kidney cancers expressed high levels of c-*myc* mRNA.[168] The majority (over 70%) of human colon adenocarcinoma cell lines were found to express high levels of c-*myc* RNA and protein during all phases of growth in culture.[169] No amplification or rearrangement of the c-*myc* gene was detected in the colon carcinoma cell lines expressing high levels of c-*myc* products and the mechanisms involved in upregulation of the gene remained uncharacterized. In an independent study, three of six human colon adenocarcinoma cell lines expressing high levels of c-*myc* transcripts contained amplification of c-*myc* gene sequences.[170] Relatively high levels of expression of three protooncogenes whose products possess tyrosine-specific protein kinase activity, the genes *lck*, *fyn*, and c-*yes*-1, were detected in several human colon carcinoma cell lines.[171]

The human c-*erb*-B/EGF receptor gene was found to be overexpressed, without gene amplification, in four human pancreatic carcinoma cell lines.[172] High levels of EGF receptors are present in human cell lines derived from nonsmall-cell lung cancers but not in small-cell lung cancer.[173] These results suggest that EGF receptors may represent a biological marker for the differential diagnosis in some cases of human lung cancer.

High levels of c-*myc* transcripts associated with an apparent activation of the c-*raf*-1 gene were detected in cell lines derived from the radioresistant skin fibroblasts of patients with the Li-Fraumeni syndrome.[174] This syndrome is inherited in a dominant manner and is characterized by a constellation of cancers (sarcomas, breast and other carcinomas, brain tumors, and leukemias) that tend to arise in young people and as multiple primaries in the same individual.

High levels of transcriptional expression of c-*myc* have been observed in some but not all immortalized cell lines derived from human urothelium.[175] A single treatment with phorbol ester (TPA) markedly induced both c-*fos* and c-*myc* expression in the mortal cell line HU 1752 from the same origin. In contrast, TPA induced only c-*fos* expression in the immortalized urothelial cell lines, either tumorigenic or not, which suggests that the normal regulation of c-*myc* may be altered in immortalized cells irrespective of their tumorigenic properties. The levels of c-H-*ras* were unaffected by the TPA treatment in all of these human urothelial cell lines.

Transcripts of the c-*sis* gene were detected in 8 of 23 human tumor cell lines derived from sarcomas and glioblastomas, although the levels showed marked variation among different cell lines; c-*sis* transcripts were not detected in cell lines derived from carcinomas, melanomas, or other human tumors, and were also undetectable in human embryonic fibroblasts.[164] Multiple forms of c-*sis* transcripts, as well as a variety of PDGF-like polypeptides, have been detected in certain tumor cell lines, like the U-2 OS human osteosarcoma line, whereas no c-*sis* mRNA and no PDGF immunoreactivity were detected in other tumor cell lines, including the MG-63 human osteosarcoma line.[176]

Variable levels of c-*myc* transcripts were detected in cell lines derived from human sarcomas, carcinomas, and lymphomas, as well as in normal human fibroblasts and hematopoietic cells.[164] There was no apparent correlation between c-*sis* and c-*myc* transcription rates in different human cell lines. The levels of c-*myc* transcripts are elevated in Daudi cells (a line of lymphoblastoid cells derived from an African Burkitt's lymphoma) and these levels can be reduced by more than 75% when the cell growth is inhibited by treatment with human IFN-β.[177] The protooncogene c-*myb* was expressed in form of 3.5- and/or 2.4-kb mRNA transcripts in the majority of seven cell lines derived from human small-cell lung carcinoma.[178] No expression of c-*myc* protein was detected in a cell line (H69) derived from a human small-cell lung carcinoma, while three other cell lines derived from other human tumors exhibited high levels of the c-*myc* protein.[179] Small-cell lung carcinoma is an aggressive tumor that is unusual for its frequent neuroendocrine activity and for its frequent change towards other histological types of lung cancer.

Expression of c-*myc* is growth related in mouse cell lines, either nontransformed or transformed by chemical carcinogens or ionizing radiation.[180] Some protooncogenes are apparently inactive in tumors and tumor cell lines. For example, c-*fos* transcripts could not be detected in more than 20 tumor cell lines established from different types of mouse tumors, although high levels of these transcripts were present in the amnion and in differentiated bone marrow cells of the same animals.[181] No transcripts of c-*sis*, c-*fms*, c-*rel*, c-*src*, and c-*myb* were detected in C3H/3T1/2 mouse embryo cell lines and in eight chemically and radiation-transformed lines derived from the same cells.[182] Other protooncogenes (c-*abl*, c-*fos*, c-H-*ras*, and c-*myc*) were expressed both in the transformed cells and in the nontransformed C3H/10T1/2 cells as well as in mouse embryo tissue and adult mouse liver. In general, the levels of expression of these genes were similar in the C3H/10T1/2 cells and in whole embryo mouse tissue, although c-*myc* was expressed at somewhat higher levels in six transformed cell lines. No major rearrangements or amplification of the c-*myc* gene were detected in the transformed cell lines overexpressing this gene. The c-*fos* protooncogene was expressed in the nontransformed C3H/10T1/2 cells but its level of expression was very low or not detectable in the transformed cells.[182] The malignant conversion of myogenic cell lines and the progression of their tumorigenic properties correlate not with activation but with the transcriptional inactivation of a set of protooncogenes.[183]

In different clones from a cell line derived from a spontaneous rat mammary tumor, metastatic ability after subcutaneous inoculation into SHR rats was correlated to expression of the c-*fos* gene.[184] The amounts of c-*fos* mRNA in the weakly metastatic clones were markedly lower than those in the highly metastatic clones. However, the levels of expression of c-*fos* gene among highly metastatic clones did not completely parallel the number of metastatic nodules in the lungs after inoculation, which suggests that other cellular genes are involved in the expression of the metastatic capacity. The amounts of c-*myc* mRNA were similar in all the cell clones, either metastatic or nonmetastatic, whereas the amounts of N-*ras* mRNA were somewhat higher in the metastatic clones.[184] No expression of c-H-*ras* was detected in any of these cell clones.

Complex patterns of transcription of several protooncogenes, including c-H-*ras* and c-*abl*, have been observed in many different human tumor cell lines as well as in normal human fibroblasts.[164,165] Studies with a flow cytometric immunofluorescence assay indicate that in different human hematopoietic cell lines, including two leukemia cell lines, $p21^{c-ras}$ proteins are equally expressed in all phases of the cell cycle.[185] No increased expression of six different protooncogenes (c-*myc*, c-*myb*, c-K-*ras*, c-H-*ras*, N-*ras*, and B-*lym*), and no amplification or rearrangement of these genes, was found in EBV-immortalized human lymphocytes which were converted into aneuploid cells capable of inducing high-grade immunoblastic lymphomas upon injection into athymic mice by treatment with N-acetoxy-2-acetylaminofluorene.[186]

Variants of the HeLa cell line, which was originally established from a human uterine cervix carcinoma, express variable levels of transcripts from different protooncogenes. The c-H-*ras* gene is expressed in HeLa-S3 cells, but the protooncogene DNA sequences are located in chromatin regions distal to sites of chromatin modification usually associated with activation of the protooncogene.[187] Abundant transcripts of 13 of 21 protooncogenes examined were detected in the cell line D98, which was derived from HeLa cells (a cell line which was initially established from a human uterine cervix carcinoma).[188] Despite the high levels of protooncogene-specific RNAs detected in D98 cells, transfection of NIH/3T3 cells with DNA from these cells did not give positive results for the appearance of transformed foci. The tumorigenicity of D98 cells in nude mice is suppressed when hybrids are made by fusing these cells with normal human diploid cells, and the nontumorigenic somatic hybrids express decreased levels of c-*fos* and c-*ets*-2 and increased levels of c-*myb*, compared with D98 parental cells.[189] The relationship between these changes in protooncogene expression and the abrogation of tumorigenicity in the hybrid cells is unclear.

Both c-*myc* and c-*ras* genes were expressed in a malignant human trophoblast cell line (BeWo), as well as in hydatiform moles and early villous normal human placenta.[190] Protooncogene transcripts with different sizes were detected in both malignant and normal human hematopoietic cells but a consistent pattern of transcription could not be discerned. No significant difference in the level of expression of 11 different protooncogenes was detected between two mast cell lines derived from murine bone marrow, one of them normal, nontumorigeni, and growth factor dependent, and the other malignant, tumorigenic, and growth factor independent.[191]

Large amounts of c-H-*ras* and c-*myc* transcripts were detected in four different human prostatic carcinoma cell lines, one of which (PC82 cell line) was androgen dependent.[192]

Transcripts of c-*fes*, c-*abl*, and c-*int*-1 were not detected in these cell lines, but in some lines the presence of N-*ras*, c-K-*ras*, c-*myb*, c-*fos*, c-*fms*, and c-*sis* mRNAs was observed. The PC82 cell line showed, in addition to high levels of c-H-*ras* and c-*myc* transcripts, high levels of c-*fos* expression. Inhibition of tumor cell proliferation by withdrawal of androgen in the PC82 androgen-sensitive cells was accompanied by a tenfold reduction of the c-*fos* mRNA level and a twofold reduction of c-H-*ras* transcripts, whereas, in contrast, the level of expression of c-*myc* was not changed by the hormone manipulation.[192]

Constitutively high expression of c-*myc* transcripts and overexpression and twofold amplification of the c-K-*ras*-2 gene was detected in human fibroblast cells transformed *in vitro* by γ-irradiation.[193] Significantly elevated transcript levels of c-K-*ras*, c-*myc*, and c-*fos* were detected in the undifferentiated and malignant murine teratocarcinoma cell line PCC4 in comparison to the levels of the differentiated, nonmalignant cell line PCD1.[194] The higher protooncogene expression of PCC4 cells may reflect the augmented proliferative capacity of these cells compared to the mature PCD1 cells.

In a human hepatoma cell line (PLC/PRF/5) the protooncogenes c-*abl*, c-*fes*, c-*fms*, c-*myc*, c-H-*ras*, and c-*sis* were expressed, whereas c-K-*ras* was not expressed.[195] However, no protooncogene was specifically expressed in the hepatoma cells, and the Daudi cell line, used as a positive control, showed stronger signals than the hepatoma cell line in every protooncogene expression. c-*myc* transcripts were found to be increased in other human hepatoma cell lines when compared with a normal human liver sample.[196] N-*ras* transcripts were not elevated in these hepatoma cell lines and c-H-*ras* expression was not detected in the same cells.

Overexpression of 4 protooncogenes (c-*abl*, c-*erb*-B, c-*myc*, and c-H-*ras*), from 11 protooncogenes analyzed, was found in the HeRo cell line, which was derived from a human glioblastoma.[197] N-*myc* transcripts are frequently elevated in human neuroblastoma cell lines with or without N-*myc* gene amplification.[198] The neuroblastoma cell line SK-N-SH expresses high levels of c-*myc* mRNA in the absence of c-*myc* or N-*myc* amplification.[199] Altered levels of expression of the c-*src*, c-*sis*, and c-*myb* protooncogenes have also been detected in human cell lines derived from neuroblastomas and neuroepitheliomas.[200]

Increased expression of several protooncogenes from a set of six (c-*abl*, c-H-*ras*, c-K-*ras*, c-*fos*, c-*myc*, and c-*sis*) was detected in some established cell lines from spontaneous and radiation-induced murine osteosarcomas, as well as in transplanted tumors of the same type.[201] However, no clear patterns of altered protooncogene expression, of the type "one protooncogene-one tumor" or "two protooncogenes-one tumor" emerged from this study. A relatively frequent increase in the expression of c-*myc* and c-*ras* genes was observed in this study, but there was no indication that any particular protooncogene, or combination of protooncogenes, was associated with murine osteosarcomas.

Teratomas represent an interesting system for the examination of protooncogene expression since the malignant stem cells (embryonal carcinoma cells) undergo differentiation, becoming nonmalignant and highly specialized. Four protooncogenes (c-*myc*, c-*ras*, c-*abl*, and c-*sis*) were found to be expressed in cell lines derived from transplantable mouse teratomas, both in the embryonal carcinoma cells and in the differentiated cell types formed from these cells.[202] Transcripts of other six protooncogenes (c-*myb*, c-*fes*, c-*mos*, c-*erb*-A, c-*erb*-B, and c-*src*) were not detected in the teratoma cell lines. In some of these cell lines there was no strict correlation between growth rate and c-*myc* and c-K-*ras* expression. Terminal differentiation of teratoma-derived myoblasts to myotubes was associated with a reduction of the expression of c-*myc* and c-K-*ras*, which was paralleled by an increased level of creatine kinase activity and a shift from β- and γ-actin to α-actin.[202]

In conclusion, the level of expression of different protooncogenes is frequently altered in tumor cell lines, but no clear-cut patterns of protooncogene alteration in a given type of tumor cell line, or in tumor cell lines in general, can usually be discerned. Human tumor cell lines show great variation in the levels of expression of different protooncogenes, and in some lines the levels may be normal. In any case, the biological significance of altered levels of protooncogene expression in tumor cell lines is not understood at present.

B. EXPRESSION OF PROTOONCOGENES IN PRIMARY HUMAN TUMORS

The study of protooncogene activity in biopsy specimens and fresh samples from tumors may be more informative than the study of cell lines since many of these lines have been maintained for years in an artificial environment and their biochemical and functional properties may be different from those existing in primary tumors. Expression of protooncogenes may be maintained relatively altered in xenografts of primary human tumors, for example, in renal carcinomas transplanted in nude mice.[203]

1. Expression of c-*ras* Genes in Human Solid Tumors

The levels of expression of p21$^{c\text{-}ras}$ proteins have been assessed in 52 fresh specimens of human tumors of different types and sites using antibodies generated to different domains of p21$^{c\text{-}ras}$ proteins.[204] Although 90% of the tested tumors were positive for proteins related to c-*ras* genes, all of nine normal gastrointestinal tissues of different sites were also positive for the same proteins. Moreover, only 21% of the tumors exhibited elevated levels of p21 and there was no clear correlation between the increased levels of p21 and particular histological features.

Variable results have been obtained in different studies evaluating the expression of p21$^{c\text{-}ras}$ proteins in a spectrum of benign and malignant human mammary tissues. 1.2-kb c-H-*ras* transcripts were found to be elevated between 2.5 to 15 times above the normal level in 12 malignant human breast tumors, whereas the c-*sis* gene was not expressed at significant levels in either malignant or normal human mammary tissue.[205] Overexpression of c-H-*ras*, but not c-K-*ras* or N-*ras*, was detected in 16 of 22 invasive ductal carcinomas of the breast.[206] In a series of 62 specimens of benign and malignant breast tissues excised from 50 patients, the levels of expression of c-H-*ras*, c-K-*ras*, and N-*ras*, as well as the expression of c-*myc*, were significantly greater in breast carcinoma than in benign breast tissue (fibroadenomas and benign fibrocystic breast tissue).[207] However, some fibrocystic specimens having prominent hyperplastic features also exhibited enhanced protooncogene expression and, conversely, protooncogene expression was undetectable in some malignant breast tumors. Moreover, the normal breast tissues surrounding tumors usually expressed the same protooncogenes as the tumor.[207] In an independent series it was found that 37 of 54 (69%) human breast cancers contained p21$^{c\text{-}ras}$ levels two- to tenfold greater than those of control breast tissues and that an excessive increase of p21 (five- to tenfold over the control value) occurred more frequently in advanced stage tumors.[208] No correlation was detected in this series between p21 levels and histological grade.

A monoclonal antibody (RAP-5) generated against a synthetic oligopeptide corresponding to amino acid positions 10 to 17 of the p21^{ras} product recognized the normal cellular component, p21$^{c\text{-}ras}$, the expression of which was not enhanced in various hyperplastic or neoplastic conditions of the human mammary gland in comparison with the normal gland.[209] The immunohistochemical study of c-*ras* protein expression showed similar staining intensity and intracellular distribution of RAP-5 in biopsy specimens of normal, benign, and cancer breast tissue. Thus, p21$^{c\text{-}ras}$ is apparently a normal component of the epithelium and other cell types of the human breast and is neither limited to normal epithelial cells undergoing proliferation nor to their neoplastic, malignant counterparts. On the contrary, mammary carcinomas may show a more variable staining pattern of p21$^{c\text{-}ras}$ expression, with weak staining observed in some cases.[209]

These conclusions should be tempered by the fact that RAP-5 is apparently not specific for p21$^{c\text{-}ras}$ protein. More recently, the p21$^{c\text{-}ras}$-specific monoclonal antibody Y13-259 has been used to determine the expression of p21$^{c\text{-}ras}$ in different human breast lesions.[210,211] Widespread positive staining of p21 was observed in both benign and malignant, including metastatic, breast diseases as well as in the adjacent normal epithelium. The authors concluded that "the presence of *ras* p21 protein as demonstrated by this antibody (Y13-259) is not a useful marker of malignancy or of proliferating epithelium but is rather a normal feature of certain cell types."[210] Moreover, the results of these studies do not support a correlation between p21 expression and tumor invasion. Thus, "elevated expression of *ras* genes is not necessarily abnormal."[211]

Elevated expression of p21$^{c\text{-}ras}$ may occur in hormone-dependent mammary carcinomas. Estrogen and progesterone receptor-positive human mammary carcinomas may contain levels of c-H-*ras* p21 protein as much as tenfold higher than those found in normal mammary tissue, whereas the receptor-negative tumors contain much less elevated levels of the same protooncogene protein product.[212] However, these results were not confirmed in an independent study where no significant difference was found in p21 expression between estrogen-receptor-rich and estrogen-receptor-poor mammary carcinomas.[213] In the latter study, the expression of p21, as assessed with two specific monoclonal antibodies, was highly heterogeneous among primary as well as metastatic mammary carcinomas, and in every case examined at least one metastatic mammary carcinoma showed a lower level of p21 than the respective primary carcinoma. The authors conclude that p21$^{c\text{-}ras}$ expression is probably not involved in the maintenance of the transformed phenotype.[213]

Increased levels of expression of p21$^{c\text{-}ras}$ protein were detected in 10 of 23 samples of fresh primary human lung tumors, in comparison with adjacent normal lung tissues from the same patients.[214] Most of the lung tumors with elevated levels of p21 protein expression were squamous cell carcinomas and, in contrast, adenocarcinomas and small-cell lung carcinomas were infrequently associated with high levels of p21 expression. There was no correlation between increased p21 expression and tobacco exposure of the patient or extent of disease at the time of diagnosis. In an immunohistochemical analysis of 187 lung epithelial tumors using the RAP-5 monoclonal antibody, approximately half of the tumors (97/187) expressed p21$^{c\text{-}ras}$ protein.[215] Certain morphological types of lung neoplasms immunostained more frequently and stronger than others. The majority of squamous carcinomas, bronchioalveolar carcinomas, carcinoids, well-differentiated neuroendocrine carcinomas, and intermediate cell neuroendocrine carcinomas displayed immunoreactivity, whereas adenocarcinomas showed only focal immunostaining and small-cell lung carcinomas were not stained. Only 3 of 26 malignant pleura mesotheliomas analyzed in this study were immunostained.

Expression of c-*ras* p21 product may be increased in premalignant lesions and high-grade bladder carcinomas.[216] Enhanced expression of p21$^{c\text{-}ras}$ proteins was detected in four of seven human bladder cancers associated with bilharziasis caused by *Schistosoma haematobium* in Egypt.[217]

An immunohistochemical assay with the monoclonal antibody RAP-5, which is directed against the p21$^{c\text{-}ras}$ product, was unable to detect p21 expression in normal or hyperplastic (benign) human prostatic epithelium, but increased expression of p21 was found in human prostatic carcinomas, especially in highly advanced stages of the disease.[218] No differences have been detected in the DNA methylation pattern of the c-H-*ras* gene in normal and neoplastic samples from the prostate of patients with prostatic cancer.[219]

Transcripts related to c-K-*ras* and c-H-*ras* were observed to be elevated in some human malignant tumors of the colorectum as compared to the levels present in the normal colorectal mucosa but similar or even higher elevations were found in adenomatous polyps of the large bowel.[220] The latter are considered as potential premalignant lesions but the fact that only a small fraction of them progress to frank malignancy indicates that an elevated protooncogene expression is in itself not sufficient to produce malignant change. However, immunohistochemical studies have indicated that the amount of p21$^{c\text{-}ras}$ may increase with the malignant potential of benign human colonic conditions, suggesting that the c-*ras* products may play a role in the malignant transformation of benign lesions of the human colon.[221] In another study, 9 of 17 primary human colorectal tumors exhibited elevated levels of p21$^{c\text{-}ras}$ expression when compared to normal tissue adjacent to the tumor.[222] Most of the tumors with elevated levels of c-*ras* expression were from either Dukes' B- or C-stage, thus representing relatively early stages of the disease. In contrast, advanced colorectal tumors exhibited no elevated levels of p21[c-ras], and substantially reduced levels of the same protein were found in metastatic lesions of the primary tumors.[222]

The expression of c-*ras* genes has been compared to the conventional staging criteria and clinical outcome in colorectal carcinomas.[223] Studies on immunohistochemical detection of p21[c-ras] using a specific monoclonal antibody demonstrated that human colonic adenocarcinomas show a similar staining intensity to that seen in normal colon mucosa, whereas colonic adenomas show consistently high p21 expression as indicated by staining intensity.[224,225] Metastatic carcinoma of colorectum in the liver showed a similar staining pattern albeit less intense than in the surrounding normal hepatocytes. The results suggest that the presence of p21[c-ras] is a widespread feature of normal metabolic processes in certain cell types and is not restricted to those actively involved in cell proliferation. The results further demonstrated that immunohistochemical studies of p21 distribution with the monoclonal antibody contribute little or nothing to a more accurate assessment of the different stages of carcinogenesis or of variations of the malignant phenotype.[225] In a recent study, c-*ras* genes were found to be expressed at highest levels in the most differentiated cells of the human colonic mucosa, at the top of the colonic crypts, and it was concluded in this study that c-*ras* expression does not correlate with proliferation or malignancy of the colon mucosa cells.[226]

Expression of the c-H-*ras* gene was studied in a total of 121 human gastric carcinomas, including 27 cases of early carcinoma and 144 cases of advanced carcinoma, and its possible correlation with invasiveness, metastasization, and prognosis was evaluated.[227] Immunoreactivity for c-H-*ras* p21 was observed in 3 of the 27 early gastric carcinomas (11.1%) and in 63 of the 144 advanced carcinomas (43.8%). Higher degrees of reactivity were observed in deeply invasive carcinomas than in the superficially invasive ones, and out of 50 metastatic tumor cases, 34 (68.0%) had p21 reactivity which was distributed diffusely within metastatic tumors of perigastric lymph nodes. The prognosis of patients with p21-positive gastric carcinomas was apparently worse than that of patients with p21-negative tumors.

Expression of c-*ras* was studied with the monoclonal antibody RAP-5 in brush smears obtained from suspected human gastric and colonic lesions with the aid of fiberoptic endoscopy.[228] Whereas most benign lesions from the stomach and colon were negative for p21[c-ras] expression, all of 20 smears from gastric carcinoma and all of 20 smears from colonic carcinoma contained cells that stained positively for p21. Considerable heterogeneity of p21 expression was observed among the cells from each gastric or colonic carcinoma, and no correlation was observed between pattern of staining for p21, the histologic type of tumor, or its degree of differentiation.

Immunohistochemical study of normal, benign, and malignant human thyroid tissues using the monoclonal antibody RAP-5 demonstrated that papillary adenocarcinomas showed moderate to intense stainings for p21[c-ras] in most cases and that cytoplasmic and apical surface stainings were the most common patterns of immunoreactivity.[229] Thyroid adenomas showed variable p21 positivity in cytoplasm, and apical surface stainings were negative or weak in most adenomas. The cytoplasm of normal thyroid tissue tissues from Hashimoto's thyroiditis or Graves' disease were uniformly positive for the presence of p21 but, in contrast to the malignant tissues, the apical cell surface was nonreactive for p21 in the benign thyroid tissues.

Elevated levels of c-*ras* expression may be associated not with a bad but with a good prognosis in patients with certain types of neural tumors. An immunohistochemical study on the expression of c-H-*ras* p21 in e7 primary human neuroblastomas demonstrated a significant correlation between the amount of the p21 product and early stages of disease at diagnosis.[230] Stratification of the tumors by patient's age at diagnosis failed to show significant difference in the amount of p21 in tumor cells. The data from this study suggest an inverse correlation between p21 expression and aggressiveness of neuroblastoma cells *in vivo*. Due to the possibility of spurious results, the studies performed with immunologic methods should be confirmed, whenever possible, by methods working at the RNA level for determination of c-*ras* gene expression in normal and malignant tissues. A combination of PCR and molecular hybridization techniques may give reliable results for the evaluation of protooncogene expression.

2. Expression of c-*myc* and N-*myc* in Human Solid Tumors

Increased level of expression of the c-*myc* gene was found in 7 of 10 human mammary adenocarcinomas from patients with 3 or more lymph node metastases, but only in 5 of 22 mammary carcinomas from patients without lymph node metastases or with metastases invading less than three nodes.[231] In a study with immunohistochemical analysis using a monoclonal antibody specific for c-*myc*, elevated levels of p62^{c-myc} protein were found in the majority of human breast carcinomas as well as in benign mammary lesions such as cystic disease and hyperplastic fibroadenomas, as compared to normal adjacent tissue.[232]

Overexpression of c-*myc* RNA was found in 25 of 72 specimens of early (stage I or II) squamous cell carcinoma of the human uterine cervix.[233] Patients whose tumors showed c-*myc* overexpression (4 to 20 times higher than in normal tissue) had an 8-fold greater incidence of relapse than other patients. However, in an independent study with flow cytometric quantitation of DNA and c-*myc* protein in archival biopsies of human uterine cervix neoplasms, no correlation was found between the levels of c-*myc* protein and grade or stage of disease, age of the patient, or prognosis.[234]

Expression of the c-*myc* gene in gastrointestinal cancers is variable. In an immunohisto-chemical study of archival specimens of human gastric carcinomas using a c-*myc*-specific monoclonal antibody, less than 40% of the tumors contained cells which stained positively.[235] In the tumors with positive staining for p62^{c-myc} expression, there was no correlation between this expression and the degree of differentiation. Moreover, staining was common in benign lesions including chronic superficial gastritis, active superficial gastritis with foveolar hyperplasia, and atrophic gastritis with metaplasia. Similar results were obtained in an independent study.[236] Analysis of c-*myc* transcripts in gastric cancer also showed variable results, and subnormal levels of these transcripts were found in esophageal cancer.[237]

Expression of the c-*myc* gene may be altered in human colon premalignant and malignant lesions. In all tissue samples from advanced colon tumors, the levels of c-*myc* transcripts were found to be elevated.[170,237] Altered patterns of distribution and abundance of the p62^{c-myc} product were detected by immunohistochemical staining using monoclonal antibodies in the premalig-nant and malignant lesions of patients with familial adenomatous polyposis.[238] This disease is characterized by the presence of numerous adenomatous polyps which develop throughout the large intestine and whose malignant transformation is inevitable, unless treated by radical surgery in the premalignant state. Studies with flow cytometric quantitation of the p62^{c-myc} protein in populations of individual nuclei extracted from archival biopsies indicated that the nuclear p62^{c-myc} levels increase progressively from normal mucosa through polyps to carcino-mas, although the difference between normal mucosa and polyps was not highly significant.[239]

Elevated expression of c-*myc* was detected in 21 of 29 (72%) primary human colon adenocarcinomas in comparison with the normal colonic mucosa.[240] For an unknown reason, tumors of the left side of the colon (rectum, sigmoid, and descendent colon) would have a significantly higher level of c-*myc* expression than tumors of the right side (caecum and ascending colon).[241] However, survival of individuals with elevated levels of c-*myc* gene expression in primary colorectal carcinoma tissue is not significantly different from that of individuals whose tumors do not express the gene at abnormally high levels.[242] Moreover, there is no significant correlation between c-*myc* expression and recurrence of the disease. No amplification or other genetic changes of c-*myc* were detected in the human colon carcinomas that exhibited high levels of c-*myc* mRNA. The c-*myc* product may also be elevated in colonic polyps.[243] Increased levels of c-*myc* expression are present in inflammatory disorders of the colon including Crohn's disease and ulcerative colitis as well as in celiac disease, which is characterized by villous atrophy of the small intestine.[236,244] It may be concluded that increased levels of c-*myc* expression are not specific for malignant colon diseases and that measurement of c-*myc* RNA or protein levels in primary human colorectal carcinomas is not useful in relation to clinical profiles or prognosis. Transcript levels of c-*fos*, c-*myc*, c-H-*ras*, and c-K-*ras* were studied in 39 tissue samples obtained from 17 patients undergoing surgery for colon carcinoma and other colon diseases.[245] Only half of the colon carcinomas exhibited increased mRNA levels (above twofold) of one or more of the four protooncogenes studied relative to normal mucosa but all deaths occurred within this group.

Expression of the c-*myc* protooncogene in human hepatomas was either slightly higher or lower than in the normal human liver tissue, but in some of these tumors a marked reduction of c-*myc* transcripts was observed.[246] These results suggest that c-*myc* gene expression is not required for the maintenance of the tumor state in human hepatomas. In three human hepatomas examined in another study, the levels of expression of several protooncogenes (c-H-*ras*, c-*fms*, c-*erb*-B, c-*myc*, and c-*fos*) were higher in the hepatoma tissue than in normal adult liver.[247] Expression of the same protooncogenes, as well as of the AFP gene, was also elevated during certain stages of normal human fetal liver development, with a peak between 4 to 6 months of gestation. Other protooncogenes (c-*rel*, c-*mos*, c-*sis*, c-*bas*, and c-K-*ras*) did not show any clear changes during fetal liver development and in hepatoma.

Monoclonal antibodies against synthetic oligopeptides corresponding to the predicted amino acid sequence of the human c-*myc* protein have been used to localize primary human bronchial carcinomas.[248] Good tumor localization was observed in 12 out of 14 patients, but only when the tumors were 3 cm or more in diameter.

The c-*myc* protooncogene was found to be expressed in both benign and malignant human prostatic tissue.[249] The levels of c-*myc* expression were significantly higher in adenocarcinoma of the prostate than in benign prostate hypertrophy, but there was extensive overlapping in the levels detected in both groups of patients. The levels of prostatic acid phosphatase (a good marker for prostatic carcinoma) did not correlate with the levels of c-*myc* gene expression and no clear correlation was observed with the staging of clinical disease.[249] In an independent study, elevated levels of c-*myc* transcripts were found in 6 of 9 specimens of human prostatic carcinoma, compared with 19 specimens of benign prostate hypertrophy.[250] The prostatic carcinomas with elevated levels of c-*myc* expression corresponded to a more aggressive type of behavior. Expression of the c-*myc* protein, as assessed by a monoclonal antibody binding p62^{c-myc}, showed wide variation among different types of human testicular tumors and only small amounts of the c-*myc* protein were seen in the tumors of five patients who subsequently died from their malignant disease.[251]

Elevated levels of c-*myc* and c-*fos* mRNAs were found in 13 of 23 and 14 of 23 thyroid carcinomas, respectively.[252] High levels of c-*myc* transcripts were more frequently found in the thyroid tumors with unfavorable prognosis. High levels of c-*myc* and c-*fos* mRNA were also found in a number of tissue samples from some thyroid adenomas, Graves' disease, and normal thyroid glands. The structure of c-*myc* and c-*fos* protooncogenes was not altered in the thyroid tumors and these genes were neither amplified nor rearranged.

High levels of N-*myc*, but not c-*myc*, expression were detected in tumors arising from primitive cell precursors, including Wilms' tumor (a neoplasm which arises in children from embryonal kidney cells), medulloblastoma, and hepatoblastoma.[253] The enhanced expression of N-*myc* in these tumors was not associated with amplification of the protooncogene sequences.

Quantitation of p62^{c-myc} protein in nuclei isolated from wax-embedded human testicular tumors by using a monoclonal antibody (Myc 1-6E10) showed not a decreased but a significantly increased expression of the protein with increasing differentiation in testicular teratomas.[254] Patients with intermediate and undifferentiated teratomas who developed recurrence had lower p62^{c-myc} levels than those who were disease free since their initial treatment. Patients with seminoma had high levels of expression of p62^{c-myc} in the tumor. Thus, quantitative studies of c-*myc* gene expression could provide prognostic indices for patients with testicular cancer. In any case, the results of this study show that increased expression of a protooncogene is not necessarily correlated to increased malignant behavior of human tumors.

An immunohistochemical study of 60 mucinous ovarian tumors using the monoclonal antibody Myc 1-6E10 showed that the staining intensity of $p62^{c-myc}$ protein varied most in the malignant mucinous tumors and that the least differentiated neoplasms stained most weakly.[255] However, it was concluded that standard histological criteria are more accurate indicators of ovarian tumor behavior than an assessment of c-myc expression.

3. Expression of the c-*src* Gene in Human Solid Tumors

Tyrosine-specific protein kinase activity associated with expression of the c-*src* gene product was detected in all human skin tumor analyzed.[256] The specific activity of $pp60^{c-src}$ was elevated between 4- to 20-fold in all primary human melanomas as compared to the normal skin. Quantitative variation of the activity was observed in the melanoma extracts of different patients and in the different metastases from the same patient and no correlation was detected between the $pp60^{c-src}$ kinase activity and the pathological type of the melanoma. Wide variation in the expression of $pp60^{c-src}$ kinase activity was also found in several established human melanoma cell lines.[256] The question about whether an increased $pp60^{c-src}$ kinase activity in human tumors is a cause or consequence of neoplastic transformation cannot be answered as yet.

High levels of $pp60^{c-src}$-associated tyrosine-specific protein kinase activity were detected in human tumors of neuroectodermal origin exhibiting a neural phenotype (neuroblastomas, neuroepitheliomas, medulloblastomas, pheochromocytomas, and retinoblastomas), but not in those that do not express neural characteristics, such as melanomas and glioblastomas.[257] Cell lines established from these tumors, as well as those derived from some pediatric tumors (osteogenic sarcoma, Ewing's sarcoma, and rhabdomyosarcoma), also exhibited high levels of $pp60^{c-src}$ kinase activity. However, in all of these tumors and tumor cell lines there was no strict correlation between the kinase activity observed in immune-complex kinase assays and the amount of $pp60^{c-src}$ protein in the respective cells and tissues.[257] The biological significance of this dissociation is not understood. Analysis of human tumor cell lines derived from tissues other than those of neuroectodermal origin revealed that $pp60^{c-src}$-associated kinase activity was low in most cases.

4. Expression of the c-*erb*-B Gene in Human Solid Tumors

The c-*erb* B/EGF receptor protooncogene is expressed in a number of primary human breast tumors. In a study of 95 human breast cancers, about half showed EGF receptor expression as measured by the presence of specific, high-affinity EGF binding sites.[258] An inverse correlation between EGF receptor values and low content of estradiol receptors was found in this series. Similar findings were obtained in other clinical studies.[259-261] The prognosis of breast cancer patients with EGF receptor-positive tumors may be worse, as determined by relapse-free survival and overall survival, than that of EGF receptor-negative patients.[262,263]

Overexpression of the c-*erb*-B/EGF receptor gene, frequently associated with amplification of the gene, has been found in many primary human squamous cell carcinomas from the skin, the oral cavity, the esophagus, the vulva, and the uterine cervix as well as in cell lines derived from these tumors.[264-267] EGF has inhibitory effects on the growth and colony formation of squamous cell carcinoma cells at doses that are mitogenic in other cells, including epidermal keratinocytes and dermal fibroblasts.[268]

Elevated expression of the EGF receptor may occur in primary human lung tumors.[269] Immunohistochemical analysis using monoclonal antibodies against the EGF receptor indicates that the elevated expression of the receptor is limited to nonsmall-cell lung carcinomas and is not found in small-cell lung carcinomas, suggesting that the study of EGF receptor expression may be useful for the differential diagnosis of human lung tumors.[270] Moreover, the intensity of staining for EGF receptor may be related to the stage of spread of the tumors.

Expression of the EGF receptor has been detected in the normal parietal cells of the human gastric mucosa as well as in over half of primary human gastric carcinomas, but it is not correlated with the histologic differentiation or potentiality for lymph node metastases of such carcinomas.[271] Increased expression of the EGF receptor may also occur in human bladder cancer, where it may be correlated to tumor invasiveness.[272] Soft parts sarcomas, including epithelioid sarcomas and synovial sarcomas, may also express increased levels of EGF receptors.[273]

Tumors of the human nervous system may express increased levels of the EGF receptor. High levels of the EGF receptor kinase activity were detected in samples derived from human brain tumors of nonneuronal origin such as glioblastomas (glioblastoma multiforme/astrocytoma) and meningiomas.[274] Human meningioma biopsy specimens may contain a mixed population of EGF binding sites.[275] The increased levels of EGF receptors expressed by human gliomas are frequently associated with EGF receptor gene amplification.[276,277] While EGF receptors are present in the normal human pituitary gland, no EGF receptors are present in either hormone-secreting or -nonsecreting human pituitary adenomas.[278] The reason for this absence is unknown.

5. Expression of the c-*neu*/*erb*-B-2 Protooncogene in Human Solid Tumors

Immunohistochemical study of 41 human malignant tumors using an antibody raised in rabbits by immunization with a synthetic peptide corresponding to a part of the intracytoplasmic domain of the predicted product of the human c-*neu*/*erb*-B-2 gene gave positive results in only 4 tumors.[279] All of the positive tumors were adenocarcinomas. Among normal human tissues, epithelial cells in stomach as well as in small and large intestine were faintly stained. The c-*neu*/*erb*-B-2 protooncogene may be overexpressed in primary human mammary carcinomas that contain amplified DNA sequences of the protooncogene.[280] This overexpression correlates with parameters used in the prognosis of breast cancer. However, in an independent study it was concluded that in breast cancer there is no association between c-*neu*/*erb*-B-2 overexpression and lymph-node status or tumor recurrence.[281]

6. Expression of the p53 Gene in Human Solid Tumors

Immunohistochemical analysis of the expression of the gene encoding the p53 nuclear antigen in fresh biopsy specimens from 200 patients with breast cancer indicated that p53 is associated with estrogen receptor-negative, EGF receptor-positive, high-grade tumors.[282] No difference in age of the patient, number of involved nodes, tumor size, ploidy, or labeling index scores were evident between p53-positive and p53-negative mammary carcinomas.

7. Expression of Multiple Protooncogenes in Human Solid Tumors

Multiple transcriptional activation of c-*onc* genes has been found in several human head and neck solid tumors.[283,284] Expression of c-H-*ras*, c-K-*ras*, and c-*myc* was significantly elevated (between 2- and 16-fold) in both premalignant lesions (pleiomorphic salivary adenomas) and malignant lesions (squamous cell carcinomas) of the head and neck in comparison with normal mucosa of the oral and pharyngeal regions and the parotid gland. The mechanisms involved in these activations were not characterized. No correlation was found between the levels of expression of c-H-*ras*, c-K-*ras*, and c-*myc* and sex, age, site of primary tumor, level of differentiation of the tumor, previous radiotherapy, or fate. However, a significant increase was found for c-*myc* expression in TNM stages III and IV as compared to the combined stages I and II.[284] There was a very wide range of expression of the three protooncogenes in the different head and neck tumors when compared with normal tissue. Levels of expression of three other protooncogenes (c-*sis*, c-*fes*, and c-*abl*) were all found very low in the head and neck tumors. Enhanced expression, amplification, or rearrangement of the c-*erb*-B/EGF receptor gene is uncommon in head and neck tumors.[285]

In a study of the expression of 15 different protooncogenes in fresh human tumor specimens from 54 patients, representing 20 different tumor types, more than one protooncogene was transcriptionally active in all of the tumors examined.[45,286] In many patients the transcriptional activity of particular protooncogenes was greater in the malignant than in the normal tissue, and the c-*fes* gene, not previously known to be transcribed in mammalian tissues, was found to be active in lung and hematopoietic malignancies. Summarizing the results of his study, the author states that "there seems to be a moderate elevation in the expression of some cellular oncogenes in tumor tissue as compared with normal tissue, but this phenomenon is by no means universal."[45]

In general, the results of the study just discussed were confirmed by another group of investigators who studied the expression of nine different protooncogenes (c-*src*, c-*mos*, c-*fps*, c-*sis*, c-*fos*, c-*fes*, c-H-*ras*, c-*myb*, and c-*myc*) in primary tissues obtained directly after surgery from a total of 24 different human solid tumors, as well as in 4 human tumors passaged in nude mice.[287] No specificity of the type "one type of tumor/one type of protooncogene" was observed and no consistently increased expression of definite protooncogene, or protooncogene subsets, was detected in tumors of particular histological types at advanced stages of the disease, when surgery is usually performed. Expression of c-*src*, c-*fps*, c-*mos*, and c-*abl* was not observed in human tumors of any kind, whereas expression of c-*myc*, c-*myb*, c-*fos*, and c-*ras* was frequently observed in different tumors. Expression of c-*sis* was detected only in nodes. The authors considered the possibility that protooncogene expression "may reflect tumor cell differentiation rate, and expression may not be related directly to cancerogenesis."[287]

8. Expression of Protooncogenes in Human Hematopoietic Malignancies

The transcriptional activity of different protooncogenes (c-*myc*, c-*myb*, c-H-*ras*, N-*ras*, c-*rel*, c-*erb*, and c-*src*) was tested in biopsy specimens or fresh cells from a variety of human leukemias and lymphomas and no consistent differences were observed between the tumor cells and their normal counterparts.[288-291] Similar results were obtained in another study of human leukemia where the transcriptional activities of eight different protooncogenes (c-*abl*, c-*erb*, c-*fes*, c-*fps*, c-H-*ras*, c-K-*ras*, c-*myc*, and c-*sis*) were examined and no evidence was obtained in favor of the hypothesis that a single protooncogene would be responsible for a given type of leukemia.[292] The author of the latter study concludes that "since the quantity of oncogene expression was not markedly different in leukemic cells over normals, in many cases these results suggest that other genes may be responsible for the malignant change."[292]

In an independent study, fresh human leukemia cells from different types of leukemia were obtained from leukapheresis in a total of 26 patients and human c-*onc* probes, not v-*onc* probes, were used for determining the expression of different protooncogenes by molecular hybridization.[293] It was found that "different (proto-)oncogenes are expressed in the different leukemic types and that the transcript copy number varies from one type of leukemia to another and within a given individual leukemic type."[293] The c-*myc* gene was expressed at detectable levels in all leukemia samples analyzed and the c-*myb* gene was expressed in all samples except in B-cell malignancies. A single 1.5-kb transcript of c-H-*ras* was present at low levels in all acute and chronic leukemias examined whereas c-*sis* was expressed only in the sample from one patient with CML in blast transformation. This was the first reported case of c-*sis* transcriptional activity in human malignant diseases. The protooncogene c-*abl* was expressed at very low levels in a fraction of all leukemia types analyzed and the transcript sizes and levels were the same in CML (where the c-*abl* gene is translocated) as in other forms of leukemia. However, in some samples of CML an aberrant 8.0-kb transcript was detected in addition to the normal 6.4- and 7.2-kb transcripts contained in control samples. The *src* and *erb* protooncogenes were not expressed in the fresh human leukemia cell samples.[293]

In a study of the transcriptional expression of 11 protooncogenes in primary cells from 51 patients with ALL or AML, the following results were obtained: (1) both c-*myc* and c-*myb* were expressed in all the leukemic cells, (2) expression of c-*fos* was confined to AML of monocytic type, (3) of the genes from the *src* family, only c-*fes* and c-*abl* were transcribed at detectable levels in leukemic cells, (4) expression of c-H-*ras* and N-*ras* was very low in all samples, and (5) the protooncogenes c-*sis* and c-*erb*-B were apparently not transcribed in leukemic cells.[294-296] The authors concluded that "cellular oncogene expression in specific subtypes of leukemic cells may relate to either the proliferative activity (c-*myc*, c-*myb*) or the differentiation state (c-*fos*) of the cells." In other series of 20 leukemia patients, elevated levels of c-*abl* transcripts were found in two cases where the leukemic cell type was derived from B-lymphocytes.[297] In these two cases the cells involved represented an early stage of B-lymphoid differentiation and the high levels of c-*abl* transcription observed may be a reflection of the state of differentiation of the leukemic cells.

The c-*myb* protein was found to be expressed within the nucleus of fresh leukemic cells (three cases of AML and two cases of ALL), where it was apparently associated with the nuclear matrix.[298] Expression of c-*myc* and c-*myb* was widely variable in a study of fresh leukemic cells of both lymphoid and myeloid cell lineages obtained from a total of 29 patients.[299] Expression of c-*myc* occurred in many neoplastic lymphoid cell populations, albeit at very different levels, and in some cases no detectable c-*myc* mRNA was detected. Increased expression of c-*myb* was detected in the malignant cells of only 2 out of 14 patients with different types of lymphoid malignancies, whereas in all other cases studied c-*myb* mRNA levels were either low or undetectable. In different cell populations obtained from patients with myeloproliferative disorders, mainly acute and chronic myeloid leukemias, c-*myc* expression was found to occur in 7 out of 12 patients, although usually at rather low levels, and c-*myb* expression was detectable only in some of the acute leukemias studied, while no c-*myb* expression was found in cases of CML.[299] In another study from the same investigators on 11 cases of AML, 6 cases showed high expression of both c-*myc* and c-*myb*, 2 cases a high expression of c-*myc* and low expression of c-*myb*, and the remaining 3 cases a low or absent expression of both c-*myc* and c-*myb*.[300] Only six patients with acute leukemias exhibited markedly high ratios of c-*myc*/H3, c-*myc*/p53, and c-*myc*/c-*myb* mRNA expression.[301] It is thus clear that such heterogeneity makes very difficult any speculation about the possible role of these protooncogenes in the pathogenesis of human hematopoietic malignancies.

Expression of c-*myc* was studied in 51 fresh samples from human lymphoid tumors, including most histological types commonly seen, using monoclonal antibodies raised to different synthetic peptides which reacted monospecifically with the p62[c-*myc*] product.[302] This product was detected in only a minority of malignant lymphomas, principally in those containing cells with immunoblastic characteristics, and was predominantly localized to the cytoplasm. In the majority of cases, especially follicle center cell tumors, the intensity of p62[c-*myc*]-specific staining was very weak relative to that seen in some normal tissues including normal lymphoid tissues. These results did not lend support to the view that elevated expression of c-*myc* is a common or necessary feature of human malignant lymphomas.

In another study, the relative abundance of c-*myc*-related RNA in the total cellular RNA of peripheral blood leukocytes from 36 patients with different forms of leukemia (ANLL, CML, ALL, and CLL) was compared with those in normal peripheral blood cells and in HL-60 cells.[303] Varying amounts of c-*myc*-related RNA were found in the leukocytes from patients with ANLL, CML, and ALL, and in all of the five cases of CLL (B-cell type) the concentrations of these transcripts were virtually identical to those of normal leukocytes. In the non-ALL leukemias, the relative abundances of c-*myc* RNA were variable; high concentrations (between 0.5 and 4.0 times that of HL-60 cells) were detected in 13 (36%) of the leukemias. A correlation, though incomplete, was found between elevated levels of c-*myc* RNA and the occurrence of higher proportions of blast cells in the particular cases. One possible interpretation of these results is that "overexpression of c-*myc* may only be a consequence of maturation arrest of transformed cells at particular stages of differentiation as a result of carcinogenic events that do not involve the c-*myc* gene directly."[303]

The products of the 3 c-*ras* genes (c-H-*ras*, c-K-*ras*, and N-*ras*) were detected in the fresh cells from all of 33 specimens of human acute leukemias.[304] The normal c-K-*ras* and N-*ras* proteins were substantially more abundant than the c-H-*ras* p21 product in all of these samples. The level of total p21^{c-ras} products varied about 20-fold among patient specimens, but in three fourths of cases studied the abundance was significantly greater than in several lymphoblastoid and leukemia cell lines. In this study, the level of c-*ras* expression did not correlate simply with clinical parameters.

The c-*fps/fes* protooncogene is normally expressed in immature cells from the human bone marrow. Expression of this gene is detected in the primary tumor cells from different types of human leukemias as well as in leukemic cell lines but the levels of c-*fps/fes* expression in the tumor cells are similar to that of the respective immature hematopoietic cells.[305]

Increased expression of p53 protein has been detected in fresh bone marrow or peripheral blood cells of approximately one fourth (8/33) of patients with leukemia, preleukemia, or other hematopoietic disorders.[306] In the same study, negligible levels of p53 mRNA and protein were found in a variety of human myeloid leukemia cell lines blocked at different stages of differentiation. The p53 protein is expressed in B-type lymphoproliferative diseases and in the tumor cells of the majority of ALL patients as well as in lymphoid cell lines of both the T and B cell origin but is not expressed in AML, myeloproliferative diseases, and myeloid leukemic cell lines.[307] The p53 protein was detected in the blast cells of 19 out of 34 patients with AML and a highly significant correlation was found between p53 protein expression in leukemic blast cells and the secondary plating efficiency of these cells.[308] Since this efficiency provides an estimate for the self-renewal capacity of progenitor cells in the blast population, these results suggest that p53 may be involved in leukemic stem cell renewal.

9. Conclusion

In conclusion, the results of different studies performed with fresh specimens of human tumors indicate that some protooncogenes may be transcribed at elevated levels in some types of tumors, or in individual tumors, but activation of specific protooncogene is usually not characteristic of a particular type of neoplasm. Although it is conceivable that some kind of hierarchical activation of different oncogenes could critically participate in the origin and/or development of malignant diseases, the results obtained in many studies do not lend support to the existence of such a phenomenon. However, these findings should be interpreted with caution because it is difficult to obtain from the same patients normal tissue adequate to be used for control, and the tumors represent late stages of evolution of a long process of carcinogenesis and are constituted by highly heterogeneous cell populations. In any case, the unpredictable and sometimes small or nonexisting differences in the levels of expression of different protoonco-gene protein products between normal and malignant cells frequently make these products unsuitable for an efficient targeting of drug-carrying monoclonal antibodies to tumor cells for cancer treatment.[309]

C. EXPRESSION OF PROTOONCOGENES IN NONHUMAN SPONTANEOUS AND EXPERIMENTAL TUMORS

The study of protooncogene expression (as well as the expression of other genes) in experimental or spontaneous tumors occurring in different nonhuman animal species may contribute to define the possible role of these genes in malignant processes.

1. Fish Tumors

Increased levels of pp60^{c-src}-associated kinase activity were found in a variety of tumors induced with carcinogens in *Xiphophorus* fishes.[310] Whereas in fish bearing hereditary tumors the elevation of pp60^{c-src} kinase activity was also present in normal tissues like the brain, in the fish with experimentally induced tumors the elevation was present only in the tumor cells.

2. Bird Tumors

In the chicken, RNA transcripts of different protooncogenes (c-*erb*, c-*myb*, c-*myc*, and c-*src*) were not elevated after transformation by either acute transforming retroviruses or chemical carcinogens.[311] In cell lines derived from ALV-induced bursal lymphomas the level of c-*myc* transcriptional activity may be increased 30- to 60-fold over normal cells.[312] c-*myc* transcripts were elevated in two of five cell lines derived from fibrosarcomas induced with 20-methylcholanthrene in Japanese quails, and this phenomenon was associated with hypomethylation of the c-*myc* locus.[313] The expression of two other protooncogenes (c-*myb* and c-*erb*) was normal in all of the latter quail cell lines.

3. Mouse Tumors

Experimental induction of a transformed phenotype in murine cells *in vitro* may be associated with altered expression of particular protooncogenes. Calcitriol induces anchorage-independent growth of BALB/c 3T3 and NIH/3T3 cells and this is accompanied by elevated levels of expression of the c-K-*ras* protooncogene, but not of c-H-*ras* or c-*myc*.[314] These effects are mediated by the calcitriol receptor but other cultured cells (mouse embryo fibroblasts in secondary cultures, NRK cells, and human diploid fibroblasts) do not form colonies in soft agar or express increased levels of c-K-*ras* mRNA in the presence of calcitriol in spite of the fact that they contain calcitriol receptors. In other cellular systems, especially in leukemic cells, calcitriol can act as a differentiation inducer.

Treatment of the phorbol ester-sensitive murine epidermis-derived cell line JB6 with TPA results in morphological transformation associated with changes of cytoskeletal components and enhanced expression of the c-H-*ras* protooncogene.[315] Normal levels of expression of c-H-*ras*, c-K-*ras*, and c-*myc* transcripts were found in epidermal cell lines established from mouse skin papillomas induced by a single topical dose of DMBA followed by 10 weeks of promotion with TPA.[316] All of these cell lines were negative for the presence of activated protooncogenes in the NIH/3T3 DNA transfection assay but three of them showed an enhanced capacity to proliferate after transfection with a mutant EJ c-H-*ras* gene and were then capable of forming rapidly growing, anaplastic carcinomas in nude mice.

Studies on the expression of the c-H-*ras* protooncogene in a two-stage mouse skin carcinogenesis model have yielded most interesting results.[317] Papillomas were induced with DMBA as an initiating agent, followed by promotion with phorbol ester (TPA), merezein, or benzoyl peroxide (a free radical generator that is widely used in the clinical treatment of acne). Early papillomas produced by the combination of DMBA with any of the three promoting agents contained significantly elevated levels of c-H-*ras* mRNA, as compared to the normal skin surrounding the tumors. Moreover, 9-week-old papillomas induced by DMBA, but not by a BP-derivative, contained a point mutation at the 61st codon of one allele of the c-H-*ras* gene.

Mouse thymomas induced with a carcinogen (*N*-nitrosomethyl urea) or γ-radiation showed increased expression (and amplification) of the N-*ras* and c-K-*ras* protooncogenes, respectively.[318,319] An active c-*ras* gene was also detected in fetal guinea pig cells transformed by four different chemical carcinogens, including nitroso compounds and polycyclic hydrocarbons.[320] About a quarter of retrovirus-induced murine T-cell lymphomas involve activation of c-*myc*, not by promoter insertion, but via the LTR enhancer or other mechanisms.[321,322] In murine erythroleukemias induced in mice by the retroviruses F-MuLV and SFFV there was no evidence for enhanced expression of c-H-*ras* and c-K-*ras* but increased levels of normal (2.3 kb) and short (1.8 kb) c-*myc* transcripts were detected in both early preleukemic and late leukemic phases of the disease.[323] In two mouse myelomas induced by pristane and mineral oil, respectively, transcription of the c-*mos* protooncogene was activated by insertion of movable LTR sequences from an endogenous retrovirus (IAP).[324-326]

A clonal cell line of low tumorigenicity, derived from a mouse embryo mouse culture, was used as a model system for the selection of rare, highly tumorigenic, malignant variant cells that were selected out efficiently by a single *in vivo* transplantation step into syngeneic animals.[327] There was no evidence for expression of protooncogenes in the highly tumorigenic clones.

Active protooncogenes may be present not only in mouse experimental tumors but also in spontaneous tumors of the same species.[158] The N-*myc* protooncogene may be active in mouse teratocarcinoma stem cells as well as in mouse embryos.[328] Differential expression of c-*myc* and c-*myb* is observed when chemically induced and spontaneous thymic lymphomas are compared in RF and AKR mice.[329] A near 100% incidence of thymic lymphomas occurs in RF mice 2 to 5 months after skin painting treatment with 3-methylcholanthrene (MCA). In contrast, untreated RF mice do not develop thymic lymphomas prior to 10 months of age and only show 25% incidence of the disease between 12 and 24 months of age. Another inbred mouse strain, AKR, shows an almost 100% incidence of spontaneous thymic lymphomas at 7 to 12 months of age. The expression of 11 protooncogenes (c-*abl*, c-*mos*, c-*fes*, c-*rel*, c-H-*ras*, c-K-*ras*, N-*ras*, c-*sis*, c-*erb*-B, c-*myc*, and c-*myb*) was determined in normal vs. lymphomatous thymus tissues of RF and AKR mice; only c-*myc* and c-*myb* transcripts were detected in an age-inappropriate pattern in thymomas. More than 90% of thymomas occurring in RF mice after MCA treatment contained c-*myc* transcripts, and 70% of the tumors contained c-*myb* transcripts. Among 11 spontaneous thymomas occurring in AKR mice only 2 showed detectable levels of c-*myc* and c-*myb* transcripts, and 2 more expressed c-*myc* or c-*myb* transcripts but not both.[329] No evidence of rearrangement or amplification of c-*myc* or c-*myb* genes was found in the same tumors. It may be concluded that inappropriate expression of c-*myc* and/or c-*myb* genes is, in marked contrast to RF MCA-induced thymomas, relatively infrequent in spontaneous thymomas of AKR mice. Thus, although these two classes of thymomas are indistinguishable at gross autopsy, they are not identical at the molecular level. A hypothetical single dominant gene, termed *Tbm-1*, would be involved in determining spontaneous development of lymphoma in particular rat strains, for example, in the BUF/Mna strain.[330] A gene homologous to *Tbm-1* could exist in mouse.

Progression of certain tumors is accompanied by a change from growth factor dependence to growth factor independence. In order to evaluate the possible role of protooncogene expression in this change, the differential expression of a series of 18 different protooncogenes was examined in a group of cultured murine T-cell lymphomas that were induced following virus inoculation into, or X-irradiation of, C57BL/6 mice.[331] Two classes of T lymphoma cell lines were studied: growth factor-dependent cells and growth factor-independent cells. Of the 18 protooncogenes studied, 5 (c-*myc*, c-*myb*, c-*abl*, c-H-*ras*, and c-K-*ras*) were consistently expressed in all cell lines tested. The results indicated no significant differences in protooncogene expression between growth factor-dependent and growth factor-independent cells, which demonstrates that protooncogene expression is in itself not sufficient to induce progression of T lymphoma cells to growth factor independence.[331] The results further suggest that expression of other cellular genes, which may not be protooncogenes, is required for the progression of tumors from growth factor dependence to growth factor independence.

4. Rat Tumors

The protooncogene c-H-*ras* was found to be expressed at tenfold higher levels in DMBA-induced rat mammary tumors in comparison with the virgin mammary gland.[332] The levels of p21[c-*ras*] in hormone-dependent rat mammary tumors were much higher than in hormone-independent tumors.[212] Tumor regression induced by hormone withdrawal (ovariectomy) was preceded by decrease in the c-H-*ras* expression, which suggests that an elevated expression of the protooncogene may contribute to the maintenance of tumor growth. Enhanced expression of the c-H-*ras* gene was detected by immunohistochemical methods in 3 of 17 MNNG-induced stomach carcinomas in rats and in 21 of 33 colon carcinomas induced by 2-dimethylhy-drazine.[333] In the colon carcinomas, the number and intensity of c-H-*ras* p21 immunoreactivity foci were greater in the tumor cells of deeply invasive tumors than in those affecting only the superficial layers. All the metastatic colon carcinomas had c-H-*ras* p21 immunoreactive tumor cells.

The Morris hepatomas are a series of transplantable tumors which were originally induced in rats by chemical carcinogens. Different Morris hepatomas maintained by transplantation in inbred rat strains are characterized by different rates of cell proliferation. Elevated levels of c-H-*ras*, c-K-*ras*, and c-*myc*, but not c-*src*, transcripts were observed in several types of rapidly growing rat Morris hepatomas as compared to normal liver.[334,335] Enhanced expression of c-H-*ras* and c-*myc* genes, but not N-*ras* and c-*fos* genes, was found in seven hepatocellular carcinomas induced in rats by treatment with the potent hepatocarcinogen aflatoxin B$_1$.[336] Amplification of the c-*myc* gene (two- to fourfold) was detected in one of these tumors. In rat liver tumors induced by a diet containing 3′-methyl-4-diethylaminoazobenzene and in established hepatoma cell lines, the expression of c-H-*ras* was found to be high in the primary tumors, in nontumorous parts of the 3′-Me-DAB-treated livers, and in the hepatoma cell lines, whereas an increased expression of c-*myc* was found only in the primary liver tumors and hepatoma cell lines. [334,337] Increased expression of c-H-*ras* was also observed in the regenerating and fetal liver, which suggests that it is associated with the increased proliferation of hepatocytes. The mouse c-H-*ras* protooncogene is also early activated in chemically induced benign skin papillomas but only a minority (5 to 7%) of these tumors progress to carcinomas, which suggests that this progression may be determined by another genetic event not involving the c-H-*ras* gene.[16]

In rat liver tumors induced by a short treatment with diethylnitrosamine (DENA), 2- to 25-times higher levels of c-*ras* genes transcripts have been found.[338] The increase of expression is parallel for the three c-*ras* genes (c-H-*ras*, c-K-*ras*, and N-*ras*) and it is observed not only in the tumor cells but also in the surrounding cells, and in some cases the levels of c-*ras* expression were higher in the perinodular tissue than in the tumor itself. These results, especially the coordinated expression of the three c-*ras* genes, are difficult to reconcile with structural changes at the DNA level, such as protooncogene amplification or protooncogene translocation, and are more easily explained by epigenetic, regulatory changes occurring in both the foci of neoplastic cells and the surrounding, apparently normal cells.[338] Administration of DENA to rats fed methyl-deficient diets results in hypomethylation of both c-H-*ras* and c-K-*ras* genes in the neoplastic and preneoplastic liver lesions.[339] However, similar hypomethylation of c-*ras* genes is observed in rats fed methyl-deficient diets without DENA administration and the significance of this hypomethylation in relation to the tumorigenic process is not understood. An immunohistochemical study of c-H-*ras* expression in rats treated with DENA indicated that the p21 product is present in foci of phenotypically altered liver cells, neoplastic nodules, and malignant liver lesions (hepatocellular carcinomas), whereas the surrounding histologically normal parenchyma does not exhibit any detectable reactivity with the antibody.[340] The results of the latter study suggest that increased c-H-*ras* expression is an early and stable event in liver lesions associated with hepatocarcinogenesis.

Administration of DENA to rats also induced an increase in c-*fos* mRNA concentration in the liver after 8 d, but the maximal increase (five- to sixfold) was observed after 70 weeks and was found in liver cancer nodules as well as in perinodular hepatocytes.[341] Expression of the c-*myc* gene product, as assessed in a histochemical study using a specific monoclonal antibody, is significantly increased in hepatic preneoplastic lesions (hyperplastic nodules) induced by DENA administration to rats.[342] The levels of expression of c-*myc* and N-*myc* genes also exhibit striking biphasic changes during DENA-induced hepatocarcinogenesis in rats.[343] Expression of c-*fos*, c-*myc*, and N-*myc* genes is also markedly enhanced during liver regeneration, which indicates that the products of these protooncogenes may be related to cell proliferation even in nontransformed cells.

In other experiments, administration of DENA or 2- acetylaminofluorene (AAF) to rats resulted in increased expression of c-*ras*, c-*myc*, and c-*abl* in the liver.[344] In this study, after single DENA doses, increased c-*ras* expression was seen from 12 h postinjection, peaking at 24 to 36 h and declining thereafter, whereas c-*myc* and c-*abl* expression occurred within 1 h after DENA administration and showed no time course. For chronic administration of AAF and DENA, increased expression of the three protooncogenes was observed within 1 week of administration, and also after 1 month, but the expression was normalized by the time of tumor development. These results are consistent with the hypothesis that different protooncogenes may be activated at various discrete steps in the multistage development of tumors.[344] However, the liver is a complex organ constituted by different types of cells and the expression of different protoon-cogenes (c-K-*ras*, c-H-*ras*, and c-*myc*) may be related to specific types of cells during hepatocarcinogenesis.[345]

In an independent study, hepatic focal lesions induced by DENA and detected histochemi-cally by their enhanced enzymatic activity of γ-glutamyl transpeptidase (GGT) were examined for the amounts and size of c-H-*ras* and c-*myc* protooncogene mRNA transcripts.[346] GGT-positive cells isolated from the liver of animals 6 or 11 months after an initiation/promotion regime with DENA and phenobarbital did not show significant differences from other hepato-cyte populations in either size or amount of mature mRNAs for the protooncogenes examined. The results suggest that elevated expression of the c-H-*ras* and c-*myc* protooncogenes eventu-ally observed in liver nodules or tumors may represent a secondary alteration in the regulation of the level of expression of these genes during the multistage process of carcinogenesis. The immunohistochemical analysis of DENA-induced rat liver lesions indicated that c-*myc* and c-*src* proteins were present in nearly all tumors and nodules, but were also present to various degrees in normal areas of the liver from both treated and untreated animals.[347] Moreover, the expressions of c-*myc* and c-*src* were heterogeneous within any tumor or nodule.

In another study with DENA-induced hepatocarcinogenesis in rats, no transcriptional overexpression of several protooncogenes (c-*ras*, c-*fos*, c-*myc*, c-*myb*, c-*mos*, c-*sis*, and c-*abl*) was detected.[348] Eight clones corresponding to mRNAs much more expressed in the induced hepatomas than in hepatocytes from normal liver tissue were isolated, but none of these clones exhibited any homology with known protooncogenes. In an independent study, the translational expression of several protooncogenes (c-*ras*, c-*myb*, c-*myc*, c-*erb*-B, c-*src*, and c-*sis*) was analyzed in the normal rat liver and in the liver of rats fed AAF alone or in combination with DENA.[349] Radioimmunoassays were performed with plasma membrane fractions and total soluble subcellular extracts of the tissues, and immunoperoxidase staining was carried out on frozen tissue sections. Immunohistology revealed significant staining of normal liver by five of the six antibodies (the exception was anti-*src*), and only minor qualitative differences of the staining pattern in some tumors and hyperplastic nodules. The conclusion from this study was that the oncogene-specific monoclonal antibodies do not consistently distinguish between normal rat liver, liver from carcinogen-treated rats, and preneoplastic lesions or tumors.[349] Therefore, these antibodies cannot be used reliably to define the precursor cells of malignant tumors.

In developing rat livers, c-K-*ras*, c-H-*ras*, and c-*myc* transcript levels were found to be high at 17 d of gestation but reached the low levels characteristic of adult rat livers between 20 d of gestation and 3 d after birth.[345] At 2 weeks after the start of a carcinogenic diet containing 0.1% ethionine in adult rats, an increase in the abundance of transcripts of the same three protoonco-genes occurred. Expression of c-K-*ras* and c-*myc* remained elevated during the 35 weeks of the diet, whereas c-H-*ras* transcripts increased transiently. A primary liver tumor sampled at 35 weeks after the carcinogenic diet was started contained high levels of both c-K-*ras* and c-*myc* mRNA. The abundance of c-*src* transcripts was unchanged during hepatocarcinogenesis, whereas c-*abl* and c-*mos* transcripts were not detected in either preneoplastic or neoplastic rat livers.[345] Since the transforming capacity of protooncogenes was not examined, the results do not permit to dissociate the possible contributions of enhanced cell division and cell transfor-mation to the increase in the expression of some protooncogenes during carcinogenesis and in tumors.

Three of five cell lines derived from primary rat tracheal epithelial cells transformed with MNNG *in vitro* expressed elevated levels of 9.5-kb transcripts from a c-*fms*-related gene.[350] The gene expressed in the transformed tracheal epithelial cells may be distinct from the gene coding the CSF-1 receptor, whose transcripts in the rat are 3.8-kb long. No amplification or rearrangement of the c-*fms* gene was detected in the cell lines expressing high levels of c-*fms*-related transcripts.

D. PROTOONCOGENE EXPRESSION IN METASTATIC TUMORS

The study of both human and experimental tumors has not demonstrated a clear correlation between levels of protooncogene expression and the occurrence of metastasis. For example, in one study using transfected NIH/3T3 cells and NMU-induced tumors containing the activated c-H-*ras* gene, it was shown that *ras* gene amplification or increased *ras* expression was apparently not important in metastasis formation.[351]

E. EXPRESSION OF GENES OTHER THAN PROTOONCOGENES IN TUMORS

Gene expression may be altered in different types of spontaneous and experimental tumors but a clear general pattern of alteration of gene expression in cancer cells has not emerged in spite of the efforts of numerous investigators. However, a frequent phenomenon observed in tumor cells is the reexpression, or enhanced expression, of sets of genes that are normally active at embryonic stages of development of the respective tissue. A typical example of this situation is the reexpression of oncofetal antigens observed in a diversity of spontaneous and experimental tumors.[352-355]

1. Human Tumors

The proportion of cellular genes whose transcriptional activity is changed in premalignant and malignant lesions, in comparison with the respective normal tissue, may be rather small. From about 4000 sequences examined in the form of a cDNA library derived from the normal human colon and screened with probes derived from normal colon mucosa, familial polyposis mucosa, colonic adenocarcinomas, and the colon tumor cell line HT29, over 99% showed very little change in molecular hybridization levels when the normal and abnormal tissue samples were compared.[356] Of the remaining 1% of sequences, amounting to some 40 clones, which showed a clear change upon premalignant or malignant transformation, only 9 exhibited an increased level of transcription, while 28 exhibited decreased transcription. The sequences with an altered transcriptional activity in the premalignant or malignant colonic lesions were not characterized in this study.

In a study based on the screening of cDNA libraries derived from transcripts expressed in the normal human stomach and in human gastric carcinoma, three genes were identified as selectively expressed in the neoplastic tissue.[357] These genes did not exhibit structural homology with known viral oncogenes and the functions of their products are unknown. Genes that are expressed exclusively or preferentially in tumor cells may be clinically useful as tumor markers.

2. Tumor Cell Lines

A set of genes has been found to be universally active in mouse cells transformed by DNA oncogenic viruses (SV40 and polyoma virus), transforming retroviruses (RSV and A-MuLV), and chemical carcinogens (MCA and MCA epoxide).[358-360] This set, which is also transcriptionally active in mouse embryonic cells and in normal adult thymus, is not related to 12 different oncogenes (*src*, *erb*, H-*ras*, K-*ras*, *mos*, *abl*, *myc*, *fes*, *fps*, *myb*, *fos*, and *rel*) but corresponds to a gene from the major histocompatibility complex (MHC) which encodes for a *Qa/Tla* class I MHC antigen expressed at the cell surface.[360] The apparent universal expression of this gene in transformed cells suggests its possible role in oncogenic processes.

In an independent study, the level of expression of ten cellular oncogenes was examined in a normal rat fibroblast cell line (F-11) and in transformants derived from it by infection with either polyoma virus (six cases) or SV40 (seven cases).[361] Detectable levels of transcripts were found in the normal fibroblast cell line for nine of the ten protooncogenes tested (c-*myc*, c-*sis*, c-*erb*-B, c-*erb*-A, c-K-*ras*, c-H-*ras*, c-*src*, c-*fps*, and c-*abl*), but no expression of c-*mos* was detected. In none of the wide variety of papovavirus-induced transformants was the expression of any of the tested protooncogenes higher than the constitutive level detected in the parental cell, with one possible exception (a slight increase of c-*sis* expression). In this study it is concluded that "although it is known that a variety of cellular genes are induced in polyoma and SV40 transformants, of which some seem to be directly under large T-antigen control, it appears that none so far encodes for a known (proto)-oncogene."[361]

3. Experimental Tumors

Recombinant DNA techniques were used to isolate sequences that are activated during multistage carcinogenesis in the mouse skin.[362] It was found that between 0.24 and 1.4% of the screened genes are activated during multistage carcinogenesis, but none of these genes showed homology to probes corresponding to 16 different protooncogenes (c-*abl*, c-*erb*-A, c-*erb*-B, c-*fes*, c-*fms*, c-*fos*, c-*mos*, c-*myb*, c-H-*ras*, c-K-*ras*, N-*ras*, c-*rel*, c-*sis*, c-*src*, and c-*yes*). In an independent study, no significant increase in the level of expression of six protooncogenes (c-H-*ras*, c-K-*ras*, c-*fos*, c-*myc*, c-*abl*, and c-*raf*) was found in tumors chemically induced *in vivo* in the mouse skin after treatment with a tumor promoter (TPA).[363] Treatment of primary mouse epidermal cells with TPA *in vitro* also failed to induce any marked alterations in protooncogene expression. Thus, an increased expression of protooncogenes is apparently not required for tumor induction in the mouse skin. It may be concluded that there is no evidence for a critical participation of altered protooncogene expression in experimental multistage carcinogenesis.

F. CONCLUSION

In spite of a number of studies on human and experimental tumors, as well as on tumor cell lines, no clear general pattern of alteration of gene expression in tumor cells has emerged. Moreover, only a very small fraction (less than 1%) of the total genes contained in mammalian cells would display an altered transcriptional activity after neoplastic transformation, and this alteration is more frequently represented by a diminished, rather than an increased, level of expression. The possible relationship between these genes and particular protooncogenes remains to be elucidated. Overexpression of particular protooncogenes is occasionally detected in some spontaneous and experimental tumors. On the basis of the available evidence, it may be concluded that overexpression or altered expression of specific protooncogenes is not crucially involved in the origin or development of spontaneous or experimental tumors.

G. EXPRESSION OF PROTOONCOGENES IN NONMALIGNANT DISEASES

Altered patterns of protooncogene expression may be observed in nonmalignant diseases. Increased expression of c-*myb*, c-*myc*, c-*ras*, and c-*abl* genes has been found in the lymph nodes and the spleen of mice with different forms of genetically determined autoimmune syndromes.[364-366] Greatly elevated expression of c-*myb* and c-*raf* genes was observed in T-cell lines and clones derived from autoimmune MRL-*lpr*/*lpr* mice.[367,368] Mice homozygous for the *lpr* gene spontaneously develop massive lymphoproliferation and an associated lupus-like autoimmune disease characterized by autoantibody production, vasculitis, glomerulonephritis, arthritis, splenomegaly, and generalized lymph node enlargement. The c-*myb* protein produced at high levels by the lymph node cells of *lpr*/*lpr* mice is of apparently normal structure, and the c-*myb* gene in the same cells shows no rearrangement or amplification.[369] However, the c-*myb* gene of these mice is undermethylated relative to c-*myb* of normal lymph node cells, which may explain its high level of transcriptional expression.

Peripheral blood mononuclear cells from human patients with systemic lupus erythematosus

(SLE) and other autoimmune diseases express significantly elevated levels of c-*myc* mRNA, and a subset of these patients with active SLE express increased levels of N-*ras* mRNA.[370] Expression of the c-*myc* protein can also be observed within mononuclear cells of renal disease tissues, but not in the immune complex deposits, in SLE patients.[371] In addition to c-*myc*, the protooncogenes c-*myb* and c-*raf*-1 may also be expressed in the activated B and T cells of patients suffering from SLE, rheumatoid arthritis, and other autoimmune diseases.[366] On the other hand, the levels of expression of c-*myb* and c-*fos* were decreased in the same cells from these patients. No protooncogene rearrangements were detected in the patients. B and T lymphocytes purified from samples donated by normal volunteers and stimulated by mitogens *in vitro* exhibited changes in the pattern of protooncogene expression that resembled those found in freshly isolated SLE cells.[370] Since SLE is a disease characterized by excessive B lymphocyte proliferation, the results of these clinical studies suggest that the differences detected in the expression of protooncogenes by patients with SLE may be due to the abnormal activation of their B cells *in vivo*.

Elevated levels of N-*ras* and decreased levels of c-*fos* mRNA are present in the peripheral blood mononuclear cells of patients with angioimmunoblastic lymphadenopathy (AILA), a relatively uncommon disease of probable autoimmune origin.[372] Expression of N-*ras* and c-*fos* mRNA was most abnormal in AILA patients with the most severe disease and this abnormality was corrected by treatment with cyclophosphamide. The levels of c-*myc* mRNA were not increased in AILA. A putative protooncogene of the *src* family, termed *pks*, was found to be expressed at very high levels in two AILA patients.[373]

Increased expression of the c-*myc* gene was observed with immunohistochemical techniques using a monoclonal antibody specific for p62[c-*myc*] in inflammatory lesions of the stomach and colon, including Crohn's disease and ulcerative colitis.[236] The c-*myc* gene is also expressed at relatively high levels in the intestinal mucosa lesion of patients with celiac disease.[244] This disease is characterized by a small intestinal villous atrophy of unknown etiology. Extremely high levels of c-*myc* transcripts have been observed in a mouse model of polycystic kidney disease with autosomal recessive inheritance, suggesting that the protooncogene may have a role in the pathogenesis of the human counterpart of this disease.[374]

It may be concluded that protooncogene activation *in vivo* is not necessarily associated with malignant diseases and that altered protooncogene expression may be observed in certain nonmalignant diseases.

H. BIOLOGICAL SIGNIFICANCE OF ALTERED PROTOONCOGENE EXPRESSION

The interpretation of findings related to levels of RNA and/or protein protooncogene products in either primary tumors or tumor cell lines may be difficult, especially when there are changes of small magnitude. Even when marked increases are observed, the levels of protooncogene expression may be simply similar to those occurring in embryonal or fetal stages of development of the respective cell or tissue. Reexpression of sets of developmental phase-specific genes is observed in cancer cells under either natural or experimental conditions. The increased levels of protooncogene products could correspond, at least in some cases, to a general phenomenon of dedifferentiation or retrodifferentiation occurring in the tumor cells. Thus, it may be similar to the reexpression of oncofetal antigens and other biochemical changes occurring in many types of human tumors, as well as in tissue and organ regenerative processes. The molecular mechanisms involved in the regulation of oncofetal antigen expression are apparently not specific for these antigens but may include regulation of other unlinked and unrelated structural genes.[375]

Expression of protooncogenes, or other cellular genes, may show important variation in conditions associated with accelerated cell proliferation, such as regenerative or neoplastic processes. Stimulation of cells, e.g., normal erythrocytes, by mitogenic agents results in increased level of expression of protooncogenes, including c-*myc* and c-*myb*.[299,376] Higher levels of protooncogene expression in neoplastic cells may not be causally related to the process of neoplastic transformation but may only reflect the increased rate of proliferation which is characteristic of tumor cells. Certain normal proliferating cells may exhibit levels of expression of particular protooncogenes as high as those observed in tumor cells. Moreover, terminally differentiated cells such as neurons may exhibit the highest level or expression of some protooncogene products, e.g., p21[c-*ras*] and pp60[c-*src*], found in any normal or neoplastic mammalian tissue. Increased protooncogene expression may also occur in nonmalignant diseases.

Changes in the pattern of DNA methylation may influence the expression of protooncogenes, or other genes, in either normal or tumor cells.[377,378] Hypomethylation of DNA sequences is frequently associated with transcriptional activation of the same sequences. The c-H-*ras* gene was found to be hypomethylated in six of eight primary human colon and lung carcinomas and the c-K-*ras* gene was hypomethylated to a lesser extent in two human colon adenocarcinomas.[379] Hypomethylation of the c-*myc* gene was detected in human hepatocellular carcinomas as well as in fetal liver.[380] However, undermethylation of the 5′ portion of the c-H-*ras* gene may be a general feature of eukaryotic cells and the undermethylated state of this gene often observed in tumor cells should be simply considered as a marker of the overall DNA methylation of the tumor cells analyzed, rather than as a specific signal of transcriptional activation.[381] Treatment of K562 cells with the demethylating agent 5-azacytidine induces undermethylation of the c-H-*ras*-1 protooncogene without major differences in the accumulation of c-H-*ras*-1 mRNA transcripts as compared to untreated cells.

In tumor cell populations, marked differences may occur in the expression of certain protooncogenes, both from one tumor to another and within different cells from a given tumor. The general physiological conditions of the patient and the local conditions of the tumor tissue may have influence on the expression of genes present in the tumor cells, including the protooncogenes. Most probably, particular protooncogenes participate, in conjunction with other cellular genes, in the complex, multistage processes related to tumorigenesis, which are associated with manifold changes in the expression of different genomic functions. Protooncogenes could contribute to the biochemical phenomena associated with progression of certain tumors. However, a correlation between increased transcriptional activity of particular protooncogenes, or protooncogenes in general, and tumor progression has not been demonstrated. In fact, such a correlation may not exist. The amounts of transcripts of c-K-*ras*, which is the major protooncogene expressed in B16 melanoma and UV-2237 fibrosarcoma tumor systems, are similar in the low- and high-metastatic variants of the tumors.[382] Expression of c-*abl* and other protooncogenes is independent of metastatic potential in A-MuLV-transformed malignant murine large cell lymphoma.[383]

I. SUMMARY

The levels of expression of one or more protooncogenes may be increased in tumor cell lines, and also, although not so frequently, in the primary tissue from spontaneous and experimental tumors. However, overexpression a particular protooncogene, or a set of protooncogenes, is apparently not a universal characteristic of specific types of tumors or of tumors in general. In some tumors the levels of expression of one or more protooncogenes may be normal, or may be rather diminished in comparison with the respective normal tissue. The biological significance of altered protooncogene expression in tumors is unknown. Altered patterns of protooncogene expression may be observed in nonmalignant diseases as well as in normal cells subjected to a diversity of endogenous or exogenous stimuli. Further studies are needed for a better understanding of the role of altered protooncogene expression in malignant and nonmalignant diseases.

IV. AMPLIFICATION OF PROTOONCOGENES IN TUMORS

Amplification of DNA sequences, including protooncogene sequences, can occur in eukaryotic cells under certain physiological conditions.[384] Amplification of genes related to drug resistance is frequently observed in cells cultured in the presence of a diversity of cytotoxic agents, including agents used in cancer chemotherapy. Protooncogene amplification may be observed *in vivo* independently of drug resistance and has been suggested as a model for the general process of carcinogenesis.[385] This phenomenon could occur through a series of unequal sister chromatid exchanges in different cell cycles. Moreover, chromosome rearrangement may be an essential and intimate step in the amplification process.[386] Another possible mechanism for generation of amplified genomic sequences is disproportionate replication, which means that there can occur more than a single initiation of replication in a portion of a chromosome within a single S phase of the cell cycle.[387] Several experimental results support the latter model of gene amplification. The amplification unit, called amplicon, usually shows a unique pattern for each individual cell line or tumor.[388] In contrast to drug resistance-associated gene amplification, protooncogene amplification occurring in tumor cells independently of drug resistance is characterized by its relatively homogeneous structure within a given tumor and the occurrence of only few DNA rearrangements. The presence of gene (including protooncogene) amplification can be detected in certain cases by cytogenetic methods. Cytogenetic changes associated with gene amplification include homogeneously staining regions (HSRs), double minutes (DMs), and abnormal banding regions (ABRs).[389] Molecular hybridization methods can be used to recognize DNA amplifications not reflected in cytogenetic alterations.

Amplification of cellular genes in eukaryotic cells may occur either chromosomally or extrachromosomally.[384] Protooncogene amplification seems to occur by a chromosomal mechanism, but in at least one case the amplification appeared to involve an extrachromosomal pathway with formation of covalent closed circular DNA.[390]

Amplification of protooncogenes, or other cellular genes, might be related to some stages of the oncogenic process because during the process of gene amplification multiple DNA rearrangements occur that generate new combinations of DNA sequences.[391] Each amplified unit has a unique structure and, at the time of formation of the units, pieces of DNA from different parts of the genome are joined together to form novel structures. Thus, gene amplification could contribute to the production of DNA molecular rearrangements that occur in many tumor cells. Amplified protooncogene sequences can be integrated at sites other than the native gene locus and different integration sites may occur in different lineages of the same tumor.[392] In general, gene amplification may constitute an example of accelerated evolution occurring in tumor cells.[393]

A. AMPLIFICATION OF PROTOONCOGENES IN HUMAN TUMOR CELL LINES AND TRANSPLANTED HUMAN TUMORS

Various protooncogene sequences have been found to be amplified in different tumor cell lines, in particular sequences related to c-*myc*, N-*myc*, c-*myb*, and c-*ras*.[394-396]

1. Amplification of c-*myc*, N-*myc*, and L-*myc*

Amplification of c-*myc*, or c-*myc*-related sequences, such as N-*myc* and L-*myc*, has been found in different human tumor cell lines,[397] including the myeloid leukemia cell line HL-60,[392,398-400] retinoblastoma cell lines,[401,402] some neuroblastoma cell lines,[403-405] a glioblastoma multiforme cell line,[406] breast carcinoma cell lines,[407-409] ovarian tumor cell lines,[410] osteosarcoma cell lines,[411] colon carcinoma cell lines,[170] and some lung cancer cell lines.[412-416] Double minutes as well as an abnormally banded region (ABR) present in HL-60 cells contain amplified c-*myc* sequences.[417]

In a study of 18 human lung cancer cell lines tested, 8 showed c-*myc* amplification, and 5 of them, which had a high degree of c-*myc* DNA amplification (20- to 76-fold) and greatly increased levels of c-*myc* RNA, were derived from patients with a variant class of small-cell lung carcinoma with very malignant behavior.[412] In other study, amplification of c-*myc*, but not N-*myc* or c-*myb*, was detected in two of six cell lines derived from human small-cell lung carcinoma.[413] Amplification of N-*myc* gene sequences (5- to 170-fold) was found in 6 of 31 independently derived small-cell lung carcinoma cell lines, as well as in tumor tissues harvested directly from 3 of these patients.[418] The c-*myc*-related gene, L-*myc*, was also found to be amplified in some human small-cell lung carcinoma cell lines as well as in one specimen of this tumor taken directly from a patient.[419] Gene mapping studies assigned L-*myc* to human chromosome region 1p32, the same region where the protooncogene B-*lym*-1 is located.[419] From two L-*myc* alleles defined by RFLP, either allele can be amplified; in heterozygotes only one of the two alleles is amplified. None of the small-cell lung carcinoma cell lines with L-*myc* amplification had either c-*myc* or N-*myc* amplification and, conversely, none of the cell lines from this type of tumor previously shown to be amplified for c-*myc* or N-*myc* was amplified for the L-*myc* gene.[419] In general, these findings suggest that *myc*-related protooncogenes may have a role in the origin and/or progression of some human small-cell lung carcinomas.

Amplification of c-*myc* and c-K-*ras* genes was observed in a cell line (Lu-65) derived from a human lung giant cell carcinoma,[420] as well as in some cell lines derived from human colon carcinomas.[421-423] Amplification of c-*myc* sequences in a human colon carcinoma cell line (COLO 320) is associated with rearrangement at the 5' end and abnormal transcription.[424] This cell line carries 15 to 20 copies of an apparently normal c-*myc* allele and 1 or 2 copies of an apparently abnormal c-*myc* allele lacking exon 1, and the cells express high levels of a normal c-*myc* mRNA 2.5 kb in size. Amplification of c-*myc* was detected in 3 of 16 human gastric adenocarcinoma samples maintained as solid tumors in nude mice.[425] In two of these samples with high degree (15- to 30-fold) amplification of c-*myc* sequences, double minute chromosomes were observed in karyotype analysis. The level of c-*myc* mRNA was variable in the tumors with c-*myc* amplification; whereas it was markedly elevated in a rapidly growing and poorly differentiated tumor, it was only slightly elevated in a slowly growing and more differentiated tumor. The c-*myc* gene was found to be amplified (about 20-fold) and overexpressed in the human choriocarcinoma cell line JEG-3, and treatment of these cells with mithramycin (a ribonucleic acid synthesis inhibitor) resulted in a marked and selective decrease of c-*myc* expression.[426]

Amplification of N-*myc* has been detected in different human neuroblastoma cell lines.[403,427-431] The N-*myc* gene product has been identified and characterized in human neuroblastoma cells by monoclonal antibodies with defined specificities.[432] Normal expression of this product occurs predominantly in immature human neural cells and disappears with differentiation but it does not show correlation with cell division.[433] In human neuroblastoma cell lines in which the N-*myc* gene is present as a single copy, the expression of N-*myc* as mRNA may be increased relative to that in nonneuroblastoma cell lines and tumors.[198] N-*myc* amplification can also occur in some human retinoblastoma cell lines.[402]

The organization and nucleotide sequence of the human N-*myc* gene are closely related to those of human c-*myc*.[434] Human neuroblastoma amplification units containing N-*myc* sequences are usually larger in size (290 to 430 kb) than those in other human tumors that contain amplified c-*myc* sequences (90 to 300 kb).[435] Amplification of N-*myc* and its neighboring sequences in human neuroblastoma cell lines may be associated with extensive DNA rearrangement which can occur during the process of amplification.[436] The N-*myc* gene was also found to be amplified in eight of nine human neuroblastoma xenografts maintained in nude mice.[437] Amplification of N-*myc* was associated with HSRs in each neuroblastoma xenograft and in one of the xenografts the gene was rearranged.

2. Amplification of c-*myb*

Amplification of the c-*myb* protooncogene was found in three cell lines which were separately cultured from the tumor cells of a patient with acute myelogenous leukemia.[438] Amplification and aberrant expression of c-*myb* has also been detected in two cell lines derived independently from the ascites fluid of a single patient with adenocarcinoma of the colon.[439,440] The amplified c-*myb* gene in one of these colon carcinoma cell lines (COLO 205) is no longer situated on its normal chromosome localization at 6q22-24, but the amplified copies reside in the subproximal part of the long arm of a large marker chromosome 1, which occurs in two copies, and a marker chromosome 2, which exists as one copy. It is possible that after amplification *in situ* in the chromosome region 6q22-24, c-*myb* became a part of the marker chromosome, perhaps through isochromosome formation followed by duplication. An enhanced frequency of SCEs was detected at the site of amplified c-*myb* in COLO 205. Amplification of c-*myb* is apparently infrequent because it was observed in only 1 additional example among 20 different human colon carcinoma cell lines examined. Moreover, in the cell lines where c-*myb* was originally found to be amplified, the domain of amplified DNA was presumably large enough to harbor a number of genes, any of which might be responsible for the origin and maintenance of amplification. In any case, a comparison of the cell lines in which gene amplification is observed and a fresh sample of the respective tumor would be necessary for a conclusive determination of the origin of the genetic change. Moreover, it would be required that the patient had not received chemotherapy since it is known that cytotoxic agents may create, either *in vitro* or *in vivo*, the conditions that favor amplification of specific genes.

3. Amplification of c-*ras* Genes

Amplification of c-K-*ras* was found in PCC4 murine embryonal carcinoma cells.[194] The c-K-*ras*-2 protooncogene has been found to be amplified (about tenfold) and rearranged, but not mutated, in two human teratocarcinoma (embryonal carcinoma)-derived cell lines (Tera-1 and Tera-2).[441,442] Other protooncogenes examined (c-*fos*, c-*mos*, c-H-*ras*, N-*ras*, c-*abl*, c-*myc*, c-*fes*, and c-*sis*) were not amplified in the Tera-1 and Tera-2 cell lines. Amplification and enhanced expression of c-K-*ras*-2 was also found in the human epidermoid lung carcinoma KT883 transplanted into athymic nude mice.[443] Amplification of c-K-*ras* associated with aberrant expression of c-*myc* was found in WI-38 cells transformed *in vitro* by γ-irradiation.[193]

Amplification of c-*ras* gene sequences is relatively rare among human malignant cell lines of different origin. Varying degrees of amplification of the N-*ras* protooncogene were detected in the human breast cancer cell line MCF-7.[408] It is interesting to look for the possible presence of activating point mutations in amplified c-*ras* genes detected in tumor cells. Mutation at codon 12 of c-K-*ras*-2, associated with amplification and overexpression of the protooncogene sequences, was detected in the human osteosarcoma cell line OHA.[444] One exceptional human breast cancer cell line (MDA-MB231) contained amplification of c-K-*ras* sequences associated with a point mutation at codon 13 of the protooncogene.[445]

Amplification of protooncogenes in human ovarian cancer is apparently rare. From five ovarian tumor cell lines and seven noncultured ovarian tumors screened from different patients for amplification of seven different protooncogenes (c-*myc*, c-*myb*, c-H-*ras*, c-K-*ras*, N-*ras*, c-*fos*, and c-*erb*-B), only in one case was the amplification of a protooncogene, c-K-*ras*, detected.[446,447] Amplification of N-*ras* was found in the human breast carcinoma cell line MCF-7, but sublines of MCF-7, serially passaged in different laboratories, showed marked variation in the degree of N-*ras* amplification.[408] Moreover, N-*ras* amplification was not detected in other breast cancer cell lines or in primary human mammary carcinomas. These results suggest that N-*ras* amplification may occur during laboratory passage of cultured tumor cells. Amplification, overexpression, and mutation of c-K-*ras* were detected in a human pancreas carcinoma cell line (T3M-4).[448] Another cell line (PSN-1), established from a human pancreatic adenocarcinoma, contains amplification of both c-*myc* and c-K-*ras*, the latter carrying an activating point mutation.[449] Amplification and point mutation of c-H-*ras* were detected in the human melanoma strain SK-2 maintained in nude mice.[450]

4. Amplification of c-*abl*

Amplification of c-*abl*, as well as of adjacent sequences corresponding to the locus for Ig lambda light-chain constant region, has been detected in the human chronic myeloid leukemia cell line K562.[451-454] In addition to two normal c-*abl* transcripts, which were approximately 6 and 7 kb long, respectively, a novel c-*abl* transcript of approximately 9 kb is present in K562 cells.[454] A double Ph-positive cell line, KBM-5, that was established from a patient with CML in the blast-transforming phase, exhibited an eightfold amplification of c-*abl*, as well as of *bcr* and C-lambda genes, but no amplification of these genes was present in the fresh uncultured cells from which KBM-5 was derived.[455] Analysis of 70 other fresh CML samples also gave negative results for c-*abl* amplification. In an independent study, no amplification of the c-*abl* gene was detected in fresh blood samples of 42 CML patients.[456] In fact, c-*abl* amplification *in vivo* has never been reported.

5. Amplification of c-*erb*-B

The c-*erb*-B protooncogene encodes a polypeptide corresponding to a portion of the EGF receptor.[457] Human epidermoid carcinoma A431 cells have 30 times more EGF receptors than normal fibroblasts and the results of molecular hybridization studies demonstrated amplification of DNA sequences related to both a v-*erb*-B probe and an EGF receptor cDNA probe.[458] The c-*erb*-B/EGF receptor gene was found to be amplified in other human breast cancer cell lines, e.g., in the lines MDA-468 and BT20.[459,460] The growth of cell lines with a high level of EGF receptor amplification and overexpression is inhibited by EGF at concentrations that stimulate most other cell lines. EGF-resistant variants isolated from A431 cells that express fewer EGF receptors have a greater potential for differentiation *in vitro* than parental cell.[461]

Amplification of the c-*erb*-B/EGF receptor gene was detected in two human lung adenocarcinoma cell lines, whereas other three lung adenocarcinoma cell lines, as well as two lines of squamous cell carcinoma and one line of small-cell lung carcinoma, did not exhibit amplification of the gene.[462] Moreover, two of these human lung carcinoma cell lines were negative for EGF receptor expression. Human cell lines derived from non-small-cell lung carcinoma, but not those derived from small-cell lung carcinoma, express elevated levels of EGF receptors.[173]

High incidence of amplification of the c-*erb*-B/EGF receptor protooncogene has been detected in different human squamous carcinoma cell lines.[264,266] The amplification is much less frequent in primary squamous and nonsquamous cell human carcinomas. Malignant cells with amplified c-*erb*-B/EGF receptor genes may adapt more readily to growth in tissue culture, leading to establishment as cell lines, than those without this amplification. Overexpression of EGF receptors was found in 15 cultured human squamous carcinomas of the skin, oral cavity, and esophagus.[268] In these cells EGF action is associated not with stimulatory but with growth inhibitory effects.

A cloned human hepatoma cell line (LKi-7A) exhibits a very high number of EGF receptors per cell and its growth is inhibited by EGF.[463] The EGF receptor gene was found to be overexpressed, but without amplification, in four different human pancreatic carcinoma cell lines.[172]

Amplification of the c-*erb*-B gene has been detected in some cell lines derived from human neural tumors. The human astrocytoma cell line SK-MG-3 contains an amplified, overexpressed, and rearranged EGF receptor gene but no similar alterations were observed in 21 other astrocytoma cell lines.[459] Polysomy of chromosome 7 was correlated with overexpression of the c-*erb*-B gene in seven permanent human glioblastoma cell lines.[464] In some of these cell lines the level of c-*erb*-B mRNA found was higher than to be expected from the increased numbers of chromosome 7 but there was no direct linear correlation between the number of chromosome 7 (up to 6 chromosomes) and the amount of c-*erb*-B mRNA (which was elevated up to 13.5 times in a line containing 5 copies of chromosome 7).

6. Amplification of c-*neu*/*erb*-B-2

The c-*neu*/c-*erb*-B-2 protooncogene was found to be amplified approximately 30-fold in a human gastric carcinoma cell line (MKN-7).[465,466] No amplification of this protooncogene was detected in 29 additional human cancerous cell lines examined. However, some human adenocarcinoma cell lines contain amplified c-*neu*/*erb*-B-2 sequences and protein.[279] The c-*neu*/*erb*-B-2 protooncogene is amplified in some human breast cancer cell lines as well as in primary human mammary tumors.

7. Double Minutes and Homogeneously Staining Regions

Numerous double minute chromosomes (DMs) and homogeneously staining regions of chromosomes (HSRs) are observed in some tumor cell lines. Since such cytogenetic abnormalities are present in a number of tumor cell lines, as well as in direct preparations of tumor specimens,[467-472] they might correspond to amplification of certain protooncogenes, and perhaps also of other genes. In some tumor cell lines no DMs or HSRs have been observed in spite of the presence of amplification of protooncogenes,[439] but in other cell lines an association between these cytogenetic abnormalities and amplification of specific oncogene has been established. For example, the c-*myc* gene was found to be amplified in cell lines derived from human neuroblastomas, and by means of *in situ* molecular hybridization it was demonstrated that HSRs are the chromosomal sites of amplified DNA.[403] However, the degree of amplification varied considerably between different human neuroblastoma cell lines (from 5- to 8-fold to 12- to 140-fold), and in one cell line no such amplification was detected (it was also not detected in cell lines derived from human melanoma, retinoblastoma, and colon carcinoma).

Amplified protooncogene sequences may be located at chromosomal sites other than the respective locus of the normal protooncogene. In several human neuroblastoma cell lines, each with multiple HSRs, all detectable HSRs represented chromosomal sites of N-*myc* amplification, but the HSRs were located on different chromosomes and none of the sites corresponded to the normal location of the N-*myc* gene on chromosome 2p23-24.[429,430] DMs could be involved in DNA transposition contributing to generate multiple HSRs, but no DMs were detected in these neuroblastoma cell lines. In two human colon carcinoma cell lines containing c-*myc* amplification there was evidence that the amplified protooncogene appeared first as DMs and was subsequently transposed to engender HSRs on an X chromosome.[423]

8. Conclusion

It is uncertain whether the amplified genomic sequences present in certain tumor cell lines are causally related to the oncogenic process or whether they are the result of the establishment of such continuous lines in an artificial environment.[388] Cytogenetic abnormalities associated with protooncogene amplification, i.e., DMs and HSRs, are observed in certain tumor cell lines but are apparently rare in tumor cells *in vivo*.[394] Amplification of genes other than known protooncogenes has been detected in different human tumor cell lines.[473]

B. AMPLIFICATION OF PROTOONCOGENES IN PRIMARY HUMAN TUMORS

The incidence of protooncogene amplification in biopsy specimens from human tumors, though highly variable, is usually rather low, and for the majority of protooncogenes has not been observed.[474] There may be, however, a tendency toward associations between amplification of specific protooncogenes and particular types of tumors.[475] For example, c-*myc* amplification occurs mainly in adenocarcinomas, squamous cell carcinomas, and sarcomas, but not in hematologic malignancies, whereas c-*neu* amplification is observed in adenocarcinomas, particularly breast cancer, and N-*myc* amplification occurs most frequently in neuroblastomas. Protooncogene amplification is apparently very rare in untreated human leukemias.[476] However, in isolated cases of leukemia amplification of a particular protooncogene, e.g., c-*myb*, could confer a growth advantage to the original leukemic clone.[477] Protooncogene amplification has been sporadically detected in benign human tumors. For example, the c-*fos* gene was found to be amplified in one prolactinoma.[478]

DMs have been detected in 15 of 22 human breast tumor specimens and in 34 of 55 human malignant effusions but their possible relation to amplification of protooncogene sequences was not characterized.[479] DMs, HSRs, and other similar cytogenetic alterations observed in human tumors may represent not only protooncogene amplification but also amplification of other unidentified gene sequences.[480]

1. Amplification of Protooncogenes of the c-*myc* Gene Family

Amplification of the c-*myc* protooncogene and other members of the *myc* gene family has been detected in primary human neuroblastomas and some other human tumors, including lung tumors.[397]

Neuroblastoma is a malignant tumor of the autonomic nervous system and is the most common solid tumor in childhood. In contrast to children with localized neuroblastoma, which may have a good chance of cure, only very few children with disseminated tumor and older than 1 year at diagnosis will eventually survive.[481] N-*myc* was found to be amplified in primary neuroblastoma tissue from 24 of 63 untreated patients, the amplification being present only in patients with advanced stages of the disease.[428] This amplification spans DNA sequences of different length in the neighborhood of the N-*myc* gene and is frequently associated with DNA rearrangements which may occur during the amplification process.[436] The N-*myc* sequences amplified in human neuroblastomas may be located not on the normal chromosome region of this gene, at 2p23-24, but may be found in other chromosomes, for example, on the short arm of chromosome 15.[482] It is conceivable that this translocation might be related to N-*myc* activation and subsequent amplification.

Chromosome abnormalities occurring in human neuroblastomas may be studied either directly in tumor specimens or in tumors xenografted in nude mice.[483] Early stage tumors are cytogenetically characterized by modal chromosome numbers in the triploid range, few structural abnormalities, and absence of DMs and HSRs. In contrast, advanced stage tumors, mostly occurring in children 1 year old or older, are characterized by modal chromosome numbers in the diploid or hypotetraploid range, numerous structural abnormalities, including those of 1p, and frequent presence of DMs and HSRs.[484] In this study no tumors with near-tetraploidy showed an increased N-*myc* copy number, but the majority of the tumors with near- or pseudodiploidy or with hypotetraploidy showed N-*myc* gene amplification, and the amplified N-*myc* sequences were apparently present in DMs or HSRs. The latter patients had a poor prognosis. N-*myc* copy number is consistent not only within a tumor, but also in tumor tissues obtained from different sites and at different times from a given patient.[485] Both untreated and drug-treated neuroblastomas may contain amplified N-*myc* gene sequences.[486] In all of five Japanese patients with primary neuroblastoma, N-*myc* amplification was associated with a specific allele, S2, detected with the *Sph*I restriction enzyme.[487] The same association was found in three human neuroblastoma cell lines. Enhanced expression of the N-*myc* gene consequent to amplification is probably not related to the origin of neuroblastoma but may contribute to progression of these tumors.[488-490] Evaluation of N-*myc* amplification and overexpression may be clinically useful for the prognosis of neuroblastomas.[491]

Detection of N-*myc* gene expression in human neuroblastomas by *in situ* molecular hybridization and blot analysis may be used for establishing correlations with clinical outcome. In four of six neuroblastomas studied with these methods, representing advanced stages of the disease (stage IV), there was increased N-*myc* gene expression (15 to 45% of positive cells).[492] Other tumors (ganglioneuromas, neurofibrosarcoma, teratoma) did not exhibit increased N-*myc* expression. Amplification of N-*myc*, greater than tenfold, was found in an undifferentiated renal neoplasm occurring in a young boy, which exhibited histologic features of both Wilms' tumor and neuroblastoma.[493]

Amplification of N-*myc* was detected in two human retinoblastomas.[401] One of these two tumors contained 100- to 200-fold amplified N-*myc* sequences and the other tumor, which had been subcutaneously passaged in nude mice, contained 10- to 20-fold amplification of the same sequences. No amplified N-*myc* sequences were found in other eight retinoblastoma tumor tissues, which included four primary tumors and four tumors passaged in nude mice, but some of these tumors expressed elevated levels of N-*myc* transcripts.[401] In another study, 7 of 23 retinoblastomas, either familial or sporadic, contained 1.9- to 2.3-fold amplification of N-*myc* gene sequences.[494] The N-*myc* gene was found to be amplified about sixfold in one of three embryonic rhabdocarcinomas.[495] An advanced Wilms' tumor that appeared in a 2-year-old boy was found to contain an amplified N-*myc* gene,[496] but this amplification is usually not present in patients with less advanced stages of the tumor.[253]

A minority of human lung tumors exhibit amplification of genes from the *myc* family. No amplification of c-*myc* was found in 25 human lung tumors of different histopathological classes.[497] The L-*myc* gene was also not amplified in clinical tumor material of ten specimens of small-cell lung carcinomas.[416] However, in other studies amplification of c-*myc* and N-*myc* genes was observed in tumor samples from some human small-cell lung carcinomas. The c-*myc* gene was found to be amplified in 3 of 21 primary nonsmall-cell lung cancers.[498] N-*myc* amplification was detected in the tumor tissues harvested directly from three patients with small-cell lung carcinoma, including one from an untreated primary tumor.[418] L-*myc* was found to be amplified in one small-cell lung carcinoma tumor specimen taken directly from a patient.[419] Amplification of either c-*myc* or N-*myc* was found in both the primary tumor and the metastases of 5 out of 45 patients with small-cell lung carcinoma.[499] The results of these and other studies suggest that amplification and/or overexpression of c-*myc*-related gene sequences may be in some way advantageous for the growth of small-cell lung carcinomas as well as for other tumors of neuroectodermal origin, like neuroblastomas and retinoblastomas. Recently, a close correlation was detected between RFLPs of the L-*myc* gene and metastases of human lung cancer to the lymph nodes and other organs.[500]

Amplification of c-*myc* associated with the presence of DMs has been observed in some patients with AML.[501] No rearrangement or amplification of c-*myc* was found in the primary tumor cells of 21 multiple myelomas, but 2 of 3 cases of plasma cell leukemia showed amplification and enhanced expression of the gene.[502] In another study, none of the fresh leukemia samples from a large series of patients with different forms of leukemia (ALL, ANLL, and CML) had a noticeable amplification or rearrangement at the c-*myc* locus.[290]

Amplification of the c-*myc* protooncogene, albeit rare in leukemias and lymphomas, may be something more frequent in carcinomas and sarcomas. This type of alteration was found in 8/71 fresh specimens of different human carcinomas and 2/9 specimens of human sarcomas.[474] The amplification of c-*myc* is apparently associated with aggressive primary or disseminated, advanced stages of these tumors. Amplification of c-*myc* was detected in two of nine primary human colon tumors.[503] A rather high incidence of c-*myc* amplification was detected in 35 fresh tumor samples of the human uterine cervix.[504] Elevated amplification (up to 60-fold) and/or rearrangement of c-*myc* were detected in approximately 90% of the uterine cervix tumor samples, 48% showing amplification and 43% presenting both amplification and rearrangement. Most of these tumors were stage II cervical carcinomas but a correlation between the alterations of c-*myc* and the clinical manifestations of the disease was not established.

Amplification of c-*myc* was found in 2 of 11 samples of DNAs from human stomach cancer transplanted into nude mice but no amplification of c-*myc* was detected in 19 primary stomach cancers, 11 metastatic lymph node tumors from stomach cancers, or 20 samples of normal stomach mucosa.[505] These results suggest that amplification of c-*myc* may occasionally occur during passage of human tumors in nude mice. In another series of 14 human primary stomach cancer tissues screened by Southern blot hybridization using six oncogene probes (*myc*, *myb*, H-*ras*, K-*ras*, *abl*, and *mos*), the only protooncogene amplification detected was one of c-*myc*, which was present in one tissue.[506] In still another study, amplification (4- to 5-fold) of the protooncogene c-*yes*-1 was detected in 1 of 22 primary human gastric carcinomas.[507] In the same study, 15 other protooncogenes examined (c-*src*, c-*fps*, c-*ros*, c-*myc*, c-*myb*, c-*fos*, N-*myc*, c-*abl*, c-*fgr*, c-*mos*, c-H-*ras*, c-K-*ras*, N-*ras*, c-*sis*, and c-*rel*) did not show amplification. It may be concluded that c-*onc* amplification in human primary stomach cancer is a rare event.

Amplification of c-*myc* (3- to 30-fold) was detected in 3 of 32 mammary adenocarcinomas and only 1 of the patients with c-*myc* amplification had lymph node metastases.[231] However, in another study amplification of c-*myc* (2- to 15-fold) was found in 38 of 121 (32%) primary human breast carcinomas.[508] All of the breast tumors tested corresponded to an advanced stage of the disease and the c-*myc* alteration showed a significant correlation with patients over 50 years of age at surgery. In an independent study of 41 breast carcinomas, 22% of 37 infiltrating ductal breast carcinoma samples contained 2- to 10-fold amplified c-*myc* gene sequences, and the amplification was found to be associated with a very poor short-term prognosis.[487] One aggressive primary breast carcinoma from the same series contained a rearranged c-*myc* gene with a deletion of approximately 5 kb within the third exon.[509]

Overexpression of c-*myc* has been found in human prostatic cancer tissue when compared to prostatic benign hyperplasia.[249] However, the c-*myc* protooncogene was not found to be amplified in primary prostatic cancer tissues, and other protooncogenes examined (c-K-*ras*, c-H-*ras*, N-*myc*, c-*sis*, and c-*fos*) were also not amplified in these tumors.

2. Amplification of the c-*ras* Gene Family

The human c-K-*ras*-2 protooncogene was found to be amplified and overexpressed in the metastatic tissues from five of nine human embryonal carcinomas (teratocarcinomas).[442] The degree of amplification varied with each tumor examined and no correlation was found between the presence of c-K-*ras*-2 gene amplification and the patient's age or history of chemotherapy.

Amplification (and rearrangement) of c-H-*ras*-1 sequences was found in only one from seven biopsied specimens of human bladder carcinoma.[510] In a series of human urinary tract tumors, 0/17, 0/19, and 1/21 were positive for amplification of c-H-*ras*, N-*ras*, and c-K-*ras*, respectively.[90] Amplification of c-K-*ras* (between 3- and 6-fold), with a point mutation at codon 12, and amplification of c-*myc* (about 50-fold) was detected in a primary pleomorphic adenocarcinoma of the pancreas and its metastatic tumors in lymph nodules.[511] None of 25 primary human lung tumors of different histopathological classes showed amplification of c-K-*ras*, but DNA isolated from the lymph node metastases of one of these patients showed a considerably elevated c-K-*ras* copy number.[497]

3. Amplification of the c-*erb*-B Gene

Amplification of the c-*erb*-B/EGF receptor protooncogene may occur in some types of human neural tumors. Four of ten primary brain tumors of glial origin which expressed high levels of EGF receptors contained an amplified c-*erb*-B gene.[276] In another study, amplification of the c-*erb*-B/EGF receptor gene was found in 27 of 63 (43%) primary malignant gliomas.[277] All 24 tumors with amplification of the c-*erb*-B/EGF receptor gene had high levels of expression of this gene, while none of the 39 tumors without amplification had increased levels. Thus, in human gliomas large increases in the c-*erb*-B/EGF receptor gene are invariably associated with alterations in gene structure. The cells of two cases of human glioblastoma multiforme containing amplified c-*erb*-B/EGF receptor genes exhibited EGF receptors about 30 kDa shorter than the normal 170-kDa receptor due to short deletions within the c-*erb*-B/EGF receptor DNA sequences.[512] The 140-kDa abnormal EGF receptor contained in these cells showed a significant constitutive elevation of tyrosine kinase activity in the absence of its ligand, which may have contributed to the tumorigenic process.

Amplification of the c-*erb*-B/EGF receptor protooncogene, without gene rearrangement, was detected in 3 of 21 uncultured tissue samples from human breast carcinomas.[513] Overexpression of the EGF receptor protein and elevated levels of the kinase activity associated with this protein were present in the three cases with gene amplification.

Amplification (20- to 30-fold) and overexpression of the c-*erb*-B/EGF receptor gene, associated with unbalanced chromosome translocation t(1;7), was detected in both peripheral blood and bone marrow cells of 3 patients with myelodysplastic syndromes.[514] The origin of this gene amplification was not clear because these patients had received treatment with cytostatic and antiinflammatory drugs, and it is known that drugs blocking DNA synthesis can cause gene amplification. Overexpression, amplification, or rearrangement of the c-*erb*-B gene was not detected in 17 fresh, uncultured human tumor samples obtained from patients with various forms of head and neck cancer.[285] Of 21 patients with nonsmall-cell lung cancers, 5 had c-*erb*-B amplification in their primary tumor cells.[498] Expression of the EGF receptor in human lung carcinomas can be determined by immunohistochemical methods using a monoclonal antibody.[515] Application of this method may allow the identification of clinically significant subtypes of human lung carcinomas.

4. Amplification of c-*neu*/*erb*-B-2 Gene

The c-*neu*/*erb*-B-2 protooncogene was found to be amplified in some primary adenocarcinomas, including a salivary gland adenocarcinoma where a 30-fold amplification of the gene was detected.[516,517] Among 21 primary nonsmall-cell lung carcinomas, 1 adenocarcinoma of the lung examined exhibited amplification of c-*neu*/*erb*-B-2.[498] Amplification of the same gene was detected in 5 of 101 fresh samples of 21 different types of human malignant tumors examined by molecular hybridization analysis using a c-*neu* complementary DNA probe.[517] All of the tumors with c-*neu* amplification detected in this series were adenocarcinomas (two out of nine of the stomach, one out of four of the kidney, and two out of ten of the breast). In one of the two breast tumors, c-*neu* was fond to be amplified in a metastasis but not in either the primary tumor or the homologous normal breast tissue. Amplification of the c-*neu*/*erb*-B-2 gene was detected in another case of human mammary carcinoma, but analysis of DNAs from ten additional mammary carcinomas did not reveal amplification of this gene.[518] In an independent study using a specific cDNA probe to explore the c-*neu* protooncogene in normal tissue and in adenocarcinomas of different sources, only 6 of 109 adenocarcinomas contained an amplified c-*neu* gene.[519] The tumors positive for c-*neu* amplification were 2 of 24 gastric adenocarcinomas, 2 of 45 colon adenocarcinomas, and 2 of 21 breast adenocarcinomas. Adenocarcinomas from other sites (rectum, kidney, ovary, endometrium, and thyroid), as well as 29 additional primary nonadenocarcinomatous tumors, were negative for c-*myc* amplification. These results indicate that amplification of the c-*neu* gene is an infrequent event that occurs in about 5 to 6% of human adenocarcinomas.

Higher incidence of c-*neu* gene amplification has been found in other studies. In a series of 95 malignant human mammary tumors and 10 established mammary tumor-derived cell lines, c-*neu* gene was found to be amplified in 15 of the primary tumors and 1 of the cell lines.[520] Overexpression of c-*neu* mRNA was found in the mammary tumors with c-*neu* amplification from which intact RNA could be isolated. In a series of 36 human breast tumors, c-*neu* overexpression associated with amplification of the protooncogene was found in 12 cases.[280,521] No significant correlation was found in this series between c-*neu* expression and lymph node involvement, EGF receptor status, or estrogen receptor levels. Amplification of the c-*neu* gene was detected in 7 of 37 infiltrating ductal mammary adenocarcinomas and the amplification was found to correlate with poor short-term prognosis.[487] In another series, 13 of 51 primary human breast tumors contained multiple copies of the c-*neu* gene.[281] In this series there was a statistically significant correlation between c-*erb*-B protein expression and parameters used in breast cancer prognosis. A correlation appears to exist between amplification of the c-*neu* gene and relapse and survival of human breast cancer.[522] A positive correlation was found in this group of patients between c-*neu* amplification in primary human breast cancer and the presence of axillary lymph node metastases.[523] These results suggest that amplification and overexpression of the c-*neu* gene may have a role in the progression of some human tumors, especially breast carcinomas. Moreover, these alterations could have a prognostic value in certain types of cancer, especially in human breast carcinoma.

Immunohistochemical methods using an antibody staining technique with specificity for the c-*neu* protein on paraffin-embedded sections of tumors can be used for the study of c-*neu* expression in human breast tumors.[524] Application of this method confirmed that only breast tumors with c-*neu* gene amplification express elevated levels of c-*neu* protein.

5. Amplification of the c-*myb* Gene

Amplification of c-*myb* has been rarely detected in primary human tumors. Among 21 primary nonsmall-cell lung cancers examined, 1 adenocarcinoma of the lung contained an amplified c-*myb* gene.[498]

6. Amplification of the c-*ets*-1 Gene

The c-*ets*-1 protooncogene, which is normally located on human chromosome region 11q23-q24, was found to be rearranged and amplified 30-fold in 1 case of acute myelomonocytic leukemia in which an HSR occurred on the same chromosome region.[525] The c-*ets*-1 gene was also rearranged and was amplified tenfold in a case of small lymphocytic cell lymphoma associated with an inverted insertion that involved chromosome region 11q23.

7. Amplification of the *int*-2 and *hst*-1 Genes

The human *int*-2 gene, which is homologous to the murine *int*-1 and *int*-2 genes that are frequently involved in MMTV insertion during mouse mammary tumorigenic processes,[526] has been mapped to human chromosome region 11q13 and its restriction map was determined.[527] The *int*-2 locus was found to be amplified 7- to 25-fold in 4 of 46 infiltrating ductal breast cancers and 30- to 60-fold in 2 of 8 squamous carcinomas of the head and neck region, but not in other cancers.[528] All the tumors containing *int*-2 gene amplification had metastasized to regional lymphatics at the time of the analysis and 5 of the 6 tumors positive for *int*-2 amplification exhibited clinically aggressive behavior. These results suggest that amplification of *int*-2 DNA sequences may contribute to the progression of some specific human tumors. The *int*-2 gene is structurally related to the growth factor FGF, and another member of the FGF family, the *hst* gene, which is located on the same chromosomal band, 11q13, was found to be coamplified with *int*-2 in 1 of 8 human primary melanomas.[151] Primary human bladder and esophageal cancers and renal cell carcinomas were found to contain coamplified *int*-2 and *hst*-1 genes.[529]

C. PROTOONCOGENE AMPLIFICATION AND TUMOR PROGRESSION

Amplification of particular protooncogene sequences may be associated with the progression of certain tumors. A positive correlation has been observed between amplification of the c-*neu*/*erb*-B-2 protooncogene in primary human mammary cancer and the presence of axillary lymph node metastases.[523] A positive correlation may also exist between amplification of *int*-2 gene sequences and the progression of certain breast carcinomas or cancers of the head and neck region.[528] In a patient with Ph chromosome-positive CML, promyelocytic transformation of the disease was associated with 8- to 16-fold amplification of c-*myc* sequences, and subtle rearrangements of these sequences were detected in the neoplastic cells.[530]

Amplification (3- to 30-fold) of c-*myc* and c-H-*ras* was detected in advanced stages of invasive squamous cell carcinomas of the human uterine cervix associated with the presence of papillomavirus genomes (HPV16 or HPV18).[531] Since amplification of N-*myc* is not found in the tumor tissue of patients with stages 1 and 2 of neuroblastoma but is present in 50% of patients with stages 3 and 4 of the same tumor,[428] this amplification could be associated with progression of neuroblastomas.[489] Amplification of N-*myc* in a rat neuroblastoma cell line was associated with down modulation of class I MHC antigen expression, which may contribute to tumor progression by helping the tumor cells to escape the immunological reactions of the host.[532] Down modulation of the expression of class I MHC antigen in this tumor cell line was reversed by treatment with IFN-γ, but the steady-state level of N-*myc* mRNA was not affected by the treatment.

In tissues of human primary stomach cancer no amplification of c-*myb*, c-H-*ras*, c-K-*ras*, c-*abl*, and c-*mos* was detected but in 1 of 14 of these tissues the c-*myc* gene was found to be amplified.[506] The patient with c-*myc* amplification has a moderately differentiated gastric adenocarcinoma and no clear distinction was found between this patient and the other gastric cancer patients with respect to clinical stage or course of the disease. Thus, the results of this study did not lend support to the hypothesis that amplification of c-*myc*, or other protoonco-genes, may be involved in tumor progression.

The level of protooncogene amplification may show variation depending on the growth condition of the malignant cells. Amplification of c-*myc* was observed in a human breast carcinoma cell line (SW 613-S) and the level of amplification increased in lines derived from tumors that were induced in mice with the same cells.[409] Inoculation into syngeneic mice of cell clones containing low copy number of mutant c-*ras* genes was accompanied by amplification of the mutant oncogenes in the resulting tumors.[36] Sincer cancer chemotherapy may induce DNA alterations, it is important to examine tumor samples from untreated patients. The study of lung tumor specimens with Southern blotting analysis showed that protooncogene amplification is a rare event in untreated lung cancer patients.[533]

D. AMPLIFICATION OF PROTOONCOGENES IN NONHUMAN TUMORS, EXPERIMENTAL TUMORS, AND TUMOR CELL LINES

Protooncogene amplification has been detected in murine tumor cell lines. Amplification and overexpression of the *met* gene occurs in spontaneously transformed NIH/3T3 fibroblasts.[534] A highly amplified c-K-*ras* gene of rat origin was detected in NIH/3T3 transformants derived from 8 tumors induced in rats by repeated intraperitoneal injections of aflatoxin B_1.[110] However, the amplified gene was apparently not present in the original tumor. A 30- to 60-fold amplification of c-K-*ras* was detected in a mouse adrenocortical tumor cell line (Y1), which contained chromosomes with HSRs or DMs and expressed high levels of c-K-*ras*-specific mRNA and p21 protein.[535] The amplified c-K-*ras* sequences present in Y1 mouse adrenal tumor cell line have been isolated as cDNA complementary copies and homologous sequences have been localized to mouse chromosome 6.[536] There is no evidence for the presence of point mutations capable of activating the oncogenic potential of p21^{c-ras} proteins in the amplified c-K-*ras* gene of Y1 cells.[537]

Amplification (10- to 20-fold) of c-H-*ras* was detected in murine teratocarcinoma cells PCC4, which are highly undifferentiated and malignant and express elevated levels of c-H-*ras*, c-*myc*, and c-*fos* transcripts.[194] In spite of the protooncogene amplification, no HSRs or DMs were detected in PCC4 cells. Amplification of N-*ras* was found in mouse thymomas induced by the carcinogen, NMU, and amplification of c-K-*ras* occurred in similar tumors induced by γ-radiation.[318] A transient twofold amplification of two c-*ras* genes (c-H-*ras* and c-K-*ras*) was detected in SV40-transformed Chinese hamster cell lines exposed to ^{125}I β particles but not after exposure to ^{60}Co γ-rays, ^{241}Am α particles, or UV light.[538,539] Amplification and mutation of c-H-*ras* was found in carcinomas induced in the mouse skin by treatment with DMBA.[540]

Amplification of c-*myc* has been detected in some experimental rodent tumors and in cell lines derived from rodent tumors. It was observed, for example, in a Morris hepatoma (hepatoma 7794A) but was absent in all other hepatomas examined, although these tumors, as well as primary liver tumors induced in rats by hepatocarcinogens and different hepatoma cell lines, express high levels of c-*myc* transcripts.[541] Amplification and enhanced expression of the c-*myc* gene associated with the presence of DMs and HSRs was detected in mouse SEWA cells,[542] which are cells derived from a polyoma virus-induced mouse osteosarcoma. The c-*myc* gene was found to be amplified, but not clearly overexpressed, in 10 of 12 rat skin tumors induced by ionizing radiation.[104] In each of three clear cell carcinomas observed in these animals, the alteration of c-*myc* was associated with activation of c-K-*ras*, as assessed in the NIH/3T3 DNA transfection assay. The c-*myc* gene was amplified and overexpressed in a chemically induced transplantable mouse colon carcinoma.[543]

The c-*erb*-B/EGF receptor gene was found to be amplified and overexpressed in tumors induced in the chick pouch of the Syrian hamster with DMBA as well as in a cell line established from one of these tumors.[390] Interestingly, the protooncogene amplification appeared to involve an extrachromosomal pathway with formation of covalent closed circular DNA.

E. AMPLIFICATION OF OTHER GENES IN TUMORS

Amplification of nonprotooncogene, or not characterized, DNA sequences may occur during tumorigenic processes. In essentially all of the cases of protooncogene amplification described in tumor cells or tumor cell lines, the amplified unit has been estimated to be in the order of 1000 to 3000 kb of DNA and it is therefore likely that, in addition to protooncogenes, other cellular genes were also amplified.[395]

Amplification of undetermined DNA sequences has been detected in some human retinoblastoma cell lines.[402,544] Differential amplification, assembly, and relocation of multiple DNA sequences may be observed in human primary neuroblastomas and neuroblastoma cell lines.[545] Human melanoma cell lines exhibiting a significant increase in the number of DMs per cell may acquire enhanced capability for the invasion through basement membranes.[546] The human colon carcinoma cell lines COLO 320 and COLO 321 contain DMs and HSRs corresponding to unidentified genes other than the c-*myc* protooncogene.[480] In addition to N-*myc* gene amplification, nononcogene-like DNA sequences were found to be amplified up to 400-fold in the neuroblastoma cell line NB1, the retinoblastoma cell line Y79, and the small-cell lung carcinoma cell line H69.[473] A spontaneously transformed derivative of the mouse 3T3 cell line contains 25 to 30 DMs per cell, corresponding to nononcogene-like DNA sequences which are amplified and overexpressed in these cells.[547]

Reiterated DNA sequences may be amplified in some human primary tumors and tumor cell lines. Reiterated DNA restriction fragments detected with the enzyme *Eco*RI were found to be amplified in a primary neuroblastoma and two gliomas.[548] Amplified repetitive DNA sequences from the *Kpn* I family were found in a human melanoma cell line, where they appear microscopically as HSRs.[549,550] An amplified DNA sequence detected in two human melanoma cell lines showed partial homology with the human papillomavirus HPV-9 genome as well as with the third internal repeat array IR3 of the EBV antigen EBNA-1.[551]

Amplification and/or rearrangement of repetitive DNA sequences may occur not only in the tumor cells but also in normal cells from cancer patients. A variable tandem repeat locus mapped to human chromosome band 10q26 was found to be amplified and rearranged in leukocyte DNAs of two cancer patients.[552] The function of such amplified sequences is unknown but they may be inherited or may be originated, at least partially, from selective pressures existing either *in vivo* or in the conditions of *in vitro* culture. Experiments involving selective killing of carcinogen-treated SV-40 transformed Chinese hamster cells by a defective parvovirus (AAV-5) suggest that gene amplification is an adaptive cellular response to initiating events resulting in enhanced cell survival.[553]

F. SUMMARY

Amplification of protooncogenes, or protooncogene-related sequences, has been detected in some tumor cell lines as well as, albeit much less frequently, in primary tumors. In established cell lines this amplification may represent only a consequence of different genetic and/or epigenetic changes that may occur during cell culture. Only a small fraction of the total primary human tumors is associated with amplification of specific protooncogenes and most of the protooncogenes have never been found to be amplified in human primary tumors. Genes other than known protooncogenes have been found to be amplified in different human tumor cell lines.[473] However, there are some interesting associations between amplification of specific protooncogenes and types of human tumors: N-*myc* amplification in neuroendocrine tumors, c-*neu*/*erb*-B-2 amplification in adenocarcinomas, c-*erb*-B/EGF receptor gene amplification in squamous carcinomas, and *int*-2 amplification in ductal breast carcinomas and cancers of the head and neck.[475,528] Such associations suggest that amplification of particular protooncogene sequences may implicate an advantage for the growth of particular types of tumors. In the human melanoma cell line MeWo there is a positive correlation between the presence of amplified DNA sequences in the form of HSRs and the capacity for the induction of spontaneous metastasis in nude mice.[554]

Amplification of specific protooncogenes, or other genes, could be involved in the development and/or progression of certain tumors *in vivo* when these genes confer some selective advantages for tumor growth. However, protooncogene amplification and/or overexpression may not be required for the growth of tumor cells or for the maintenance of a transformed phenotype. In different sublines of the human promyelocytic cell line HL-60, the extent of amplification of c-*myc* DNA sequences was found to vary from 4- to 30-fold, which was associated with parallel variation in the levels of expression of c-*myc* mRNA, but this variation did not correlate with any obvious growth advantage and would not be necessary for the maintenance of the HL-60 phenotype.[400] Moreover, in malignant cells there may be no clear correlation between the level of protooncogene amplification and the level of expression of the respective protooncogene, which indicates that amplified protooncogene copies may be, relative to the single copy in normal cells, transcriptionally silent.[555] Thus, protooncogene amplification is not always clearly correlated with overexpression of the gene product.

Protooncogene amplification is not found exclusively in malignant cells. The protooncogenes c-H-*ras* and c-K-*ras* have been found to be amplified in normal animals from several rodent species, and some of these species contain about 10 copies of a given protooncogene in their genome.[556] Amplification and overexpression of the c-H-*ras* protooncogene can occur during the limited replicative lifespan of normal human fibroblasts.[557] Thus, it is clear that amplification of protooncogenes can occur in some malignant cell populations, but a similar amplification may be present in normal cells and may be associated with normal cellular growth.

V. TRANSLOCATION AND/OR REARRANGEMENT OF PROTOONCOGENES IN TUMORS

DNA rearrangements are intimately associated with the normal processes of differentiation occurring in different hematopoietic cell lineages, especially in the processes of functional maturation of B and T lymphoid cells. Similar rearrangements can also occur in malignant lymphomas and leukemias and may represent molecular markers that can be profited for the study and classification of lymphoid neoplasms.[558-562] Malignant diseases are characterized by the almost universal presence of cytogenetic abnormalities, including aneuploidy and structural chromosome aberrations.[563] Some malignancies, especially leukemias and lymphomas, are characterized by the regular presence of chromosome breaks, rearrangements, and translocations, not only on specific chromosomes, but, more importantly, on specific regions within chromosomes.[564-575] It has been suggested that a majority, but not all, of the known heritable and constitutional chromosomal fragile sites are associated with a higher rate of breakage and specific chromosome translocations and rearrangements in cancer.[576] However, on the basis of the available evidence it cannot be decided if there is a significant correlation between common or rare chromosomal fragile sites and cancer-specific chromosome breakpoints.[577] The chromosome translocations associated with malignant diseases may be conveniently represented in the form of a circular chromosome translocation map which may facilitate the appreciation of their peculiarities.[578] Numerical and structural chromosome aberrations may be present not only in the fully developed hematologic malignancies but also in a proportion (usually less than 50%) of preleukemic or myelodysplastic syndromes.[579] Small chromosome translocations and DNA rearrangements may be difficult to recognize by cytogenetic methods alone but may be identified by molecular hybridization analysis. In the last years, the study of these structural chromosome abnormalities and their possible relation to protooncogene changes yielded very interesting observations. Some definite relationships between specific chromosome rearrangements and translocations involving protooncogene loci, and neoplastic diseases, especially malignant diseases of the hematopoietic system, have been described and characterized.[580-593] Chromosome regions corresponding to the loci of c-*abl*, c-*myc*, and other protooncogenes are frequently involved in the chromosomal aberrations associated with malignant hematologic diseases.

A. CHRONIC MYELOID LEUKEMIA AND TRANSLOCATION OF THE C-*ABL* PROTOONCOGENE

Chronic myeloid (or myelogenous) leukemia (CML) is a human disease characterized by a clonal proliferation and accumulation of myeloid cells and their progenitors.[594] The primary abnormality of the disease is a marked increase in the stem cell compartment of bone marrow committed to myelopoiesis. CML is a typical multistage malignant human disease in which an initially, relatively benign chronic phase is followed to a more aggressive, usually lethal, blast crisis phase. The combined efforts of cytogeneticists and molecular biologists have provided important and fundamental insights into the origin and nature of CML.[595-602]

1. The Philadelphia Chromosome Translocation and the c-*abl* Protooncogene

The first structural chromosome abnormality described as consistently associated with a human malignant disease was the Philadelphia chromosome (Ph[1], Ph', or Ph chromosome),[603] which is a deleted autosome 22, i.e., a 22q- chromosome.[604] This abnormal chromosome is present in over 90% of CML patients. The Ph chromosome is not generated by a simple chromosome deletion but is formed by a translocation that occurs between the autosome 22 and other chromosome(s). In CML the translocation usually occurs between chromosome 22q- and chromosome 9q, in particular t(9;22)(q34;q11).[605] The use of high-resolution banding techniques, with chromosomes at the prometaphase stage, allowed the precise localization of the breakpoints in the Ph translocation to chromosome regions 9q34.11 and 22q11.21.[606] The Ph chromosome involves a reciprocal translocation in which the protooncogene c-*abl*, normally located on human chromosome region 9q34.1, is translocated to chromosome 22q.[607] The breakpoints are situated in *Alu* repetitive sequences either on chromosome 22 or on chromosome 9, and the t(9;22) translocation is associated with deletion of small or large DNA sequences on both chromosomes.[608] The Ph chromosome translocation could alter the structure and/or expression of the c-*abl* gene, as well as the expression of the C_{lambda} Ig light-chain gene, which is adjacent to the translocation site on human chromosome 22q-.[451] The latter gene cluster can also be interrupted by a chromosome 22q11 breakpoint occurring in Ph-positive ALL.[609]

The mouse c-*abl* protooncogene is located on chromosome 2. This gene is apparently not implicated in the pathogenesis of radiation-induced murine leukemias associated with translocations or rearrangements that involve the mouse chromosome 2.[610]

2. Variants of the Ph Chromosome in CML

Variant translocations are present in less than 10% of patients with Ph-positive CML.[611,612]

The prognostic and hematologic features of CML patients with variant translocations are not significantly different from those of CML cases with the typical t(9q;22q) translocation.[613] Almost all chromosomes may be involved in such variant translocations. The distribution of chromosome breakpoints in Ph-positive variant translocations clearly exhibits a nonrandom pattern with preference for light-staining chromosome bands, but the distribution of the translocations does not show any correlation with known chromosome fragile sites or with known protooncogene locations.[611,612,614,615] However, the analysis of 325 aberrant breakpoints in CML with Ph chromosome revealed that 7 out of 8 highly involved chromosome bands corresponded to protooncogene-carrying bands and/or to bands involved as primary breakpoints in cancer, while bands carrying fragile sites were involved only twice.[616] The interpretation of these findings is obscured by the imprecise localization of both breakpoints and protooncogene localization as well as for the fact that there is a great disproportion between band size and gene size.

Chromosome band 9q34 is always rearranged in the variant Ph translocations. Variants of Ph chromosome in CML may be divided in two groups: "simple" (two-way) translocations, involving chromosome 22 and a chromosome other than 9, and complex (three- or four-way) translocations, involving chromosomes 9, 22, and at least one other chromosome. Using high-resolution R-banding methods and *in situ* molecular hybridization techniques, it has been demonstrated that c-*abl* sequences are present in all Ph chromosome variants where a segment of chromosome region 9q34 is translocated to the Ph chromosome.[617-620] These results lend support to the hypothesis that "translocation of the c-*abl* protooncogene to a specific region of chromosome 22 is essential for the development of CML."[617]

3. Translocation and Expression of c-*sis* in CML

The protooncogene c-*sis*, which is normally located on human chromosome region 22q13.1, may be translocated to chromosome 9q in the Ph translocation.[621] The c-*sis* gene segregates with the translocated part of chromosome 22 to different chromosomes, (most frequently to chromosome 9q+, in some cases to 11q–) in Ph chromosome-positive CML cells.[622] Normal (4.0 kb) c-*sis* transcripts were detected in 7 of 24 fresh blood samples obtained from patients with CML, as well as from patients with chronic myelomonocytic leukemia.[623] However, expression of the c-*sis* gene is of low level and is found only in the blast, accelerated phase of the disease. Probably, the c-*sis* gene is not critically involved in the origin or development of CML. However, this point is still under discussion and it has been proposed that increased expression of the c-*sis* gene product (which is closely related to the growth factor PDGF), as well as of a specific platelet DNA polymerase which has properties similar to that of viral reverse transcriptase, are important in the initial phases of CML development.[624]

Translocation of human c-*sis* from chromosome 22 to chromosome 11 has been observed in Ewing sarcoma-derived cell lines, but c-*sis* is apparently not rearranged or activated in this tumor.[625,626] The behavior of c-*sis* was also studied in a pedigree with familial meningioma and chromosome translocation t(14;22).[627] The breakpoints of the translocation in this family were not located near the c-*sis* gene but in regions coding for ribosomal RNA, in which polymorphisms are frequently found in normal persons. Further studies are required to characterize the possible role of c-*sis* in human tumors.

The c-*sis* protooncogene is located on the distal third of mouse chromosome 15, at region 15E.[627] Other genes located on mouse chromosome 15, not far from the c-*sis* locus, include c-*myc* and *int*-1. Murine chromosome 15 is frequently involved in tumorigenic processes.

4. Chromosome Abnormalities other than Ph in CML

Karyotype abnormalities other than the Ph chromosome may occur in CML patients, especially during the final blastic phase of the disease.[629] These changes consist of numerical chromosome abnormalities, including trisomy of chromosomes 8, 17, 19, and 21, as well as duplication of the Ph chromosome. In addition, there may be structural chromosome aberrations, most of which are represented by random structural rearrangements. Less than 10% of CML patients retain the Ph as the only chromosome abnormality to the end of the disease without further karyotype evolution. In all CML patients, independently of the chromosome abnormalities, the average survival from the beginning of the blastic phase is around 6 months.

5. Expression of the Fused P210 Protein in CML

The site of breakage is variable among different cases of Ph chromosome-positive CML.[451] Only about 15% of CML samples exhibit breaks on chromosome 9 within 18 kb of the v-*abl* homologous human DNA sequences and there is no particular "hotspot" for chromosome breakage 5′ to the c-*abl* protooncogene.[630] The breakpoints on chromosome 9q may be distributed over a relatively large region of up to 100 kb or more 5′ to c-*abl* sequences. One of the alternative 5′ exons of the c-*abl* gene lies at least 200 kb upstream of the remaining c-*abl* exons and this exon is disrupted in the human CML cell line K562.[631] In the BV173 cell line, which was established from the malignant cells of a patient with CML in blast crisis, studies using pulse-field gel electrophoresis demonstrated that the chromosome 9 breakpoint occurred within the c-*abl* intron which is located 160 kb upstream of the v-*abl* homologous sequences, but still 35 kb downstream of the 5′-most c-*abl* exon.[632] Fusion genes *bcr*/c-*abl* and c-*abl*/*bcr* were detected on the Ph and 9+ chromosomes, respectively, and both of these genes were expressed in BV173 cells. These results suggest that the t(9;22) breakpoints in CML consistently occur within the limits of the large c-*abl* gene and that RNA splicing, sometimes of very large regions, appears to compensate for the variability in the breakpoint location.

On the other hand, the breakpoints on chromosome 22q- are distributed within a limited break cluster region (*bcr*) of up 5.8 kb.[633] There are four *bcr*-related loci on human chromosome 22, all of them located at chromosome region 22q11.2, but only one of these related loci, designated *BCR1*, contains the full gene sequence and is involved in the CML-associated Ph chromosome translocation.[634] In one study, 19 of 21 patients with CML exhibited a chromosome break within the 5.8-kb *bcr* region.[635] It is thus possible that DNA sequences from the *bcr* region on chromosome 22q- may contribute to the tumorigenic properties of Ph chromosome-positive cells in CML. In contrast to human normal c-*abl* transcripts that are expressed as 6- and 7-kb mRNA species which direct the synthesis of a 145-kDa protein (p145$^{c\text{-}abl}$), chimeric (fused) 8.2-kb transcripts of c-*abl* and *bcr* are generated as a product of the specific chromosome translocation in CML, and such transcripts are translated into hybrid polypeptides of approximately 210 kDa (p210$^{bcr\text{-}abl}$ or P210) which have been detected in cell lines derived from CML bone marrow and in tumor cells of CML patients.[633-644]

The human *bcr* gene has been cloned and it was determined that *bcr* codes for a protein of 1271 amino acids.[645] The product of the normal *bcr* gene may have an important function since the gene is evolutionarily conserved and is expressed in a wide variety of actively proliferating and nonproliferating vertebrate tissues.[646] The normal function of the *bcr* gene is not understood, but a truncated *bcr* mRNA has been detected in normal chick testes. The gene contained in the *bcr* region, termed *phl*, encodes a 160-kDa phosphoprotein with an associated serine or threonine kinase activity.[647] The hybrid polypeptide product of the Ph translocation could thus also be designated as *phl*/c-*abl* P210. This protein appears to possess both tyrosine- and serine/threonine-specific kinase activities.

Molecular probes containing *bcr* sequences are commercially available and can be conveniently used for the diagnostic evaluation of CML patients, especially in cases when cytogenetic analysis is inconclusive.[648] These probes may also have a potential diagnostic value for the early detection of leukemic relapse in Ph-positive CML following bone marrow transplantation.[630,649] Minimal residual *bcr*/c-*abl* transcripts can be detected in remission samples from CML patients by a modified polymerase chain reaction (PCR) analysis.[650] Both *bcr* and *bcr*/c-*abl* transcripts are expressed at similar levels in CML cells, and within individual CML samples the relative amounts of *bcr*/c-*abl* hybrid transcripts and normal *bcr* transcripts from chromosome 22 are similar.[646]

A single *bcr* restriction pattern has been observed in human CML cell lines containing multiple copies of the Ph chromosome, which suggests that these copies are generated by duplication of a single Ph chromosome, rather than by independent translocation events.[651] DNA rearrangements involving the *bcr* locus are not present in T cells from CML patients, which indicates that these cells are not involved in the pathogenesis of CML.[652]

The quantitative aspects of altered gene expression related to the Ph translocation are little known. Variable levels of expression of the qualitatively altered protein product of the translocated *c-abl* gene are observed in Ph chromosome-positive B-lymphoid cell lines established from CML patients.[653] The translocated *c-abl* protooncogene is transcribed at variable levels in fresh cells from human CML, and in some cases the levels may be similar to those present in other forms of leukemia where *c-abl* is not translocated.[293] Qualitatively altered *bcr*/*c-abl* transcripts may be detected in high amounts in some fresh samples of CML cells, especially during the blast crisis stage of the disease.[454,623,654-656] Similarly altered transcripts are present in patients during the chronic phase of CML, but there may be no significant increase in *c-abl* expression in CML cells compared to normal bone marrow.[654] Direct comparison of the expression of *bcr*/*c-abl* transcript levels in fresh blood samples from CML patients in different stages of the disease indicated that, while all chronic phase patients had relatively low amounts of the aberrant transcript, only four of ten patients in blast crisis expressed elevated levels of the transcript, and the remaining exhibited levels comparable to those of chronic phase patients.[657] These results suggest that increased expression of aberrant *bcr*/*c-abl* transcripts is not absolutely necessary for blast transformation to occur.

Fused *bcr*/*c-abl* transcripts are apparently not present in human hematologic malignancies lacking the Ph chromosome and in normal human bone marrow cells. In a patient in the acute phase of a CML, a modified 10.3-kb *c-abl* transcript was found to replace the 8.2-kb transcript usually detected in the chronic phase.[658] However, a similar 10.3-kb transcript was not detected in three additional patients with similar characteristics.

6. Biological Significance of the p210 Product in CML

The biological role of the molecular alterations observed in CML is not understood at present. Rearranged *bcr*/*c-abl* DNA sequences are apparently not required for progression of CML since deletion of these sequences was detected in a patient with CML who entered blast crisis.[659] Only normal *bcr* and *c-abl* RNA species were detected by Northern blot analysis in the blastic cells from this patient, which indicates that the altered product is of subordinate importance for the maintenance and progression of the leukemic state. These results also indicate that in most cases the acceleration from chronic towards acute phase of Ph-positive CML is not linked to alterations within *c-abl* or *bcr* sequences.

The study of *ts* mutants of the v-*abl* oncogene product has demonstrated that the tyrosine-specific kinase activity of the product is crucial to the transforming function.[660] The v-*abl*-associated specific kinase activity is required to maintain the transformed phenotype. Cells transformed with *ts* kinase mutants revert back to normal morphology shortly after a shift to the nonpermissive temperature. Tyrosine-specific protein kinase activity is present in the altered P210 product as well as in the p160$^{gag-v-abl}$ product of the acute retrovirus A-MuLV,[636-638,661-663] but the same specific activity is present in the normal *c-abl* protein.[662,664] Thus, it is clear that a qualitative difference in the kinase activities of v-*abl* and *c-abl* protein products is not responsible for the different oncogenic potentialities of these products. However, the hybrid proteins p160$^{gag-v-abl}$ and p210$^{bcr-c-abl}$ may have a greater stability than the normal p145^{c-abl} protein.[646,661,665] Quantitative differences could exist between the specific kinase activities of the v-*abl* and *c-abl* products, as well as between the normal *c-abl* protein and the fused *phl*/*c-abl* protein. Moreover, the fused *phl*/*c-abl* P210 protein could possess both tyrosine- and serine/treonine-specific kinase activity.[647] It is also conceivable that the cellular substrates of these different kinases may be different, although no definite evidence exists in favor of this possibility.

7. Multiple Ph Chromosomes

Some CML patients exhibit multiple Ph chromosomes per metaphase after entering blast crisis. These extra Ph chromosomes most likely arise from a duplication of preexisting Ph chromosome rather than from new t(9;22) translocation events.[630] Amplified and rearranged c-*abl*-related fragments can be detected in such cases. The presence of amplified c-*abl* sequences within the genome of CML cells does not necessarily lead to enhanced expression of these sequences.[666] Thus, genomic amplification of a translocated c-*abl* protooncogene cannot, by itself, be the sole genetic event giving rise to CML blast crisis. Some Ph-positive CML patients may lose the Ph chromosome after entering blast crisis.

8. Ph-Negative CML

Between 5 and 10% of patients with CML are negative for the presence of a Ph chromosome, and in these cases the protooncogenes c-*abl* and c-*sis* are not translocated.[622,667] Most probably, Ph-positive and Ph-negative CMLs are different clinical entities, the latter group of cases having a poorer prognosis.[668] However, rearrangement of c-*abl* has been detected in some Ph-negative CML patients by molecular approaches, which suggests that karyotypic analysis is not sufficient to identify individuals with rearranged *bcr*/c-*abl* sequences and that a subset of Ph-negative patients may in fact belong to the clinical entity of Ph-positive CML.[669-672] Thus, Ph-negative CML patients carrying rearranged *bcr*/c-*abl* sequences may have a prognosis and clinical course similar to that of Ph-positive CML patients. Other Ph-negative CML patients lack rearranged *cr*/c-*abl* sequences and still other patients may have *bcr* rearrangement without involvement of c-*abl* sequences.[670,673,674] In one study it was concluded that the clinical heterogeneity of CML may be based on factors other than *bcr*/c-*abl* rearrangements.[675] The possible role of P210-associated tyrosine protein kinase in Ph-negative CML patients is unknown. No P210-associated kinase has been detected in Ph-negative CML patients in blast crisis.[644]

9. Relationship between c-*abl* Protooncogene Translocation and CML Development

The precise relationship between the Ph translocation, the c-*abl* and c-*sis* protooncogenes, the *bcr*/*phl* gene, and the origin of CML is not understood. Despite the fact that the Ph chromosome can be observed in the vast majority of CML patients, it is uncertain whether this chromosome is present in all of the malignant cells and whether the acquisition of the Ph chromosome is the seminal oncogenic event for the origin of the disease.[594] The target cell for the Ph-positive leukemia is apparently a multipotential cell, i.e., a stem cell.[582] Acquisition of the Ph chromosome may not be the primary event in the development of CML but may, at least in some cases, be acquired later in the course of the established disease.[676] Patients with typical Ph chromosome-positive CML may enter blast crisis with blast cells lacking the Ph chromosome.[677] These observations suggest a multistep pathogenesis for CML, in which the acquisition of the Ph chromosome is a second or subsequent event in the oncogenic process.[594] Spontaneous regression of cytogenetic and hematologic abnormalities was observed in a patient with Ph chromosome-positive CML, and this regression, which lasted for over 3 years, occurred in spite of the persistent presence of Ph-positive cells.[678] A trisomy 8, which was initially present in the same patient, disappeared without therapy. Thus, the continued presence of Ph-positive cells in CML patients may be compatible with spontaneous regression of the disease as well as with the initiation of a final blast crisis.

Hybrid *bcr*/c-*abl* transcripts have not been detected in some Ph-positive cell lines derived from CML patient, e.g., in the PB-1049 cell line.[679] Thus, the presence of a Ph chromosome may not ensure the production of the hybrid *bcr*/c-*abl* mRNA. Treatment of Ph-positive CML cells with IFN-α_2 at doses which inhibit CML cell proliferation does not decrease expression of the *bcr*/c-*abl* fusion gene or modulate expression of the normal *bcr*/*phl* gene in CML blast crisis cell lines.[680] Therefore, the antiproliferative effect of IFN-α_2 on these cells is not mediated through modulation of *bcr*/c-*abl* gene transcription. These results render unlikely the possibility that expression of the *bcr*/c-*abl* fusion gene is crucially involved in the persistence of abnormal cell proliferation associated with CML.

The P210 protein is not myeloid cell specific since it has also been expressed in somatic cell hybrids between a mouse fibroblast cell line and two human CML-derived cell lines which carry the Ph chromosome.[681] Autophosphorylation of the P210 protein at tyrosine has been detected in blast cells from CML patients regardless of whether these blasts were of the myeloid, the lymphoid, or the undifferentiated morphology.[644] Since the P210 kinase is expressed not only in myeloid cells but also in Ph-positive B lymphocytes of CML patients, the proliferative advantage of Ph-positive myeloid cells over the Ph-positive lymphoid cells in benign phase CML patients cannot be attributed only to the presence of this kinase in the myeloid cells of CML patients.[644] The presence of the P210 hybrid protein would not interfere with the possibility of cell differentiation, since both Ph-positive and Ph-negative human lymphoblastoid cell lines can be equally induced by treatment with phorbol ester (TPA) to differentiate towards plasma cells.[682] Expression of *bcr*/c-*abl* transcripts does not change during TPA-induced megakaryocytic differentiation and decreased proliferation of the human K562 cell line, which contains a Ph chromosome and a rearranged and amplified c-*abl* protooncogene.[683] However, the high tyrosine kinase activity of the P210 protein of K562 cells is strongly reduced during the initial 24 hours of TPA treatment.[684] Induction of differentiation of K562 cells by treatment with hemin is apparently associated with reduction in the level of *bcr*/c-*abl*-associated tyrosine kinase.[685] The reason for the discrepant results obtained in different studies is not clear at present.

10. Conclusion

The Ph chromosome translocation is considered as a hallmark of human CML, being present in over 90% of CML patients. The Ph translocation involves the c-*abl* protooncogene and *bcr* DNA sequences, containing the *phl* gene, located on human chromosome 22q, which may result in the generation of *bcr*/c-*abl* fused transcripts and a hybrid p210$^{bcr/c-abl}$ protein containing both *phl* and c-*abl*-encoded amino acid sequences. The altered hybrid protein possesses tyrosine-specific protein kinase activity. However, the same activity is present, albeit at lower levels, in the normal c-*abl* protein product. In comparison to the normal levels of c-*abl*-encoded protein, the hybrid P210 protein may not be produced in excessive amounts in CML cells, and it is usually absent in Ph-negative CML cases. However, P210 may possess both tyrosine- and serine/threonine-specific protein kinase activities, which could result in the recognition of different substrates or an altered pattern of substrate phosphorylation. In any case, "the question remains open whether the translocation product of this (*bcr*/c-*abl*) mRNA is the cause or merely a consequence of transformation in CML."[608] In contrast to the v-*abl* oncogene product, the oncogenic potential of P210 seems to be rather low; recombinant retroviruses coding for the hybrid *bcr*/c-*abl* product do not transform NIH/3T3 cells or B lymphocytes *in vitro*.[686]

In conclusion, the precise role of either qualitative or quantitative alterations of c-*abl*-related protein products in the origin and/or development of CML is not clearly understood at present. Analysis of the effect of the hybrid P210 protein on normal hematopoietic cell proliferation and differentiation by using gene-transfer techniques, or the alternative inhibition of the chimeric *bcr*/c-*abl* mRNA with specific antisense RNA, is needed to define the precise role of P210, and hence the Ph translocation, in the pathogenesis of CML.[599] The demonstration of molecular heterogeneity at the DNA, RNA, and protein levels in both Ph-positive and Ph-negative CML patients could eventually contribute to a better definition and classification of this group of leukemias.[673] In any case, it is clear that PCR analysis and molecular hybridization studies with probes containing *bcr*/c-*abl*-specific sequences are most useful for the diagnosis and following-up of CML patients.

B. B-CELL LYMPHOMAS AND TRANSLOCATION OF THE C-*MYC* PROTOONCOGENE

Immunoglobulin (Ig) genes involved in the synthesis of antibody molecules are organized as discontinuous, separated DNA segments in the germ line and DNA rearrangements are critically involved in the processes of lymphoid B-cell differentiation leading to the generation of different types of Igs.[558,687] Important studies revealed an association between the c-*myc* gene, the loci corresponding to Ig genes, and the development of human lymphomas, especially B-cell lymphomas.[580-582,585-587,688-695] The human genes coding for Ig heavy, light-kappa and light-lambda chains are located on specific regions of chromosomes 14, 2 and 22, respectively, and these regions are involved in chromosome translocations occurring in malignant B lymphocytes.[696-701]

1. Chromosome Translocations in Human B-Cell Lymphomas

In biopsies and cultured cells derived from the tumor tissue of patients with Burkitt's lymphoma, an extra band was detected in chromosome 14 by Giemsa and quinacrine mustard staining techniques.[702] The extra band in the marker chromosome corresponds to a (8;14) translocation.[703] It was shown that in the tumor cells of 75 to 90% of patients with Burkitt's lymphoma a small region from the long arm of human chromosome 8 (8q24-qter), containing the c-*myc* gene, is translocated to chromosome region 14q32, which corresponds to the locus of heavy-chain Ig genes.[704-706] In 10 to 25% of Burkitt's lymphomas translocations occur between the same region of chromosome 8 and chromosome regions 2p12 and 22q11, which correspond to regions containing the loci of light-kappa and light-lambda Ig genes, respectively.[586] Thus, the chromosome translocations characteristically associated with Burkitt's lymphoma are (8;14)(q24;q32), (2;8)(p12;q24), and (8;22)(q24;q11), the first one being much more frequent than the other two, but all of them involving the c-*myc* protooncogene and the loci of either the heavy or light chains of Igs. The chromosome translocations associated with Burkitt's lymphoma are so characteristic that their presence in a bone marrow aspirate may allow to make an appropriate diagnosis and staging of the disease, even in patients whose bone marrow does not show typically abnormal cells.[707]

Chromosome alterations associated with c-*myc* translocation or rearrangement are present in the enlarged nodes that occur in patients with AIDS.[708,709] These nodes are frequently associated with EBV infection but are free from HIV-related sequences, which suggests that HIV is not directly involved in the development of such lymphomas. Clonal expansions of altered B cells residing in these nodes may lead to development of non-Hodgkin's lymphomas.

2. Chromosome Translocations in Murine Plasmacytomas

Plasmacytomas can be induced in mice by different types of experimental manipulations, including a variety of solids and liquids, when implanted or injected into the peritoneal cavity. The most used plasmacytoma-inducing agent is pristane (2,6,10,14-tetramethylpentadecane), which is obtained from biogenic sources (whale and shark livers). Probably, pristane is metabolically inert and it does not appear to be capable of inducing DNA damage. Only a few selected strains of mice are susceptible to experimentally induced plasmacytomagenesis, namely, the strains BALB/c and NZB, while most of the common strains are resistant. Such differences are obviously of genetic origin, but the number and identity of the responsible genes is unknown.[710]

Murine plasmacytomas are characterized by structural chromosome abnormalities usually involving translocations of chromosome 15 to chromosome 6 and 12, which carry the loci of light-kappa and heavy chain Ig genes, respectively.[711-714] Translocation involving the Ig heavy-chain gene, located on chromosome 12, and the c-*myc* gene, located on the distal third of chromosome 15,[628,715] i.e., rcpt(12;15), have been observed in the majority of mouse plasmacytomas.[705,714,716-720] The Ig heavy-chain switch region ($S\alpha$) constitutes the target of most of these recombinations, particularly in IgA-producing murine plasmacytomas.[721] Usually, the involved c-*myc* gene is translocated and resides on the 12q+ chromosome in mouse plasmacytomas, adjacent to the Ig C_{alpha} DNA sequences, whereas the V_H and J_H sequences are translocated to the involved mouse chromosome 15q-.[722,723]

A minority of murine plasmacytomas exhibits translocation of a portion of chromosome 15 to chromosome 6, at the region corresponding to the gene coding for the Ig light-kappa chain. In such cases the breakpoint is distal to the c-*myc* locus and the c-*myc* gene remains on chromosome 15, while the kappa-chain gene, C_{kappa}, is translocated from chromosome 6 to chromosome 15 and is recombined with a chromosome 15 segment, termed plasmacytoma variant translocation locus 1 (*pvt*-1).[724,725] It has been suggested that in the mouse t(6;15) translocation the *pvt*-1 locus, but not c-*myc*, is implicated, either directly or indirectly, in the transformation of lymphoid cells.[726] The normal function of the *pvt*-1 locus is unknown. A *pvt*-1 homologous gene, termed *Mis*-1, exists in the rat, where it has been associated with the development of M-MuLV-induced thymomas.[727]

The two DNA strands of the rearranged and truncated c-*myc* gene can be transcribed in murine plasmacytomas.[728] However, transcription of both the coding and noncoding strands of c-*myc* may also occur in some normal cells.[729] Moreover, the coding and noncoding strands of the c-*myc* gene are subjected to independent transcriptional regulation. The biological significance of these differences is unknown.

In some (5 from a total of 39) murine plasmacytomas no chromosome translocations were detected in the tumor cells but 1 of every 2 chromosomes 15 was shortened in all of three translocation-negative tumors examined.[730,731] A murine plasmacytoma was originally classified as translocation negative, but the cloning and extensive molecular analysis of the rearranged c-*myc* gene demonstrated that the tumor had undergone a hemizygous interstitial deletion of chromosome 15 followed by a series of switch (S) region-mediated recombinations between chromosomes 12 and 15, which resulted in leaving the IgH enhancer approximately 2.5 kbp 5′ of c-*myc*.[732] The results suggest that a *cis*-acting regulatory element normally located 5′ of exon 1 of c-*myc* was lost and that heavy-chain constant region or enhancer sequences may exert similar *cis* effects on translocated c-*myc* loci. In B-cell lymphomas induced in mice with Rauscher MuLV (R-MuLV), the transformed cells may belong to five stepwise stages of the B-cell differentiation lineage, characterized by different types of rearrangements of the Ig genes, and rearrangement of the c-*myc* gene is restricted to a particular stage of this developmental process.[733] No evidence of c-*myc* or c-*myb* rearrangement or amplification was obtained in thymomas occurring in RF mice after treatment with 3-methylcholanthrene.[329] In the rat, the c-*myc* gene is located on chromosome 7 and rearranges in immunocytomas with t(6;7) chromosomal translocation.[734]

3. Chromosome Translocations in Rat Immunocytomas

Spontaneously arising immunocytomas in Lou/Wsl rats contain a consistent translocation between chromosomes 6 and 7.[735] Sequence analysis revealed that the t(6;7) translocation must have involved multiple DNA rearrangements in the tumor. One event juxtaposes the c-*myc* gene and the switch mu region of Ig locus in a head-to-head (5′-to-5′) orientation, whereas another rearrangement lead to transposition of sequences upstream from the switch gamma-1 region to the c-*myc* distant end of the switch mu region in a tail-to-tail (3′-to-3′) configuration.

In the IgE-producing rat immunocytoma IR162, the c-*myc* gene recombined with the excluded allele of the nonfunctional epsilon heavy-chain Ig gene.[736] This recombination resulted in the loss of 5′-proximal DNA of the c-*myc* gene via joining to the epsilon heavy-chain switch region in a head-to-head configuration.

4. Activation of c-*myc* in Canine Transmissible Venereal Tumor

Canine transmissible venereal tumor (CTVT) is a naturally occurring neoplastic disease of uncertain histologic origin that affects the external genitalia of both sexes. CTVT is transmitted during coitus. The etiologic agent of this tumor is unknown but cytogenetic and immunologic studies strongly suggest that the tumor is transmitted from one animal to another by transplantation of the transformed cells, which are characterized by extensive and specific chromosome aberrations.[737]

Insertion of a retroposon can occur into the c-*myc* oncogene in some cases of a CTVT.[738] Retroposons are defined as a class of dispersed repeated sequences present in mammalian DNA that share common properties which imply that they are derived from RNA by a process of reverse transcription.[739-741] Retroposons are tailed by an adenine-rich segment and flanked by a 7- to 21-bp duplication of the insertion site, implying a common mechanism of insertion. The retroposon inserted in CTVT shows 62% homology to the monkey *Kpn* family of repetitive DNA sequences.[738] These LINE sequences behave like mobile elements that transpose to the vicinity of structural genes and may contribute to their transcriptional activation. Analysis of four CTVTs from individual dogs from various geographical locations indicated that in all tumors the same LINE insert was present upstream to c-*myc*, which suggests that CTVTs in various dogs may have a common cellular origin.[742] The levels of c-*myc* mRNA were found to be increased in CTVT cells as compared with liver cells, but it is not known whether this comparison is valid.

5. Activation of c-*myc* in Avian Bursal Lymphomas

In ALV-induced bursal lymphomas of chickens activation of c-*myc* may occur not by chromosome translocation but by insertion of viral sequences, including the LTR, near the c-*myc* protooncogene.[743-746] Activation of c-*myc* gene expression by an insertional mechanism is also observed in chicken bursal lymphomas induced by the CSV isolate of REV.[747] On the other hand, an insertional activation mechanism involving the c-*myc* gene is much more less frequent in M-MuLV-induced murine lymphomas.[748] This topic is discussed in detail in Chapter 3, Volume I.

6. Role of c-*myc* in B-Cell Lymphomas

In the most frequent type of translocation observed in human B-cell lymphoma, i.e., t(8;14), there is marked variability among patients in the chromosome breakpoints on both chromosomes, 8q and 14q.[706] In such tumors the breakpoint on chromosome 14q is usually within the Ig heavy-chain locus and may occur at the mu- or gamma-switch regions, often resulting in the Ig heavy-chain genes and the rearranged c-*myc* gene occurring in opposite transcriptional orientations. The breakpoints on chromosome 8q span a wide range and have been found at positions both 3′ and 5′, as well as within the first intron, of c-*myc*.[719] Chromosome translocation can occur on either side of the c-*myc* gene in Burkitt's lymphoma cells but the general rule is that the c-*myc* gene becomes situated at the 5′ side of the Ig constant region.[749,750] The region of chromosome 8 involved can recombine with a J region of the Ig heavy-chain on chromosome 14, which may be due to the action of a V-D-J recombinase that is normally involved in the rearrangement of the Ig locus during B-cell maturation.[751,752] Abnormalities of Ig heavy chain synthesis have been detected in human B lymphoid cell lines of malignant origin carrying the 8;14 translocation.[753] Genes distal to c-*myc* on human chromosome 8, like the thyroglobulin gene, are translocated with c-*myc* to chromosome 14 in the Burkitt's lymphoma 8;14 translocation.[754]

Translocation of the c-*myc* gene to the Ig heavy-chain locus in murine plasmacytomas is also an imprecise reciprocal exchange, implicating the frequent occurrence of deletions, insertions, and duplications.[755] A variant t(6;15) translocation detected in a murine plasmacytoma occurred near a kappa light Ig chain but more than 20 kb away from the c-*myc* protooncogene.[724,756]

In the variant t(8;22) and t(2;8) translocations of Burkitt's lymphoma, the c-*myc* gene is not translocated but remains in its germ-line configuration on the involved chromosome 8.[586,756,757] In the (2;8) translocation the constant region of the kappa-light chain Ig gene (C-kappa) may be translocated from chromosome 2 to chromosome 8 in the tumor cells, and the C-kappa gene may then end up adjacent to the 3′ side of c-*myc*.[758] In these variant translocations the c-*myc* gene is located on the 8q+ chromosome, proximal to the breakpoint in band 8q24. In (2;8) translocations the cluster of kappa variable genes may remain on the 2p− chromosome whereas the constant kappa light chain gene has been found on the 8q+ chromosome.[749] In a (2;8) translocation detected in a Burkitt's lymphoma variant, the 2p breakpoint interrupted the variable kappa light chain of the Ig locus.[759] In most cases with variant translocations the breakpoint are distantly located from the c-*myc* gene, but in an exceptional t(8;22) variant the translocation placed the Ig genes 3' to the c-*myc* in Burkitt's lymphoma.[760] In all other t(8;22) translocations, no DNA rearrangement could be detected within 20 kb 3' of c-*myc*.[761,762] The structural gene coding for transforming growth factor alpha (TGF-α) is located on human chromosome 2, close to the breakpoint of the Burkitt's lymphoma t(2;8) variant translocation.[763] The biological significance of this association, if any, is not understood. No protooncogenes were involved in a reciprocal translocation t(6;14)(q15;q32) observed in a variant cell line originated from an EBV-transformed human B cell precursor.[764]

Molecular probes specific for particular subtypes of DNA rearrangements occurring in human B cell lymphomas have been constructed from clones derived from human T-cell lymphoma sublines,[765] but the usefulness of such probes for the detection of DNA rearrangements in human T-cell malignancies is limited by the molecular heterogeneity of these diseases. The only general rule including the common t(8;14) and the variant t(2;8) and t(8;22) translocations is that after translocation the human c-*myc* gene ends up adjacent to the Ig constant gene region, either H, kappa, or lambda, and that the breakpoint falls within the Ig locus.[758]

7. Somatic Mutations of c-*myc* and Ig Genes

Somatic point mutations are present in some bursal lymphomas induced in chickens by ALVs.[766] Mutations have also been observed in the coding and noncoding region of the c-*myc* gene in some Burkitt's lymphoma cell lines.[757,762,767-769] Somatic mutations in the 5' exon of the c-*myc* gene have been detected in 9 of 15 Burkitt's lymphoma cell lines associated with t(8;22), in which the gene remains on chromosome 8.[770] It has been suggested that the first exon of the human c-*myc* gene contains a coding sequence,[771] but this point is still under discussion. Mutations associated with amino acid changes of the c-*myc* protein have been detected in the primary tumor cells of some cases of human acute B-cell leukemia.[772]

The possible role of somatic mutations of c-*myc* in the origin and/or development of B-cell lymphomas and leukemias is unknown. In principle, somatic mutations in the noncoding sequences of the gene could contribute to deregulation of its expression. The coding sequence of the translocated c-*myc* gene was found to be altered in the Ly65 Burkitt's lymphoma cell line, which contains several point mutations giving origin to amino acid substitutions as well as a frameshift mutation in the second exon.[769] Despite these changes, the translocated gene retained reduced transforming ability in a REF focus assay. In other Burkitt's lymphoma cell lines, including the AW-Ramos line,[690] the c-*myc* gene nucleotide sequences are completely normal. Clusters of extensive somatic mutations have been found not in c-*myc* but in the variable region of the IgH gene from a human B cell lymphoma.[773]

8. Expression of c-*myc* in Lymphomas

The role that the complex molecular changes occurring in B-cell lymphomas may have in the process of lymphomagenesis is not clear. B-cell lymphomas are apparently not originated by a simple activation mechanism of the translocated c-*myc* gene.[774,775]

Expression of the c-*myc* gene in B-cell tumors could be quantitatively and/or qualitatively altered upon chromosome translocation. Regulation of the transcriptional activity of both normal and chromosomally translocated c-*myc* genes depends on the chromatin structure of the c-*myc* locus, which is related to alterations in the chromatin-associated proteins and the local physical state of the DNA.[776] Translocation has little or no effect on the usual patterns of DNase I hypersensitive sites near to the c-*myc* gene but new hypersensitive sites can be observed in some cases in the Ig gene region near to the breakpoint.[777] In murine plasmacytomas, the translocated c-*myc* gene may have a more open chromatin structure, as evidenced by DNase I sensitivity, than that of the untranslocated allele.[778] Expression of the normal c-*myc* allele in murine plasmacytomas is apparently repressed by a specific protein that recognizes a single binding site 290 bp 5′ to the transcription start site P1 within the c-*myc* promoter.[779]

DNA sequences including promoters located upstream of the c-*myc* gene may play a central role in the regulation of c-*myc* expression.[780] The germ-line c-*myc* gene is regulated by specific positive and negative factors that bind to multiple sites near and within the gene.[781] The putative positive regulatory factors bind to two distinct regions near the promoters and the negative factors bind to an upstream site as well as to sites within the c-*myc* gene. Transcription depending on the P0 promoter of the c-*myc* locus may be associated with the synthesis of a 12.5-kDa protein which is distinct from the p62[c-myc] protein. The 12.5-kDa protein corresponds to the first ORF of the c-*myc* locus but its function is unknown. Enhanced transcription of c-*myc* in bursal lymphoma cells requires continuous protein synthesis.[782]

In some, but not all, human and mouse B-cell lymphoma cell lines, as well as in chicken bursal lymphoma cell lines, high levels of c-*myc*-related transcripts are observed.[690,783-785] Elevated levels of c-*myc* RNA associated with t(8;14) translocation involving the c-*myc* gene were also detected in fresh uncultured cells obtained from a patient with rapidly progressive and fatal ALL.[786] In some Burkitt's lymphoma cell lines, as well as in fresh biopsies from Burkitt's lymphoma and mouse plasmacytomas, c-*myc* transcripts are present in normal or only slightly elevated concentrations.[165,290,714,787-789] In some Burkitt's lymphoma cell lines the total steady-state level of c-*myc* RNA is rather low.[790] The tumor cells of a patient with ALL type L3, which represents the leukemic counterpart of Burkitt's lymphoma, contained a t(8;14) translocation similar to that present in the non-Hodgkin's lymphoma cell line Manca, juxtaposing the enhancer element of the IgH locus to the c-*myc* gene sequences interrupted within the first intron, but, in contrast to the Manca cell line, the leukemic cells of the patient expressed low amounts of c-*myc* transcripts.[791] It is thus clear that a high level of expression of the translocated c-*myc* gene is not a general characteristic of B-cell lymphomas and leukemias and that, in contrast to cell lines, the primary blast cells of these malignant diseases may frequently express normal or low amounts of c-*myc* transcripts.

Activation of the translocated c-*myc* gene may depend on the stage of differentiation of the cells harboring the translocated gene and not on alterations in the structure of the gene.[792] Analyses of steady-state levels of c-*myc* mRNA in Burkitt's lymphoma cell lines with t(8;22) translocation and chromosomal breakpoints ranging from 10 kb to greater than 47 kb 3′ of c-*myc* showed large variation in the specific mRNA levels (from 0.5 to 10 times the levels in lymphoblast controls).[793] The different levels of c-*myc* transcripts in the different cell lines did not correlate with the distance between the c-*myc* gene and the translocated Ig light-chain locus. In some Burkitt's lymphoma cells, e.g., in the cell line BL2 which contains a t(8;22), all of the genomic regions that have been suggested to play a role in the regulation of c-*myc* expression are normal.[794] Since the normal c-*myc* allele is transcriptionally silent in BL2 cells, as it is in other Burkitt's lymphoma cells, it may be suggested that the *de novo* association of c-*myc* with an activated Ig locus results in deregulated c-*myc* expression.

Translocation may affect normal c-*myc* promoter usage and may activate several cryptic transcription start sites in murine plasmacytomas.[795,796] In some of these tumors, translocation activates heterogeneously initiated, bipolar transcription of the c-*myc* gene.[797] In the mouse variant t(15;6) translocation, the chromosome breakpoint may be situated more than 50 kbp away from the c-*myc* promoter, which suggests that c-*myc* transcriptional activation should occur by different mechanisms in the classic t(15;12) and the variant t(15;6) types of translocation.[798]

Allelic exclusion and deregulated c-*myc* expression may be associated with translocations involving the c-*myc* gene in B-cell lymphomas. The c-*myc* gene remains on the 8q+ chromosome in Burkitt's lymphoma associated with t(8;22) translocation but, as a result of translocation, transcriptional activation of the c-*myc* gene on the rearranged chromosome 8q+ may occur, while the c-*myc* gene in the normal chromosome 8 is transcriptionally silent.[799,800] Allelic exclusion of c-*myc* expression in B-cell lymphomas may be caused by a repression of transcription which is specific to the P1 and P2 promoters of the c-*myc* gene, while transcription controlled by the P0 promoter of the gene may persist on the untranslocated allele of some human B-cell lymphoma cell lines, e.g., in the Manca cell line.[780] In mouse plasmacytomas both the translocated and the normal positioned c-*myc* alleles may be transcribed but the specifically associated chromosome translocations would result in deregulation of c-*myc* protooncogene expression.[510,720,732] Not only the rearranged c-*myc* but also the nonrearranged c-*myc* is unresponsive to serum stimulation and temperature changes in the S194 mouse plasmacytoma cell line, even though cell growth rate is markedly changed.[801]

Suppression of the expression of a normal murine c-*myc* gene is observed in hybrids between a Burkitt's lymphoma cell line and bacterial lipopolysaccharide (LPS)-stimulated mouse spleen cells (in which the murine c-*myc* gene is actively transcribed).[802] In contrast, when Daudi Burkitt's lymphoma cells (which express only the translocated c-*myc* gene) are hybridized with human lymphoblastoid cells (which express the normal c-*myc* gene), the hybrids are phenotypically lymphoblastoid and express both the translocated and the normal c-*myc* gene.[803] On the basis of these results it has been suggested that human B-cell neoplasms carrying t(8;14) may represent a heterogeneous group of diseases in which related mechanisms result in a transcriptional deregulation of the c-*myc* protooncogene that leads to its constitutive expression in the B cells.[803]

A transcriptional enhancer identified near the human Ig heavy chain gene may be unavailable to the translocated c-*myc* gene in some Burkitt's lymphomas,[804] but in other cases of the tumor the c-*myc* gene may be activated by the enhancer.[805] Transposition of the Ig heavy chain enhancer was also detected in a mouse plasmacytoma.[806] However, transcriptional activation of translocated c-*myc* genes in murine plasmacytomas may occur in the absence of strong promoters or detectable enhancers.[807] Ig heavy chain gene antisense transcripts may contribute to the expression of translocated c-*myc* genes in murine plasmacytoma cell lines, where such chimeric transcripts comprise 5 to 50% of steady-state c-*myc* mRNA.[808]

Increased c-*myc* mRNA levels are found in some mouse lymphomas without proviral integration near c-*myc*, but in a few lymphomas c-*myc* transcripts are hardly detectable.[322] Increased expression of c-*myc* and c-*myb* was observed in 90 and 70%, respectively, of thymic lymphomas induced in RF mice by treatment with MCA.[329] In contrast, among 11 spontaneous thymic lymphomas occurring in AKR mice, only 2 showed detectable levels of c-*myc* and c-*myb* transcripts, and 2 more expressed c-*myc* or c-*myb* but not both.[329] No indication of rearrangement or amplification of these protooncogenes was obtained in the tumor cells of the same animals. Increased levels of c-*myc* transcripts can be produced upon transposition of Ig enhancers but, when biopsy specimens or fresh blood cells (not cell lines) of human B-cell malignancies and other types of human hematopoietic tumors are studied, only a few or none of the total neoplasms show high levels of c-*myc*-related transcripts.[66-68] Expression of the c-*myc* protein may also be rather low in lymphoma cells. In the majority of fresh tumor samples from the most common types of human lymphomas, including not only B-cell lymphomas but also a variety of histological types, the expression of c-*myc* protein, as detected by using p62[c-myc]-specific monoclonal antibodies, was found to be very weak relative to that seen in normal human lymphoid tissues.[302] It is thus clear that an increased level of c-*myc* RNA and protein expression is not a universal characteristic of lymphoma cells. To the contrary, decreased levels of c-*myc* gene expression are frequently detected when fresh samples of lymphoma tissues are analyzed.

The translocated c-*myc* gene in Burkitt's lymphomas and mouse plasmacytomas may show structural changes as a consequence of recombination.[768,809] The c-*myc* gene may be broken within a 5'-nontranslated exon, thereby separating the promoter region of the normal c-*myc* gene from its protein coding sequences.[810,811] High levels of truncated c-*myc*-related RNAs, corresponding to the decapitated c-*myc* gene remaining at its normal locus, may be produced as a consequence of c-*myc* gene breakages occurring during the process of translocation.[799] c-*myc* mRNAs of different sizes produced in Burkitt's lymphomas are translated with comparable efficiency.[812] In a Burkitt's lymphoma cell line (BL67), two classes of c-*myc* mRNA (2.4 and 3.5 kb) were detected and, interestingly, transcription of the 3.5-kb mRNA was found to be initiated within the Ig heavy chain locus on chromosome 14, and the transcription occurred from the Ig antisense strand towards and across the breakpoint of the chromosomal translocation into the first exon of the c-*myc* gene.[790]

Truncation of the 5' region of the c-*myc* gene occurring as a consequence of its translocation in Burkitt's lymphomas and murine plasmacytomas would be responsible for the deregulation of c-*myc* expression observed in the respective neoplastic cells. However, it has been demonstrated that treatment of Burkitt's lymphoma cells with sodium butyrate (a potent inducer of differentiation in various cellular systems) leads to a rapid decrease of c-*myc* transcripts, irrespective of the type of translocation, the location of the breakpoint relative to the c-*myc* gene, or the association with EBV infection.[813] That sodium butyrate is capable of down regulating a truncated c-*myc* gene indicates that an important target site for its transcriptional regulation is located outside the region encompassing the upstream regulatory sequences, the dual promoters, and the leader region of the gene.

Posttranscriptional mechanisms could play a significant role in the accumulation of truncated c-*myc* mRNAs in murine plasma cell tumors.[814] Altered c-*myc* transcripts could be translated with different efficiency than normal c-*myc* transcripts. Transcripts of c-*myc* containing a shorter 5' noncoding region (as a structural result of translocation with loss of the noncoding first exon) may be more efficiently translated *in vitro* than normal c-*myc* transcripts.[815] Such a difference might depend on the secondary structure at the 5' noncoding region of the c-*myc* mRNA and would result in the synthesis of high amounts of the c-*myc* protein. However, these explanations are untenable since it has been conclusively demonstrated by means of expression vectors that exon 1 has no effect on the translational efficiency of c-*myc* mRNA transcripts in COS cells.[816] Moreover, changes in translational control mechanisms cannot explain all malignant transformations in which c-*myc* appears to be implicated since in many Burkitt lymphoma cell lines and mouse plasmacytomas c-*myc* transcripts with an apparently normal structure are produced.

In spite of the above-mentioned structural alterations, the coding sequences and the protein products of the translocated and rearranged c-*myc* gene in Burkitt's lymphomas and murine plasmacytomas may be identical to that of the respective normal gene sequences and polypeptide products.[698,817-819] The chromosomal breakpoint in the t(8;14) translocation associated with Burkitt's lymphoma may lie far away 5' to the c-*myc* coding sequences. For example, in the EBV-negative cell line EW-36, derived from an American case of undifferentiated lymphoma, the region of chromosome 8 involved in the translocation is situated approximately 50 kb 5' to the c-*myc* gene.[820] No structural alteration of the c-*myc* transcriptional unit was observed in EW-36 cells.

Chromosome translocation frequently breaks the c-*myc* gene within the first exon or intron but the exon that may be lost by breakage would be noncoding and the c-*myc* polypeptide product remains qualitatively intact. Recent evidence indicates that the synthesis of one of the two proteins encoded by the human c-*myc* gene (the larger protein, c-Myc-1) is initiated within the first exon of the gene and is abolished as a consequence of structural alterations (removal or mutations) affecting the first exon of the gene.[789] It was suggested that protein c-Myc-1 may normally exert a regulatory action on the expression of the smaller protein, c-Myc-2, and that the lack of c-Myc-1 expression in Burkitt's lymphoma cells may result in deregulation of the expression of c-Myc-2, which is apparently the most abundant and functionally important product of the human c-*myc* gene. Studies with constructed retroviral vectors have indicated that truncation of the first exon of the chicken c-*myc* gene is not necessary to convert the normal protooncogene into a transforming gene.[821] This conversion can be achieved by substitution of a retroviral LTR for the native c-*myc* promoter and for as yet poorly defined, untranslated regulatory elements of the protooncogene.

Aberrant c-*myc* mRNAs of Burkitt's lymphoma cells may have longer half-lives than their normal counterparts,[790,822] but the biological significance of this phenomenon is unclear. In spite of such longer half-lives, the steady-state concentration of c-*myc* mRNA may be rather low and, conversely, a high steady-state level of c-*myc* RNA may be found in some Burkitt's lymphoma cell lines in which the half-life of c-*myc* RNA is normal. These facts indicate that mechanisms other than RNA half-lives, including variation in transcriptional rates, RNA processing and transport, and efficiency of translation may contribute significantly to the steady-state level of c-*myc* mRNA in the cytoplasm.[790]

In avian bursal lymphoma cell lines, the sizes of c-*myc*-related products are highly variable, and it has been suggested that transformation-associated polypeptides may be truncated versions of the normal c-*myc* gene product.[823] According to the promoter insertion model of oncogenesis, LTR sequences contained in AVL would be inserted 5′ to the c-*myc* gene and would act as promoters for increasing the transcription of the protooncogene.[743,744] The viral insertion would lead to formation in high amounts of hybrid RNA molecules containing both viral LTR and cellular *myc* sequences. However, in some chicken bursal lymphoma cell lines the viral LTR is integrated downstream to c-*myc* sequences and would act only as an enhancer of c-*myc* transcription.[312] Thus, the transcripts produced in the latter manner are not hybrid molecules containing LTR sequences fused with c-*myc* sequences and the LTR promoter function is not required for the maintenance of the transformed in these cell lines. Moreover, in many virus-induced chicken bursal lymphomas no viral insertion occurs near the c-*myc* protooncogene.

9. Conclusion

The relationship between the c-*myc* gene, its RNA and protein products, its translocation, and the origin and development of B-cell neoplasms is difficult to assess at present. The normal function(s) of the c-*myc* protein is unknown but its predominant location in the nucleus suggests a possible role in genome regulation. Chromosome translocation involving the c-*myc* gene is apparently not associated with a permanent block of B-cell differentiation.[824] No characteristic chromosome translocation is observed in certain Burkitt's lymphoma cell lines, e.g., in the BJAB cell line.[774,825] Moreover, rearrangements of c-*myc* may be absent when fresh cells isolated from the blood of Burkitt's lymphoma patients, not established tumor cell lines, are analyzed with modern techniques including Southern blot analysis.[826] An intriguing finding is that in fresh tissue samples from human B- and T-cell lymphomas analyzed with these techniques rearrangement of c-*myc* is observed in only a small proportion of the cells from a given tumor.[827] In addition, there is no clear correlation between c-*myc* rearrangement and clinical behavior of the lymphoid tumor. In certain primate species specific types of chromosome translocations are apparently not required for the origin of B cell neoplasms, which may arise from different cell clones even in the same animal.[828]

DNA rearrangements involving the c-*myc* and Ig loci associated with expression of aberrant transcripts of the c-*myc* gene have been detected in patients with cryoglobulinemia, a nonmalignant monoclonal disease.[829] This finding indicates that rearrangement of the c-*myc* gene may not represent a final step in malignant cell transformation, although it may be related to the clonal expansion of these cells and the high rate of cryoglobulin synthesis.

The c-*myc* protein is of normal structure and may be produced in normal amounts after translocation of the c-*myc* gene in at least some human and murine B-cell lymphomas. Moreover, rather low amounts of c-*myc* RNA and protein have been detected in human and murine lymphoma cells when fresh tumor tissue samples, not tumor cell lines, have been compared with normal lymphoid tissue. There may be little doubt, however, that the c-*myc* gene is involved in some way in lymphomagenesis. The chromosome translocations associated with human and murine B-cell lymphomas place the c-*myc* gene near genetic elements whose expression is strictly controlled in a B-cell-specific fashion, which may result in a constitutive deregulation of the c-*myc* gene expression. This deregulation may play an essential role in the pathogenesis of B-cell lymphomas. Recent evidence indicates that the synthesis of c-Myc-1, the larger of the two protein products of the human c-*myc* gene, may be abolished as a consequence of the structural alterations of c-*myc* gene sequences occurring in Burkitt's lymphoma cells.[789] The synthesis of c-Myc-1 is initiated within the first exon of c-*myc*. The lack of c-Myc-1 expression could contribute, in principle, to deregulate the expression of the other product of the gene, the c-Myc-2 protein, whose synthesis is initiated within the second exon of the c-*myc* gene.

It has been demonstrated that the c-*myc* protooncogene driven by Ig enhancers is capable of inducing lymphoid malignancy in transgenic mice.[830] However, the deregulated B-cell-specific expression of c-*myc* occurring in the transgenic mice is insufficient by itself to precipitate neoplasia. Moreover, the altered expression of c-*myc* in these mice does not establish a complete barrier to B cell differentiation.[831] The primary consequence of the enhanced c-*myc* expression in the transgenic mice is a benign polyclonal proliferation of B cells and progression to clonal malignant B cell tumors from this population may require the operation of at least a second genetic accident.[832,833] Most probably, the origin of B-cell neoplasms is complex, involving several successive critical steps in addition to c-*myc* translocation and deregulated c-*myc* expression. Genes other than c-*myc*, e.g., *bcl-2*,[834] may be involved in the origin and/or development of lymphomas. Further studies are required for a better definition of the genetic and nongenetic factors related to lymphomagenesis.

C. TRANSLOCATION AND/OR REARRANGEMENT OF PROTOONCOGENES IN OTHER MALIGNANCIES

Particular types of chromosome translocations and/or rearrangements occur frequently in hematologic malignant diseases other than CML and B-cell lymphomas.

1. Acute Myeloid Leukemia

A segment of human chromosome 21q may be translocated to chromosome 8q in acute myelogenous (myeloblastic) leukemia (AML), but no translocation of c-*mos* occurs in AML associated with t(8;21).[835] However, a genomic rearrangement resulting in the loss of an *Eco* RI cleavage site next to the 3′-end of the c-*mos* locus was detected in certain cases of human myeloid leukemia as well as in some established hematopoietic cell lines.[836]

The c-*ets*-2 protooncogene may be involved in the translocation t(8;21)(q22;q22) associated with human AML, but it is not rearranged and its expression in these cases may be much lower than that observed in control lymphocytes.[837,838] Thus, the possible role of c-*ets*-2 translocation in the pathogenesis of AML, if any, is not understood. Translocation t(7;11)(p15;p15), involving the c-H-*ras*-1 gene, was found in a patient with AML.[839] The c-H-*ras*-1 gene was not involved in another patient with CML that exhibited the same type of translocation.

Human chromosome 17q contains the protooncogenes c-*erb*-A, which is located on region 17q11.2,[840] and c-*neu*/*erb*-B-2, which is located on region 17q21. Both protooncogenes are proximal to the chromosome breakpoint occurring in translocation t(15;17)(q22;q21) and remain on chromosome 17 in APML cells.[841-843] Their possible role in APML development is not understood. The gene coding for p53 antigen is located on chromosome band 17p13, but it is not altered by the APML-associated translocation.[844] Another gene located on the same chromosome region, at 17q11.2-q21, is that encoding the hematopoietic growth factor, granulocyte colony-stimulating factor (G-CSF), but it is not rearranged or disrupted in the tumor cells of APML patients.[845]

The putative protooncogene *pim*-1 is located on human chromosome region 6p21, which is cytogenetically rearranged in the K562 erythroleukemia cell line.[846] High levels of 3.2-kb *pim*-1 transcripts are expressed in K562 cells. A reciprocal translocation t(6;9)(p21,q33) has been described in human myeloid leukemias and could involve the *pim*-1 gene.

The incidence of the Ph chromosome in AML is less than 1% and is restricted to the M1 subtype.[602] The breakpoint locations are heterogeneous in Ph-positive AMLs and in at least some of these cases the tumor cells may contain only c-*abl* product of normal size.[847]

2. Acute Monocytic Leukemia

The protooncogenes c-*ets*-1 and c-*ets*-2 are located on human chromosomes 11 and 21, respectively, and may be transposed in acute leukemias with (4;11) and (8;21) translocations.[848] The c-*ets*-1 gene may be translocated from its normal place on chromosome 11q23-q24 to chromosome 9p, adjacent to the interferon (IFN) genes, in cases of acute monocytic leukemia (AMOL) associated with t(9;11)(p22;q23).[849] However, less than 10% of patients with AMOL have this type of translocation and the possible role, if any, of c-*ets* and IFN genes in AMOL remains undetermined. The c-*ets*-1 protooncogene may be translocated in AMOL to human chromosome region 4q21, a region which contains the gene coding for IP-10, an IFN-induced polypeptide showing homology to some chemotactic and mitogenic proteins.[850]

3. Acute Myelomonocytic Leukemia

Specific rearrangements of human chromosome 16 occur in a subgroup of patients with acute myelomonocytic leukemia (AMML). These rearrangements are clustered in chromosome band 16q22, which contains the loci for metallothionein genes, and the breakpoint at 16q22 may split the metallothionein gene cluster.[851] However, no protooncogenes have been assigned to human chromosome 16. A rare fragile site, *FRA16B*, is located on human chromosome region 16q22.1. However, the specific breakpoint associated with AMML is proximal to *FRA16B* as well as to a common fragile site, *FRA16C*, located on the same chromosome band.[852] These results remove some of the support for a relationship between chromosome fragile sites and malignant diseases.

4. Acute Promyelocytic Leukemia

Translocation t(15;17)(q22:q11.2) is regularly associated with acute promyelocytic leukemia (APML).[568,853] The protooncogenes c-*erb*-A and c-*neu*/*erb*-B-2 as well as the NGF receptor gene are located on human chromosome region 17q21-q22, but they are apparently not involved in the development of APML. The gene coding for the hematopoietic growth factor G-CSF is located on human chromosome region 17q11-q22,[854] more precisely at 17q11, proximal to the breakpoint of the translocation t(15;17) associated with APML.[855] No rearrangement of the G-CSF gene occurs in APML cells. The gene encoding myeloperoxidase (MPO), an enzyme whose synthesis is restricted to the promyelomonocytic stage of myeloid differentiation, is also located in the human chromosome region 17q22-q23, near the breakpoint site characteristic of APML.[856] Intense MPO activity is observed in azurophilic granules that are abundantly present in APML cells. The use of cDNA clones complementary to the *MPO* gene and *in situ* hybridization analysis indicated that the *MPO* gene is translocated to chromosome 15 in the t(15;17)(q22;q11.2) associated with APML.[857] It is thus possible that this rearrangement activates an as yet unknown protooncogene on human chromosome 15.

5. Acute Lymphocytic Leukemia

Acute lymphocytic (lymphoblastic) leukemia (ALL) is frequently associated with the presence of a diversity of numerical and structural chromosome abnormalities, including different types of translocations.[858] The presence of chromosome translocations in ALL, either random or nonrandom, is associated with poor prognosis and frequent therapeutic failure.[859] The Ph chromosome is usually considered as a hallmark of CML, but it is present in about 20% of adult patients with ALL and much less frequently (about 3%) in pediatric ALLs.[671] The Ph chromosome is an unfavorable prognostic variable in adult patients with ALL.[860] A small proportion of adult patients with AML also have a Ph chromosome. Since the majority of Ph-positive adult ALLs exhibit a *bcr*/c-*abl* DNA rearrangement and express the 8.2-kb hybrid transcripts, the question arises as to whether these cases may not represent acute phases of Ph-positive CMLs in which the chronic phase remained clinically silent.[861] Rearrangements involving the *bcr* and c-*abl* loci, 8.2-kb *bcr*/c-*abl* hybrid transcripts, and P210 fused protein are not present, however, in some Ph-positive acute leukemias characterized by the t(9:22) translocation.[862-865] However, these patients may be characterized by the presence of an altered c-*abl* mRNA of about 7 kDa that codes for an aberrant c-*abl* protein of 190 kDa, p190[c-abl].[866-870] The molecular analysis of Ph-positive ALLs revealed that breakpoints on chromosome 22 may be scattered through a relatively large region of DNA upstream of the *bcr* coding sequence, but still within the *bcr* gene.[871] A fusion point which is still within the *bcr* gene, but upstream of the region characteristic of CMLs, may contribute to the creation in ALLs of an aberrant 7-kDa *bcr*/c-*abl* transcript and p190[c-abl] protein.[872] The altered p190[c-abl] protein present in Ph-positive ALL patients could possess an altered tyrosine kinase activity which may be involved in the leukemogenic process. Given the large size of the *bcr* gene and the heterogeneity in breakpoint location, detection of *bcr* rearrangement by standard Southern blot analysis is difficult, and pulsed-field gel electrophoresis may be used more conveniently for the detection of these changes at the DNA level, thus allowing clinical correlation of the breakpoint location with prognosis.[871] In a case of ALL exhibiting *bcr* rearrangement, only c-*abl* transcripts of normal size were detected in the tumor cells.[847] In some cases of Ph-positive ALL the DNA rearrangement on chromosome 22 may lie outside the *bcr* locus.[873] In one Ph-positive ALL patient the c-*abl* translocation breakpoint was localized within the Ig C_{lambda} locus on chromosome region 22q11.[609]

In a series of 122 children with ALL, 36 cases disclosed chromosome translocation and in 8 of these cases a t(8;14) was present.[874] Presumably, the c-*myc* locus was involved in this minority of ALL cases with t(8;14) but the data did not support a proliferative advantage for all leukemic cells with a translocation. Translocation and rearrangement of c-*myc* into Ig alpha heavy chain locus associated with enhanced c-*myc* expression was detected in the primary tumor cells from another patient with ALL.[875] In a case of ALL with t(8;14) the c-*myc* gene was at least 35 kb distant from the chromosome breakpoint.[751] Thus, translocation-induced activation of the c-*myc* locus is apparently not important in the pathogenesis of ALL.

The protooncogene c-*ets*-1 is located on human chromosome region 11q23 but it was not found to be altered in ALLs associated with translocations involving this region.[876] However, in another study rearranged c-*ets*-1 sequences were detected in 2 of 7 cases of ALL.[877]

An inversion of chromosome 14 present in the tumor cells of a patient with childhood ALL of B-cell lineage was shown to be the result of a site-specific recombination event between the Ig heavy-chain variable gene and the joining (J) segment of a T-cell receptor alpha chain.[878] This rearrangement resulted in the formation of a hybrid gene, part Ig and part T-cell receptor, which was transcribed into mRNA with a completely open reading frame.

6. Acute Nonlymphocytic Leukemia

Chromosome abnormalities have been detected in 48 to 61% of adults with acute nonlymphocytic leukemia (ANLL).[879] The disease is frequently associated with a translocation between the short arm of chromosome 6 and the long arm of chromosome 9, t(6;9)(p23;q34). In ANLL associated with this translocation, the c-*abl* protooncogene is not translocated from chromosome 9, the breakpoint does not reside within the c-*abl* DNA sequence but is on its 3′ side, and an abnormal hybrid protein product containing c-*abl* sequences is not observed.[880] In one patient with ANLL an extra copy of c-*abl* was found to be inserted at the junction of a reciprocal translocation involving chromosomes 4 and 10.

The FAB-M2 subtype of human ANLL is associated with the translocation t(8;21)(q22.1;q22.3). Since the c-*mos* protooncogene is located on human chromosome region 8q22, it may be suspected that c-*mos* is involved in the ANLL-associated translocation. However, the available evidence indicates that c-*mos* is not translocated in the FAB-M2 subtype of ANLL, which suggests that it is not involved in the pathogenesis of this hematological disorder.[835,881,882]

7. Diffuse Large-Cell Lymphoma

Diffuse large-cell lymphoma is different from Burkitt's lymphoma in biological and clinical characteristics. The primary tumor from one of ten patients with this subtype of lymphoma examined with Southern blot analysis revealed a rearrangement of the c-*myc* gene which apparently did not involve the Ig loci.[883] No rearrangement of c-*myc* was detected in 28 additional patients with other subtypes of non-Hodgkin's lymphoma examined in this study.

The putative protooncogene *bcl*-2 was found to be translocated in form of t(14;18)(q32;q21) in 8 of 20 cases of human diffuse large-cell lymphomas.[834] The translocation resulted in a hybrid *bcl*-2/J-H gene in head-to-tail juxtaposition, similar or identical to that found in follicular lymphomas. In an independent series, 11 of 58 (19%) diffuse lymphomas of follicular center cell lineage contained a rearranged *bcl*-2 gene.[884] Non-Hodgkin's lymphomas, both with and without a follicular morphology, can be associated with t(14;18) involving the *bcl*-2 gene.[885]

8. Follicular Lymphoma

A genetic locus, termed *bcl*-2, located on chromosome 18q21, was detected in an acute B-cell leukemia cell line from a young patient with t(14;18) translocation.[886] The *bcl*-2 locus may be involved in the pathogenesis of follicular lymphoma. A cytogenetic study of 71 patients with follicular lymphoma showed that a translocation t(14;18) occurred in 85% of the total cases.[887] In another series, 18 of 26 (69%) follicular lymphomas had a t(14;18)(q32;q21) translocation associated with *bcl*-2 rearrangement.[834] A lower incidence of *bcl*-2 rearrangement (30%) was found in an independent series of 37 patients with follicular lymphoma.[884] A similar rearrangement occurs, although at lower frequency, in diffuse large-cell lymphomas, but the rearrangement is not present in lymphomas not derived from follicle center cells (diffuse lymphomas of B lymphocytes, B-cell chronic lymphocytic leukemia, and T-cell neoplasms).[884,885] Preferential DNA amplification by means of the highly sensitive polymerase chain reaction (PCR) technique has been applied to the detection of minimal residual cells carrying the t(14;18) in patients with follicular lymphoma during remission.[888]

The *bcl*-2-associated translocation involves the IgH locus, which is juxtaposed to the *bcl*-2 gene. The hybrid *bcl*-2/J-H gene is in head-to-tail juxtaposition and the *bcl*-2 gene is 5′ to the J-H gene component. Most of the breakpoints on human chromosome 18 are clustered within a short stretch of DNA, approximately 2.1 kb in length, which contains a *bcl*-2 gene that is interrupted by the translocation and which produces 6-kb RNA transcripts.[889] The coding regions of the *bcl*-2 gene are left intact in the t(14;18) translocation associated with follicular lymphoma. The association of the *bcl*-2 gene with the IgH locus may result in high levels of expression of *bcl*-2 transcripts which are inappropriate for a mature B-cell stage of development.[890]

Most frequently, the IgH locus, including the IgH enhancer sequence, is 3′ to the involved *bcl*-2 ORFs, suggesting that the IgH locus is responsible for the *bcl*-2 activation in the follicular lymphomas, However, in some cases of follicular lymphoma the analysis with molecular probes indicates that DNA rearrangements may also occur 5′ to the involved *bcl*-2 gene.[891] The c-*yes*-1 protooncogene is located on chromosome band 18q21.3, which corresponds to the break point of chromosome 18 in the t(14;18) associated with follicular lymphoma, but c-*yes*-1 is not rearranged or overexpressed in the cells of this tumor.[892] Thus, c-*yes*-1 is apparently not involved in the pathogenesis of human follicular lymphoma.

The *bcl*-2 locus was cloned and no sequences homologous to known oncogenes were present in the isolated probe. However, the *bcl*-2-encoded protein shows homology to a predicted EBV-encoded protein, BHRF-1.[893] The biological significance of this homology, if any, and the function of the *bcl*-2-encoded protein are unknown. Transcripts of the *bcl*-2 gene are expressed in mouse B-cell lymphomas, but only in tumors consisting of pre-B and follicular center mature B cells, not in pro-B or plasma cell tumors.[894] These results suggest that the product of the *bcl*-2 gene may represent a B-cell differentiation marker that is expressed only in committed B cells but is shut off in end stage plasma cells. It is possible that tumors of B cells that represent less mature stages of differentiation remain at this stage because *bcl*-2 cannot be turned off in lymphomas secondarily to translocation.

The human t(14;18) translocation can result in the production of hybrid *bcl*-2/Ig heavy chain transcripts which consist of the 5′ half of the *bcl*-2 mRNA fused to a decapitated Ig heavy-chain mRNA.[893] The results of these studies suggested that t(14;18) translocations associated with human follicular lymphoma may alter the expression of the putative *bcl*-2 protooncogene both by transcriptional activation and by abnormal posttranscriptional regulation of *bcl*-2 mRNA.

The chromosome translocations and DNA rearrangements occurring in follicular lymphomas may be used as markers for the study of clonality of these tumors.[895] A 2.8-kb DNA region, termed major breakpoint region (*mbr*), that is located on human chromosome 18 and rearranges with Ig gene sequences from chromosome 18 in the t(14;18)(q32;q31) translocation observed in the majority of human follicular lymphomas was used as a marker to demonstrate that the translocation breakpoint is conserved in each individual case of the tumor, which indicates that evolving neoplastic subpopulations of the tumor (which may exhibit additional rearrangements) arise from a common clonal progenitor cell.

9. T-Cell Leukemias

Specific DNA rearrangements involving the T-cell antigen-specific receptor (T-cell receptor) gene occur in human T-cell leukemia.[560,561,896-899] The T-cell receptor gene is a polymorphic disulfide-linked heterodimer consisting of α and β subunits encoded by distinct genes and has a structure which is similar to that of the Ig genes, with variable (V), diversity (D), joining (J), and constant (C) region elements.[900] In addition to the α and β chains, the T-cell receptor complex contains another polypeptide chain, the γ chain. The genes encoding the different polypeptides constituting the T-cell receptor are located on human chromosomes 7, 11 and 14, and these chromosomes are frequently involved in translocations occurring in abnormal human T cells.[897,901] There is a striking homology at both the DNA and chromosomal levels, including the production of particular types of DNA rearrangements, between B- and T-cell hematologic neoplasms.[902,903] The unique DNA rearrangements involving the T-cell receptor gene in human T-cell leukemias can be used to establish the monoclonality of T-cell expansions as well as DNA-level markers of T-cell lineage commitment and tumor-specific markers to monitor therapy.[898]

Translocation t(8;14)(q24;q11) occurring in human T-cell lymphomas can involve breakpoints that produce a physical proximity between the gene coding for the constant region of the α chain (C_{alpha}) of the T-cell receptor protein and the 3′ side of the c-*myc* protooncogene.[902] Fresh leukemic cells from a patient with T-cell ALL exhibited a t(8;14) translocation involving the c-*myc* and T-cell receptor genes.[904] Interestingly, the translocation was not found in the initial stages of the disease but was present in all the cells collected during relapse, which suggests that it could contribute to the selection of a leukemic cell subclone. In human T-cell leukemia cell lines, translocation t(8;14) involving the gene coding for the alpha subunit of the T-cell receptor 3′ to the c-*myc* gene could result in transcriptional deregulation of c-*myc* expression.[905-907] The possible role of such deregulation in the origin and/or development of primary human T-cell leukemia is unknown but only some of human T-cell leukemia cell lines are associated with this type of translocation. Rearrangement of c-*myc* associated with overexpression of the gene, but not with chromosome translocation, was detected in the human leukemic T-cell line Hut 78, derived from a patient with Sézary syndrome.[908] No overexpression of c-*myc* was detected in four other leukemic T-cell lines (CEM, CCRF-CEM, Jurkat, and JM).

Translocations other than t(14;18) may be associated, although less frequently, with the development of human T- cell leukemias. Two regions of chromosome 7 containing the β-chain (region 7q35-36) and the γ-chain (region 7p15) of the T-cell receptor may be affected in T-cell leukemias. The T-cell receptor beta gene, which is located on human chromosome region 7q32-q36, was the site of breakpoints in 4 of 31 cases of T-cell ALL but was not involved in any of 166 ALL cases originating from B-cell precursors.[909] A T-cell leukemia that occurred in a patient with ataxia-telangiectasia was associated with translocation t(7;14)(q35;q32), which involved a breakpoint in the T-cell receptor β chain locus on chromosome 7 and another breakpoint on chromosome 14, proximal to the IgH locus.[910] Translocation of the reciprocal joint-containing segment of the T-cell receptor from chromosome 7 to chromosome 6 was observed in cells from one patient with T-cell ALL.[911] The possible role of the c-*myb* protooncogene, normally located on human chromosome 6, in this translocation and in the neoplastic disease that occurred in the patient remained undetermined. The RPMI 8402 cell line, which was established from the leukemia cells of a patient with ALL, contains a translocation involving chromosomes 11 and 14, t(11;14)(p15;q11), in which the breakpoint at 14q11 occurs within the variable sequences of the T-cell receptor antigen (V_{alpha}) and the breakpoint at 11p15 occurs between the c-H-*ras*-1 gene and the genes for insulin and the related growth factor IGF-2.[912]

10. Chronic Lymphocytic Leukemia

Chromosomal aberrations are present in a number of patients with chronic lymphocytic leukemia (CLL).[913-915] This disease is a neoplasm characterized by proliferation and accumulation of mature-appearing lymphocytes.[916] In the majority of patients with CLL the neoplastic cells contain B-cell markers and only less than 5% have monoclonal T-cell markers. Structural and/or numerical chromosome abnormalities have been found in up to 74% of the patients with chronic B-cell lymphocytic leukemia, the most frequent abnormality consisting in the presence of an extra chromosome 12. Trisomy 12 in CLL is limited to the neoplastic B cells and is absent in the normal T cells.[917] This finding provides an explanation for the presence of normal karyotypes in the peripheral blood cells of one third to one fourth of the patients with CLL, since such normal metaphases would correspond to T cells. Furthermore, the results demonstrate that the cytogenetic changes in CLL, characteristically represented by trisomy 12, occur after the differentiation of a lymphoid precursor into B cells.[917] An extra chromosome 12 is associated with a more aggressive behavior of CLL and two protooncogenes have been assigned to this chromosome, namely, c-K-*ras* and c-*int*-1, but their possible participation in the pathogenetic phenomena of the disease is unknown.

In some cases of CLL a 14q+ marker chromosome is detected. An established cell line (SKW-3) derived from the malignant cells of a patient with T-cell CLL contains a t(8;14) translocation in which the constant region of the T-cell receptor α-chain gene, which is normally located on chromosome region 14q11-q12, was translocated to the 8q+ chromosome, distal to the c-*myc* gene.[905] Two rare cases of CLL in children were associated with t(2;14) translocation which involved the variable heavy-chain region of the Ig locus on chromosome 14 and an unidentified locus on chromosome 2.[918] Translocation t(14;19)(q32;q13.1) found in some (3 of 30) cases of CLL, especially in those associated with poor prognosis, may involve rearrangement of the IgH locus.[919] In a human CLL cell line (CLL-271), a reciprocal translocation was observed between chromosomes 11q13 and 14q32 and it was suggested that a new putative protooncogene, termed *bcl*-1, located on chromosome 11q13, would contribute, after translocation to the rearranged Ig variable heavy-chain locus on chromosome 14+, to the neoplastic transformation of B-cells.[920-922]

11. Myelomas and Myeloproliferative Disorders

No evidence for c-*mos* rearrangement was detected in cell lines or fresh cells from several types of human myelomas and lymphoproliferative disorders.[835,881,923] A cell line established from the malignant pleural effusion of a patient with plasma cell myeloma contained a complex translocation which resulted in the formation of a chimeric mRNA that included 5′ sequences of the c-*myc* gene.[924] No gross rearrangements of DNA sequences close to or within the c-*myc* and c-*mos* genes were detected in 16 patients with myeloproliferative disorders associated with trisomy 8.[925]

12. Solid Tumors

No regular reciprocal chromosome translocations, involving or not protooncogenes, are usually observed in common human solid tumors (carcinomas and sarcomas).[926] There are some exceptions to this general rule, however. Translocation of c-*myc* was found in a rare hereditary renal cell carcinoma associated with a t(3;8)(p14.2;q24.13) translocation.[927] In two of six renal cell carcinomas associated with 3p- deletions, chromosomal hybridization *in situ* with a c-*raf*-1 protooncogene probe demonstrated that this gene, which is normally located on chromosome region 3p25, had shifted to 3p14 as a result of an interstitial deletion.[928]

Rearrangement of c-*myc* was detected in one of two human cell lines of giant cell carcinoma of the lung (line C-Lu65) as well as in one of two human primary tumors of the same type.[929] The rearrangements occurred in chromosome regions located about 7.5 and 6 kb, respectively, upstream from the c-*myc* transcription initiation site. No rearrangements of c-*myc* were detected in 48 human primary lung tumors of other histological types. Giant cell carcinomas of the lung are aggressive tumors characterized by a short survival time and by their resistance to various kinds of therapy. Rearrangement of c-*myc* was also detected in 5 of 121 human primary breast carcinomas corresponding to advanced stages of the disease in patients over 50 years old.[508] The tumor tissue, but not the normal tissue, of a patient with ductal adenocarcinoma of the breast contained a c-*myc* gene rearranged as the consequence of the insertion of a long interspersed repetitive element (LINE-1 sequence or L1) within the second intron of the gene.[930] Two colon adenocarcinomas, from a series of 109 primary human adenocarcinoma tumors, exhibited a rearranged c-*neu*/*erb*-B-2 gene and expressed aberrant polypeptide product of this gene.[519] A rearranged c-*myb* gene was found in 1 of 22 human melanoma cell lines, but it could not be ascertained if the rearranged gene was transcriptionally active.[931] The structure of 28 other genes, including many protooncogenes, was unaltered in the melanoma cell lines, with the exception of one cell line which contained a homozygous deletion of a protein kinase C exon.

Reciprocal chromosome translocations, either acquired or constitutional, involving human chromosomes 11 and 22 may occur in Ewing sarcoma, peripheral neuroepithelioma, and Askin tumor (a malignancy of the thoracopulmonary region).[932-936] Although these translocations may be similar at the cytogenetic level, they are distinguishable at the molecular level.[935] The breakpoint is proximal to the C_{lambda} locus and the c-*ets*-1 protooncogene in the constitutional type of t(11;22) translocation, whereas it is distal to the same loci in the tumor cell lines examined. However, the c-*ets*-1 gene is not rearranged in these cases and its possible role, if any, in t(11;22) translocations, both constitutional and tumor-related, is not clear.

Translocation of the c-*sis* protooncogene was detected by *in situ* hybridization in two human neuroepithelioma cell lines carrying a t(11;22)(q24;q12) translocation.[937] However, the translocation was not associated with rearrangement or amplification of c-*sis* DNA sequences and no c-*sis* RNA transcripts were detected in the tumor cells. Thus, although c-*sis* may be translocated in neuroepitheliomas, there is no evidence for its involvement in the pathogenesis of this tumor.

D. REARRANGEMENT OF NONPROTOONCOGENE GENES IN HEMATOLOGIC MALIGNANCIES

The Ig and T-cell antigen receptor genes are composed of multiple, separated gene subsegments within their germline or embryonic configuration, and during the development of lymphoid cells a DNA recombination process assembles the components of Ig genes in B cells and the components of T-cell receptors in T cells.[560] Rearrangements of the Ig heavy- and light-chain genes and the T-cell receptor β-chain gene may represent highly sensitive markers of lineage and clonality in human lymphomas and lymphoid leukemias.[938] The type of gene rearrangement correlates well with the cell lineage of lymphoid neoplasms. Illegitimate clonal rearrangements at the Ig heavy-chain (IgH) and/or T-cell receptor β-chain genes can also occur in a proportion of patients with acute myeloid leukemia.[939,940]

E. REARRANGEMENT OF PROTOONCOGENES IN EXPERIMENTAL TUMORS

Rearrangement occurring at the 5′ side of the protooncogene c-*mos* was detected in a mouse myeloma (XRPC24) originally induced by treatment with pristane.[325,941,942] The rearranged c-

mos gene contained a segment where c-*mos* sequences were substituted by an insertion sequence (IS-like element) from an endogenous retrovirus (intracisternal A particle), and transcripts of the altered c-*mos* gene were detected in the tumor cells. A similar rearrangement and transcriptional activation of c-*mos* was detected in the cell line P3-X63-Ag8-653, a derivative of the mouse myeloma MOPC 21, which was originally induced by treatment with mineral oil.[923] The biological significance of rearrangements and activation of c-*mos* are unknown but this protooncogene is transcriptionally silent in the majority of normal cells, and in most mouse plasmacytomas c-*mos* is not rearranged. When the viral LTR of M-MuSV is covalently linked to the 5' region of a cloned c-*mos* protooncogene, the transcriptional activity of the cloned c-*mos* gene is enhanced and the activated gene efficiently induces transformation when transfected into NIH/3T3 cells.[7] The results suggest that occasional rearrangements occurring between promoter sequences from endogenous retroviruses and c-*onc* genes may contribute to the origin and/or progression of some experimental tumors.

The mouse plasmacytoma XRPC24 contains, in addition to the rearranged c-*mos* gene, a translocation of c-*myc* into the Ig C-alpha gene.[943] The translocated part of c-*myc*, which contains only the second and third exons of the gene, was isolated and cloned in a molecular vector under the control of an SV40 promoter. Cotransfection of this construct with an activated EJ c-H-*ras* gene into rat embryo fibroblasts resulted in a high level of transformation.[943] These results, when considered in the context that translocation of c-*myc* is a regular feature of mouse plasmacytomas, suggest that it is this translocation, and not the casual rearrangement of c-*mos*, which is the crucial oncogenic event in the development of the XRPC24 plasmacytoma. However, it is possible that the presence of both activated c-*mos* and c-*myc* may affect the growth of particular types of cells.

Protooncogenes other than c-*mos* may be rearranged in experimentally induced tumors as well as in animal tumor cell lines. DNA rearrangement and increased transcriptional activity of the protooncogene c-*myb* was observed in plasmacytoid lymphosarcomas induced in mice by treatment with pristane and A-MuLV, and increased transcriptional activity of c-*myc* was found in plasmacytomas induced in mice by similar experimental procedures.[944,945] In a rat leukemia cell line (K3D), secondary activation of c-*abl* may be related to translocation of the protooncogene to the nucleolar organizer chromosome region.[946]

An apparent rearrangement of the human *met* protooncogene, which is normally located on human chromosome 7q21-q31, with another locus, termed *tpr*, located on human chromosome 1, would result in the generation of hybrid 5.0 kb RNA transcripts which are detected in a human osteosarcoma cell line (MNNG-HOS) treated with the chemical carcinogen, N-methyl-N-nitronitrosoguanidine (MNNG).[140,141] The hybrid 5-kb mRNA transcripts contain 5' sequences derived from *tpr* and 3' sequences from the *met* gene as a consequence of a recombinational event.[142] The activated *met* gene encodes 60- and 65-kDa proteins that can catalyze autophosphorylation on tyrosine, but the same protein-tyrosine kinase activity is present in the normal *met* protein.[947] The possible role of hybrid *tpr/met* transcripts an altered *met* proteins in neoplastic transformation is unknown, but DNA from MNNG-HOS cells is capable of inducing oncogenic transformation in the NIH/3T3 DNA transfection assay.

F. BIOLOGICAL SIGNIFICANCE OF PROTOONCOGENE TRANSLOCATION AND/OR REARRANGEMENT IN RELATION TO NEOPLASIA

DNA recombinations and gene rearrangements may play a central role in the normal processes of cellular differentiation,[948] and this is probably also true in abnormal cell differentiation leading to neoplasia. DNA rearrangements may be involved in tumorigenic processes occurring even in plants, for example, in the integration of the T-DNA which is contained in the Ti plasmid of *Agrobacterium tumefaciens*, which is associated with the induction of plant crown gall tumors.[949]

The possible role of specific chromosome translocations, either involving or not protooncogenes, in the origin and/or development of hematologic malignant diseases and solid tumors remains undetermined but the high frequency of their occurrence in hematologic malignancies suggest that these translocations are important for the pathogenesis of these diseases. However, the translocations observed in hematologic malignant diseases are heterogeneous at the molecular level and they are not present in all cases of the particular diseases. With the exception of the production of fused *bcr/c-abl* transcripts and hybrid p210$^{bcr/c-abl}$(P210) protein in CML, and the assumed deregulation of c-*myc* expression in Burkitt's lymphoma cells, few consistent patterns of altered expression of translocated protooncogenes have been found in tumor cells. Moreover, the exact role of these alterations in the origin and/or development of tumors remains to be determined.

Although it is frequently assumed that chromosome translocations can cause cancer through activation of protooncogenes, there are at least three good reasons for caution in generalizing this deduction: (1) activation of a protooncogene as a result of translocation has yet to be demonstrated as a general phenomenon, (2) even if it were, it would be premature to accept it as the cause of malignant transformation *in vivo,* and (3) the specificity of many of the chromosome abnormalities reported in leukemias and lymphomas is not absolute.[950] Protooncogenes are relatively evenly distributed among the different types of human chromosomes and their involvement in chromosome translocations or DNA rearrangements may be casual in some cases.[892] Moreover, rearrangement and/or overexpression of the translocated protooncogene is not always observed in chromosome translocations involving protooncogenes and some translocated protooncogenes are expressed at low levels. Furthermore, in some types of hematologic malignancies the specific translocations involving protooncogenes are observed in only a minority of the total cases. The possibility should be considered that at least certain associations between a numerical and/or structural alteration of a particular chromosome and a given type of tumor may be independent of the presence of protooncogene(s) in the chromosome.

In human ANLL, normal-appearing granulocyte/macrophage colonies can form *in vitro* from progenitors carrying chromosomal abnormalities as well as from progenitors with a diploid chromosome complement.[951] It is thus apparent that the presence of leukemia-associated chromosomal abnormalities in granulocyte-macrophage progenitors does not hinder their capacity to form normal cell colonies *in vitro,* and that specific chromosome translocations themselves may not induce irreversible leukemic transformation. Chromosome translocations are apparently not present in an important proportion of patients with CLL and ALL.[913,952] In a cytogenetic study of 941 consecutive patients with suspected neoplastic hematologic disorders, only 50% of the patients with hematologic malignancies exhibited an acquired clonal chromosome abnormality.[953] However, some chromosome abnormalities may involve small chromosome portions that cannot be detected by the usual cytogenetic techniques. Studies with polymerase chain reaction (PCR) and molecular hybridization methods should contribute to a better characterization of submicroscopic genomic alterations with hematologic malignant diseases.

No specific and consistent chromosome translocations involving protooncogenes are observed in many hematopoietic neoplasms or in the common solid tumors (carcinomas and sarcomas). Rather, solid tumors are characterized by the intratumoral heterogeneity of karyotypes which may be a consequence of the karyotype instability occurring *in vivo* during tumor progression.[954] It seems thus clear that mechanisms other than chromosome translocations and protooncogene rearrangements are involved in the origin of the most common types of solid tumors. In any case, it is not known if there exists a general correlation between particular types of structural chromosome abnormalities and alterations of protooncogene functions that would be crucially involved in neoplastic transformation and/or tumorigenicity. Further studies are required for a better characterization of the relationships between chromosome translocations, protooncogene alterations, and cancer.

VI. MUTATION OF PROTOONCOGENES IN TUMORS

The hypothesis that the origin of neoplastic transformation involves somatic cell mutation has been widely accepted, but specific genes responsible for the phenomenon of malignant transformation have not been identified. Recently, much interest has arisen from the possibility that altered polypeptides produced by mutant protooncogenes could be related to the origin of some human tumors, particularly bladder, lung and colon cancer. The vast majority of mutants detected in tumor cells are from the c-*ras* protooncogenes.[46,955-958]

A. DETECTION OF PROTOONCOGENE MUTATIONS IN TUMORS

Tumor cell populations that give positive results in the NIH/3T3 DNA transfection/ transformation assay are highly suspicious of carrying a mutated c-*ras* protooncogene. A part of all the theoretically possible mutations occurring in protooncogene sequences can be detected by DNA RFLP analysis or by alterations in the electrophoretic mobility of the protein product. Other c-*ras* mutations can be detected by molecular hybridization with specific synthetic oligonucleotide probes. Recently, the polymerase chain reaction (PCR) method has contributed to a better knowledge of protooncogene mutations associated with tumors.

1. Restriction Endonucleases

Studies using specific restriction endonucleases (RFLP analysis) can be applied to the detection of some mutations affecting c-*ras* genes. In addition, the interesting possibility that polymorphic changes in protooncogene sequences could be related to an increased susceptibility to neoplastic processes is suggested by the finding of unique allelic restriction fragments of the human c-H-*ras* locus in DNAs from both normal leukocytes and tumor cells in cancer patients.[959,960] Different restriction endonucleases (*Bam*HI, *Msp*I/*Hpa*II, *Ava*II, and *Taq*I) have been used to detect DNA polymorphisms associated with the human c-H-*ras*-1 gene. A detected allelic RFLP associated with this locus consists of variation in the number of variable tandem repeats (VTRs) of 28 bp, 3' to the c-H-*ras* coding sequences.

Restriction enzyme analysis of the DNA from 104 breast cancer patients and 56 unaffected individuals indicated a significantly increased frequency of rare c-H-*ras*-1 alleles in the breast cancer population.[961] A significantly increased frequency of an allelic variant, termed Tp, associated with the human c-H-*ras*-1 gene and detected by digestion with the *Taq*I restriction enzyme, was found in a series of 55 melanoma patients, in comparison with a group of 53 healthy individuals.[962] The frequency of unusual alleles of the human c-H-*ras*-1 gene in 35 patients with bladder cancer was significantly greater than in controls.[963] However, no significant differences in the distribution of different c-H-*ras* allelic restriction fragments between patients with tumors and normal individuals were found by other investigators.[964,965] The association of a predisposition to melanoma or the precursor lesion, the dysplastic nevus syndrome, with the inheritance of the c-H-*ras*-1 locus, or the segment of chromosome 11 on which it is located, was excluded in a clinical study.[966] Further studies are required for a proper assessment of the possible relationship between RFLP of c-*ras* protooncogene DNA sequences and susceptibility to malignant diseases.

2. Synthetic Oligonucleotide Probes

Taking profit of the fixed position of c-*ras* mutations, mutations of these genes that have weak transforming capacity in the NIH/3T3 DNA transfection assay have been detected by means of synthetic oligonucleotide probes.[967-970] The analysis is based on the fact that a fully matched DNA hybrid has a higher thermal stability than a hybrid with a mismatch pair. Using a set of synthetic oligonucleotide probes, mutation at codon 13 of the N-*ras* gene was detected in the tumor cells of patients with AML. Less than one fourth of AML patients have N-*ras* gene mutations and the possible role of these mutations in the pathogenesis of tumors is unknown.

3. RNAse A Mismatch Cleavage Analysis

RNAse A mismatch cleavage analysis is a sensitive method for detecting point mutations. The use of this method has indicated that c-*ras* mutations may be more frequent in certain types of primary human tumors than previously suspected by the results of DNA transfection assays.[971,972] Almost 40% of point mutations within the 12th codon of c-K-*ras* was detected in a large panel of primary human colon carcinomas which had given only 20% positive results in the NIH/3T3 DNA transfection assay. No clear differences were found in the levels of expression of both normal and mutant c-K-*ras* alleles in these tumors. No significant differences were found between the mutation frequency at position 12 of the c-K-*ras* gene and the degree of differentiation or stage of progression of the tumors. On the other hand, a striking difference was apparent between the nucleotide position of the mutations at codon 12 of the gene and the degree of invasiveness of the tumors, with 16 of 18 mutations at the second position of the triplet being present in the gene of tumors displaying more invasive properties (tumor grades B, C, and D). Evidence was also obtained for c-*ras* mutational activation in premalignant lesions of the human colon.

4. Combined DNA Amplification-Direct Sequencing Method

Inclusion of an *in vitro* amplification step of *ras*-specific sequences in the procedure, based on selective hybridization of mutation-specific oligodeoxynucleotide probes to genomic DNA, may greatly increase the sensitivity of the method for the detection of c-*ras* mutations associated with tumorigenic processes.[973] Moreover, paraffin-embeded material may be a suitable source for DNA, which enables the analysis of archival material in retrospect. Primer-directed enzymatic amplification of DNA combined with direct sequencing of amplified DNA derived from a specific gene region has been successfully applied. This method may provide a rapid means of detecting and characterizing mutations of c-*ras* genes or other genes. By combining the polymerase chain reaction (PCR) technique with a liquid hybridization and gel retardation assay, c-*ras* (or other) DNA sequences can be detected at the single cell level.[974] The PCR protocol can be modified by the use of mismatched primers. This approach allowed the detection of c-*ras* genes in the presence of 10^5 normal cells.

5. Altered Electrophoretic Mobility of p21$^{c\text{-}ras}$ Proteins

Mutant proteins frequently exhibit altered electrophoretic mobilities that can be detected by electrophoresis in sodium dodecyl sulfate (SDS)-polyacrylamide gels. Among 52 fresh specimens of different types of human cancers and 9 samples of normal human fresh tissues, a single rapidly migrating electrophoretic variant of c-H-*ras* p21 protein was observed, which corresponded to a malignant fibrohistiocytoma.[204] In another study, only 1 of 23 fresh samples of primary human bronchogenic carcinoma contained a p21$^{c\text{-}ras}$ protein that migrated in SDS-polyacrylamide gel electrophoresis differently (more slowly) than the normal.[214] Mutations of c-*ras* genes, as detected by altered mobility in electrophoretic analysis of the p21 protein products, appear to be rare in human primary tumors.

6. Antibodies to Mutant p21 Proteins

Antisera raised in rabbits to a set of chemically synthesized peptides spanning position 12 of p21^{ras} protein (residues 5 to 17) are able to distinguish between different forms of p21 according to the amino acid substituting glycine at 12th codon position (serine, arginine, valine, or aspartate).[975] Monoclonal antibodies with specificity for activated c-*ras* proteins have also been developed. However, spurious results may be obtained with at least some of the immunologic methods using either polyclonal or monoclonal antibodies for the detection of normal or mutated p21$^{c\text{-}ras}$ proteins.[976] Immunohistochemical studies of c-*ras* proteins should thus be accompanied, whenever possible, by other analyses such as RNA *in situ* hybridization. PCR and synthetic oligonucleotide probes are most useful for the detection and characterization of mutant protooncogenes.

B. MUTANT C-*RAS* PROTOONCOGENES IN HUMAN TUMOR CELL LINES

Mutations of the three c-*ras* genes (c-H-*ras*, c-K-*ras,* and N-*ras*) have been identified in different human tumor cell lines.

1. Mutation of c-H-*ras*-1

A biologically active protooncogene, with high oncogenic capacity in DNA transfection experiments with the NIH/3T3 assay system, was initially detected in the T24 and EJ human bladder carcinoma cell lines.[977-979] The protooncogene was cloned in molecular vectors and was identified as c-*ras* or c-*bas*, cellular homologs of the Harvey- and BALB-MuSV oncogenes.[980,981] It was demonstrated thereafter that the 21-kDa (p21) polypeptide product of the T24/EJ c-H-*ras*-1 protooncogene is different from the respective p21 product present in normal human cells, the difference consisting in substitution of a single amino acid. Whereas human p21^{ras} has glycine at position 12, EJ/T24 p21^{ras} has valine at this position, which would correspond to a single G-T nucleotide change at the DNA level.[982-984] This nucleotide change was later confirmed by DNA sequence analysis.[985-987] The complete sequence of the T24 gene was determined and a single point mutation residing within the first exon distinguished the coding region of this gene from the sequence of its normal counterpart, c-H-*ras*-1. Mutations at two different exon sites of the c-H-*ras*-1 gene, determining single amino acid substitutions at positions 12 and 61 of the respective p21 product, may not be associated with enhanced capability for transformation in DNA transfection assays.[988] A c-H-*ras* gene activated by mutation at codon 61 was detected in the human squamous-cell lung carcinoma cell line QG56.[989] Protooncogene c-H-*ras* was found to be activated by mutation at codon 12 in the human gastric carcinoma cell line BGC-823.[990] Other two gastric carcinoma cell lines (PACM-82 and MGC 80-3) were negative for this mutation.

2. Mutation of c-K-*ras*-2

Similar qualitative changes were detected in c-*ras* protooncogenes from some human lung, colon, and pancreas carcinoma cell lines.[420,449,991-996] The activated transforming gene of these lines corresponds to the protooncogene c-K-*ras*-2 and its mutational change may also determine single amino acid substitutions at position 12 or 61 of the protein. Mutation of the c-K-*ras*-2 gene consisting of a single nucleotide transition from G to T at the 12th codon was detected in the DNA of a cell line derived from a colon carcinoma that arose in a patient with familial polyposis coli.[997] Thus, single amino acid substitutions at either position 12 or position 61 of p21$^{c\text{-}ras}$ proteins may represent a common mechanism of transforming activation depending on somatic mutation of c-*ras* genes, as detected by transfection into NIH/3T3 cells.[94,994] Moreover, at least two different mutational changes of the c-K-*ras*-2 gene have been observed in two human lung tumors which were propagated in nude mice and were introduced into NIH/3T3 cells by DNA transfection experiments, and these mutations also determined amino acid substitutions at positions 12 and 61 of the p21 product.[998,999]

In the human pancreas carcinoma cell line T3M-4, mutation of c-K-*ras* at codon 61 was found to be associated with amplification and overexpression of either the same mutated allele or its normal allele.[448] Mutation of c-K-*ras* at codon 12 associated with amplification and overexpression of the protooncogene was found in the human osteosarcoma cell line OHA.[449] Among 10 different human mammary tumor cell lines, only one was scored as positive in the NIH/3T3 DNA transfection assay and, interestingly, the positive tumor cell line (H-466B), established from an ascitic effusion of a woman with an adenocarcinoma of the breast, contained a double mutation in codon 12 of c-K-*ras*-2, leading to the replacement of the normal glycine by phenylalanine.[95] An exceptional human breast carcinoma cell line (MDA-MB231) contains a mutation at codon 13 of the c-K-*ras* gene, resulting in a substitution of glycine by aspartic acid in the p21 protein.[445] The mutation was associated with amplification of the protooncogene sequences.

3. Mutation of N-*ras*

Mutation of N-*ras*, determining amino acid substitution at position 61 of the protein product, has been detected in several human tumor cell lines,[86] including lines derived from neuroblastoma,[1000] lung carcinoma,[1001] fibrosarcoma,[1002] melanoma,[1003] rhabdomyosarcoma,[83] and rectal carcinoma.[1004] In three human tumor cell lines (HT1080, HL-60, and RD301) different mutations at the three possible codon positions of codon 61 of the N-*ras* gene were detected by molecular hybridization with synthetic oligonucleotide probes.[968] These cell lines contained, in addition to a mutated N-*ras* allele, a normal allele, which demonstrates the dominant character of the protooncogene mutation.

Mutation of N-*ras* affecting amino acid position 61 of p21 was detected in a cell line derived from mouse Lewis lung carcinoma.[1005] Five tumorigenic guinea pig cell lines that were initiated with diverse carcinogens were found to contain an activated N-*ras* gene with identical mutation (AT-TA transversion) at the third position of codon 61.[1006] Both the mutated N-*ras* gene and its normal allele were up-regulated in these cell lines.[1007] Mutational activation and transcriptional down regulation were limited to the tumorigenic guinea pig cell lines; preneoplastic progenitors of these cells were unaffected, suggesting that the changes occurred at a late stage of carcinogenesis, closely associated with acquisition of tumorigenicity.

4. Conclusion

Analysis of a diversity of human tumor cell lines has demonstrated that codons 12 and 61, and less frequently codon 13, of the c-*ras* protooncogenes are hot spots for mutagenesis resulting in acquisition of enhanced transforming capability by the encoded p21 protein products, at least when NIH/3T3 cells are used as a test system in DNA transfection assays.

C. BIOLOGICAL SIGNIFICANCE OF C-*RAS* MUTANT GENES PRESENT IN HUMAN TUMOR CELL LINES

The possible relationship between point mutations of c-*ras* genes observed in human cell lines and the origin of human tumors is difficult to evaluate. Human tumor cell lines may have suffered different changes after many years in culture, and cross-contamination of cell cultures is a persistent problem in laboratories.[1008] Moreover, since changed protooncogenes are cloned from transformed cell lines, specific point mutations could have been selected for growth in tissue culture and, therefore, may be an artifact of cell culture systems.[1009] In general, DNA transfected into mammalian cells suffers an extraordinarily high mutation frequency,[1010] which may explain, at least in some cases, the detection of activated c-*ras* genes after transfection of DNA from tumor cells. Tumor cells are characterized by genomic instability and the increased susceptibility of the c-*ras* genes derived from tumor cells for mutagenesis could be attributed to some chromatin conformational changes present in them, perhaps related to increased transcriptional activity, which would then be followed by *in vitro* selection of cells carrying the c-*ras* mutation.

The NIH/3T3 assay system used in transfection experiments is apparently biased for the detection of altered products from mutant c-*ras* genes, and fibroblast immortality is a prerequisite for transformation by mutant c-*ras* genes.[1011] Moreover, there is evidence that some protooncogene mutations may be induced during the experimental procedures used for their detection or during prolonged cell culture *in vitro*. Spontaneous activation of a human c-*ras* protooncogene, associated with a point mutation at position 35 of the first exon, occurred during a transfection experiment.[987] Interestingly, the mutation produced a change of aspartic acid instead of glycine at position 12 of the p21^{ras} protein, i.e., at the same position altered in T24 and EJ human bladder carcinoma cell lines. A similar phenomenon was observed in the human teratocarcinoma cell line PA1, where activation of the protooncogene N-*ras*, associated with mutation in the codon corresponding to amino acid 12 of the p21^{ras} protein arose during prolonged cell culture *in vitro* (after more than 100 passages).[118] The reasons for the apparently very high susceptibility of specific sites of the c-*ras* genes for point mutational events are unknown.

D. MUTATION OF PROTOONCOGENES IN PRIMARY TUMORS

Detection of mutant protooncogenes in fresh tumor samples may be more relevant for understanding their possible role in tumorigenic processes. Mutant c-*ras* protooncogenes with increased transforming potential are present in a minority of the total tumors occurring under natural conditions, including human tumors. However, a relatively high incidence of c-*ras* mutations has been found in some common types of human tumors by using highly sensitive detection procedures.[956,958]

1. Mutation of c-H-*ras*

A study of 29 patients with bladder, lung, and colon cancer, including analysis of 20 primary tumor tissues (biopsy specimens), was negative for the presence of mutations producing substitutions of the 12th amino acid in the p21 product of the c-H-*ras* gene.[1012] Mutation of c-H-*ras* resulting in substitution of leucine for glutamine at amino acid residue 61 of the p21 protein was detected in a melanoma isolated from a Japanese patient and maintained in nude mice.[1013] In a series of 38 randomly selected specimens of primary human tumors of the urinary tract, only 2 cases were positive in the DNA transfection assay and in both positive tumors a single point mutation was localized at codon 61 of c-H-*ras*.[35] None, or perhaps only one, of nine squamous cell carcinomas of the bladder surgically obtained in Egypt from patients with bilharziasis caused by *Schistosoma haematobium* contained mutations of the c-H-*ras* gene.[217] No mutated c-*ras* genes were detected by DNA transfection or RFLP assay in two series of primary human mammary carcinomas.[94,206] Mutations of the c-H-*ras* gene were detected by using synthetic oligonucleotide probes in 2 of 24 tissue samples from human breast carcinomas.[1014] In summary, point mutations of c-H-*ras* are detected in a small minority of human solid tumors. A mutated c-H-*ras* gene was detected in a human keratoacanthoma, which is a benign, self-regressing tumor.[1015]

Progression of Ph chromosome-positive CML from the chronic phase to blast crisis may be associated with mutation of c-*ras* genes. Three of six patients with CML in blast crisis had mutations at codon 12 of c-*ras* genes (two in c-H-*ras* and one in N-*ras*).[1016] In contrast, only one of six patients in the chronic phase of CML had a mutation at codon 12 of a c-*ras* gene (c-H-*ras*).

2. Mutation of c-K-*ras*

Mutation at the 12th codon of the c-K-*ras* protooncogene was detected in some primary human lung tumors, for example, in the primary tumor tissue of a squamous cell lung carcinoma removed from a 66-year-old man.[1017] The mutation present in this patient was of a somatic origin since it was present in the tumor tissue but not in normal tissue from the same patient. None of 24 primary or metastatic human lung tumors tested for mutation of c-K-*ras* by using the RFLP method exhibited GGT-CGT mutation at codon 12.[1018] Only 1 of 23 human lung tumors studied by immunoblotting analysis exhibited abnormal migration of the p21 protein suggesting a mutational event.[214] A possible point mutation of c-K-*ras* was detected in the tumor from a patient with serous cystadenocarcinoma of the ovary by DNA transfection assay and demonstration of an altered electrophoretic mobility of the respective p21 protein product.[1019] A human gastric carcinoma was found to possess a single mutated c-K-*ras* allele (glycine-12 to serine) as well as a 30- to 50-fold amplified normal allele.[970] Activation of c-K-*ras* by mutation at codon

12 was also observed in a human pancreas carcinoma.[511] Mutation of c-K-*ras* or N-*ras* is rarely found in human hepatocellular carcinomas. Among 34 primary hepatocellular carcinoma specimens obtained from 30 patients and examined with PCR and oligonucleotide hybridization techniques, only 2 contained c-*ras* mutations, one case in c-K-*ras* and the other in N-*ras*.[1020]

A relatively high incidence of c-*ras* mutations has been found in some human tumors by using modern methodology. A combination of DNA hybridization analysis and tissue sectioning techniques allowed the demonstration of c-*ras* gene mutation in 11 of 27 human colorectal cancers.[1021] Of the 11 mutations found in this series, 10 were in the c-K-*ras* gene, and 9 of these were at codon 12 of the gene. Mutation of codon 12 of the N-*ras* gene was found in one tumor of the same series. Interestingly, in five of six colorectal cancers with c-*ras* mutations the same mutation was found in adenomatous (benign) and carcinomatous (malignant) regions of the tumor, suggesting that the mutation preceded the development of malignancy.[1021] In an independent study of human colorectal cancer using RNAse a mismatch analysis, 26 of 66 primary human colon tumors scored positive for c-*ras* mutations, most of them affecting codon 12 of the c-K-*ras* gene.[971,972] A striking high incidence of mutant c-K-*ras* genes was found in tumors originating in villous adenomas and villoglandular polyps, which are relatively common types of benign tumors that can develop malignant behavior. In a study of 51 primary lung, colon, and breast carcinomas using a panel of specific oligonucleotide probes, 4 of 16 colon carcinomas, 2 of 27 lung carcinomas, and 1 of 8 breast carcinomas were found to contain mutations at codon 12 of the c-K-*ras* gene.[1022] No mutations at position 61 of c-K-*ras* were found in this study. Apparently, mutations at position 61 of c-K-*ras* are very rare in primary human tumors.

Using the highly sensitive assay based on oligonucleotide hybridization following an *in vitro* amplification step with PCR, mutations of c-K-*ras* at codon 12 were detected in five of ten adenocarcinomas of the human lung.[1023] This mutation apparently occur very infrequently or not at all in other types of non-small-cell lung carcinomas. Activation of c-H-*ras* or N-*ras* were not detected in this series of 39 lung cancer specimens.

The use of a combination of techniques, including the aplication of PCR to small sections of formalin-fixed, paraffin-embedded tissue and the detection of mutation by cleavage at single base mismatches by RNAse A in DNA:RNA and RNA:DNA heteroduplexes, allowed the detection of mutations at codon 12 of c-K-*ras* in 21 of 22 primary human carcinomas of the exocrine pancreas.[1024] The ubiquitous presence of the mutant c-K-*ras* gene (in different tumor regions, in the majority of the tumor cells, and in both primary tumors and their corresponding metastases, either from autopsies or from surgical specimens, suggests that c-K-*ras* mutational activation is an early event in cancer of the exocrine pancreas and that it may contribute to the progress of this tumor, including metastasization.

3. Mutation of N-*ras*

Mutation of the N-*ras* gene has been detected mostly in hematologic malignancies. Mutations at codon 12, 13, or 61 of N-*ras* are present in myeloid and lymphoid leukemias as well as in myelodysplastic syndromes.[1025] Mutations at codon 12 of N-*ras* have been detected in the tumor cells from a relatively high proportion of patients with AML.[78,1026-1028] Mutations at codon 12 of N-*ras* were also detected in the fresh bone marrow cells of 2 out of 32 patients with a diversity of leukemias.[87] One of the two positive cases had CML and the other ALL, and both mutations consisted in a G-T transversion determining the substitution of cysteine for glycine in the p21 protein.

Some patients with myelodysplastic syndromes, which are characterized by a high risk for leukemia, contain in their peripheral blood cells with N-*ras* genes mutated at codon 12, in spite of the fact that these cells do not exhibit morphological characteristics of neoplastic transformation.[1027] Other patients with myelodysplastic syndromes may have mutations of the c-K-*ras* gene, including mutations occurring at codon 13 of this gene.[1029]

Point mutations at codon 12 of both N-*ras* and c-K-*ras* genes were detected in the fresh leukemic cells from an AML patient as well as in an AML cell line.[1030] However, it could not be determined whether the cell samples investigated consisted of two different cell types, one with an N-*ras* and another with a c-K-*ras* mutation or both mutations affected the genome of a clonal cell population. In an independent study of 33 specimens of fresh leukemic cells using immunoprecipitation with monoclonal antibodies, abnormal p21 products of the N-*ras* gene were detected in 6 of 11 samples of AML and 1 of 20 samples of ALL, but in every case the mutant protein comprised only a minority of the total p21[c-*ras*] protein.[304] Similar results were obtained in another study of 22 AMLs in which 4 samples contained an N-*ras* gene mutated at codon 12 or 13 and 2 samples contained a c-H-*ras* gene mutated at codon 12, but the mutations were present in only a minor proportion of the cells from the major leukemic clone.[1031] These findings imply that only a small fraction of the leukemic cells in an individual patient may carry the mutant c-*ras* gene, suggesting that the c-*ras* mutations occur relatively late during the leukemogenic process and may not be responsible for the initial neoplastic transformation.

Using synthetic oligonucleotide probes, mutation of N-*ras* was detected in 5 of 18 cases of ANLL.[1032] The mutation consisted in GGT-GAT transition at codon 12 (four cases) and CAA-AAA transversion at codon 61 (one case). In this study, none of 14 ALL patients exhibited N-*ras* mutations.

Upon examination of fractionated mononuclear cells from bone marrow or peripheral blood from 9 cases of overt ANLLs and preleukemias causally related to intensive cancer treatment with alkylating agents, only one case showed N-*ras* mutation, which consisted in a GGT-TGT change at codon 13.[1033] These results seem to rule out point mutation of c-*ras* genes as causally related to the high risk for ANLL following chemotherapy with alkylating agents.

Mutations occurring at sites other than codons 12 or 61 of c-*ras* genes may remain undetected in the NIH/3T3 DNA transfection assay. Mutations of the N-*ras* protooncogene at codon 13 were detected by means of synthetic oligonucleotide probes in the tumor cells of four out of five patients with AML.[968] The mutations substituted asparagine or valine for glycine at this codon but such mutations are relatively weak for inducing foci of transformed cells in the NIH/3T3 assay. However, from 37 additional AML patients studied by the same group of investigators, only one contained a mutation at codon 13 of the N-*ras* gene.[1034] In this AML series, mutations in codon 61 of N-*ras* were detected in four cases and a mutation in codon 12 of c-K-*ras* in two cases. Mutation of N-*ras* did not correlate with the cytological features or the differentiation level of the immature AML cells.

Mutation at codon 13 of N-*ras* was detected in the tumor cell DNA from a patient with a non-Hodgkin's T-cell lymphoma.[1035] In two patients with myelodysplastic syndromes and chromosome 5 deletion, point mutation of N-*ras* at codon 13 was detected during the neoplastic progression of the disease.[1036]

Mutations of the N-*ras* gene have been detected in a few cases of solid human tumors, especially in gastrointestinal cancers. Only a very small fraction of these tumors would contain N-*ras* mutations. Only 1 of 35 human colorectal cancers that occurred in Japanese patients contained a mutation (G-C transversion) at codon 13 of the N-*ras* gene.[1037] N-*ras* mutation was detected in a fresh human gastric adenocarcinoma tumor tissue and the analysis revealed a single base change in codon 61 of the gene, resulting in the substitution of an arginine in place of glutamine at this position of the protein.[996] Mutation at codon 13 of N-*ras* was also detected in a surgically removed stomach cancer with the histological diagnosis of poorly differentiated adenocarcinoma.[1038] The mutation resulted in the substitution of arginine for glycine at the respective position of the p21 protein. Differences in the transforming activities of mutants at codon 13 of N-*ras* genes could be related to the particular type of amino acid substitution, but the mechanisms involved in the oncogenic potential of mutant c-*ras* proteins remain elusive.

4. Conclusion

Somatic mutations of c-*ras* protooncogenes occur apparently randomly among different types of human malignant diseases. At least in some cases, only a minority of the tumor cells contain the mutation. These mutations are selectively localized at codon 12, 13, or 61 of the genes. The altered protein products of mutant c-*ras* genes could have a role in the origin and/ or progression of certain tumor cell populations *in vivo*. Mutations of c-*ras* gene do not usually correlate with known biological parameters or with the clinical behavior of human tumors. These mutations may be present in benign, self-regressing tumors such as human keratoacanthomas, and they are apparently not necessary or sufficient to develop and maintain the expression of a transformed phenotype.[1015] Most probably, c-*ras* mutations constitute only one of the several steps required by certain human cells to express a fully malignant phenotype. Further studies are required for establishing the exact role of mutant c-*ras* genes in human tumorigenic processes.

E. MUTATION OF PROTOONCOGENES IN EXPERIMENTAL TUMORS

As stated in a previous section of this chapter, activated protooncogenes have been detected by DNA transfection assays in different types of experimental tumors. However, the molecular changes involved in this activation were characterized in only a part of these cases. The use of modern biochemical methods has allowed the characterization of protooncogene mutations associated with experimentally induced animal tumors.[100]

1. Mutation of c-*ras* Genes

A DNA fragment cloned from a mouse tumor induced by γ-radiation contained a single base pair difference (G-A) in the exonic sequence of c-K-*ras*, determining a change of glycine to aspartic acid in the transformed cell.[1039] Direct mutagenesis of c-H-*ras*-1 genes can occur during initiation of mammary carcinomas induced in rats by *N*-nitroso-*N*-methylurea (NMU).[1040] G-A transition, the type of mutation induced by NMU, occurs in c-H-*ras*-1 genes present in the mammary tumors induced by this carcinogen. Of 48 NMU-induced tumor DNAs, 36 (75%) were positive for the appearance of foci in the NIH/3T3 assay and each of 36 NMU-induced tumors carried the same activating mutation (G-A transition) in an c-H-*ras*-1 protooncogene.[1040] NMU is also capable of inducing thymic tumors in mice. In one of these tumors, a C-A transversion in the first base of codon 61 of the N-*ras* gene associated with deletion of the normal allele was detected.[1041] A significant percentage of thymic lymphomas induced in mice by either NMU or γ-radiation contain activated protooncogenes of the c-*ras* family (c-K-*ras* and N-*ras*) and cloning and sequencing of the activated genes showed that they contain single base substitutions which result in amino acid changes at either codon 12 or 61 of the p21 protein.[99]

Activating mutations of the c-H-*ras* gene were observed in each of 25 hepatomas induced in male B6C3 F1 mice by administration of a single dose of three structurally different carcinogens (*N*-hydroxy-2-acetylaminofluorene, vinyl carbamate, and 1′-hydroxy-2′,3′-dehydroestragole).[1042] The majority of these mutations were localized in codon 61 of the c-H-*ras* gene. In contrast, only 14 of 33 liver tumors induced in B6C3F1 mice and 1 of 28 liver tumors induced in Fischer 344 rats by a single injection of *N*-nitrosodiethylamine were positive in the NIH/3T3 transfection assay.[112] The mouse tumors positive in the transfection assay contained transition or transversion mutations at the first or second base of codon 61 of c-H-*ras*. Most of the tumors induced in mice and rats with *N*-nitrosodiethylamine may involve genetic targets other than c-H-*ras* genes.

Furan and furfural are two compounds that have hepatocarcinogenic activity in mice but that are negative for induction of mutations in the commonly used *Salmonella* assay (Ames test). Liver tumors induced in mice with furan and furfural frequently give positive results in the NIH/3T3 DNA transfection assay.[1043] Of 10 hepatocellular carcinomas, 4 induced by furan and 11 of 13 hepatocellular carcinomas induced by furfural were positive in the NIH/3T3 assay system. Benign liver adenomas induced by the same compounds were also frequently positive in the assay. Both the adenomas and the carcinomas that appeared in the mouse liver after treatment with furan or furfural and which were positive in the NIH/3T3 DNA transfection assay contained mutations in the c-H-*ras* or c-K-*ras* protooncogenes. While spontaneous liver tumors appearing in mice contain only mutations at codon 61 of c-H-*ras*, the furan- and furfural-induced tumors frequently contain point mutation affecting other codons of either c-H-*ras* or c-K-*ras* genes (codons 13 and 117). Although the biological significance of such mutations is not clear, the results may provide a basis for risk assessment of potential carcinogenic compounds.[1043]

G-T transversion in codon 12 was detected in the c-K-*ras* gene of 1 of 7 fibrosarcomas induced in rats by 1,8-dinitropyrene.[1044] Activated c-K-*ras* and N-*ras* genes have been detected in primary renal mesenchymal tumors induced in F344 rats by methyl(methoxymethyl)nitrosamine.[1045]

DMBA-induced mouse mammary tumors may be associated with specific mutational activation of the c-H-*ras* protooncogene.[1046] This activation consists in an A-T transversion at the middle nucleotide of codon 61 and it is apparently specific for DMBA, not being found in spontaneous tumors or in tumors induced in the same animals by X-irradiation. DNA isolated from carcinomas induced in the mouse skin by DMBA or dibenz(*c,h*)acridine, but not benzo(*a*)pyrene, frequently contain amplified c-H-*ras* genes mutated at the 61st codon.[1047] Over 90% of tumors, including papillomas, initiated in the mouse skin with DMBA have a specific A-T transversion at the second nucleotide of codon 61 of the c-H-*ras* gene.[540,1048] The frequency of this mutation depends on the initiating agent used, but not on the promoter, suggesting that the mutation occurs at the time of initiation. The mutation was found to be heterozygous in most papillomas, but was homozygous or amplified in some carcinomas. Similar results were obtained in an independent study with a two-stage mouse skin carcinogenesis model.[317] The conclusion is that c-H-*ras* point mutation can occur very early in the development of carcinogen-induced mouse papillomas, perhaps immediately following carcinogen application. Interestingly, several cell lines established from papillomas induced in mice by the DMBA/TPA initiation-promotion protocol did not contain a point mutation in codon 61 of the c-H-*ras* gene, and the p21[c-ras] product of these lines did not exhibit altered electrophoretic migration.[1049] The reason for such a discrepancy between the primary tumor cells and the cell lines is not clear.

An A-T transversion detected in codon 61 of a c-H-*ras* gene contained in a mouse skin squamous cell carcinoma induced by topical application of the direct-acting alkylating agent β-propiolactone could be caused by a direct alkylation of the middle adenine of the codon by the β-propiolactone-DNA adduct.[1050] It seems likely that activated oncogenes found in other experimental tumors may also contain mutated c-*ras* genes.

The efficiency and selectivity of certain mutagenic agents for inducing a specific protooncogene mutation is striking. Single doses of NMU activated c-H-*ras* by a G to A base change in all of 61 rat mammary tumors that gave positive results in the NIH/3T3 DNA transfection assay.[957] Natural selection for mutations that impart growth advantages to the cells is the explanation given for this positional bias,[1051] but this explanation is inconsistent with the efficiencies of transformation of NIH/3T3 cells by mutations at other positions in c-H-*ras*.[1052] Alternative explanations are that some DNA sequences may present particular base positions as easy targets to the mutagen or that some DNA sequences may hide mutagenic lesions from repair activities so that the molecular lesions persist.

Because there is usually a long delay (several months) between administration of the carcinogen and appearance of the tumor, the possibility should be considered that the carcinogen is not acting directly to induce point mutations in the c-*ras* protooncogenes. However, it has been shown that plasmids containing the human c-H-*ras*-1 protooncogene can be modified *in vitro* by treatment with ultimate carcinogens.[115-117] The modified plasmids contain mutations at either codon 12 or codon 61 of the protooncogene protein product and exhibit transforming activity upon transfection into NIH/3T3 cells.

Experiments involving chronic exposure of animals to compounds that are potentially carcinogenic to humans are important for the evaluation of occupational cancer risks. Rats and mice chronically exposed to tetranitromethane, a highly volatile compound used in several industrial processes, develop lung tumors of varied histological types, similar to lung tumors occurring in humans. Transfection of tumor cell DNA into NIH/3T3 cells gave results positive for neoplastic transformation in 14 of 19 rat lung tumors and 4 of 4 mouse lung tumors.[1053] The tumors positive in the DNA transfection assay contained mutation (GC to AT transition) at codon 12 of c-K-*ras*.

The exact relationship between specific mutations of c-*ras* genes and experimental carcinogenesis remains to be elucidated but the available evidence suggests that mutation of c-*ras* gene at specific sites may represent one important step in the multistage process leading to the formation of tumors induced by treatment with particular carcinogenic agents. Transfection of first passage rat embryo cells with a plasmid construct containing a mutated EJ c-H-*ras* gene results in a rapid conversion to a tumorigenic but not metastatic phenotype; cotransfection of the cells with both EJ c-H-*ras* and c-*myc* genes induces the expression of both tumorigenic and metastatic capabilities.[25]

The reason for the apparently very high sensitivity of c-*ras* gene to carcinogen-induced mutation at specific codon sites is not clear at present. Furthermore, in contrast to the rather high incidence of c-*ras* mutations detected in experimental systems using rodent cells, no evidence of c-*ras* mutation or activation was found with a system using human epidermal keratinocytes immortalized by Ad12 and SV40 and transformed thereafter with chemical carcinogens.[1054] About 60% of keratoacanthomas induced in rabbits by repeated applications of DMBA contained a c-H-*ras* gene mutated at codon 12.[1015] However, karatoacanthomas occurring in both rabbits and humans are benign, self-regressing tumors, which indicates that the expression of a mutated c-*ras* gene may be insufficient to develop and/or maintain a malignant phenotype. Thus, the general importance of c-*ras* mutations in experimental carcinogenic processes is not readily apparent.

2. Mutation of the c-*neu* Gene

Oncogenic activation of the c-*neu* gene may be associated with neurogenic tumors (schwannomas) induced in rats with *N*-ethyl-*N*-nitrosourea.[1055,1056] The cells of these tumors contain in their DNA a T to A transversion which affects the transmembrane domain of the p185^{c-neu} product.

F. MECHANISMS RESPONSIBLE FOR THE INCREASED TRANSFORMING POTENTIAL OF MUTANT P21^{c-ras} PROTEINS

The mechanisms responsible for the increased transforming potential of mutant c-*ras* genes remain little understood. Phenotypic alterations induced *in vitro* by mutant c-*ras* alleles may not represent, however, a discrete qualitative event but a continuum according to the amounts of altered p21^{c-ras} products present within the cells. The malignant transformation of cultured rat fibroblasts induced by transfection of mutant c-*ras* genes is a gradual but reversible process that depends on the relative abundance of mutant c-*ras* sequences and their corresponding transcripts.[36,37] Clonal NIH/3T3 cell lines expressing multiple copies of a mutant c-H-*ras* gene with valine substitution at codon 12 have a more transformed phenotype than cells expressing only a single copy of the mutant gene.[34] The results of these experiments indicate that a minimum level of mutant c-*ras* gene products may be critical for the expression of a malignant phenotype and that the continuous presence of the mutant c-*ras* gene is necessary not only for the initiation but also for the maintenance of the transformed phenotype.

Human cells are generally considered as resistant to transformation by mutant c-*ras* genes, but normal diploid human fibroblasts in culture can be transformed *in vitro* into morphologically altered, focus-forming, and anchorage-independent cells following transfection with a T24 c-H-*ras* gene exprssed at high levels by a plasmid vector.[1057] However, the transfected human cells are nontumorigenic in nude mice and they revert to a normal phenotype as the cells are passaged in culture. It may be concluded that normal human cells are rather resistant to transformation induced by mutant c-*ras* genes.

Experiments with transgenic mice support the notion that tumorigenesis associated with the expression of mutated c-*ras* genes is a multistage process protracted over a long period of time and that additional genetic changes are crucially required in order for tumor formation to occur. Mammary gland-specific, hormone-dependent expression of an EJ c-H-*ras* gene introduced into the germ line of transgenic mice resulted in the formation of mammary tumors in only a few of the animals and after a long latency period.[41]

The molecular mechanisms responsible for the increased transforming potential of mutant p21[*ras*] products altered at specific positions (codons 12 or 61 in human cells), as tested in the NIH/3T3 assay or other assay systems, are unknown. Not only the mammalian proteins carrying mutation at either codons 12 or 61 have an increased transforming potential on NIH/3T3 cells but also yeast proteins encoded by *ras*-related genes, normally present in the yeast genome, have the same oncogenic potential when point mutations are introduced into the regions coding for the corresponding amino acids in the yeast DNA sequences.[1058] It is thus apparent that these sites are of critical importance for some functional property of the *ras* gene products.

The reasons for the apparently very high susceptibility of particular sites of c-*ras* gene sequences to point mutational events are unknown. Studies on experimental mutagenesis with the benzo(*a*)pyrene metabolite *anti*-BPDE suggest that particular DNA sequences, such as alternating sequences of CGs, may be prone to strand scissions by some chemical carcinogenic agents, and these sequences have been found in the DNA region of codon 12 of the c-H-*ras* protooncogene.[1059] It is not clear at present, however, whether there are specific DNA sequences that act as hot spots for different types of DNA-reacting carcinogens. Mutagenic agents such as NMU have a strikingly high efficiency for inducing selective base substitutions in c-H-*ras* genes,[957] but the molecular basis of this property is not clear,[1052] and the general validity of this mechanism for c-*ras* mutation occurring under natural conditions is not apparent.

DNA fragments from normal human lymphocytes may acquire transforming activity in the NIH/3T3 assay as a consequence of spontaneous activation (mutation at codon 12) of c-*ras* genes.[1060,1061] Studies with random bisulfite-induced mutagenesis on the cloned wild-type human c-H-*ras* gene indicate that, although most mutations are not activating, mutations that specify single amino acid substitutions at positions 12, 13, 59, or 63 of the encoded protein do activate the transforming potential of the c-H-*ras* protooncogene.[1062] However, only mutations specifying amino acid substitutions at position 12, 13 or 61 have been found in human tumor cells. The reasons of this discrepancy are unknown.

1. Structural and Functional Alterations of Mutant p21 Proteins

In DNA transfection assays the cloned mutant c-*ras* genes have a transforming potency that is several orders of magnitude greater than that of cloned nonmutant c-*ras*, and models for explaining the detected enhanced activity have been proposed.[1063-1067] The biochemical, antigenic, and biological properties of the normal and mutant human c-*ras* p21 proteins may be different.[1068-1071] Human p21[c-*ras*] products activated by mutations at codon 12 or 61 can be distinguished from one another by differences in the electrophoretic mobilities under reducing and nonreducing conditions, which suggests that intramolecular disulfide bonds affect native p21[c-*ras*] conformation.[1072] Substitution of valine in EJ c-H-*ras* for the glycine in normal c-H-*ras* results in the production of antisera of considerably divergent reactivities.[1073]

Marked functional alteration of the mutant p21[c-*ras*] products has been predicted from three dimensional models of the protein.[987,1063-1067,1074] Substitution of any L-amino acid for the normal glycine at position 12 of p21[c-*ras*] would cause major structural changes in the polypeptide, resulting in enhanced capacity for inducing malignant transformation.[1066] By use of site-directed mutagenesis it has been shown that different deletions and insertions of amino acid residues in the region of residue 12 are effective in conferring oncogenic activity on the p21 product of c-H-*ras*.[1075] Common to these various alterations is the disruption that they create in this domain of the protein, which may result in the inactivation of a normal function of p21. The loop of the mutated c-*ras* protein that binds the β-phosphate of the guanine nucleotide is enlarged.[1067] This change in the "catalytic site" conformation may explain the reduced GTPase activity of the mutant, which would keep the protein in the GTP-bound "signal on" state for a prolonged period of time, ultimately leading to neoplastic transformation.

2. Autophosphorylation of p21

Autophosphorylation of the v-H-*ras* p21 protein is modulated by amino acid residue 12 and microinjection of the mutant T24 p21^{ras} protein results in rapid proliferation of quiescent cultured cells.[1076,1077] The p21 product of the viral H-*ras* oncogene has greater auto-phosphorylating activity with a valine at residue 12 than with a glycine,[1078] but the possible relation of this change to the acquisition of increased cell transforming activity is not understood. It is noticeable that the same mutation, AGT at codon 12 of the p21 protein, is also present in human c-H-*ras*-2, which is a processed pseudogene inactivated by numerous base substitutions.[1079] There is evidence that p21-induced oncogenic transformation occurs by mechanisms not necessarily involving the autophosphorylating activity of p21.[1080]

3. GTP Binding and GTPase Activity of p21

The purified p21 product of human c-H-*ras* possesses intrinsic GTPase activity and this activity is decreased by a valine at residue 12 or a threonine at residue 59 of the mole-cule.[1068,1078,1081] The normal p21^{c-ras} protein may exhibit between five and ten times higher GTPase activity than the "activated" mutant protein.[1068,1082] Recombinant plasmids carrying the human c-H-*ras* gene with two point mutations in codons 12 and 61 have the same transforming activity in the NIH/3T3 DNA transfection assay as the genes with single mutations.[988] Thus, a single point mutation of c-*ras* would be enough to reduce the GTPase activity of p21 and activate the oncogenic potential of the gene. The severalfold reduction of p21^{ras}-associated GTPase activity observed in the T24 mutant product in comparison to the normal human c-H-*ras* p21 product may result in prolonged stimulation of an otherwise regulatable activity within the cell.[1082] A diminished ability to hydrolize GTP efficiently could result in persistent activation of the system, which could be responsible for the uncontrolled cell division and transformation ability associated with p21^{c-ras} proteins containing mutations at some particular positions of the amino acid chain (codons 12 or 61 of human cells). However, there is clear evidence that activation of efficient transforming properties by p21^{c-ras} can occur by mechanisms which are independent of a reduced p21 GTP binding and GTPase activity.[1083-1085]

An antibody that specifically recognizes an epitope of p21^{ras} including amino acid 12 blocks binding of GTP to p21 and, conversely, guanine nucleotides prevent interaction of the antibody with p21.[1086] Transient reversion of *ras* oncogene-induced cell transformation can be obtained by antibodies specific for amino acid 12 of the p21 protein.[1087] This antibody inhibits binding of GTP to the v-K-*ras* p21 product. These results would support the hypothesis that interaction of p21^{ras} with guanine nucleotides at a region including amino acid 12 of p21 is required for the transforming function of the protein. However, amino acid substitution at position 12 of p21^{ras} does not modify the GTP or GDP binding ability of the protein, which makes the possibility of a direct contribution of this residue to the binding site unlikely.[1083]

The protein products of constructed *ras* mutant genes containing amino acid substitutions at *ras* codon 83, 119, or 144 show decreased affinity for GTP binding by a factor of 25 to 100, primarily as a consequence of increased rates of dissociation of GTP from p21.[1088] Nevertheless, these artificial mutant genes induce transformation of NIH/3T3 cells with efficiencies compa-rable to that of the v-H-*ras* oncogene. Single amino acid substitutions introduced by site-directed mutagenesis into a region of p21^{c-ras} which is homologous to a variety of GTP-binding proteins (amino acid residues 116, 117, and 119) result in p21 proteins with 10- to 5000-fold reduction in GTP binding activity but with unaltered ability to morphologically transform NIH/3T3 cells.[1089] A constructed p21 mutant with a substitution of valine for glycine at position 10 did not exhibit ability to bind GTP and had lost autokinase activity but was fully capable of transforming

NIH/3T3 cells to a tumorigenic phenotype.[1090] Thus, a role for GTP binding and hydrolysis in *ras*-induced oncogenic transformation is not readily apparent on the basis of the results obtained in such experiments.

Normal (glycine-12) and two mutant (asparagine-12 and valine-12) forms of human N-*ras* proteins have no significant differences in their affinities for GTP or GDP but the mutant proteins have a significantly reduced GTPase activity.[1085] The valine-12 mutant retains only 12% of wild-type GTPase activity, whereas the asparagine-12 mutant retains 43%. Both mutants, however, were equally potent in causing transformation after their microinjection into NIH/3T3 cells. In general, there is a lack of correlation between the guanine nucleotide binding or GTPase activity of p21 proteins and their transforming potency.

Recent studies suggest the existence of a cytoplasmic protein, called GTPase activated protein (GAP), that stimulates the hydrolysis of GTP by normal p21[c-ras] more than 200-fold *in vitro*, but that has no effect on position-12 p21 mutants.[1091] The major effect of mutations at position 12 of p21 would be to prevent GAP from stimulating p21 GTPase activity, thereby allowing these mutants to remain in the active, GTP-bound state. The possible relationship between this alteration and neoplastic transformation has not been determined.

4. Mitogenic Activity of p21 Proteins

Nuclear microinjection of c-H-*ras* DNA is capable of inducing DNA synthesis in nonproliferating, quiescent human diploid fibroblasts but the normal and mutated (EJ/T24) forms of c-H-*ras* are equally effective inducers of mitogenesis.[1092] Senescent nondividing normal human cells do not respond to the mitogenic effects of c-H-*ras* either alone or in combination with the adenovirus E1A gene.

5. Regulation of G Proteins by p21 Proteins

Hormone-stimulated adenylate cyclase activity is reduced in NIH/3T3 cells expressing high levels of the EJ-*ras* gene product.[1093] Proteins p21[ras] share sequence homology with the α subunit of G proteins and may be involved in regulation of G proteins. Mutations that activate p21 products can produce an altered regulation of particular cellular systems associated with G protein activity. G proteins regulate the activity of phospholipases A2 and C and the activity of these enzymes may be deregulated by the presence of mutant p21 products, which may result in reduced production of PGE_2 and arachidonate.[1094]

6. Metabolic Turnover of p21 Proteins

The metabolic turnover of normal and mutant (EJ) c-H-*ras* p21 proteins is similar (intracellular half-life of 20 h), but the v-H-*ras* p21 protein, which differs from the c-*ras* protooncogene by mutation at the 12th codon and other structural changes, is more stable in cells (half-life of 42 h), apparently due to differences in phosphorylation.[1095] It is unlikely that the different transforming capabilities of p21 proteins are due to differences in their respective metabolic turnover.

7. Adenylate Cyclase Activity and p21-Induced Transformation

The adenylate cyclase system may have a role in transformation induced by either v-*ras* proteins or mutant c-*ras* proteins. Adenylate cyclase activity is depressed in C127 mouse fibroblasts infected with wild-type K-MuSV but the activity increases when cells infected with a *ts* mutant of K-MuSV are shifted from the permissive temperature to the nonpermissive temperature.[1096] Reduced hormone-stimulated adenylate cyclase activity is observed in NIH/3T3 cells expressing the mutated EJ human c-*ras* gene.[1093] However, the possible relationship between cellular adenylate cyclase activity and p21-induced transformation is not understood.

Activity of cAMP-dependent protein kinase is decreased in the soluble fraction, but not in the particulate fraction, of NIH/3T3 cells transformed by either a v-H-*ras* oncogene or an activated c-H-*ras* gene, as compared with the level of activity present in unaltered NIH/3T3 cells.[1097] The decrease of cAMP-dependent protein kinase activity found in the transfected cells may be indirectly induced by the v-H-*ras* or the activated c-H-*ras* genes since the p21 products of these genes have no direct effects on the enzyme. Proteolytic cleavage of the regulatory subunit of cAMP-dependent protein kinase is inhibited by p21 proteins.[1098] In any case, the possible significance of the detected alteration is unknown.

8. Activation of Phosphatidylinositol Turnover

Activated c-*ras* proteins may be involved in modulation of phosphatidylinositol turnover with increased production of inositol trisphosphate, which would lead to increased generation of 1,2-diacylglycerol, mobilization of intracellular Ca^{2+}, and activation of protein kinase C.[1099,1100] These effects may be achieved through the coupling of surface receptors to phospholipase C. Mutant c-*ras* proteins would inactivate the phospholipase C constitutively, thus enhancing the basal level of inositol phospholipid breakdown.[1101] However, NIH/3T3 cells transformed by the EJ c-H-*ras* gene have markedly reduced PDGF-stimulated phospholipase C activity and PGE_2 biosynthesis.[1094] Chinese hamster lung fibroblasts (CCL39 cells) transfected with T24 c-H-*ras* or v-K-*ras* genes are highly tumorigenic in nude mice, but a constitutive activation of phospholipase C is not observed in these cells.[1102] Thus, the role of phosphoinositide metabolism and protein kinase C activity in neoplastic transformation associated with mutant c-*ras* genes or v-*ras* oncogenes is not clear.

9. Alteration of Glycolipid Metabolism

Transfection of NIH/3T3 cells with activated c-*ras* genes results in decreased levels of particular gangliosides (GM1 and GD1a), as compared to logarithmically growing normal NIH/3T3 cells.[1103] Similar alterations occur in MuSV-transformed mouse fibroblasts.

10. Interaction of p21 with other Cellular Proteins

Activation of c-*ras* genes in human tumors does not affect subcellular localization, posttranslational modification, or guanine nucleotide binding properties of p21.[1104] Thus, the mutational activation of p21$^{c\text{-}ras}$ may be a consequence of alterations in the interaction of p21 with other cellular proteins rather than a change in the intrinsic biochemical activity of p21. An intact cysteine residue at position 186 of the p21^{ras} gene product is required for both membrane localization and transforming ability of the protein.[1105] Deletion of the 23 carboxy-terminal part of oncogenic p21^{ras} proteins (p21$^{v\text{-}ras}$ or mutated p21$^{c\text{-}ras}$) results in a drastic reduction of their transforming capacities.[1106] Thus, both the amino-terminal part of p21^{ras} molecules, involved in guanine nucleotide binding, and the carboxyl-terminal part, involved in their localization to the inner face of the cell membrane, are necessary for the expression of a transforming capacity.

Recent evidence indicates that p21$^{c\text{-}ras}$ protein possesses inhibitory activity against cathepsin L, a proteinase involved in the degradation of the EGF receptor.[1107] These results suggest the possibility that p21 proteins can suppress the degradation of growth-related proteins such as EGF receptors and thereby affect cell proliferation and/or differentiation. However, the presence of a functional EGF receptor is apparently not required for *ras*-mediated neoplastic transformation. Murine NR6 cells, which lack functional EGF receptors, acquire a fully transformed phenotype upon transfection with a plasmid carrying an activated EJ c-H-*ras* gene.[1108]

11. Accelerated Rate of Glucose Transport

An accelerated rate of glucose transport is among the most characteristic cellular alterations occurring in neoplastic transformation. The rate of glucose uptake is markedly increased in rat fibroblasts transfected with an activated EJ c-H-*ras* gene.[1109] A similar increase is observed in cells transfected with a v-*src* oncogene as well as in cells exposed to phorbol ester (TPA), but not in cells transfected with an activated c-*myc* gene. The increased transport of glucose into the cell is paralleled by a marked increase in the amount of glucose transporter mRNA and protein.

12. Alteration of Intracellular Communication

Cells neoplastically transformed by oncogenes or other agents may exhibit a selective blockage of functional intercellular communication. BALB/c 3T3 cells transformed by transfection of the EJ c-H-*ras* gene show a lack of communication with nontransformed cells, as assessed by microinjection of a fluorescent dye.[1110] This lack of intercellular communication may contribute to maintain autonomous growth in transformed cells.

13. Reduction of Collagen Production

Basement membranes are thin layers of extracellular matrix that separate epithelial structures from the surrounding stroma and that may function as a barrier to the passage of both epithelial and mesenchymal cells.[1111] The basement membrane appears to play a crucial role during the progression of invasive tumors and during hematogenous dissemination.[1112] A characteristic of some malignant tumors is a loss of basement membrane in areas of invasion, but the mechanisms responsible for this loss are not well understood. Transformation of a mouse mammary epithelial cell line (NMuMg) with a mutated EJ c-H-*ras* gene results in a marked reduction in the capacity of cells to produce collagen when the cells are grown on collagen gels.[1111] This alteration may facilitate the invasion of the stroma by cells carrying mutated c-*ras* genes.

14. Alteration in Gene Expression

The effects of mutated c-*ras* gene products on the expression of other cellular genes is little known. Expression of a cloned inducible T24 c-H-*ras* gene in cultured rat liver epithelial cells increases the steady-state RNA levels of γ-glutamyltransferase and glutathione transferase-P.[1113] The level of activity of these two enzymes is also altered in carcinogen-induced rat liver tumors, suggesting that both activated oncogenes and chemical carcinogens may produce similar biochemical alterations in relation to neoplastic transformation. Expression of a T24 c-H-*ras* gene in cultured rat fibroblasts (aneuploid cell line 208F) was associated with enhanced expression of c-*abl* and c-*fos* genes, whereas the expression of seven other protooncogenes analyzed was not altered.[1114]

15. Cell Susceptibility to Transformation Induced by *ras* Protein Products

Mutant p21[c-*ras*] products, as well as mutant products of other protooncogenes, are apparently unable to induce by themselves neoplastic transformation of normal cells since immortality of the mouse fibroblasts or other cells used for *in vitro* tests is a prerequisite for the occurrence of transformation.[1011]

The susceptibility to transformation by c-*ras* genes may be markedly different in cells from different species, or in different types of cell from a given species. Human cells are generally more resistant to transformation than are rodent cells. Cultured rodent fibroblasts (NIH/3T3 cells) can be transformed by a normal human c-H-*ras* protooncogene ligated to a control element (LTR) from a murine or feline retrovirus.[1115] Early passage hamster and rat cells can be completely transformed by the mutant c-H-*ras*-1 gene from T24 human bladder carcinoma when linked to a transcriptional enhancer, but the normal c-H-*ras*-1 protooncogene is only capable of inducing immortalization, not transformation, in the same system.[1116] Transfection of mutated EJ c-H-*ras* gene, under the transcriptional control of its own promoter, is able to induce the malignant transformation of a preneoplastic cell line established after treatment of hamster epidermal cells with the carcinogen, *N*-methyl-*N*'-nitro-*N*-nitrosoguanidine (MNNG).[108] Human cells are generally resistant to c-*ras*-induced tumorigenic transformation.

Cultured normal human cells (FS-2 diploid, neonatal human fibroblasts) are not transformed by the cloned EJ gene in spite of the presence of increased levels of the mutant p21 product.[1117]

16. Cooperation between Mutant c-*ras* Genes and other Protooncogenes

While the expression of a mutant c-*ras* gene alone may not be sufficient to induce the expression of a transformed phenotype, coexpression of c-*ras* and other oncogene or protoon-cogene may induce this expression, which supports the multistep hypothesis of neoplastic transformation. The mouse embryonic fibroblast cell line C3H/10T1/2 is only partially trans-formed after transfection with a T24 c-H-*ras* gene, but cotransfection of these cells with the T24 c-H-*ras* gene and a v-*myc* oncogene results in the appearance of a large number of foci of morphologically transformed cells that show anchorage-independent growth in soft agar.[1118] Cooperation between the mutant c-H-*ras* oncogene and other protooncogenes such as c-*myc* or N-*myc*, may be important for the expression of tumorigenic properties in secondary REF cells after transfection with molecular vectors expressing the oncogene sequences.[1119,1120] Augmented expression of a normal cloned c-*myc* protooncogene may be sufficient for cotransformation of REF cells with a mutant EJ/T24 c-*ras* gene.[1121,1122] In a human lung cancer cell line (Lu-65) point mutation of c-K-*ras* was combined with amplification of c-*myc*.[420] Multiple protooncogene alteration may be more frequent than suspected previously. From 12 human tumors and tumor cell lines examined, 3 tumor cell lines and 2 primary solid tumors contained an amplification of c-*myc* (5- to 10-fold) and a third protooncogene was found to be amplified and rearranged in the two primary solid tumors.[1123] The possible role of dual or multiple protooncogene alterations in the general mechanisms of carcinogenesis remains undetermined, but the results obtained in these studies suggest that protooncogenes may participate through different alterations in the multistage genetic processes that lead to tumorigenic processes.

Previous immortality required for expression of the oncogenic potential of a T24 c-H-*ras* oncogene can be conferred to cells with a definite lifespan (cultured adult rat chondrocytes) by transfection of cloned cDNA sequences encoding antigen p53 of murine origin.[1124] The results obtained in these experiments suggest that expression of p53 is associated with the acquisition of cellular immortality and that the immortalized cells are susceptible to transformation by a mutated c-*ras* oncogene. However, expression of a mutated c-*ras* gene in certain types of cells may also be associated with immortalization rather than with proliferation. For example, transfection of BRK cells with a vector plasmid carrying the EJ c-H-*ras* gene leads to immortalization and not to transformation, although this immortalization renders the transfected cells more susceptible to other transforming factors.[1125] Interestingly, even low levels of expression of the mutated c-H-*ras* gene induce deregulation in the expression of the endogenous c-*myc* gene and increased sensitivity to growth factors, which may contribute to the acquisition of neoplastic properties.

Primary human embryonic kidney (HEK) cells are capable of growth in soft agar after transfection with a combination of the human papovavirus BK and the mutant EJ c-H-*ras*-1 gene.[1126] Thus, it is evident that genetic and/or epigenetic changes in addition to the presence of an activating c-*ras* mutation are required for the malignant transformation of susceptible cells. However, mutant c-*ras* genes, in conjunction with other genes, which may or may not be protooncogenes, could contribute to the neoplastic progression of transformed cells.

17. Production of Chromosome Aberrations

Numerical and/or structural chromosome aberrations are almost universally present in tumor cells. Transformation induced by *ras* oncogenes of either viral or cellular origin may be, however, independent of chromosome abnormalities. Early passage diploid rat embryo cells transformed by cloned *ras* genes (v-H-*ras* of EJ c-H-*ras*) acquire tumorigenic properties and are capable of developing metastases after injection into nude mice without the appearance of any chromosome changes or increased rates of SCE.[1127,1128] These studies demonstrate that *ras* oncogenes can lead to transformation with tumorigenic and metastatic potential without the requirement for selection of karyotypically abnormal clones.

18. Autocrine Mechanisms

Several human tumor cell lines producing TGFs contain mutant c-*ras* genes. Transfection of these mutant c-*ras* genes into the genome of normal rodent cells results in the induction of TGFs, accompanied by morphological transformation and *in vivo* tumorigenicity of these recipients.[1129,1130] The induction of TGF-α expression occurs at the level of transcription. Reversion to a normal phenotype by deletion of the exogenous c-*ras* genes is also accompanied by loss of the ability to produce TGFs. These results suggest that at least one of the pathways by which mutant c-*ras* genes induce malignant transformation of established rodent fibroblasts may be the activation of TGF production by these cells, especially the production of TGF-α. However, it is rather unlikely that neoplastic transformation induced by v-*ras* oncogenes or activated c-*ras* genes is universally mediated by the endogenous production of TGFs or other growth factors by an autocrine type of mechanism. In contrast to the susceptibility of some established rodent cell lines to transformation induced by c-*ras* genes containing activating mutations, normal human cells (cultured mesothelial cells and fibroblasts) are resistant to neoplastic transformation induced by introduction of these gene and remain dependent on the exogenous supply of serum factors for their growth *in vitro*.[11]

19. Suppression of Transformation Induced by c-*ras* Genes

The continued presence of a mutant p21^{ras} product may be compatible with reversion of the transformed phenotype. Tumorigenicity was suppressed in EJ bladder carcinoma cells after fusion with normal human fibroblast cells in spite of the continued expression of the mutated c-H-*ras* protooncogene.[1131] The fusion resulted in hybrid cells that behaved as transformed cells in culture but failed to form tumors in nude mice. After repeated cell passage, two tumorigenic segregants of the hybrids arose in culture, but the levels of mRNA and protein expression of the mutated c-H-*ras* gene were similar in the tumorigenic progenitor EJ cell line, the nontumorigenic cell hybrids, and the tumorigenic segregants. Thus, the expression of an activated, mutated c-*ras* protooncogene may be insufficient for inducing the malignant transformation of cells.

In a similar manner, a Chinese hamster embryo fibroblast (CHEF) cell line transformed by transfection of a mutant EJ c-H-*ras* gene exhibited a normal phenotype after fusion to normal CHEF cells.[14] Rat-1 cells transformed by transfection with a mutated EJ c-H-*ras* gene can also be suppressed in their transformed properties by hybridization with early-passage embryonic rat cells.[1132,1133] These suppressions occurred without interfering with the transcription or translation of the mutant c-*ras* protooncogene, which suggests that some products of normal cells can interact, modulate, or compete with the altered protooncogene product, or may act at a different point within a chain of events leading to transformation or tumorigenicity.

The results of these experiments are compatible with the existence of tumor suppressor genes, antioncogenes, or emerogenes, i.e., genes capable of suppressing the neoplastic transformation induced by oncogenes of either viral or cellular origin. However, other hypotheses may be equally plausible for explaining the results obtained in such experiments. The results suggest a recessive behavior of the mutant c-*ras* gene, which is in apparent contradiction with the usual dominant behavior of oncogenes. In any case, it is clear that the continued expression of a mutated, oncogenically activated c-*ras* gene is compatible with suppression of tumorigenic properties.

20. Continued Expression of Tumorigenicity in Cells that have Lost a Mutant c-*ras* Gene

For an unknown reason, NIH/3T3 cells transfected with a mutant T24 c-H-*ras* gene acquire a normal phenotype and subsequently lose the protooncogene when cultured in the presence of nonlethal concentrations of methionine.[1134] However, a substantial proportion of subclones from the cells that have lost the mutant protooncogene are still capable of giving rise to tumors, which indicates that the mutant c-H-*ras* gene is not responsible for the tumorigenic properties of these cells.

21. Mutant c-*ras* Genes and Expression of Differentiated Functions

The mutated, oncogenic forms of p21$^{c\text{-}ras}$ proteins may interfere with the normal processes of cell differentiation or may block the expression of differentiated functions. Transfection of the skeletal mouse muscle cell lines C2 and BC$_3$H1 with oncogenic N-*ras* or c-H-*ras* alleles completely suppresses expression of muscle-specific genes after withdrawal of myoblasts from the cell cycle in medium without mitogens.[1135,1136] In contrast, the normal c-*ras* protooncogenes do not have apparent effects on the ability of C2 cells to differentiate into muscle cells. These results suggest that mutated c-*ras* gene can inhibit myogenic processes through a mechanism independent of cell proliferation and can preclude activation of genes whose up regulation normally accompanies mitogen withdrawal.

Transfection of a mutated EJ c-H-*ras* gene into P19 embryonal carcinoma cells does not interfere with differentiation induced by retinoic acid.[1137] The transfected cells develop in response to retinoic acid into the same spectrum of neuroectodermal cell types as the parental P19 cells, which suggests that p21$^{c\text{-}ras}$ is probably not a component of the cellular machinery involved in the initiation of differentiation or the choice between different cell lineages. However, although neurons and glial cells developed normally after exposure to the differentiation-inducing agent, cells with fibroblast-like morphology appeared as transformed, displaying characteristics of immortality and anchorage-independent growth. Since transfection of the mutant c-*ras* gene into fibroblasts formed from P19 cells does not result in transformation, the results suggest that there is a discrete period or "window of sensitivity" during differentiation of the fibroblast lineage when cells are susceptible to transformation by expression of the mutated EJ c-H-*ras* gene.[1137]

22. Interaction between Mutant c-*ras* Genes and Serum Factors or Tumor Promoters

Interaction between mutated c-*ras* genes and tumor promoters in the multistage processes leading to tumorigenesis is suggested by the fact that potent tumor promoters such as TPA and teleocidin cause an approximately fivefold increase in the number of transformed foci obtained in C3H 10T1/2 cells transfected with the T24 oncogene.[1138,1139] An even higher increase in T24 gene-induced neoplastic transformation *in vitro* was obtained with the addition of fetal calf serum to the culture medium.[1140] The molecular mechanisms involved in such interactions are unknown but it has been demonstrated that protein kinase C can act as a cellular receptor for phorbol esters and that TPA causes a rapid decrease in soluble protein kinase C associated with the particulate membrane fraction of cells.[1141]

23. Role of Mutant c-*ras* Genes in Tumor Progression and Metastasization

Experimental and clinical evidence indicate that mutant c-*ras* genes may be involved in the progression mechanisms of at least certain tumors. Expression of a T24 c-H-*ras* gene in both early and late passage cultured rat fibroblasts (aneuploid cell line 208F) confers to the aggressive properties of the cell, with capacity to form rapidly growing tumors capable of producing metastases.[1114] Transfection of the mouse mammary adenocarcinoma cell line SP1 with an activated T24 c-H-*ras* gene, but not with the normal c-H-*ras* gene, induced the metastatic phenotype in every clone expressing the mutant gene product.[24] Unlike the parental control cells, which are tumorigenic but unable to metastasize from a subcutaneous site, all SP1 transfectants expressing the T24 c-H-*ras* gene were able to metastasize, predominantly in the lung, in syngeneic CBA/J mice. Expression of the mutant c-H-*ras* gene was generally low in the transfected cells, which suggests that elevated expression of mutant c-*ras* genes is not required for the acquisition of metastatic potential. Results obtained with phenotypically transformed BALB/c cell lines in which the expression of a mutant T24 c-H-*ras* gene is regulated by zinc are consistent with the view that mutant c-*ras* genes play a role in the expression of a metastatic phenotype.[1142] Lung homing, implantation, and growth within the first 48 h of intravenous inoculation into mice of cells transformed by a T24 c-H-*ras* gene are regulated by NK cells from the host, but the expression of the mutated protooncogene leads subsequently to escape from immune attack and growth of lung metastases.[1143]

Transfection of the EJ c-H-*ras* gene into keratinocytes derived from carcinogen-induced mouse papillomas caused malignant progression with capability of the cells to form rapidly growing, anaplastic carcinomas in nude mice.[316] Mouse carcinoma cells transfected with an activated c-H-*ras* gene acquired enhanced spontaneous metastasis ability.[1144] NIH/3T3 cells transfected with DNA from malignant tumors which contain activated c-H-*ras* of N-*ras* genes are capable of producing experimental and spontaneous metastases in nude mice.[1145] Transfection of a constructed plasmid carrying a T24 c-H-*ras* gene into 10T1/2 mouse fibroblast cell lines resulted in acquisition of metastatic capacity, whose efficiency was closely correlated to the level of c-H-*ras* expression.[1146] The same type of plasmid, as well as plasmids carrying v-*ras* genes, confer to the transfected cells (NIH/3T3 mouse fibroblasts) an increased motility which is stimulated by components of the extracellular matrix such as laminin and fibronectin, as assessed in a micropore filter assay *in vitro*.[1147]

The role of mutant c-*ras* genes in tumor progression and metastasization is not totally clear. Both mutated and nonmutated c-*ras* genes were equally able to induce a rapid acquisition of a metastatic phenotype upon transfection into NIH/3T3 fibroblasts, followed by testing in experimental metastasis systems using nude mice.[1148] Thus, mutation-induced activation of c-*ras* genes is not necessarily associated with an enhanced potential for metastasization in experimental systems. Invasiveness and metastatic capability are often acquired in an apparently spontaneous way by some established cell lines but the rates of these spontaneous conversions are too large to provide definite evidence that either c-*ras* or c-*myc* activation are involved in the acquisition of such properties.[64,67] The metastatic potential of cells can be greatly enhanced by nonspecific manipulations such as those inherent to the DNA transfection assay.[1149] Only one of two cell line variants derived from a single colon adenocarcinoma induced in a rat by 1,2-dimethylhydrazine expressed tumorigenic properties when inoculated into the syngeneic host, but the two variants contained the same mutated c-K-*ras* gene and expressed the same levels of transcripts from this gene.[1150] Thus, the activated c-K-*ras* gene was not sufficient to induce tumorigenic progression of this cell line and factors other than the mutated c-K-*ras* gene were responsible for this progression. An enhancement of the metastatic behavior of the rat rhabdomyosarcoma cell line RMS/8 was observed after transfection with DNA from highly metastasizing tumor cells as well as with DNA from nonmetastasizing tumor cells and even with DNA from rat muscle or *Drosophila* cells. The treatment of cells with calcium phosphate alone can also strongly enhance their metastatic capability. These results suggest that rather unspecific destabilizations of the genome can result in an increased metastatic potential of certain premalignant cells. Genes that may be different from known protooncogenes may have an important role in tumor progression and metastasization.[1151]

Not all cell lines expressing activated, mutant c-*ras* genes are converted to the metastatic phenotype.[1152] Tumors produced by Fischer REF cells either before or after transfection with immortalizing or transforming genes, including the EJ or T24 c-H-*ras* gene, do not show differences in invasive or metastatic capability.[13] In any case, the relevance of these experimental manipulations in relation to spontaneous carcinogenic processes occurring in humans and other animals is unknown.

The biochemical mechanisms that would be responsible for the acquisition of invasive and metastatic potential in cells transformed by activated *ras* oncogenes are unknown. A factor with hemolytic properties has been purified from conditioned media produced by T24 c-H-*ras*-transformed NIH/3T3 cells,[1153] but the possible role of this factor in cancer invasion and metastasis has not been elucidated. Some structural DNA alterations may contribute to confer a metastatic potential to cells that have already suffered other neoplastic changes. A discrete DNA segment derived from a human tumor cell line was capable of conferring metastatic potential to NIH/3T3 mouse fibroblasts which had been transformed previously by an EJ c-H-*ras* oncogene, but no sequences related to c-*myc* or c-*ras* were detected in the DNA segment associated with the expression of the metastatic phenotype.[1154]

24. Antigenic Changes and Resistance to Immune Mechanisms

Antigenic changes on the cell surface may be associated with transformation induced by activated, mutant c-*ras* genes. NIH/3T3 cells transfected with a c-H-*ras* gene mutated at amino acid 61 of the p21 protein express a 74-kDa glycoprotein (gp74) antigen on the cell surface which is distinct from the p21$^{c\text{-}ras}$ product.[1155,1156] The same gp74 protein is also highly expressed by some human tumors, but is only minimally expressed by most normal adult tissues. A monoclonal antibody that recognizes gp74, when conjugated to the A chain of ricin toxin, can mediate an essentially complete inhibition of leucine and thymidine incorporation by the transfected cells prepared as simple cell suspensions from tumors grown *in vivo*.[1157] After 72-h incubation in the presence of the monoclonal antibody conjugated with the toxin, lysis of 80% of the protooncogene-transfected cells was demonstrated by tripan blue exclusion. The possible role of specific antigenic changes in the expression of tumorigenic properties in cells carrying mutated c-*ras* genes is unknown.

NIH/3T3 tertiary transfectants containing activated c-*ras* genes (N-*ras* or c-H-*ras*) are resistant to lysis by murine and human NK cells, although they are susceptible to lysis by LAK cells.[1158] Different protooncogenes, or the same protooncogene activated by different point mutations, do not specifically determine susceptibility to lysis by NK or LAK cells. Moreover, the presence of an activated protooncogene does not appear to be sufficient for inducing susceptibility to cytotoxic lymphocyte populations.[1158] The relevance of these studies *in vitro* to the clinical situation *in vivo*, in tumors containing mutant c-*ras* genes, is unknown.

25. Resistance of Cells Containing Mutated c-*ras* Genes to Chemotherapeutic Agents and Ionizing Radiation

The mechanisms involved in intrinsic acquired resistance of cancer cells to chemotherapeutic agents are obscure, but at least some of them include genetic changes. The possibility that such changes are related to structural and/or functional protooncogene alterations should be considered. Resistance to the anticancer drug *cis*-diaminedichloroplatinum(II) could be related to mutational activation of endogenous c-*ras* genes.[1159] NIH/3T3 fibroblasts transformed by either mutated c-H-*ras* and N-*ras* gene or v-H-*ras* and v-K-*ras* oncogenes are significantly more resistant to the chemotherapeutic agent than untransformed NIH/3T3 cells. In a similar way, NIH/3T3 cells transfected with mutated c-*ras* genes or infected with acute retroviruses carrying v-*ras* oncogenes exhibit increased resistance to ionizing radiation.[1160] The biochemical mechanisms by which mutated c-*ras* genes or v-*ras* oncogenes may impart resistance to anticancer drugs or ionizing radiation is obscure, and the clinical relevance of the studies performed *in vitro* to the complex situations of human tumors *in vivo* remains speculative.

26. Suppression of the Transformed Phenotype Induced by Mutated c-*ras* Genes

Cocultivation of rodent cells transformed by an expression vector carrying a T24 c-H-*ras* gene with normal rodent cells may result in suppression of the transformed phenotype in the oncogene-transformed cells.[1161] It is not known whether this suppression of the transformed phenotype by normal cells is caused by depletion of growth factors by the normal cells or secretion by them of factors that might inhibit growth of transformed cells. In any case, it is clear that the continued expression of a mutated c-*ras* gene is not necessarily accompanied by the expression of a transformed phenotype in susceptible cells and that factors from the microenvironment may be critically important for the expression or lack of expression of the oncogene-induced transformation.

Infection of cells with DNA viruses may alter the expression of the transforming potential of mutated c-*ras* genes cloned in molecular vectors. For example, infection of NIH/3T3 cells transformed by a plasmid (pJ234) carrying a T24 c-H-*ras* gene with adeno-associated virus (AAV) resulted in a decrease in their growth rate and cloning efficiency and an increase in the latent period for tumor appearance in nude mice.[1162] AAV did not affect significantly the number of transformed foci when different multiplicities of infection were used and when the virus was added to the cultures at different time intervals before or after transfection.

27. Conclusion

In spite of numerous studies with interesting results, the molecular mechanisms responsible for the oncogenic potential of c-*ras* genes containing mutations at either codon 12 or 61 remain unknown. The role of these mutant genes in the progression and metastasization of tumor cells *in vivo* has not been elucidated. The same mutations may be contained in some benign, spontaneously regressing tumors, indicating that the presence of c-*ras* mutations may be insufficient for the development and maintenance of a transformed phenotype. Most probably, c-*ras* mutations confer growing advantages to certain cells and may represent one of the multiple steps required by these cells for the expression of a transformed phenotype.

G. SUMMARY

Mutations of c-*ras* protooncogenes have been detected in a number of human tumor cell lines as well as in a proportion of primary human tumors and experimental tumors. For an unknown reason, there is an apparently very high susceptibility of c-*ras* genes to point mutational events occurring at two specific activating sites (codons 12 and 61 of the p21 protein). The mutant c-*ras* genes display an enhanced transforming capability when tested in DNA transfection assays using preneoplastic cell lines such as NIH/3T3 cells. Altered $p21^{c-ras}$ proteins are present in cells carrying mutations of c-*ras* genes. However, the mechanisms responsible for the enhanced oncogenic potential of the mutant p21 proteins are unknown.

The possible role of c-*ras* mutations in tumorigenic processes occurring *in vivo*, especially in human tumors, is not totally clear. On the ground of the available evidence it seems rather unlikely that c-*ras* mutations represent a kind of critical and universal contributing factor to the origin of spontaneous tumors. However, specific mutational events related to oncogenic activation of c-*ras* genes are frequently observed in tumors induced in animals by particular types of physical and chemical carcinogenic agents and it is plausible that c-*ras* mutations may contribute, in conjunction with other factors, to the origin and/or progression of some spontaneous tumors occurring in humans and other animals. Indeed, a rather high incidence of c-*ras* gene mutations has been found not only in cell lines but also in fresh samples from particular types of human tumors. Most probably, c-*ras* genes participate in the development of certain tumors in cooperation with other cellular genes, and this cooperation would be largely responsible for the increased rate of proliferation and altered behavior of the tumor cells.

VII. GENE DELETION OR INACTIVATION

The cytogenetic and molecular study of human tumors demonstrates that deletion of defined chromosome segments is frequently associated with certain types of human tumors. In fact, deletion is the structural chromosome abnormality most frequently detected in human solid tumors with the aid of modern cytogenetic techniques.[581] Deletion may result in the occurrence of hemizygosity or homozygosity (if duplication is associated with deletion) at particular loci.

As discussed in Chapter 1, Volume I, studies on the suppression of tumorigenicity with somatic cell hybrids suggest the existence of normal cellular genes capable of suppressing the expression of a transformed phenotype. The analysis of hybrids formed between carcinogen-transformed normal hamster embryo cells or human fibroblasts suggests the existence of tumor suppressor genes, some of which may be located on human chromosome 1.[1163,1164] However, methods of somatic cell genetics do not permit molecular analysis of genes involved in supression of tumorigenicity and the use of other methods is required for the characterization of these genes at the molecular level. The use of polymorphic DNA markers for the study of primary human colorectal carcinomas allowed the elaboration of an allelotype and demonstrated the high prevalence of allelic deletions in the tumor cells.[1165] These results suggest the existence of numerous tumor supporessor genes in the human genome. In contrast to the dominant acting oncogenes, these genes can be considered as recessive genes whose physical or functional loss may lead to the tumorigenic conversion of the cell. Two possibilities should be considered in relation to gene deletion and oncogenic processes: deletion of the normal allele of an altered protooncogene and deletion of a tumor suppressor gene (antioncogene or emerogene).[1166-1168]

In addition to the physical loss of a gene, which represents a true deletion, some point mutations or other structural alterations of the gene can result in its functional inactivation or in the abrogation of its normal function, thus producing phenotypic effects similar or identical to those associated with gene deletion. Both gene deletion (physical loss) and gene inactivation (functional loss) may lead to loss of constitutional heterozygosity at specific genetic loci. Abrogation of the homologous locus leading to loss of heterozygosity can occur by a diversity of potential mechanisms that include loss of a whole chromosome or part of a chromosome, loss of one chromosome and reduplication of the other, mitotic recombination, chromosome translocation, insertion, or inversion, gene deletion or conversion, and point mutation. Loss of tumor suppressor genes would result in the oncogenic transformation of the cell. Recent studies in *Drosophila* indicate that inactivation of specific genetic loci by homozygous mutation may lead to tumorigenic processes.[1169,1170] A 18-kb DNA restriction fragment of human origin was found to be capable of suppressing the transformed phenotype of rat FE-8 cells transformed by a cloned EJ c-H-*ras* gene.[1171] This suppression occurred in spite of the continuous expression of the activated protooncogene and the DNA fragment would contain a human tumor suppressor gene.

Microscopic or submicroscopic intercalary chromosome deletions, leading to specific hemizygosity, are associated with human syndromes characterized by cancer proneness.[1172] In individuals carrying acquired or constitutional (inherited) mutations predisposing to cancer, the malignancy would only arise following elimination of the wild-type allele.[1173,1174] The detection of deleted chromosome segments which presumably predispose to the expression of alleles with transforming potentialities may be facilitated by the recent construction of a linkage map of the human genome, based on the pattern of inheritance of 403 polymorphic loci which include 393 RFLPs distributed among the 23 human chromosomes.[1175] A catalog of genes mapped in the human genome has been published recently.[1176] A list of acquired recurring clonal structural chromosome abnormalities in human neoplasia was also published.[1177]

Besides the deletion or inactivation of antioncogenes, the possibility of protooncogene deletion or inactivation should also be considered. Protooncogene alleles may be affected by these processes, which may result in derangements in the regulation of normal cell functions that could lead, depending on the cell type and its stage of differentiation, to the malignant transformation of the cell. Deletion or inactivation of the normal allele of an heterozygously mutated recessive protooncogene may result in the activation of the oncogenic potential of the mutated allele. On the other hand, allelic deletion of protooncogenes might occur in some cancers as a consequence of random chromosome loss and may thus not have clear biological relevance for tumor development.

Human tumors most frequently associated with deletion of genes or specific genomic segments include Wilms' tumor and retinoblastoma. These tumors occur in children and their etiology is almost completely unknown. The possibility should be considered that these tumors, as well as other types of pediatric tumors, could be originated by a process of transplacental carcinogenesis due to the action of chemical carcinogens or oncogenic viruses during pregnancy in the mother.[1178] Recent studies indicate, however, that human tumors associated with gene deletion are not limited to children but may also occur in adults. In the following, some of these tumors are discussed.

A. WILMS' TUMOR AND RHABDOMYOSARCOMA

Wilms' tumor, a relatively common childhood renal tumor of embryonal origin, usually occurs in a sporadic form, but rare familial cases have been reported.[1179] Moreover, some cases are associated with aniridia, constituting the aniridia-Wilms' tumor association (AWTA). An interstitial deletion of human chromosome 11, region 11p13-p14, has been observed in Wilms' tumor, either associated or not with the AWTA anomaly.[1180,1181] The human protooncogene c-H-*ras*-1 is situated in close proximity to this region, but it is usually not deleted in patients with the AWTA anomaly.[1182,1183] Thus, the predisposition of aniridia patients to develop Wilms' tumors is not due to a constitutional deletion of one of the c-H-*ras*-1 alleles. Moreover, familial predisposition to Wilms' tumor is not linked to genetic markers located on chromosome region 11p13.[1184,1185]

The study of Wilms' tumors by cytogenetic methods alone disclose variation in the short arm of chromosome 11 in only a minority of cases.[1186] On the other hand, combination of cytogenetic methods with gene probes specific for chromosome 11 indicate that most cases of Wilms' tumors are associated with loss of 11p DNA sequences by mechanisms including somatic recombination, chromosome loss, and recombination or chromosome loss and duplication.[1187] Examination of DNA samples from five patients with Wilms' tumors showed loss of chromosome 11 alleles and examination of DNA from their parents indicated that alleles lost in the tumors were of maternal origin.[1188] Thus, the parental derivation of chromosome 11 alleles lost in these Wilms' tumor is not random. Interestingly, the deletions at chromosome 11p loci are associated in some tumors with duplication of the nondeleted alleles, leading to homozygosity of the corresponding genes.[1185,1189,1190] An abnormal mitotic segregation event could occur in each predisposed kidney cell such that one chromosome 11 homolog may be lost and the remaining homolog may be reduplicated during the processes of tumorigenesis.[1191] It seems thus likely that certain abnormal mitotic events that allow the expression of recessive mutations predisposing to cancer are involved in the origin of Wilms' tumor and also in other types of tumors with similar chromosomal abnormalities.

The insulin gene (*INS*) would be proximal to the locus of c-H-*ras*-1 (*RAS*^{H}), and the β-globin (*HBB*) gene has been localized on a human chromosome region distal to 11p13.[1182,1192] The calcitonin gene (*CAL*) is also located near this site, on human chromosome region 11p13-p15, and a rearrangement of this chromosomal region has been detected in a cell line derived from a patient with medullary thyroid carcinoma,[1193] a disease in which an elevated blood calcitonin level is considered as an excellent tumor marker.[1194] The gene coding for parathormone (*PTH*) is also located on human chromosome 11, at region 11p11.21.[1195] According to an *in situ* hybridization technique, the following genes are located on human chromosome 11: *PTH* at 11p11.21, *HBB* at 11p11.22, *INS* at 11p14.1, and *RAS*^{H} at 11p14.1. Genes on human chromosome 11 appear to be arranged in the linear order cen-*PTH-HBB-RAS*^{H}-*INS*-pter.[1195,1196] Another locus which is closely linked to the putative AWTA locus is that of the gene encoding the β-subunit of follicle-stimulating hormone (FSH).[1197] However, the possible relationships, if any, between the c-H-*ras*-1 protooncogene, the genes of insulin, β-globin, parathormone, calcitonin, and β-FSH and the putative AWTA locus have not been established, and the possible role of these genes in different types of tumors associated with structural changes on the short arm of chromosome 11 remains unknown. The deletion of the affected chromosome in AWTA patients may begin distal to the locus of lactate dehydrogenase A (*LDH*^{A}) and includes band 11p13 with deletion of catalase gene (*CAT*) sequences but may not extend to *CAL, PTH,* or other genes thought to be located in the distal half of chromosome 11p, including *RAS*^{H}.[1198] The loci on chromosome 11p13 responsible for aniridia and Wilms' tumor are physically separated.[1199]

The gene coding for IGF-II is located on human chromosome region 11p14.1,[1195] which is also close to the site of deletion in Wilms' tumor. High levels of expression of IGF-II transcripts have been detected in the cells of Wilms' tumors,[1200] but the possible role of this alteration in the origin and/or development of Wilms' tumor is unknown. IGF-II transcripts are elevated in the cells of this tumor when compared with adult tissues but the levels are similar to those found in several fetal tissues including kidney, liver, adrenals, and striated muscle. Thus, it is not clear whether the high level of IGF-II expression in Wilms' tumor reflects only the stage of tumor differentiation or whether IGF-II contributes to the malignant process by its mitogenic properties through an autostimulatory action.

Rhabdomyosarcoma is another pediatric tumor which can be associated with loss of constitutional heterozygosity at a locus on chromosome 11p.[1201] The genetic association observed between Wilms' tumor and rhabdomyosarcoma could be due to the proximity of the locus corresponding to the AWTA anomaly/retinoblastoma on 11p13 and a rhabdomyosarcoma locus which appears to be localized in 11p15.5-11pter. The genetic association between the two diseases could be explained by homozygosity of an extended region of the short arm of chromosome 11 which encompasses both loci or by a rearrangement of a tumor-associated chromosome that brings the two loci in juxtaposition and subjects them to coordinate control.[1201]

Deletion 11p- with generation of homozygosity for the c-H-*ras*-1 locus was detected in an adrenal adenoma that occurred in an adult patient with Wiedemann-Beckwith syndrome.[1202] This syndrome is characterized by the association of multiple congenital anomalies including exophalos, macroglossia, visceromegaly, and gigantism, as well as by a high risk for the development of embryonal neoplasms (Wilms' tumor, rhabdomyosarcoma, and hepatoblastoma) and neoplasms of the adrenal cortex.

B. RETINOBLASTOMA AND OSTEOSARCOMA

Retinoblastoma, the most common intraocular tumor, occurs in children in both heritable and sporadic forms. Most familial retinoblastomas are bilateral and most of the sporadic forms of the tumor are unilateral. The tumor originates from a primitive bipotential or multipotential neuroectodermal cell. Retinoblastoma is associated with a diversity of chromosome aberrations.[1203-1205] The cytogenetic abnormalities observed in a series of 77 cases of retinoblastoma involved chromosomes 13 (21% of cases), additional 1q material (44%), isochromosome 6p (45%), monosomy 16 (18%), marker 1p+ (13%), and HSRs and DMs (9%).[1206] Amplification of the N-*myc* gene has been found in 30% of retinoblastomas (both familial and sporadic) and is frequently associated with double minutes.[494] An isochromosome 6p is not frequently observed in other tumors, but can occur in as much as 60% of retinoblastoma tumors.[1207]

Retinoblastoma represents an excellent model for the study of genetic alterations associated with tumorigenesis.[1208] Deletion of human chromosome 13, region 13q14, is observed microscopically in a minority of children with retinoblastoma.[1209-1214] However, this deletion may be present in a higher proportion of retinoblastoma patients because it can occur at a submicroscopical level, as can be determined by DNA hybridization methods.[1173,1215,1216] The same deletion at human chromosome region 13q14 may occur in the tumor cells of human osteosarcoma, a tumor that may appear in patients surviving heritable retinoblastoma as a consequence of surgery and radiotherapy.[1217] These facts suggest that some gene(s) related to the origin of retinoblastoma and osteosarcoma may be located in human chromosome 13, at region 13q14. This region would contain a putative retinoblastoma locus, *RB1*.[1218] Mutation or deletion of this locus could lead to the development of retinoblastoma or osteosarcoma.[1219] No protooncogenes have been assigned to human chromosome 13. Hypothetically, the deleted region on this chromosome would contain not an oncogene but, on the contrary, a tumor suppressor gene.[1215,1220]

1. Gene Deletion in Retinoblastoma

A phenomenon of gene deletion associated with duplication and homozygosity of nondeleted alleles, similar to that described in Wilms' tumor, occurs in the tumor cells of some cases of hereditary and nonhereditary forms of retinoblastoma.[1221,1222] Molecular hybridization studies with DNA fragments obtained from a locus spanning 29 kb within human chromosome band 13q14 detected deletions in 3 retinoblastomas out of 37 such tumors examined.[1223] Somatically occurring, homozygous deletions spanning at least 25 kb were detected in retinoblastomas from two unrelated patients. Loss of heterozygosity related to elimination of the normal *RB1* allele at the retinoblastoma locus would occur most frequently by mitotic nondisjunction or recombination, resulting in a tumor cell that is homozygous over much of its chromosomes 13.[1224] In hereditary cases of retinoblastoma, the genetic material lost from chromosome 13 during tumorigenesis would be the one inherited from the phenotypically (and genotypically) normal parent, whereas the retained chromosome 13 material containing the *RB1* locus would be inherited from the affected parent. The *RB1* tumor suppressor gene can not only be deleted in tumor cells but can also be inactivated by single point mutations.[1219]

A cDNA fragment, termed p4.7R, is capable of detecting a locus spanning at least 70 kb in human chromosome band 13q14 representing the *RB1* gene, part or all of which is deleted in some retinoblastomas and osteosarcomas.[1225] The use of the p4.7R probe allowed the demonstration that the *RB1* locus is the target for mutations or structural alterations occurring not only in retinoblastoma (7 of 49 cases) and osteosarcoma (3 of 13 cases), but also in soft tissue sarcomas (3 of 16 cases).[1226] The latter mesenchymal tumors account for a majority of the tumors that occur at second sites in patients with an inherited predisposition to retinoblastoma. Transcripts of the *RB1* gene were found to be absent in most of primary human osteosarcomas and soft tissue sarcomas, thus indicating the occurrence of deletions or structural alterations of the gene in the tumor cells.[1227] Using a DNA probe, termed H3-8, a heterozygous deletion in chromosome 13 was detected in nearly 20% of patients with bilateral and multifocal unilateral retinoblastoma.[1228] Almost half of these deletions did not include the locus of the enzyme esterase D (*ESD* locus), which is also contained in human chromosome region 13q14, and were undetectable by conventional cytogenetic analysis. The size of these deletions was in the range of a few to several hundred kilobase pairs. The deletion detected with the H3-8 probe cosegregated with retinoblastoma in a familial case.[1228] Thus, the probe may be useful for early diagnosis and for genetic counseling. RFLPs within the retinoblastoma gene have been successfully applied to the study of families with members who had retinoblastoma.[1229] These RFLPs are valuable in the genetic counseling of patients with retinoblastoma and their relatives.

2. The *ESD* Locus

Determination of esterase D isoenzymes may be useful for the genetic study of patients with retinoblastoma.[1230] Studies of familial retinoblastoma indicate that the *ESD* locus is linked to the *RB1* locus on human chromosome 13.[1231] In fact, the *ESD* locus is known to be the closest human genetic marker to the *RB1* locus, being localized to the same subband of chromosome 13 as the *RB1* gene. *ESD* maps to human chromosome region 13q14.2-14.3.[1232] The *ESD* locus and the *RB1* locus are separated by more than 5 kb and less than 1500 kb.[1233] A cDNA clone of the *ESD* gene has been obtained.[1234] Lack of esterase D activity has been detected in retinoblastoma cells and it has been suggested that a submicroscopic deletion in these cells would have resulted in the loss of both the retinoblastoma and esterase D loci.[1215] However, no deletions or rearrangements in the coding sequences of the *ESD* gene have been detected in the tumor cells of some retinoblastomas by using specific cDNA probes.[1233,1234]

RFLP and isozymic alleles of loci on chromosome 13 have been successfully applied for the prediction of familial predisposition to retinoblastoma.[1235] Moreover, RFLP analysis has demonstrated that partial homozygosity for genetic markers located on chromosome 13 may occur in the tumor cells of about 7.5% of retinoblastomas.[1236] Thus, homozygosity or hemizygosity at the *RB1* locus occurs in the majority of retinoblastomas.

3. The Human *RB1* Gene

The human *RB1* gene has been cloned and sequenced recently.[1237] The *RB1* gene contains at least 12 exons distributed in a region of over 100 kb and a single long ORF that can encode a hypothetical protein of 816 amino acids and 94 kDa which shows no strong homology with other known proteins. The human *RB1* gene encodes a 4.6-kb mRNA which is present in normal human fetal retina and placenta, as well as in tumors such as neuroblastoma and medulloblastoma, but that was found to be absent or qualitatively altered in all of six human retinoblastomas examined.[1237] The *RB1* gene encodes a nuclear phosphoprotein with DNA binding activity.[1238] Introduction of a cloned *RB1* gene into cultured retinoblastoma and osteosarcoma cells, via retroviral-mediated gene transfer, resulted in suppression of the neoplastic phenotype.[1239] If confirmed, this result would represent the first example of gene therapy of human cancer.

C. MENINGIOMA AND ACOUSTIC NEURINOMA

Meningioma is a common benign human intracranial tumor with highest incidence during the 5th and 6th decades of life. Females are more frequently affected than males and the majority of cases are sporadic. However, there may be a hereditary predisposition to meningioma and patients with this predisposition may develop acoustic neurinoma as a second tumor.

Monosomy of chromosome 22 has been found frequently in cytogenetic studies of human meningiomas.[1240] RFLP analysis in 35 unrelated patients with meningiomas revealed that 16 tumors retained the constitutional genotype along chromosome 22, 14 tumors (40%) were associated with monosomy 22, and 5 tumors (14%) showed loss of heterozygosity in tumor DNA at one or more chromosome 22 loci and retained heterozygosity at other loci, consistent with the variable terminal deletions of one chromosome 22 in the tumor DNA.[1241] The results of this study suggest the existence of a meningioma locus, situated distal to the myoglobin locus within human chromosome region 22q12.3-qter. In addition to 22q deletions, 12 of 19 tumors exhibited losses of heterozygosity at loci on one to three other chromosomes. The loss of genes on the long arm of chromosome 22 was confirmed in other clinical studies.[1242,1243]

Gene loss on chromosome 22 was detected by a molecular genetic approach in tumor DNA from 7 of 16 patients with unilateral acoustic neurinoma and 1 of 3 patients with the bilateral form of the same tumor.[1244] Hemizygosity for genes on chromosome 22 is apparently not associated with any particular characteristic of these tumors, including the clinical course.

D. LUNG CARCINOMA

A cytogenetic deletion in human chromosome region 3p14-p23 was detected in human small-cell lung carcinoma.[1245] By using polymorphic DNA probes for chromosome 3p and comparing tumor and constitutional genotypes, loss of alleles of chromosome 3p markers was detected in the tumor cells of all of nine patients with small-cell lung carcinoma (two tumor cell lines and seven tumor tissue samples obtained directly from the patients without intervening cell culture).[1246] More recently, it has been recognized that deletion at the chromosomal region 3p21 is present not only in small-cell lung carcinoma but in all major types of human lung cancer.[1247] Abnormalities in the structure and expression of the human *RB1* gene at chromosome region 13q14 have been found in small-cell lung carcinomas.[1248]

Allelic deletion of the c-H-*ras*-1 protooncogene, which is normally located on human chromosome 11p, has been detected in some lung tumors.[498] In a series of patients with various histologic types of lung cancer analyzed for RFLPs, 17 of 41 informative tumor samples showed loss of heterozygosity on the short arm of chromosome 11.[1249] The 11p deletion was predominantly associated with the more advanced tumors, suggesting a role for the deletion in tumor progression. The 11p deletion included the c-H-*ras*-1 protooncogene, but the remaining allele did not contain activating point mutations. Thus, loss of constitutional heterozygosity at the c-H-*ras*-1 gene would not be relevant for the development of lung carcinoma. Losses of heterozygosity on loci from chromosomes 9 and 10 were also found in some patients from the same series. Although loss of alleles on chromosomes 3p, 11p, 13q, and 17p have been observed in a significant proportion of lung cancers, such losses are infrequent in non-small-cell lung carcinomas.[1250] Further studies are required for a proper evaluation of the biological and clinical significance of gene deletion in human lung cancer.

E. COLON CARCINOMA AND FAMILIAL ADENOMATOUS POLYPOSIS

Familial adenomatous polyposis, also called familial polyposis coli, is a dominantly inherited disease with very high risk for colon cancer. Interstitial deletion of human chromosome 5 at a specific locus, with the consequent loss of constitutional heterozygosity, has been detected in familial adenomatous polyposis as well as in colorectal carcinomas not associated with this disease.[1251-1253] A gene, the familial adenomatous polyposis (*FAP*) gene, located on human chromosome region 5q21-q22, may be crucially deleted in both familial adenomatous polyposis and colorectal carcinomas. Loss of genes other than *FAP* may be important for the development of colon carcinomas. Allele loss of the gene coding for the glucocorticoid receptor, which is localized on human chromosome region 5q11-q13, was detected in the fresh tumor samples from 3 out of 11 sporadic colon carcinomas.[1254] The relationship between this locus and the *FAP* gene is not understood at present. In addition to the deletion of the *FAP* and glucocorticoid receptor genes on chromosome 5q, genes located on human chromosome 6, 12, 15, and 22 may be deleted in colon carcinomas associated with familial adenomatous polyposis as well as in sporadic colorectal carcinomas. RFLP analysis demonstrated that loss of human chromosome 17p sequences occurred in over 75% of 34 human colorectal carcinomas examined.[1255] The deletions of chromosome 17p involve the gene encoding the p53 protein, and the remaining p53 allele is mutated in some colorectal carcinomas. These results suggest a tumor suppressor function for the wild-type p53 gene. The presence of numerous allelic deletions in primary colon carcinomas has been demonstrated by allelotype analysis of these tumors.[1165] Many human colorectal carcinomas would be originated from a single cell which had lost at least part of either the short arm of chromosome 17 or the whole chromosome 18.[1256] The results of these studies, as well as those related to mutation of the c-K-*ras* protooncogene,[956-958] strongly suggest that human colorectal tumors are the result of a complex multistage process involving distinct genomic changes, including deletions and mutations. The chronological and hierarchical aspects of the molecular alterations leading to the origin and development of human carcinomas remain to be elucidated.

F. LEUKEMIA

Monosomy or partial deletion of human chromosome 7 is frequently observed in acute nonlymphocytic leukemia (ANLL).[567] The oncogene c-*erb*-B is located on the same chromosome, at region 7p11-13, but the chromosomal breakpoint in ANLL is usually localized far away from this site, at region 7q32-34. [1257] In three patients with myeloid disorders associated with 20q- deletion studied by *in situ* chromosomal hybridization, the c-*src* locus was consistently preserved and no major rearrangement or amplification of the c-*src* gene were detected.[1258] Loss of part of the short arm of human chromosome 9 (9p-) is significantly associated with lymphoid malignancies, especially ALL and non-Hodgkin's lymphomas.[1259] The 9p- as a single change does not appear as a specific chromosomal rearrangement and the patients with 9p- usually have high tumor load and poor outcome. Deletion of one copy of the homeobox gene Hox-4.1, located on mouse chromosome 2, has been detected in murine myeloid leukemias.[1260] The possible role of homeobox gene deletion in human and nonhuman malignant diseases is not understood.

G. THE 5q- SYNDROME

Acquired partial deletions localized to the distal portion of the long arm of human chromosome 5 occur in the 5q- syndrome, which is characterized by the existence of a transfusion-dependent refractory macrocytic of aplastic anemia.[1261,1262] The 5q- abnormality may also be associated with leukemias such as AML or ANLL as well as with myelodysplastic syndromes. The syndromes are characterized by a diversity of phenotypic manifestations with varying degrees of ineffective hematopoiesis and a high likelihood of developing into refractory anemia or ANLL. Among patients with myelodysplastic syndromes it has been observed that 5q- may be a primary event and the only cytogenetic alteration, but in some cases of these syndromes 5q- is a secondary event and may be associated with other cytogenetic abnormalities.[1263] In two patients with myelodysplastic syndrome, deletion of chromosome 5 that occurred in the early phase of the disease coexisted in later phases with mutation of the N-*ras* gene at codon 13, which may have contributed to the leukemic progression of the premalignant syndrome.[1035]

1. The c-*fms* Protooncogene and the 5q- Syndrome

The c-*fms* gene has been assigned to human chromosome region 5q34 or 5q33.[1264,1265] Studies with *in situ* hybridization localize this gene to region 5q31-q33.[1266] The protein product of this protooncogene is closely related to, or identical with, the receptor for macrophage colony-stimulating factor, CSF-1.[1267] The 5q- deletion removes the c-*fms* gene, suggesting that hemizygosity at the c-*fms* locus could lead to abnormalities in hematopoietic cell maturation.[1264,1265,1268]

2. Hematopoietic Growth Factors and the 5q- Syndrome

The c-*fms* gene is just one of several different genes involved in deletions observed in the 5q- syndrome. The gene coding for the CSF-1 itself has been mapped to human chromosome region 5q33.1, and is thus closely linked to the c-*fms*/CSF-1 receptor gene.[1269] The gene coding for another factor involved in the control of hematopoiesis, the granulocyte-macrophage colony-stimulating factor (GM-CSF), also called colony-stimulating factor 2 (CSF-2), is located on human chromosome region 5q23-31.[1265] The genes coding for interleukin 3 (IL-3) and interleukin 5 (IL-5) are located on human chromosome region 5q23-q31.[1270] Thus, the genes coding for several factors or factor receptors involved in the control of hematopoiesis (CSF-1, CSF-2, IL-3, IL-5, and CSF-1 receptor) are located on the same segment of human chromosome 5q, and these genes are lost in the 5q- syndrome associated with leukemia or refractory anemia. Other genes located on human chromosome arm 5q are those coding for the PDGF receptor and the β_2-adrenergic receptor.[1271,1272] The gene encoding the CD14 monocyte differentiation antigen is also contained in human chromosome 5q, at region 5q23-q31, and may be deleted in patients with myelodysplastic syndrome or ANLL.[1273] However, the biological significance of these genetic alterations in relation to the hematologic symptoms and other symptoms occurring in the 5q- syndrome is not understood at present.

H. MULTIPLE ENDOCRINE NEOPLASIA

Multiple endocrine neoplasia (MEN) syndromes, also called multiple endocrine adenomatosis, exhibit a characteristic combination of multiple endocrine tumors, most of them of benign nature. Hormonal studies can be used as markers for the diagnosis and following up of these tumors.[341] A familial aggregation of cases is frequently observed in these syndromes, and most of the pedigrees are compatible with autosomal dominant heredity. Variable expressivity of the symptoms occurs frequently among different affected members of the same family. Two main types of these syndromes have been described, MEN type 2 and MEN type 1.

1. MEN Type 2

MEN type 2 (MEN-2), also called Sipple's syndrome, is an autosomal dominant disease with high penetrance and variable expressivity and is characterized by the development of medullary thyroid carcinoma (almost 100% of the total cases), pheochromocytoma (about 50% of cases), and parathyroid adenoma (30% of cases). The specific association of medullary thyroid carcinoma and pheochromocytoma is referred to as MEN-2A. A small interstitial deletion of human chromosome 20, at region 20p12.2, was detected in the peripheral blood lymphocytes from patients with MEN type 2.[1274,1275] However, some control cases had a similar deletion. Deletion of genes on chromosome 1 was detected in patients with MEN-2A. In a study of Japanese patients, loss of heterozygosity at a locus on chromosome 22 was detected in one of nine medullary thyroid carcinomas and two of five pheochromocytomas.[1252] Recently, a gene closely related to MEN-2A was localized to human chromosome region 10q21.1.[1276,1277] The gene coding for the interstitial retinol-binding protein is closely linked to this region. However, deletion of the putative MEN-2A locus on chromosome 10 was detected by analysis of tumor DNA in only 1 of 42 patients with the MEN-2A syndrome.[1278]

2. MEN Type 1

MEN type 1 (MEN-2), also called Wermer's syndrome, is characterized by a combination of parathyroid adenoma, islet cell adenoma or carcinoma, and anterior pituitary adenoma. A MEN type 1 gene has been mapped to human chromosome 11 and it may be lost in patients with insulinoma.[1279]

I. GENE DELETION IN OTHER TUMORS

Loss of constitutional heterozygosity at specific chromosome loci has been detected in a diversity of childhood and adult tumors, including hepatoblastoma,[1280] transitional cell carcinoma of the bladder (chromosome 11),[1281] and renal cell carcinoma (chromosome 3).[1282] Results from recent studies indicate that alteration of the *RB1* gene may occur in human tumors other than retinoblastoma and osteosarcoma. Loss of heterozygosity indicating a recessive mutation on chromosome 13 was detected in human ductal breast tumors and inactivation of the *RB1* gene was detected in human breast cancers.[1283,1284] Deletion of the same chromosome region (11p13-14) was detected in the tumor cells of a human hepatocellular carcinoma as a consequence of HBV integration at this site, with the consequence of leaving only a single copy of the remaining normal allele.[1285] However, it is not clear whether gene loss or inactivation represents a general pathogenetic mechanism for tumorigenesis. Loss of chromosomal heterozygosity appears to be infrequent in some common human tumors, e.g., in stomach cancer.[1286]

J. SYNDROMES ASSOCIATED WITH INCREASED CHROMOSOME FRAGILITY AND HIGH CANCER RISK

There are two classes of chromosomal fragile sites: heritable and constitutive.[1287] Whereas the heritable fragile sites are rare and segregate in a simple Mendelian fashion with complete penetrance, the constitutive fragile sites are common, if not ubiquitous, and may be caused by environmental factors such as chemicals, radiations, and/or viruses. At present, the mechanisms of fragile site formation are unknown and the exact nature of the alteration at the DNA or gene level remains obscure. Increased chromosome fragility (chromosome instability) is found in several clinical syndromes associated with increased cancer risk.[1288] A similar fragility was found in patients with sporadic unilateral retinoblastoma.[1289] The chromosome fragility observed in patients with retinoblastoma would not be caused by the retinoblastoma mutation itself,[1290] but would be due to unidentified environmental agents which could be etiologically associated with the tumor. However, no significant evidence for environmental influence on the occurrence of retinoblastoma was found in an epidemiological study.[1291]

A possible relationship between chromosome fragility and neoplastic diseases may be anticipated if this fragility results in loss or alteration of genome segments involved in the transcriptional control of protooncogene expression or in deletion of antioncogenes. In general, it is interesting to look for a possible association of familial chromosome fragility at specific sites, especially those corresponding to the loci of protooncogenes or putative antioncogenes, and increased incidence of specific types of cancer segregating with the fragile site(s) in the same families.[1292] Although there is a significant association between the location of fragile sites and recurrent chromosomal breakpoints associated with different types of cancer (most frequently, hematologic neoplasms), there is no evidence in favor of a general involvement of protooncogenes in these changes. At present, the function and identity of genes located at the fragile sites remain an enigma.[1287] There is no clear general correlation between constitutive fragile sites in chromosomes and protooncogene locations.[1293]

K. PROTOONCOGENE DELETION AND TUMOR PROGRESSION

Deletion of specific protooncogenes could be correlated with the progression and metastasization of human carcinomas and sarcomas *in vivo*. Loss of one allele of the c-H-*ras* protooncogene was observed in 18% of fresh specimens from human tumors, and loss of one allele of c-*myb* was detected in 11% of these tumors, and such deletions were not found in the normal cells of the same individuals.[474] Loss of a c-H-*ras*-1 allele was detected in tumor DNA from 14 of 51 patients with primary breast carcinomas and the loss was usually associated with a highly aggressive behavior of the tumor.[206] Deletion of one c-H-*ras* allele was also detected in 1 of 9 primary human colon tumors.[503] The tumor tissue from 1 of 5 cases of bladder cancer and 2 of 3 cases of renal pelvic cancer exhibited deletion of one c-H-*ras* allele.[1294] Allelic loss of c-H-*ras*-1 was also detected in ovarian and cervical cancers as well as in kidney tumors, and in some of these cases the remaining c-H-*ras*-1 allele contained a point mutation.[1295-1297] Although the biological significance of these alterations is not understood, the allelic deletions of c-H-*ras* and c-*myb* loci may reflect loss of chromosomes or parts of chromosomes in the tumor cells during their proliferation and may be correlated with progression and metastasis of carcinomas and sarcomas.

L. GENE DELETION OR INACTIVATION IN EXPERIMENTAL TUMORS

Deletion of a normal protooncogene with preservation of the mutated respective allele may occur in experimental tumors. For example, loss of the normal N-*ras* allele was detected in a mouse thymic lymphoma induced by the chemical carcinogen *N*-nitroso-*N*-methylurea, whereas the only allele of N-*ras* present in the same tumor contained a C-A transversion in the first base of codon 61.[1041] Studies on deletion or inactivation of genes that may correspond to protooncogenes or putative antioncogenes are warranted in view of the recent evidence suggesting the importance of such alterations in human tumorigenic processes.

M. FUNCTIONAL LOSS OF GENES IN *DROSOPHILA* TUMORS

Studies performed recently in *Drosophila melanogaster* may greatly contribute to a better understanding of the important relationships existing between functional loss of genes and tumorigenic processes in general.[1169,1170] Homozygous mutations of the recessive gene *l*²*gl* in *Drosophila* cause lethal neoplasms of the imaginal discs and the brain hemispheres. Introduction into the germ line of heterozygous *l*²*gl*⁻/⁺ flies of a 13-kDa DNA segment spanning the *l*²*gl*⁺ locus inserted into a molecular vector can fully rescue the homozygous *l*²*gl* deficient animals, which would have died of brain and imaginal disc neoplasms.[1169] Thus, restoration of a normal *l*²*gl*-encoded function results in complete suppression of tumor development.

N. SUMMARY

Deletion or inactivation of specific chromosome segments is associated with a markedly increased risk for some particular types of tumors. The deleted or inactivated DNA sequences would contain putative tumor suppressor genes (antioncogenes or emerogenes). Loss of constitutional heterozygosity for specific DNA sequences containing such genes may be crucially important for certain tumorigenic processes. Inactivation of the normal allele of an activated protooncogene could also contribute, in principle, to tumorigenic processes.

VIII. CONCLUSIONS

Alterations of protooncogenes have been frequently detected in neoplastic transformation induced either *in vivo* or *in vitro* by different experimental procedures, including radiations and chemical carcinogens. In fact, some experimental systems related to oncogenic processes are associated with an almost constant activation of DNA sequences with recognized oncogenic capabilities.

The possible role of protooncogenes in the origin and/or development of tumors occurring spontaneously in humans and other animal species is difficult to evaluate at present. In spite of numerous studies, the evidence in favor of a causal association between protooncogene alterations and natural forms of cancer is only circumstantial. In any case, it must be recognized that the study of protooncogene alterations has undoubtedly contributed in a substantial manner to improve our basic knowledge about the complex mechanisms involved in oncogenic processes. From the practical point of view, however, the results of these studies have contributed very little to improve our resources for the diagnosis, prognosis, treatment, and following-up of cancer patients.

In principle, several types of alterations would be responsible for an activation of the oncogenic potential of protooncogenes. These alterations include increased expression at unscheduled times and/or sites, amplification, translocation and/or rearrangement, and mutation. Increased expression of particular protooncogenes is observed in certain natural and experimental tumors. Specific translocations and/or rearrangements involving protooncogenes occur regularly in particular types of hematologic malignancies. Amplification or mutation of protooncogenes is observed in a relatively high percentage of certain types of tumors but is rare or absent in other tumors. The biological significance of protooncogene structural and/or functional changes in the origin and/or development of the malignant disease is not understood at present. Recent evidence suggests the existence of tumor suppressor genes (antioncogenes or emerogenes), whose deletion or functional inactivation would lead to the loss of constitutional heterozygosity at the respective locus and would contribute to the malignant transformation of cells.

On the ground of the available evidence it seems plausible to accept that oncogenes, protooncogenes, and tumor suppressor genes may contribute, through different types of changes and in conjunction with other genetic and/or epigenetic changes, to the complex, multistage tumorigenic processes.

REFERENCES

1. Hanafusa, H., Cell transformation by RNA tumor viruses, in *Comprehensive Virology,* Vol. 10, Fraenkel-Conrat, H. and Wagner, R., Eds., Plenum Press, New York, 1977, 401.
2. Hines, D.L., Viral oncogene expression during differentiation of Abelson virus-infected murine promonocytic leukemia cells, *Cancer Res.,* 48, 1702, 1988.
3. Robinson, H.L., Retroviruses and cancer, *Rev. Infect. Dis.,* 4, 1015, 1982.
4. Weinberg, R.A., Oncogenes of spontaneous and chemically induced tumors, *Adv. Cancer Res.,* 36, 149, 1982.
5. Cooper, G.M., Cellular transforming genes, *Science,* 217, 801, 1982.
6. Shilo, B.-Z. and Weinberg, R.A., Unique transforming gene in carcinogen-transformed mouse cells, *Nature,* 289, 607, 1981.
7. Blair, D.G., Oskarsson, M., Wood, T.G., McClements, W.L., Fischinger, P.J., and Vande Woude, G.G., Activation of the transforming potential of a normal cell sequence: a molecular model for oncogenesis, *Science,* 212, 941, 1981.
8. Yoakum, G.H., Lechner, I.F., Gabrielson, E.W., Korba, B.I., Malan-Shibley, L., Willey, J.C., Valerio, M.G., Shamsuddin, A.M., Trump, B.F., and Harris, C.C., Transformation of human bronchial epithelial cells transfected by Harvey *ras* oncogene, *Science,* 227, 1174, 1985.
9. Tainsky, M.A., Shamanski, F., Blair, D., and Giovanella, B.C., Causal role of an activated N-*ras* oncogene in the induction of tumorigenicity acquired by a human cell line, *Cancer Res.,* 47, 3235, 1987.

10. Stevenson, M. and Volsky, D.J., Activated v-*myc* and v-*ras* oncogenes do not transform normal human lymphocytes, *Mol. Cell. Biol.,* 6, 3410, 1986.

11. Tubo, R.A. and Rheiwald, J.G., Normal human mesothelial cells and fibroblasts transfected with the *EJras* oncogene become EGF-independent, but are not malignantly transformed, *Oncogene Res.,* 1, 407, 1987.

12. Nicolaiew, N. and Dautry, F., Growth stimulation of rat primary embryo fibroblasts by the human *myc* gene, *Exp. Cell Res.,* 166, 357, 1986.

13. Gao, J., Van Roy, F., Messiaen, L., Cosaert, J., Liebaut, G., Coopman, P., Fiers, W., and Mareel, M., Pathology of tumors produced in syngeneic Fischer rats by fibroblast-like cells before and after transfection with oncogenes, *Pathol. Res. Pract.,* 182, 48, 1987.

14. Craig, R.W. and Sager, R., Suppression of tumorigenicity in hybrids of normal and oncogene-transformed CHEF cells, *Proc. Natl. Acad. Sci. U.S.A.,* 82, 2062, 1985.

15. Balmain, A. and Pragnell, I.B., Mouse skin carcinomas induced *in vivo* by chemical carcinogens have a transforming Harvey-*ras* oncogene, *Nature,* 303, 72, 1983.

16. Balmain, A., Ramsden, M., Bowden, G.T., and Smith, J., Activation of the mouse cellular Harvey-*ras* gene in chemically induced benign skin papillomas, *Nature,* 307, 658, 1984.

17. Fung, Y.-K.T., Crittenden, L.B., Fadly, A.M., and Kung, H.-J., Tumor induction by direct injection of cloned v-*src* DNA into chickens, *Proc. Natl. Acad. Sci. U.S.A.,* 80, 353, 1983.

18. Milford, J.J. and Duran-Reynals, F., Growth of a chicken sarcoma virus in the chick embryo in the absence of neoplasia, *Cancer Res.,* 3, 578, 1943.

19. Dolberg, D.S. and Bissell, M.J., Inability of Rous sarcoma virus to cause sarcomas in the avian embryo, *Nature,* 309, 552, 1984.

20. Iba, H., Takeya, T., Cross, F.R., Hanafusa, T., and Hanafusa, H., Rous sarcoma virus variants that carry the cellular *src* gene instead of the viral *src* gene cannot transform chicken embryo fibroblasts, *Proc. Natl. Acad. Sci. U.S.A.,* 81, 4424, 1984.

21. Piwnica-Worms, H., Kaplan, D.R., Whitman, M., and Roberts, T.M., Retrovirus shuttle vector for study of kinase activities of pp60[c-src] synthesized *in vitro* and overproduced *in vivo, Mol. Cell. Biol.,* 6, 2033, 1986.

22. Brown, K., Quintanilla, M., Ramsden, M., Kerr, I.B., Young, S., and Balmain, A., v-*ras* genes from Harvey and BALB murine sarcoma viruses can act as initiators of two-stage mouse skin carcinogenesis, *Cell,* 46, 447, 1986.

23. Braun, L., Goyette, M., Yaswen, P., Thompson, N.L., and Fausto, N., Growth in culture and tumorigenicity after transfection with the *ras* oncogene of liver epithelial cells from carcinogen-treated rats, *Cancer Res.,* 47, 4116, 1987.

24. Waghorne, C., Kerbel, R.S., and Breitman, M.L., Metastatic potential of SP1 mouse mammary adenocarcinoma cells is differentially induced by activated and normal forms of c-H-*ras, Oncogene,* 1, 149, 1987.

25. Storer, R.D., Allen, H.L., Kraynak, A.R., and Bradley, M.O., Rapid induction of an experimental metastatic phenotype in first passage rat embryo cells by cotransfection of EJ c-Ha-*ras* and c-*myc* oncogenes, *Oncogene,* 2, 141, 1988.

26. Samid, D., Chang, E.H., and Friedman, R.M., Biochemical correlates of phenotypic reversion in interferon-treated mouse cells transformed by a human oncogene, *Biochem. Biophys. Res. Commun.,* 119, 21, 1984.

27. Samid, D., Chang, E.H., and Friedman, R.M., Development of transformed phenotype induced by a human *ras* oncogene is inhibited by interferon, *Biochem. Biophys. Res. Commun.,* 126, 509, 1985.

28. Drebin, J.A., Link, V.C., Weinberg, R.A., and Greene, M.I., Inhibition of tumor growth by a monoclonal antibody reactive with an oncogene-encoded tumor antigen, *Proc. Natl. Acad. Sci. U.S.A.,* 83, 9129, 1986.

29. Prywes, R., Foulkes, J.G., Rosenberg, N., and Baltimore, D., Sequences of the A-MuLV protein needed for fibroblast and lymphoid cell transformation, *Cell,* 34, 569, 1983.

30. Bryant, D. and Parsons, J.T., Site-directed point mutation in the *src* gene of Rous sarcoma virus results in an inactive *src* gene product, *J. Virol.,* 45, 1211, 1983.

31. Bryan, D.L. and Parsons, J.T., Amino acid alterations within a highly conserved region of the Rous sarcoma virus *src* gene product pp60[src] inactivate tyrosine protein kinase activity, *Mol. Cell. Biol.,* 4, 862, 1984.

32. Snyder, M.A. and Bishop, J.M., A mutation at the major phosphotyrosine in pp60[v-src] alters oncogenic potential, *Virology,* 136, 375, 1984.

33. Cross, F.R. and Hanafusa, H., Local mutagenesis of Rous sarcoma virus: sites of tyrosine and serine phosphorylation of p60[src] are dispensable for transformation, *Cell,* 34, 597, 1983.

34. Sistonen, L., Keski-Oja, J., Ulmanen, I., Hölttä. E., Wikgren, B.-J, and Italo, K., Dose effects of c-Ha-*ras*[Val 12] oncogene in transformed cell clones, *Exp. Cell Res.,* 168, 518, 1987.

35. Varmus, H.E., The molecular genetics of cellular oncogenes, *Annu. Rev. Genet.,* 18, 553, 1984.

36. Winter, E. and Perucho, M., Oncogene amplification during tumorigenesis of established rat fibroblasts reversibly transformed by activated human *ras* oncogenes, *Mol. Cell. Biol.,* 6, 2562, 1986.

37. Reynolds, V.L., Lebovitz, R.M., Warren, S., Hawley, T.S., Godwin, A.K., and Lieberman, M.W., Regulation of a metallothionein-*ras*T24 fusion gene by zinc results in graded alterations in cell morphology and growth, *Oncogene,* 1, 323, 1987.

38. Paterson, H., Reeves, B., Brown, R., Hall, A., Furth, M., Bos, J., Jones, P., and Marshall, C., Activated N-*ras* controls the transformed phenotype of HT1080 human fibrosarcoma cells, *Cell,* 51, 803, 1987.
39. Quaife, C.J., Pinkert, C.A., Ornitz, D.M., Palmiter, R.D., and Brinster, R.L., Pancreatic neoplasia induced by *ras* expression in acinar cells of transgenic mice, *Cell,* 48, 1023, 1987.
40. Schoenenberger, C.-A., Andres, A.-C., Groner, B., van der Valk, M., LeMeur, M., and Gerlinger, P., Targeted c-*myc* gene expression in mammary glands of transgenic mice induces mammary tumours with constitutive milk protein gene transcription, *EMBO J.,* 7, 169, 1988.
41. Andres, A.-C., Schönenberger, C.-A., Groner, B., Henninghausen, L., LeMeur, M., and Gerlinger, P., Ha-*ras* oncogene expression directed by a milk protein gene promoter: tissue specificity, hormonal regulation, and tumor induction in trasgenic mice, *Proc. Natl. Acad. Sci. U.S.A.,* 84, 1299, 1987.
42. Sinha, S., Webber, C., Marshall, C.J., Knowles, M.A., Proctor, A., Barrass, N.C., and Neal, G.E., Activation of *ras* oncogene in aflatoxin-induced rat liver carcinogenesis, *Proc. Natl. Acad. Sci. U.S.A.,* 85, 3673, 1988.
43. Gilmer, T.M., Annab, L.A., and Barrett, J.C., Characterization of activated proto-oncogenes in chemically transformed Syrian hamster embryo cells, *Mol. Carcinogenesis,* 1, 180, 1988.
44. Cardiff, R.D., Gumerlock, P.H., Soong, M.-M., Dandekar, S., Barry, P.A., Young, L.J.T., and Meyers, F.J., c-H-*ras*-1 expression in 7,12-dimethyl benzanthracene-induced Balb/c mouse mammary hyperplasias and their tumors, *Oncogene,* 3, 205, 1988.
45. Watatani, M., Perantoni, A.O., Reed, C.D., Enomoto, T., Wenk, M.L., and Rice, J.M., Infrequent activation of K-*ras,* H-*ras,* and other oncogenes in hepatocellular neoplasms initiated by methyl(acetoxymethyl)-nitrosamine, a methylating agent, and promoted by phenobarbital in F344 rats, *Cancer Res.,* 49, 1103, 1989.
46. Pimentel, E., Oncogenes and human cancer, *Cancer Genet. Cytogenet.,* 14, 347, 1985.
47. Duesberg, P.H., Activated proto-onc genes: sufficient or necessary for cancer?, *Science,* 228, 669, 1985.
48. Duesberg, P.H., Nunn, M., Kan, N., Watson, D., Seeburg, P.H., and Papas, T., Are activated proto-*onc* genes cancer genes?, *Haematol. Blood Transfus.,* 29, 9, 1985.
49. Ratner, L., Josephs, S.F., and Wong-Staal, F., Oncogenes: their role in neoplastic transformation, *Annu. Rev. Microbiol.,* 39, 419, 1985.
50. Goldfarb, M.P., The role of cellular oncogenes in cancers of non-viral etiology, *Pharmacol. Ther.,* 29, 205, 1985.
51. Aaronson, S.A. and Tronick, S.R., Transforming genes of human malignancies, *Carcinog. Compr. Surv.,* 10, 35, 1985.
52. Pitot, H.C., Oncogenes and human neoplasia, *Clin. Lab. Med.,* 6, 167, 1986.
53. Peehl, D.M. and Stamey, T.A., Oncogenes: a review with relevance to cancers of the urogenital tract, *J. Urol.,* 135, 897, 1986.
54. Pimentel, E., Proto-oncogenes as human tumor markers, *J. Tumor Marker Oncol.,* 1, 27, 1986.
55. Garrett, C.T., Oncogenes, *Clin. Chim. Acta,* 156, 1, 1986.
56. Barbacid, M., Oncogenes and human cancer: cause or consequence?, *Carcinogenesis,* 7, 1037, 1986.
57. Klein, G. and Klein, E., Conditioned tumorigenicity of activated oncogenes, *Cancer Res.,* 46, 3211, 1986.
58. Marshall, C.J., Oncogenes, *J. Cell Sci.,* Suppl. 4, 417, 1986.
59. Colb, M. and Krontiris, T.G., Oncogenes, *Adv. Int. Med.,* 31, 47, 1986.
60. Bishop, J.M., The molecular genetics of cancer, *Science,* 235, 305, 1987.
61. Nishimura, S. and Sekiya, T., Human cancer and cellular oncogenes, *Biochem. J.,* 243, 313, 1987.
62. Der, C.J., Cellular oncogenes and human carcinogenesis, *Clin. Chem.,* 33, 641, 1987.
63. Pimentel, E., Update on proto-oncogenes and human cancer, in *Human Tumor Markers: Biology and Clinical Application,* Cimino, F., Birkmayer, G.D., Klavins, J.V., Pimentel, E., and Salvatore, F., Eds., Walter de Gruyter, Berlin, 1987, 49.
64. Herskowitz, I., Functional inactivation of genes by dominant negative mutations, *Nature,* 329, 219, 1987.
65. Duesberg, P.H., Cancer genes: rare recombinants instead of activated oncogenes, *Proc. Natl. Acad. Sci. U.S.A.,* 84, 2117, 1987.
66. Rosen, P., The significance of proto-oncogenes in carcinogenesis, *Med. Hypotheses,* 22, 23, 1987.
67. Mareel, M.M. and Van Roy, F.M., Are oncogenes involved in invasion and metastasis?, *Anticancer Res.,* 6, 419, 1986.
68. Van Roy, F.M., Messiaen, L., Liebaut, G., Gao, J., Dragonetti, C.H., Fiers, W.C., and Mareel, M.M., Invasiveness and metastatic capability of rat fibroblast-like cells before and after transfection with immortalizing and transforming genes, *Cancer Res.,* 46, 4787, 1986.
69. Shih, C., Padhy, L.C., Murray, M., and Weinberg, R.A., Transforming genes of carcinomas and neuroblastomas introduced into mouse fibroblasts, *Nature,* 290, 261, 1981.
70. Krontiris, T.G. and Cooper, G.M., Transforming activity of human tumor DNAs, *Proc. Natl. Acad. Sci. U.S.A.,* 78, 1181, 1981.
71. Perucho, M., Goldfarb, M., Shimizu, K., Lama, C., Fogh, J., and Wigler, M., Human-tumor-derived cell lines contain common and different transforming genes, *Cell,* 27, 467, 1981.
72. Krontiris, T.G., The emerging genetics of human cancer, *N. Engl. J. Med.,* 309, 404, 1983.

73. Der, C.J., Krontiris, T.G., and Cooper, G.M., Transforming genes of human bladder and lung carcinoma cell lines are homologous to the *ras* genes of Harvey and Kirsten sarcoma viruses, *Proc. Natl. Acad. Sci. U.S.A.,* 79, 3637, 1982.

74. Pulciani, S., Santos, E., Lauver, A.V., Long, L.K., Aaronson, S.A., and Barbacid, M., Oncogenes in solid human tumors, *Nature,* 300, 539, 1982.

75. Sekiya, T., Hirohashi, S., Nishimura, S., and Sugimura, T., Transforming activity of human melanoma DNA, *Jpn. J. Cancer Res.,* 74, 794, 1983.

76. Eva, A., Tronick, S.R., Gol, R.A., Pierce, J.H., and Aaronson, S.A., Transforming genes of human hematopoietic tumors: frequent detection of *ras*-related oncogenes whose activation appears to be independent of tumor phenotype, *Proc. Natl. Acad. Sci. U.S.A.,* 80, 4926, 1983.

77. Souyri, M. and Fleissner, E., Identification by transfection of transforming sequences in DNA of human T-cell leukemias, *Proc. Natl. Acad. Sci. U.S.A.,* 80, 6676, 1983.

78. Gambke, C., Signer, E., and Moroni, C., Activation of N-*ras* gene in bone marrow cells from a patient with acute myeloblastic leukaemia, *Nature,* 307, 476, 1984.

79. Marshall, C.J., Hall, A., and Weiss, R.A., A transforming gene present in human sarcoma cell line, *Nature,* 171, 173, 1982.

80. Shimizu, K., Goldfarb, M., Perucho, M., and Wigler, M., Isolation and preliminary characterization of the transforming gene of a human neuroblastoma cell line, *Proc. Natl. Acad. Sci. U.S.A.,* 80, 383, 1983.

81. Shimizu, K., Goldfarb, M., Suard, Y., Perucho, M., Li, Y., Kamata, T., Feramisco, J., Stavnezer, E., Fogh, J., and Wigler, M.H., Three human transforming genes are related to the viral *ras* oncogenes, *Proc. Natl. Acad. Sci. U.S.A.,* 80, 2112, 1983.

82. Hall, A., Marshall, C.J., Spurr, N.K., and Weiss, R.A., Identification of transforming gene in two human sarcoma cell lines as a new member of the *ras* gene family located on chromosome 1, *Nature,* 303, 396, 1983.

83. Chardin, P., Yeramian, P., Madaule, P., and Tavitian, A., N-*ras* gene activation in the RD human rhabdomyosarcoma cell line, *Int. J. Cancer,* 35, 647, 1985.

84. Janssen, J.W.G., Steenvoorden, A.C.M., Collard, J.G., and Nusse, J., Oncogene activation in human myeloid leukemia, *Cancer Res.,* 45, 3262, 1985.

85. Needleman, S.W., Kraus, M.H., Srivastava, S.K., Levine, P.H., and Aaronson, S.A., High frequency of N-*ras* activation in acute myelogenous leukemia, *Blood,* 67, 753, 1986.

86. McKay, I.A., Paterson, H., Brown, R., Toksoz, D., Marshall, C.J., and Hall, A., N-*ras* and human cancer, *Anticancer Res.,* 6, 483, 1986.

87. Hirai, H., Tanaka, S., Azuma, M., Anraku, Y., Kobayashi, Y., Fujisawa, M., Okabe, T., Urabe, A., and Takaku, F., Transforming genes in human leukemia cells, *Blood,* 66, 1371, 1985.

88. Lane, M.-A., Sainten, A., Doherty, K.M., and Cooper, G.M., Isolation and characterization of a stage-specific transforming gene, *Tlym-1*, from T-cell lymphomas, *Proc. Natl. Acad. Sci. U.S.A.,* 81, 2227, 1984.

89. Fujita, J., Yoshida, O., Yuasa, Y., Rhim, J.S., Hatanaka, M., and Aaronson, S.A., Ha-*ras* oncogenes are activated by somatic alterations in human urinary tract tumors, *Nature,* 309, 464, 1984.

90. Fujita, J., Srivastava, S.K., Kraus, M.H., Rhim, J.S., Tronick, S.R., and Aaronson, S.A., Frequency of molecular alterations affecting *ras* protooncogenes in human urinary tract tumors, *Proc. Natl. Acad. Sci. U.S.A.,* 82, 3849, 1985.

91. Raybaud, F., Noguchi, T., Marics, I., Adelaide, J., Planche, J., Batoz, M., Aubert, C., de Lapeyriere, O., and Birnbaum, D., Detection of a low frequency of activated *ras* genes in human melanomas using a tumorigenicity assay, *Cancer Res.,* 48, 950, 1988.

92. Peehl, D.M., Wehner, N., and Stamey, T.A., Activated Ki-*ras* oncogene in human prostatic adenocarcinoma, *Prostate,* 10, 281, 1987.

93. Haas, M., Isakov, J., and Howell, S.B., Evidence against *ras* activation in human ovarian carcinomas, *Mol. Biol. Med.,* 4, 265, 1987.

94. Kraus, M.H., Yuasa, Y., and Aaronson, S.A., A position 12-activated H-*ras* oncogene in all HS578T mammary carcinosarcoma cells but not normal mammary cells of the same patient, *Proc. Natl. Acad. Sci. U.S.A.,* 81, 5384, 1984.

95. Prosperi, M.-T., Even, J., Calvo, F., Lebeau, J., and Goubin, G., Two adjacent mutations at position 12 activate the K-*ras*2 oncogene of a human mammary tumor cell line, *Oncogene Res.,* 1, 121, 1987.

96. Needleman, S.W., Yuasa, Y., Srivastava, S., and Aaronson, S.A., Normal cells of patients with high cancer risk syndromes lack transforming activity in the NIH/3T3 transfection assay, *Science,* 222, 173, 1983.

97. Albino, A.P., Le Strange, R., Oliff, A.I., Furth, M.E., and Old, L.J., Transforming *ras* genes from human melanoma: a manifestation of tumour heterogeneity?, *Nature,* 308, 69, 1984.

98. Suárez, H.G., Du Villard, J.A., Caillou, B., Schlumberger, M., Tubiana, M., Parmentier, C., and Monier, R., Detection of activated *ras* oncogenes in human thyroid carcinomas, *Oncogene,* 2, 403, 1988.

99. Guerrero, I., Villasante, A., Diamond, L., Berman, J.W., Newcomb, E.W., Steinberg, J.J., Lake, R., and Pellicer, A., Oncogene activation and surface markers in mouse lymphomas induced by radiation and nitrosomethylurea, *Leukemia Res.,* 10, 851, 1986.

100. Guerrero, I. and Pellicer, A., Mutational activation of oncogenes in animal model systems of carcinogenesis, *Mutat. Res.,* 185, 293, 1987.

101. Stowers, S.J., Maronpot, R.R., Reynolds, S.H., and Anderson, M.W., The role of oncogenes in chemical carcinogenesis, *Environ. Health Perspect.,* 75, 81, 1987.

102. Knowles, M.A., Eydmann, M.E., Proctor, A., Padua, R.A., and Roberts, J., *N*-methyl-*N*-nitrosourea-induced transformation of rat urothelial cells *in vitro* is not mediated by activation of *ras* oncogenes, *Oncogene,* 1, 143, 1987.

103. Merregaert, J., Michiels, L., Van der Rauwelaert, E., Lommel, M., Gol-Winkler, R., and Janowski, M., Oncogene involvement in radiation- and virus-induced mouse osteosarcomas, *Leukemia Res.,* 10, 915, 1986.

104. Sawey, M.J., Hood, A.T., Burns, F.J., and Garte, S.J., Activation of c-*myc* and c-K-*ras* oncogenes in primary rat tumors induced by ionizing radiation, *Mol. Cell. Biol.,* 7, 932, 1987.

105. Eva, A. and Aaronson, S.A., Frequent activation of c-*kis* as a transforming gene in fibrosarcomas induced by methylcholanthrene, *Science,* 220, 955, 1983.

106. Ochiai, M., Nagao, M., Tahira, T., Ishikawa, F., Hayashi, K., Ohgaki, H., Terada, M., Tsuchida, N., and Sugimura, T., Activation of K-*ras* and oncogenes other than *ras* family in rat fibrosarcomas induced by 1,8-dinitropyrene, *Cancer Lett.,* 29, 119, 1985.

107. Ishizaka, Y., Ochiai, M., Ohgaki, H., Ishikawa, F., Sato, S., Miura, Y., Nagao, M., and Sugimura, T., Active H-*ras* and N-*ras* in rat fibrosarcomas induced by 1,6-dinitropyrene, *Cancer Lett.,* 34, 317, 1987.

108. Storer, R.D., Stein, R.B., Sina, J.F., DeLuca, J.G., Allen, H.L., and Bradley, M.O., Malignant transformation of a preneoplastic hamster epidermal cell line by the EJ c-Ha-*ras*-oncogene, *Cancer Res.,* 46, 1458, 1986.

109. Eva, A. and Trimmer, R.W., High frequency of c-K-*ras* activation in 3-methylcholanthrene-induced mouse thymomas, *Carcinogenesis,* 7, 1931, 1986.

110. McMahon, G., Hanson, L., Lee, J.-J., and Wogan, G.N., Identification of an activated c-Ki-*ras* oncogene in rat liver tumors induced by aflatoxin B$_1$, *Proc. Natl. Acad. Sci. U.S.A.,* 83, 9418, 1986.

111. Funato, T., Yokota, J., Sakamoto, H., Kameya, T., Fukushima, S., Ito, N., Terada, M., and Sugimura, T., Activation of N-*ras* gene in a rat hepatocellular carcinoma induced by dibutylnitrosamine and butylated hydroxytoluene, *Jpn. J. Cancer Res.,* 78, 689, 1987.

112. Stowers, S.J., Wiseman, R.W., Ward, J.M., Miller, E.C., Miller, J.A., Anderson, M.W., and Eva, A., Detection of activated proto-oncogenes in *N*-nitrosodiethylamine-induced liver tumors: a comparison between B6C3F$_1$ mice and Fischer 344 rats, *Carcinogenesis,* 9, 271, 1988.

113. Rhim, J.S., Fujita, J., and Park, J.B., Activation of H-*ras* oncogene in 3-methylcholanthre-transformed human cell line, *Carcinogenesis,* 8, 1165, 1987.

114. Ishizaka, Y., Ochiai, M., Ishikawa, F., Sato, S., Miura, Y., Nagao, M., and Sugimura, T., Activated N-*ras* oncogene in a transformant derived from a rat small intestinal adenocarcinoma induced by 2-aminopyrido(1,2-α:3′,2′-D)imidazole, *Carcinogenesis,* 8, 1575, 1987.

115. Marshall, C.J., Vousden, K.H., and Phillips, D.H., Activation of c-Ha-*ras*-1 proto-oncogene by *in vitro* modification with a chemical carcinogen, benzo(*a*)pyrene diol-epoxide, *Nature,* 310, 586, 1984.

116. Vousden, K.H., Bos, J.L., Marshall, C.J., and Phillips, D.H., Mutations activating human c-Ha-*ras1* protoon-cogene (*HRAS1*) induced by chemical carcinogens and depurination, *Proc. Natl. Acad. Sci. U.S.A.,* 83, 1222, 1986.

117. Hashimoto, Y., Kawachi, E., Shudo, K., Sekiya, T., and Sugimura, T., Transforming activity of human c-Ha-*ras*-1 proto-oncogene generated by the binding of 2-amino-6-methyl-dipyrido(1,2-α:3′,2′-D)imidazole and 4-nitroquinoline N-oxide: direct evidence of cellular transformation by chemically modified DNA, *Jpn. J. Cancer Res.,* 78, 211, 1987.

118. Tainsky, M.A., Cooper, C.S., Giovanella, B.C., and Vande Woude, G.F., An activated *ras*^{N} gene: detected in late but not early passage human PA1 teratocarcinoma cells, *Science,* 225, 643, 1984.

119. Vousden, K.H. and Marshall, C.J., Three different activated *ras* genes in mouse tumours; evidence for oncogene activation during progression of a mouse lymphoma, *EMBO J.,* 3, 913, 1984.

120. Smith, G.J. and Grisham, J.W., Activation of the Ha-*ras* gene in C3H 10T1/2 cells transformed by exposure to *N*-methyl-*N*′-nitro-*N*-nitrosoguanidine, *Biochem. Biophys. Res. Commun.,* 147, 1194, 1987.

121. Reynolds, S.H., Stowers, S.J., Maronpot, R.R., Anderson, M.W., and Aaronson, S.A., Detection and identification of activated oncogenes in spontaneously occurring benign and malignant hepatocellular tumors of the B6C3F1 mouse, *Proc. Natl. Acad. Sci. U.S.A.,* 83, 33, 1986.

122. Lane, M.-A., Sainten, A., and Cooper, G.M., Stage-specific transforming genes of human mouse B- and T-lymphocyte neoplasms, *Cell,* 28, 873, 1982.

123. Goubin, G., Goldman, D.S., Luce, J., Neiman, P.E., and Cooper, G.M., Molecular cloning and nucleotide sequence of a transforming gene detected by transfection of chicken B-cell lymphoma DNA, *Nature,* 302, 114, 1983.

124. Diamond, A., Cooper, G.M., Ritz, J., and Lane, M.-A., Identification and molecular cloning of the human *Blym* transforming gene activated in Burkitt's lymphomas, *Nature,* 305, 112, 1983.

125. Devine, J.M., Diamond, A., Lane, M-A., and Cooper, G.M., Characterization of the Blym-1 transforming genes of chicken and human B-cell lymphomas, *J. Cell. Physiol.,* Suppl. 3, 193, 1984.

126. Devine, J.M., Mechanism of activation of *HuBlym*-1 gene unresolved, *Nature,* 321, 437, 1986.

127. Rogers, J., Relationship of *Blym* genes to repeated sequences, *Nature,* 320, 579, 1986.

128. Cooper, G.M., Goubin, G., Diamond, A., and Neiman, P., Relationship of *Blym* genes to repeated sequences, *Nature,* 320, 579, 1986.

129. Shimizu, K., Nakatsu, Y., Sekiguchi, M., Hokamura, K., Tanaka, K., Terada, M., and Sugimura, T., Molecular cloning of an activated human oncogene, homologous to v-*raf*, from primary stomach cancer, *Proc. Natl. Acad. Sci. U.S.A.,* 82, 5641, 1985.

130. Kasid, U., Pfeifer, A., Weichselbaum, R.R., Dritschilo, A., and Mark, G.E., The *raf* oncogene is associated with a radiation-resistant human laryngeal cancer, *Science,* 237, 1039, 1987.

131. Fukui, M., Yamamoto, T., Kawai, S., Maruo, K., and Toyoshima, K., Detection of a *raf*-related and two other transforming DNA sequences in human tumors maintained in nude mice, *Proc. Natl. Acad. Sci. U.S.A.,* 82, 5954, 1985.

132. Ishikawa, F., Takaku, F., Ochiai, M., Hayashi, K., Hirohashi, S., Terada, M., Takayama, S., Nagao, M., and Sugimura, T., Activated c-*raf* gene in a rat hepatocellular carcinoma induced by 2-amino-3-methylimidazo(4,5-*f*)quinoline, *Biochem. Biophys. Res. Commun.,* 132, 186, 1985.

133. Ishikawa, F., Takaku, F., Hayashi, K., Nagao, M., and Sugimura, T., Activation of rat c-*raf* during transfection of hepatocellular carcinoma DNA, *Proc. Natl. Acad. Sci. U.S.A.,* 83, 3209, 1986.

134. Fukui, M., Yamamoto, T., Kawai, S., Mitsunobu, F., and Toyoshima, K., Molecular cloning and characterization of an activated human c-*raf*-1 gene, *Mol. Cell. Biol.,* 7, 1776, 1987.

135. Tahira, T., Ochiai, M., Hayshi, K., Nagao, M., and Sugimura, T., Activation of human c-*raf*-1 by replacing the N-terminal region with different sequences, *Nucleic Acids Res.,* 15, 4809, 1987.

136. Cooper, C.S., Park, M., Blair, D.G., Tainsky, M.A., Huebner, K., Croce, C.M., and Vande Woude, G.F., Molecular cloning of a new transforming gene from a chemically transformed human cell line, *Nature,* 311, 29, 1984.

137. Eva, A. and Aaronson, S.A., Isolation of a new human oncogene from a diffuse B-cell lymphoma, *Nature,* 316, 273, 1985.

138. Eva, A., Vecchio, G., Diamond, M., Tronick, S.R., Ron, D., Cooper, G.M., and Aaronson, Independently activated *dbl* oncogenes exhibit similar yet distinct structural alterations, *Oncogene,* 1, 355, 1987.

139. Takahashi, M., Ritz, J., and Cooper, G.M., Activation of a novel human transforming gene, *ret*, by DNA rearrangement, *Cell,* 42, 581, 1985.

140. Park, M., Dean, M., Cooper, C.S., Schmidt, M., O'Brien, S.J., Blair, G., and Vande Woude, G.F., Mechanism of *met* oncogene activation, *Cell,* 45, 895, 1986.

141. Tempest, P.R., Reeves, B.R., Spurr, N.K., Rance, A.J., Chan, A.M.-L., and Brookes, P., Activation of the *met* oncogene in the human MNNG-HOS cell line involves a chromosomal rearrangement, *Carcinogenesis,* 7, 2051, 1986.

142. Dean, M., Park, M., and Vande Woude, G.F., Characterization of the rearranged *tpr-met* oncogene breakpoint, *Mol. Cell. Biol.,* 7, 921, 1987.

143. Srivastava, S.K., Wheelock, R.H.P., Aaronson, S.A., and Eva, A., Identification of the protein encoded by the human diffuse B-cell lymphoma (*dbl*) oncogene, *Proc. Natl. Acad. Sci. U.S.A.,* 83, 8868, 1986.

144. Eva, A., Vecchio, G., Rao, C.D., Tronick, S.R., and Aaronson, S.A., The predicted *DBL* oncogene product defines a distinct class of transforming proteins, *Proc. Natl. Acad. Sci. U.S.A.,* 85, 2061, 1988.

145. Sakamoto, H., Mori, M., Taira, M., Yoshida, T., Matsukawa, S., Shimizu, K., Sekiguchi, M., Terada, M., and Sugimura, T., Transforming gene from human stomach cancers and a noncancerous portion of stomach mucosa, *Proc. Natl. Acad. Sci. U.S.A.,* 83, 3997, 1986.

146. Koda, T., Sasaki, A., Matsushima, S., and Kakinuma, M., A transforming gene, *hst*, found in NIH 3T3 cells transformed with DNA from three stomach cancers and a colon cancer, *Jpn. J. Cancer Res.,* 78, 325, 1987.

147. Yuasa, Y. and Sudo, K., Transforming genes in human hepatomas detected by a tumorigenicity assay, *Jpn. J. Cancer Res.,* 78, 1036, 1987.

148. Nakagama, H., Ohnishi, S., Imawari, M., Hirai, H., Takaku, F., Sakamoto, H., Terada, M., Nagao, M., and Sugimura, T., Identification of transforming genes as *hst* in DNA samples from two hepatocellular carcinomas, *Jpn. J. Cancer,* 78, 651, 1987.

149. Delli Bovi, P. and Basilico, C., Isolation of a rearranged human transforming gene following transfection of Kaposi sarcoma DNA, *Proc. Natl. Acad. Sci. U.S.A.,* 84, 5660, 1987.

150. Delli Bovi, P., Curatola, A.M., Kern, F.G., Greco, A., Ittmann, M., and Basilico, C., An oncogene isolated by transfection of Kaposi's sarcoma DNA encodes a growth factor that is a member of the FGF family, *Cell,* 50, 729, 1987.

151. Adelaide, J., Mattei, M.-G., Marics, I., Raybaud, F., Planche, J., De Lapeyriere, O., and Birnbaum, D., Chromosomal localization of the *hst* oncogene and its co-amplification with the *int*.2 oncogene in a human melanoma, *Oncogene,* 2, 413, 1988.

152. Ochiya, T., Fujiyama, A., Fukusige, S., Hatada, I., and Matsubara, K., Molecular cloning of an oncogene from a human hepatocellular carcinoma, *Proc. Natl. Acad. Sci. U.S.A.,* 83, 4993, 1986.

153. Martin-Zanca, D., Hughes, S.H., and Barbacid, M., A human oncogene formed by the fusion of truncated tropomyosin and protein tyrosine kinase sequences, *Nature,* 319, 743, 1986.

154. Reinach, F.C. and MacLeod, A.R., Tissue-specific expression of the human tropomyosin gene involved in the generation of the *trk* oncogene, *Nature,* 322, 648, 1986.

155. Kozma, S.C., Redmond, S.M.S., Xiao-Chang, F., Saurer, S.M., Groner, B., and Hynes, N.E., Activation of the receptor kinase domain of the *trk* oncogene by recombination with two different cellular sequences, *EMBO J.,* 7, 147, 1988.

156. Friedman, W.H., Rosenblum, B.N., Loewenstein, P., Thornton, H., Katsantonis, G., and Green, M., Oncogenes: their presence and significance in squamous cell cancer of the head and neck, *Laryngoscope,* 95, 313, 1985.

157. Hollingsworth, M.A., Rebellato, L.M., Moore, J.W., Finn, O.J., and Metzgar, R.S., Antigens expressed on NIH 3T3 cells following transformation with DNA from a human pancreatic tumor, *Cancer Res.,* 46, 2482, 1986.

158. Fox, T.R. and Watanabe, P.G., Detection of a cellular oncogene in spontaneous liver tumors of B6C3F1 mice, *Science,* 228, 596, 1985.

159. Iwamura, Y, Mitamura, K., Yanagi, K., Hashimoto, T., and Kato, K., Transforming potential of DNA of the human PLC/PRF/5 hepatoma cell line, *Intervirology,* 26, 223, 1986.

160. Borek, C., Ong, A., and Mason, H., Distinctive transforming genes in x-ray-transformed mammalian cells, *Proc. Natl. Acad. Sci. U.S.A.,* 84, 794, 1987.

161. Penn, A., Garte, S.J., Warren, L., Nesta, D., and Mindich, B., Transforming gene in human atherosclerotic plaque DNA, *Proc. Natl. Acad. Sci. U.S.A.,* 83, 7951, 1986.

162. Scott, J., Oncogenes in atherosclerosis, *Nature,* 325, 574, 1987.

163. Calabretta, B., Venturelli, D., Kaczmarek, L., Narni, F., Talpaz, M., Anderson, B., Beran, M., and Baserga, R., Altered expression of G_1-specific genes in human malignant myeloid cells, *Proc. Natl. Acad. Sci. U.S.A.,* 83, 1495, 1986.

164. Eva, A., Robbins, K.C., Andersen, P.R., Srinivasan, A., Tronick, S.R., Reddy, E.P., Ellmore, N.W., Galen, A.T., Lautenberger, J.A., Papas, T.S., Westin, E.H., Wong-Staal, F., Gallo, R.C., and Aaronson, S.A., Cellular genes analogous to retroviral *onc* genes are transcribed in human tumor cells, *Nature,* 295, 116, 1982.

165. Westin, E.H., Wong-Staal, F., Gelmann, E.P., Dalla Favera, R., Papas, T.S., Lautenberger, J.A., Eva, A., Reddy, E.P., Tronick, S.R., Aaronson, S.A., and Gallo, R.C., Expression of cellular homologues of retroviral *onc* genes in human hematopoietic cells, *Proc. Natl. Acad. Sci. U.S.A.,* 79, 2490, 1982.

166. Huber, B.E. and Thorgeirsson, S.S., Analysis of c-*myc* expression in a human hepatoma cell line, *Cancer Res.,* 47, 3414, 1987.

167. Yoshimoto, K., Hirohashi, S., and Sekiya, T., Increased expression of the c-*myc* gene without gene amplification in human lung cancer and colon cancer cell lines, *Jpn. J. Cancer,* 77, 540, 1986.

168. Kubota, Y., Shuin, T., Yao, M., Inoue, H., and Yoshioka, T., the enhanced ^{32}P labeling of CDP-diacylglycerol in c-*myc* gene expressed human kidney cancer cells, *FEBS Lett.,* 212, 159, 1987.

169. Erisman, M.D., Scott, J.K., Watt, R.A., and Astrin, S.M., The c-*myc* protein is constitutively expressed at elevated levels in colorectal carcinoma cell lines, *Oncogene,* 2, 367, 1988.

170. Untawale, S. and Blick, M., Oncogene expression in adenocarcinomas of the colon and in colon tumor-derived cell lines, *Anticancer Res.,* 8, 1, 1988.

171. Veillette, A., Foss, F.M., Sausville, E.A., Bolen, J.B., and Rosen, N., Expression of the *lck* tyrosine kinase gene in human colon carcinoma and other non-lymphoid human tumor cell lines, *Oncogene Res.,* 1, 357, 1987.

172. Korc, M., Meltzer, P., and Trent, J., Enhanced expression of epidermal growth factor receptor correlates with alterations of chromosome 7 in human pancreatic cancer, *Proc. Natl. Acad. Sci. U.S.A.,* 83, 5141, 1986.

173. Haeder, M., Rotsch, M., Bepler, G., Hennig, C., Havemann, K., Heimann, B., and Moelling, K., Epidermal growth factor receptor expression in human lung cancer cell lines, *Cancer Res.,* 48, 1132, 1988.

174. Chang, E.H., Pirollo, K.F., Zou, Z.Q., Cheung, H.-Y., Lawler, E.L., Garner, R., White, E., Bernstein, W.B., Fraumeni, J.W., Jr., and Blattner, W.A., Oncogenes in radioresistant, noncancerous skin fibroblasts from a cancer-prone family, *Science,* 237, 1036, 1987.

175. Skouv, J., Christensen, B., and Autrup, H., Differential induction of transcription of c-*myc* and c-*fos* proto-oncogenes by 12-*O*-tetradecanoylphorbol-13-acetate in mortal and immortal human urothelial cells, *J. Cell. Biochem.,* 34, 71, 1987.

176. Graves, D.T., Owen, A.J., Barth, R.K., Tempst, P., Winoto, A., Fors, L., Hood, L.E., and Antoniades, H.N., Detection of c-*sis* transcripts and synthesis of PDGF-like proteins by human osteosarcoma cells, *Science,* 226, 972, 1984.

177. Jonak, G.J. and Knigth, E., Jr., Selective reduction of c-*myc* mRNA in Daudi cells by human beta interferon, *Proc. Natl. Acad. Sci. U.S.A.,* 81, 1747, 1984.

178. Griffin, C.A. and Baylin, S.B., Expression of the c-*myb* oncogene in human small cell lung carcinoma, *Cancer Res.,* 45, 272, 1985.

179. Uchida, Y., Yamaguchi, K., Abe, K., Tsuchihashi, T., Asanuma, F., Nagasaki, K., Kimura, S., Yanaihara, N., and Track, N.S., Radioimmunoassay of c-*myc* protein, *Jpn. J. Cancer Res.,* 77, 615, 1986.

180. Billings, P.C., Shuin, T., Lillehaug, J., Miura, T., Roy-Burman, P., and Landolph, J.R., Enhanced expression and state of the c-*myc* oncogene in chemically and X-ray-transformed C3H/10T1/2 Cl 8 mouse embryo fibroblasts, *Cancer Res.,* 47, 3643, 1987.

181. Müller, R., Müller, D., and Guilbert, L., Differential expression of c-*fos* in hematopoietic cells: correlation with differentiation of monomyelocytic cells *in vitro*, *EMBO J.,* 3, 1887, 1984.

182. Shuin, T., Billings, P.C., Lillehaug, J.R., Patierno, S.R., Roy-Burman, P., and Landolph, J.R., Enhanced expression of c-*myc* and decreased expression of c-*fos* protooncogenes in chemically and radiation-transformed C3H/10T1/2 mouse embryo cell lines, *Cancer Res.,* 46, 5302, 1986.

183. Leibovitch, S.A., Leibovitch, M.P., Guillier, M., Hillion, J., and Harel, J., Differential expression of protooncogenes related to transformation and cancer progression in rat myoblasts, *Cancer Res.,* 46, 4097, 1986.

184. Yuhki, N., Hamada, J., Kuzumaki, N., Takeichi, N., and Kobayashi, H., Metastatic ability and expression of c-*fos* oncogene in cell clones of a spontaneous rat mammary tumor, *Jpn. J. Cancer Res.,* 77, 9, 1986.

185. Andreeff, M., Slater, D.E., Bressler, J., and Furth, M.E., Cellular *ras* oncogene expression and cell cycle measured by flow cytometry in hematopoietic cell lines, *Blood,* 67, 676, 1986.

186. Kessler, D.J., Heilman, C.A., Cossman, J., Maguire, R.T., and Thorgeirsson, S.S., Transformation of Epstein-Barr virus immortalized human B-cells by chemical carcinogens, *Cancer Res.,* 47, 527, 1987.

187. Kasid, U.N., Hough, C., Thraves, P., Dritschilo, A., and Smulson, M., The association of human c-Ha-ras sequences with chromatin and nuclear proteins, *Biochem. Biophys. Res. Commun.,* 128, 226, 1985.

188. O'Hara, B., Klinger, H.P., and Blair, D.G., Many oncogenes are transcribed in the D98AH2 derivative of the HeLa carcinoma cell line, *Cytogenet. Cell Genet.,* 43, 97, 1986.

189. O'Hara, B.M., Klinger, H.P., Curran, T., Zhang, Y.-D., and Blair, D.G., Levels of *fos, ets2,* and *myb* proto-oncogene RNAs correlate with segregation of chromosome 11 of normal cells and with suppression of tumorigenicity in human cell hybrids, *Mol. Cell. Biol.,* 7, 2941, 1987.

190. Sarkar, S., Kacinski, B.M., Kohorn, E.I., Merino, M.J., Carter, D., and Blakemore, K.J., Demonstration of myc and ras oncogene expression by hybridization *in situ* in hydatiform mole and in the BeWo choriocarcinoma cell line, *Am. J. Obstet. Gynecol.,* 154, 390, 1986.

191. Conscience, J.-F., Verrier, B., and Martin, G., Interleukin-3-dependent expression of the c-*myc* and c-*fos* proto-oncogenes in hemopoietic cell lines, *EMBO J.,* 5, 317, 1986.

192. Rijnders, A.W.M., van der Korput, J.A.G.M., van Steenbrugge, G.J., Romijn, J.C., and Trapman, J., Expression of cellular oncogenes in human prostatic carcinoma cell lines, *Biochem. Biophys. Res. Commun.,* 132, 548, 1985.

193. Mizuki, K., Nose, K., Okamoto, H., Tsuchida, N., and Hayashi, K., Amplification of c-Ki-*ras* gene and aberrant expression of c-*myc* in WI-38 cells transformed *in vitro* by gamma-irradiation, *Biochem. Biophys. Res. Commun.,* 128, 1037, 1985.

194. Vilette, D., Emanoil-Ravier, R., Tobaly, J., and Peries, J., Studies on four cellular proto-oncogenes and their expression in PCC4 embryonal carcinoma cells: amplification of c-Ki-ras oncogene, *Biochem. Biophys. Res. Commun.,* 128, 513, 1985.

195. Motoo, Y., Mahmoudi, M., Osther, K., and Bollon, A.P., Oncogene expression in human hepatoma cells PLC/PRF/5, *Biochem. Biophys. Res. Commun.,* 135, 262, 1986.

196. Huber, B.E., Dearfield, K.L., Williams, J.R., Heilman, C.A., and Thorgeirsson, S.S., Tumorigenicity and transcriptional modulation of c-*myc* and N-*ras* oncogenes in a human hepatoma cell line, *Cancer Res.,* 45, 4322, 1985.

197. Blin, N., Müller-Brechlin, R., Carstens, C., Meese, E., and Zang, K.D., Enhanced expression of four cellular oncogenes in a human glioblastoma cell line, *Cancer Genet. Cytogenet.,* 25, 285, 1987.

198. Kohl, N.E., Gee, C.E., and Alt, F.W., Activated expression of the N-*myc* gene in human neuroblastomas and related tumors, *Science,* 226, 1335, 1984.

199. Sadée, W., Yu, V.C., Richards, M.L., Preis, P.N., Schwab, M.R., Brodsky, F.M., and Biedler, J.L., Expression of neurotransmitter receptors and *myc* protooncogenes in subclones of a human neuroblastoma cell line, *Cancer Res.,* 47, 5207, 1987.

200. Thiele, C.J., McKeon, C., Triche, T.J., Ross, R.A., Reynolds, C.P., and Israel, M.A., Differential protooncogene expression characterizes histopathologically indistinguishable tumors of the peripheral nervous system, *J. Clin. Invest.,* 80, 804, 1987.

201. Schön, A., Michiels, L., Janowski, M., Merregaert, J., and Erfle, V., Expression of protooncogenes in murine osteosarcomas, *Int. J. Cancer,* 38, 67, 1986.

202. Sejersen, T., Sümegi, J., and Ringertz, N.R., Expression of cellular oncogenes in teratoma-derived cell lines, *Exp. Cell Res.,* 160, 19, 1985.

203. Karthaus, H.F.M., Bussemakers, M.J.G., Schalken, J.A., Kurth, K.H., Feitz, W.F.J., Debruyne, F.M.J., Bloemers, H.P.J., and Van de Ven, W.J.M., Expression of proto-oncogenes in xenografts of human renal cell carcinomas, *Urol. Res.,* 15, 349, 1987.

204. Tanaka, T., Slamon, D.J., Battifora, H., and Cline, M.J., Expression of p21 *ras* oncoproteins in human cancers, *Cancer Res.,* 46, 1465, 1986.

205. Spandidos, D.A. and Agnantis, N.J., Human malignant tumours of the breast, as compared to their respective normal tissue, have elevated expression of the Harvey *ras* oncogene, *Anticancer Res.,* 4, 269, 1984.

206. Theillet, C., Lidereau, R., Escot, C., Hutzell, P., Brunet, M., Gest, M., Schlom, J., and Callahan, R., Loss of a c-H-*ras*-1 allele and aggressive human primary breast carcinomas, *Cancer Res.,* 46, 4776, 1986.

207. Whittaker, J.L., Walker, R.A., and Varley, J.M., Differential expression of cellular oncogenes in benign and malignant human breast tissue, *Int. J. Cancer,* 38, 651, 1986.

208. Clair, T., Miller, W.R., and Cho-Chung, Y.S., Prognostic significance of the expression of a *ras* protein with a molecular weight of 21,000 by human breast cancer, *Cancer Res.,* 47, 5290, 1987.

209. Ghosh, A.K., Moore, M., and Harris, M., Immunohistochemical detection of *ras* oncogene p21 product in benign and malignant mammary tissue in man, *J. Clin. Pathol.,* 39, 428, 1986.

210. Candlish, W., Kerr, I.B., and Simpson, H.W., Immunocytochemical demonstration and significance of p21 *ras* family oncogene product in benign and malignant breast disease, *J. Pathol.,* 150, 163, 1986.

211. Agnantis, N.J., Petraki, C., Markoulatos, P., and Spandidos, D.A., Immunohistochemical study of the *ras* oncogene expression in human breast lesions, *Anticancer Res.,* 6, 1157, 1986.

212. De Bortoli, M.E., Abou-Issa, H., Haley, B.E., and Cho-Chung, Y.S., Amplified expression of p21 *ras* protein in hormone-dependent mammary carcinomas of humans and rodents, *Biochem. Biophys. Res. Commun.,* 127, 699, 1985.

213. Ohuchi, N., Thor, A., Page, D.L., Hand, P.H., Halter, S.A., and Schlom, J., Expression of the 21,000 molecular weight *ras* protein in a spectrum of benign and malignant human mammary tissues, *Cancer Res.,* 46, 2511, 1986.

214. Kurzrock, R., Gallick, G.E., and Gutterman, J.U., Differential expression of p21*ʳᵃˢ* gene products among histological subtypes of fresh primary human lung tumors, *Cancer Res.,* 46, 1530, 1986.

215. Lee, I., Gould, V.E., Radosevich, J.A., Thor, A., Ma, Y., Schlom, J., and Rosen, S.T., Immunohistochemical evaluation of ras oncogene expression in pulmonary and pleural neoplasms, *Virchows Arch.,* B53, 146, 1987.

216. Viola, M.V., Fromowitz, F., Oravez, S., Deb, S., and Schlom, J., *ras* oncogene p21 expression is increased in premalignant lesions and high grade bladder carcinoma, *J. Exp. Med.,* 161, 1213, 1985.

217. Fujita, J., Nakayama, H., Onoue, H., Rhim, J.S., El-Bolkainy, M.N., El-Aaser, A.A., and Kitamura, Y., Frequency of active *ras* oncogenes in human bladder cancers associated with schistosomiasis, *Jpn. J. Cancer Res.,* 78, 915, 1987.

218. Viola, M.V., Fromowitz, F., Oravez, S., Deb, S., Finkel, G., Lundy, J., Hand, P., Thor, A., and Schlom, J., Expression of *ras* oncogene p21 in prostate cancer, *N. Engl. J. Med.,* 314, 133, 1986.

219. Menegazzi, M., Scarpa, A., and Libonati, M., Analysis of the methylation pattern of c-Ha-ras oncogene in human prostatic cancer, *Ital. J. Biochem.,* 37, 104, 1988.

220. Spandidos, D.A. and Kerr, I.B., Elevated expression of the human *ras* oncogene family in premalignant and malignant tumours of the colorectum, *Br. J. Cancer,* 49, 681, 1984.

221. Michelassi, F., Leuthner, S., Lubienski, M., Bostwick, D., Rodgers, J., Handcock, M., and Block, G.E., ras oncogene p21 levels parallel malignant potential of different human colonic benign conditions, *Arch. Surg.,* 122, 1414, 1987.

222. Gallick, G.E., Kurzrock, R., Kloetzer, W.S., Arlinghaus, R.B., and Gutterman, J.U., Expression of p21*ʳᵃˢ* in fresh primary and metastatic human colorectal tumors, *Proc. Natl. Acad. Sci. U.S.A.,* 82, 1795, 1985.

223. Kerr, I.B., Spandidos, D.A., Finlay, I.G., Lee, F.D., and McArdle, C.S., The relation of *ras* family oncogene expression to conventional staging criteria and clinical outcome in colorectal carcinoma, *Br. J. Cancer,* 53, 231, 1986.

224. Williams, A.R.W., Piris, J., Spandidos, D.A., and Wyllie, A.H., Immunohistochemical detection of the *ras* oncogene p21 product in an experimental tumour and in human colorectal neoplasms, *Br. J. Cancer,* 52, 687, 1985.

225. Kerr, I.B., Lee, F.D., Quintanilla, M., and Balmain, A., Immunocytochemical demonstration of p21 *ras* family oncogene product in normal mucosa and in premalignant and malignant tumours of the colorectum, *Br. J. Cancer,* 52, 695, 1985.

226. Augenlicht, L.H., Augeron, C., Yander, G., and Laboisse, C., Overexpression of *ras* in mucus-secreting human colon carcinoma cells of low tumorigenicity, *Cancer Res.,* 47, 3763, 1987.

227. Tahara, E., Yasui, W., Taniyama, K., Ochiai, A., Yamamoto, T., Nakajo, S., and Yamamoto, M., Ha-*ras* oncogene product in human gastric carcinoma: correlation with invasiveness, metastasis or prognosis, *Jpn. J. Cancer Res.,* 77, 517, 1986.

228. Czerniak, B., Herz, F., Koss, L.G., and Schlom, J., ras oncogene p21 as a tumor marker in the cytodiagnosis of gastric and colonic carcinomas, *Cancer,* 60, 2432, 1987.

229. Mizukami, Y., Nomomura, A., Hashimoto, T., Terahata, S., Matsubara, F., Michigishi, T., and Noguchi, M., Immunohistochemical demonstration of *ras* p21 oncogene product in normal, benign, and malignant human thyroid tissues, *Cancer,* 61, 873, 1988.

230. Tanaka, T., Slamon, D.J., Shimoda, H., Waki, C., Kawaguchi, Y., Tanaka, Y., and Ida, N., Expression of Ha-*ras* oncogene products in human neuroblastomas and the significant correlation with a patient's prognosis, *Cancer Res.,* 48, 1030, 1988.

231. Guérin, M., Lacombe, M.-J., and Riou, G., Analyse de l'expression de l'oncogène c-*myc* dans les adémpcarcinomes mammaires humaines, *C.R. Acad. Sci. (Paris),* 301, 833, 1985.

232. Spandidos, D.A., Pintzas, A., Kakkanas, A., Yiagnisis, M., Mahera, H., Patra, E., and Agnantis, N.J., Elevated expression of the *myc* gene in human benign and malignant breast lesions compared to normal tissue, *Anticancer Res.,* 7, 1299, 1987.

233. Riou, G., Barrois, M., Le, M.G., George, M., LeDoussal, V., and Haie, C., c-*myc* proto-oncogene expression and prognosis in early carcinoma of the uterine cervix, *Lancet,* 1, 761, 1987.

234. Hendy-Ibbs, P., Cox, H., Evan, G.I., and Watson, J.V., Flow cytometric quantitation of DNA and c-*myc* oncoprotein in archival biopsies of uterine cervix neoplasia, *Br. J. Cancer,* 55, 275, 1987.

235. Allum, W.H., Newbold, K.M., Macdonald, F., Russell, B., and Stokes, H., Evaluation of p62$^{c\text{-}myc}$ in benign and malignant gastric epithelia, *Br. J. Cancer,* 56, 785, 1987.

236. Ciclitira, P.J., MacArtney, J.C., and Evan, G., Expression of c-myc in non-malignant and pre-malignant gastrointestinal disorders, *J. Pathol.,* 151, 293, 1987.

237. Tsuboi, K., Hirayoshi, K., Takeuchi, K., Sabe, H., Shimada, Y., Ohshio, G., Tobe, T., and Hatanaka, M., Expression of the c-myc gene in human gastrointestinal malignancies, *Biochem. Biophys. Res. Commun.,* 146, 699, 1987.

238. Sundaresan, V., Forgacs, I.C., Wight, D.G.D., Wilson, B., Evan, G.I., and Watson, J.V., Abnormal distribution of c-myc oncogene product in familial adenomatous polyposis, *J. Clin. Pathol.,* 40, 1274, 1987.

239. Watson, J.V., Stewart, J., Cox, H., Sikora, K., and Evan, G.I., Flow cytometric quantitation of the c-*myc* oncoprotein in archival neoplastic biopsies of the colon, *Mol. Cell. Probes,* 1, 151, 1987.

240. Erisman, M.D., Rothberg, P.G., Diehl, R.E., Morse, C.C., Spandorfer, J.M., and Astrin, S.M., Deregulation of c-*myc* gene expression in human colon carcinoma is not accompanied by amplification or rearrangement of the gene, *Mol. Cell. Biol.,* 5, 1969, 1985.

241. Rothberg, P.G., Spandorfer, J.M., Erisman, M.D., Staroscik, R.N., Sears, H.F., Petersen, R.O., and Astrin, S.M., Evidence that c-myc expression defines two genetically distinct forms of colorectal adenocarcinoma, *Br. J. Cancer,* 52, 629, 1985.

242. Erisman, M.D., Litwin, S., Keidan, R.D., Comis, R.L., and Astrin, S.M., Noncorrelation of the expression of the c-*myc* oncogene in colorectal carcinoma with recurrence of disease or patient survival, *Cancer Res.,* 48, 1350, 1988.

243. Stewart, J., Evan, G., Watson, J., and Sikora, K., Detection of the c-*myc* oncogene product in colonic polyps and carcinoma, *Br. J. Cancer,* 53, 1, 1986.

244. Ciclitira, P.J., Stewart, J., Evan, G., Wight, D.G.D., and Sikora, K., Expression of c-myc oncogene in coeliac disease, *J. Clin. Pathol.,* 40, 307, 1987.

245. Monnat, M., Tardy, S., Saraga, P., Diggelmann, H., and Costa, J., Prognostic implications of expression of the cellular genes *myc, fos,* Ha-*ras,* and Ki-*ras* in colon carcinoma, *Int. J. Cancer,* 40, 293, 1987.

246. Su, T.-S., Lin, L.-H., Lui, W.-Y., Chang, C., Chou, C.-K., Ting, L.-P., Hu, C.-P., Han, S.-H., and P'eng, F.-K., Expression of c-myc gene in human hepatoma, *Biochem. Biophys. Res. Commun.,* 132, 264, 1985.

247. Zhang, X.-K., Huang, D.-P., Chiu, D.-K., and Chiu, J.-F., The expression of oncogenes in human developing liver and hepatomas, *Biochem. Biophys. Res. Commun.,* 142, 932, 1987.

248. Chan, S.Y.T., Evan, G.I., Ritson, A., Watson, J., Wraight, P., and Sikora, K., Localisation of lung cancer by a radiolabelled monoclonal antibody against the c-*myc* oncogene product, *Br. J. Cancer,* 54, 761, 1986.

249. Fleming, W.H., Hamel, R., MacDonald, R., Ramsey, E., Pettigrew, N.M., Johnston, B., Dodd, J.G., and Matusik, R.J., Expression of the c-*myc* protooncogene in human prostatic carcinoma and benign prostatic hyperplasia, *Cancer Res.,* 46, 1535, 1986.

250. Buttyan, R., Sawczuk, I.S., Benson, M.C., Siegal, J.D., and Olsson, C.A., Enhanced expression of the c-*myc* protooncogene in high-grade human prostate cancers, *Prostate,* 11, 327, 1987.

251. Sikora, K., Evan, G., Stewart, J., and Watson, J.V., Detection of the c-*myc* oncogene product in testicular cancer, *Br. J. Cancer,* 52, 171, 1985.

252. Terrier, P., Sheng, Z.-M., Schlumberger, M., Tubiana, M., Caillou, B., Travagli, J.-P., Fragu, P., Parmentier, C., and Riou, G., Structure and expression of c-*myc* and c-*fos* proto-oncogenes in thyroid carcinomas, *Br. J. Cancer,* 57, 43, 1988.

253. Nisen, P.D., Zimmerman, K.A., Cotter, S.V., Gilbert, F., and Alt, F.W., Enhanced expression of the N-*myc* gene in Wilms' tumors, *Cancer Res.,* 46, 6217, 1987.

254. Watson, J.V., Stewart, J., Evan, G.I., Ritson, A., and Sikora, K., The clinical significance of flow cytometric c-*myc* oncoprotein quantitation in testicular cancer, *Br. J. Cancer,* 53, 331, 1986.

255. Polacarz, S.V., Hey, N.A., Stephenson, T.J., and Hill, A.S., c-*myc* oncogene product p62$^{c\text{-}myc}$ in ovarian mucinous neoplasms: immunohistochemical study correlated with malignancy, *J. Clin. Pathol.,* 42, 148, 1989.

256. Barnekow, A., Paul, E., and Schartl, M., Expression of the c-*src* protooncogene in human skin tumors, *Cancer Res.,* 47, 235, 1987.

257. Rosen, N., Bolen, J.B., Schwartz, A.M., Cohen, P., DeSeau, V., and Israel, M.A., Analysis of pp60$^{c\text{-}src}$ protein kinase activity in human tumor cell lines and tissues, *J. Biol. Chem.,* 261, 13754, 1986.

258. Pérez, R., Pascual, M., Macìas, A., and Lage, A., Epidermal growth factor receptors in human breast cancer, *Breast Cancer Res. Treat.,* 4, 189, 1984.

259. Sainsbury, J.R.C., Farndon, J.R., Sherbet, G.V., and Harris, A.L., Epidermal growth-factor receptors and oestrogen receptors in human breast cancer, *Lancet,* 1, 364, 1985.

260. Macìas, A., Azavedo, E., Pérez, R., Rutqvist, L.E., and Skoog, L., Receptors for epidermal growth factor in human mammary carcinomas and their metastases, *Anticancer Res.,* 6, 849, 1986.

261. Wyss, R., Fabbro, D., Regazzi, R., Borner, C., Takahashi, A., and Eppenberger, U., Phorbol ester and epidermal growth factor receptors in human breast cancer, *Anticancer Res.,* 7, 721, 1987.

262. Sainsbury, J.R.C., Malcolm, A.J., Appleton, D.R., Farndon, J.R., and Harris, A.L., Presence of epidermal growth factor receptor as an indicator of poor prognosis in patients with breast cancer, *J. Clin. Pathol.,* 38, 1225, 1985.

263. Sainsbury, J.R.C., Farndon, J.R., Needhan, G.K., Malcolm, A.J., and Harris, A.L., Epidermal-growth-factor receptor status as predictor of early recurrence of and death from breast cancer, *Lancet,* 1, 1398, 1987.

264. Hunts, J., Ueda, M., Ozawa, S., Abe, O., Pastan, I., and Shimizu, N., Hyperproduction and gene amplification of the epidermal growth factor receptor in squamous cell carcinomas, *Jpn. J. Cancer Res.,* 76, 663, 1985.

265. Gullick, W.J., Marsden, J.J., Whittle, N., Ward, N., Ward, B., Bobrow, L., and Waterfield, M.D., Expression of epidermal growth factor receptors on human cervical, ovarian, and vulval carcinomas, *Cancer Res.,* 46, 285, 1986.

266. Yamamoto, T., Kamata, N., Kawano, H., Shimizu, S., Kuroki, T., Tohoshima, K., Rikimaru, K., Nomura, N., Ishizaki, R., Pastan, I., Gamou, S., and Shimizu, N., High incidence of amplification of epidermal growth factor receptor gene in human squamous carcinoma cell lines, *Cancer Res.,* 46, 414, 1986.

267. Ozanne, B., Richards, C.S., Hendler, F., Burns, D., and Gusterson, B., Over-expression of the EGF receptor is a hallmark of squamous cell carcinomas, *J. Pathol.,* 149, 9, 1986.

268. Kamata, N., Chida, K., Rikimaru, K., Horikoshi, M., Enomoto, S., and Kuroki, T., Growth-inhibitory effects of epidermal growth factor and overexpression of its receptors on human squamous cell carcinomas in culture, *Cancer Res.,* 46, 1648, 1986.

269. Hwang, D.L., Tay, Y.-C., Lin, S.S., and Lev-Ran, A., Expression of epidermal growth factor receptors in human lung tumors, *Cancer,* 58, 2260, 1986.

270. Cerny, T., Barnes, D.M., Hasleton, P., Barber, P.V., Healy, K., Gullick, W., and Thatcher, N., Expression of epidermal growth factor receptor (EGF-R) in human lung tumours, *Br. J. Cancer,* 54, 265, 1986.

271. Sakai, K., Mori, S., Kawamoto, T., Taniguchi, S., Kobori, O., Morioka, Y., Kuroki, T., and Kano, K., Expression of epidermal growth factor receptors on normal human gastric epithelia and gastric carcinomas, *J. Natl. Cancer Inst.,* 77, 1047, 1986.

272. Neal, D.E., Marsh, C., Bennett, M.K., Abel, P.D., Hall, R.R., Sainsbury, J.R.C., and Harris, A.L., Epidermal growth-factor receptors in human bladder cancer: comparison of invasive and superficial tumors, *Lancet,* 1, 366, 1985.

273. Gusterson, B., Cowley, G., McIlhinney, J., Ozanne, B., Fisher, C., and Reeves, B., Evidence for increased epidermal growth factor receptors in human sarcomas, *Int. J. Cancer,* 36, 689, 1985.

274. Libermann, T.A., Razon, N., Bartal, A.D., Yarden, Y., Schlessinger, J., and Soreq, H., Expression of epidermal growth factor receptors in human brain tumors, *Cancer Res.,* 44, 753, 1984.

275. Weisman, A.S., Raguet, S.S., and Kelly, P.A., Characterization of the epidermal growth factor receptor in human meningioma, *Cancer Res.,* 47, 2172, 1987.

276. Libermann, T.A., Nusbaum, H.R., Razon, N., Kris, R., Lax, I., Soreq, H., Whittle, N., Waterfield, M.D., Ullrich, A., and Schlessinger, J., Amplification, enhanced expression and possible rearrangement of EGF receptor gene in primary human brain tumours of glial origin, *Nature,* 313, 144, 1985.

277. Wong, A.J., Bigner, S.H., Bigner, D.D., Kinzler, K.W., Hamilton, S.R., and Vogelstein, B., Increased expression of the epidermal growth factor receptor gene in malignant gliomas is invariably associated with gene amplification, *Proc. Natl. Acad. Sci. U.S.A.,* 84, 6899, 1987.

278. Birman, P., Michard, M., Li, J.Y., Peillon, F., and Bression, D., Epidermal growth factor-binding sites, present in normal human and rat pituitaries, are absent in human pituitary adenomas, *J. Clin. Endocrinol. Metab.,* 65, 275, 1987.

279. Mori, S., Akiyama, T., Morishita, Y., Shimizu, S., Sakai, K., Sudoh, K., Toyoshima, K., and Yamamoto, T., Light and electron microscopical demonstration of c-*erbB*-2 gene product-like immunoreactivity in human malignant tumors, *Virchows Arch.,* B54, 8, 1987.

280. Berger, M.S., Locher, G.W., Saurer, S., Gullick, W.J., Waterfield, M.D., Groner, B., and Hynes, N.E., Correlation of c-*erbB*-2 gene amplification and protein expression in human breast carcinoma with nodal status and nuclear grading, *Cancer Res.,* 48, 1238, 1988.

281. van de Vijver, M.J., Peterse, J.L., Mooi, W.J., Wisman, P., Lomans, J., Dalesio, O., and Nusse, R., *neu* protein overexpression in breast cancer — association with comedo-type ductal carcinomas *in situ* and limited prognostic value in stage II breast cancer, *N. Engl. J. Med.,* 319, 1239, 1988.

282. Cattoretti, G., Rilke, F., Andreola, S., D'Amato, L., and Delia, D., p53 expression in breast cancer, *Int. J. Cancer,* 41, 178, 1988.

283. Spandidos, D.A., Lamothe, A., and Field, J.K., Multiple transcriptional activation of cellular oncogenes in human head and neck solid tumors, *Anticancer Res.,* 5, 221, 1985.

284. Field, J.K., Lamothe, A., and Spandidos, D.A., Clinical relevance of oncogene expression in head and neck tumours, *Anticancer Res.,* 6, 595, 1986.

285. Eisbruch, A., Blick, M., Lee, J.S., Sacks, P.G., and Gutterman, J., Analysis of the epidermal growth factor receptor gene in fresh human head and neck tumors, *Cancer Res.,* 47, 3603, 1987.

286. Slamon, D.J., de Kernion, J.B., Verma, I.M., and Cline, M.J., Expression of cellular oncogenes in human malignancies, *Science,* 224, 256, 1984.

287. Tatosyan, A.G., Galetzki, S.A., Kisseljova, N.P., Asanova, A.A., Zborovskaya, I.B., Spitkovsky, D.D., Revasova, E.S., Martin, P., and Kisseljov, F.L., Oncogene expression in human tumors, *Int. J. Cancer,* 35, 731, 1985.

288. Rosson, D. and Tereba, A., Transcription of hematopoietic-associated oncogenes in childhood leukemia, *Cancer Res.,* 43, 3912, 1983.

289. Roy-Burman, P., Devi, B.G., and Parker, J.W., Differential expression of c-*erbB*, c-*myc* and c-*myb* oncogene loci in human lymphomas and leukemias, *Int. J. Cancer,* 32, 185, 1983.

290. Rothberg, P.G., Erisman, M.D., Diehl, R.E., Rovigatti, U.G., and Astrin, S.M., Structure and expression of the oncogene c-*myc* in fresh tumor material from patients with hematopoietic malignancies, *Mol. Cell. Biol.,* 4, 1096, 1984.

291. Rodenhuis, S., Bos, J.L., Slater, R.M., Behrendt, H., van't Veer, M., and Smets, L.A., Absence of oncogene amplifications and occasional activation of N-*ras* in lymphoblastic leukemia of childhood, *Blood,* 67, 1698, 1986.

292. McClain, K.L., Expression of oncogenes in human leukemias, *Cancer Res.,* 44, 5382, 1984.

293. Blick, M., Westin, E., Gutterman, J., Wong-Staal, F., Gallo, R.C., McCredie, K., Keating, M., and Murphy, E., Oncogene expression in human leukemia, *Blood,* 64, 1234, 1984.

294. Mavilio, F., Sposi, N.M., Petrini, M., Bottero, L., Marinucci, M., De Rossi, G., Amadori, S., Mandelli, F., and Peschle, C., Expression of cellular oncogenes in primary cells from human acute leukemias, *Proc. Natl. Acad. Sci. U.S.A.,* 83, 4394, 1986.

295. Mavilio, F., Testa, U., Sposi, M., Petrini, M., Pelosi, E., Bordignon, C., Amadori, S., Mandelli, F., and Peschle, C., Selective expression of *fos* proto-oncogene in human acute myelomonocytic and monocytic leukemias: a molecular marker of terminal differentiation, *Blood,* 69, 160, 1987.

296. Sposi, N.M., Mavilio, F., Petrini, M., Bottero, L., Zappavigna, V., Mastroberardino, G., De Rossi, G., Amadori, S., Mandelli, F., and Peschle, C., *Haematologica,* 72 (Suppl.), 23, 1987.

297. de Kretser, T., Adams, F., Devereux, L., Garson, M., Michael, P., and Savin, K., Elevation of c-*abl*-mRNA in human leukemic B lymphoblasts, *Leukemia Res.,* 10, 1391, 1986.

298. Slamon, D.J., Boone, T.C., Murdock, D.C., Keith, D.E., Press, M.F., Larson, R.A., and Souza, L.M., Studies of the human c-*myb* gene and its product in human acute leukemias, *Science,* 233, 347, 1986.

299. Ferrari, S., Torelli, U., Selleri, L., Donelli, A., Venturelli, D., Narni, F., Moretti, L., and Torelli, G., Study of the levels of expression of two oncogenes, c-myc and c-myb, in acute and chronic leukemias of both lymphoid and myeloid lineage, *Leukemia Res.,* 9, 833, 1985.

300. Torelli, U., Selleri, L., Venturelli, D., Donelli, A., Emilia, G., Ceccherelli, G., Turchi, L., and Torelli, G., Differential patterns of expression of cell cycle-related genes in blast cells of acute myeloid leukemia, *Leukemia Res.,* 10, 1249, 1986.

301. Ferrari, S., Narni, F., Mars, W., Kaczmarek, L., Venturelli, D., Anderson, B., and Calabretta, B., Expression of growth-regulated genes in human acute leukemias, *Cancer Res.,* 46, 5162, 1986.

302. Jack, A.S., Kerr, I.B., Evan, G., and Lee, F.D., The distribution of the c-*myc* oncogene product in malignant lymphomas and various normal tissues as demonstrated by immunocytochemistry, *Br. J. Cancer,* 53, 713, 1986.

303. Birnie, G.D., Warnock, A.M., Burns, J.H., and Clark, P., Expression of the *myc* gene locus in populations of leukocytes from leukaemia patients and normal individuals, *Leukemia Res.,* 10, 515, 1986.

304. Shen, W.P.V., Aldrich, T.H., Venta-Perez, G., Franza, B.R., Jr., and Furth, M.E., Expression of normal and mutant *ras* proteins in human acute leukemia, *Oncogene,* 1, 157, 1987.

305. Feldman, R.A., Gabrilove, J.L., Tam, J.P., Moore, M.A.S., and Hanafusa, H., Specific expression of the human cellular *fps/fes*-encoded protein NCP92 in normal and leukemic myeloid cells, *Proc. Natl. Acad. Sci. U.S.A.,* 82, 2379, 1985.

306. Koeffler, H.P., Miller, C., Nicolson, M.A., Ranyard, J., and Bosselman, R.A., Increased expression of p53 protein in human leukemia cells, *Proc. Natl. Acad. Sci. U.S.A.,* 83, 4035, 1986.

307. Prokocimer, M., Shaklai, M., Ben Bassat, H., Wolf, D., Goldfinger, N., and Rotter, V., Expression of p53 in human leukemia and lymphoma, *Blood,* 68, 113, 1986.

308. Smith, L.J., McCulloch, E.A., and Benchimol, S., Expression of the p53 oncogene in acute myeloblastic leukemia, *J. Exp. Med.,* 164, 751, 1986.

309. Embleton, M.J., Habib, N.A., Garnett, M.C., and Wood, C., Unsuitability of monoclonal antibodies to oncogene proteins for anti-tumour drug-targeting, *Int. J. Cancer,* 38, 821, 1986.

310. Schartl, M., Schmidt, C.-R., Anders, A., and Barnekow, A., Elevated expression of the cellular *src* gene in tumors of differing etiology in *Xiphophorus*, *Int. J. Cancer*, 36, 199, 1985.

311. Coll, J., Saule, S., Martin, P., Raes, M.B., Lagrou, C., Graf, T., Beug, H., Simon, I.E., and Stehelin, D., The cellular oncogenes c-*myc*, c-*myb* and c-*erb* are transcribed in defined types of avian hematopoietic cells, *Exp. Cell Res.*, 149, 151, 1983.

312. Linial, M. and Groudine, M., Transcription of three c-*myc* exons is enhanced in chicken bursal lymphoma cell lines, *Proc. Natl. Acad. Sci. U.S.A.*, 82, 53, 1985.

313. Saule, S., Martin, P., Gegonne, A., Begue, A., Lagrou, C., and Stehelin, D., Increased transcription of the c-*myc* oncogene in two methylcholanthrene-induced quail fibroblastic cell lines, *Exp. Cell Res.*, 155, 496, 1984.

314. Huh, N., Satoh, M., Nose, K., Abe, E., Suda, T., Rajewski, M.F., and Kuroki, T., 1α,25-dihydroxyvitamin D_3 induces anchorage-independent growth and c-Ki-*ras* expression of BALB/3T3 and HIH/3T3 cells, *Jpn. J. Cancer Res.*, 78, 99, 1987.

315. Takahashi, K., Heine, U.I., Junker, J.L., Colburn, N.H., and Rice, J.M., Role of cytoskeleton changes and expression of the H-*ras* oncogene during promotion of neoplastic transformation in mouse epidermal JB6 cells, *Cancer Res.*, 46, 5923, 1986.

316. Harper, J.R., Roop, D.R., and Yuspa, S.H., Transfection of the EJ *ras*[Ha] gene into keratinocytes derived from carcinogen-induced mouse papillomas causes malignant progression, *Mol. Cell. Biol.*, 6, 3144, 1986.

317. Pelling, J.C., Fischer, S.M., Neades, R., Strawhecker, J., and Schweickert, L., Elevated expression and point mutation of the Ha-*ras* proto-oncogene in mouse skin tumors promoted by benzoyl peroxide and other promoting agents, *Carcinogenesis*, 8, 1481, 1987.

318. Guerrero, I., Calzada, P., Mayer, A., and Pellicer, A., A molecular approach to leukemogenesis: mouse lymphomas contain an activated c-*ras* oncogene, *Proc. Natl. Acad. Sci. U.S.A.*, 81, 202, 1984.

319. Guerrero, I., Villasante, A., D'Eustachio, P., and Pellicer, A., Isolation, characterization, and chromosome assignment in mouse N-*ras* gene from carcinogen-induced thymic lymphoma, *Science*, 225, 1041, 1984.

320. Sukumar, S., Pulciani, S., Doniger, J., DiPaolo, J., Evans, C.H., Zbar, B., and Barbacid, M., A transforming *ras* gene in tumorigenic guinea pig cell lines initiated by diverse chemical carcinogens, *Science*, 223, 1197, 1984.

321. Corcoran, L.M., Adams, J.M., Dunn, A.R., and Cory, S., Murine T lymphomas in which the cellular *myc* oncogene has been activated by retroviral insertion, *Cell*, 37, 113, 1984.

322. Selten, G., Cuypers, H.T., Zijlstra, M., Melief, C., and Berns, A., Involvement of c-*myc* in MuLV-induced T cell lymphomas in mice: frequency and mechanisms of activation, *EMBO J.*, 3, 3215, 1984.

323. Robert-Lezenes, J., Moreau-Gachelin, F., Wendling, F., Tambourin, P., and Tavitian, A., Expression of c-*ras* and c-*myc* in murine erythroleukemias induced by Friend viruses, *Leukemia Res.*, 8, 975, 1984.

324. Rechavi, G., Givol, D., and Canaani, E., Activation of a cellular oncogene by DNA rearrangement: possible involvement of an IS-like element, *Nature*, 300, 607, 1982.

325. Kuff, E.L., Feenstra, A., Lueders, K., Rechavi, G., Givol, D., and Canaani, E., Homology between an endogenous viral LTR and sequences inserted in an activated cellular oncogene, *Nature*, 302, 547, 1983.

326. Gattoni-Celli, S., Hsiao, W.-L.W., and Weinstein, I.B., Rearranged c-*mos* locus in a MOPC 21 murine myeloma cell line and its persistence in hybridomas, *Nature*, 306, 795, 1983.

327. Smith, C.A.D., Winterbourne, D.J., McFarland, V.W., and Mora, P.T., Changes in heparan sulfate pattern but not in oncogene expression correlate with tumor growth in spontaneous transformation of cells, *Oncogene Res.*, 1, 325, 1987.

328. Jakobovits, A., Schwab, M., Bishop, J.M., and Martin, G.R., Expression of N-*myc* in teratocarcinoma stem cells and mouse embryo fibroblasts, *Nature*, 318, 188, 1985.

329. Chinsky, J., Lilly, F., and Childs, G., Comparison of chemically induced and spontaneous murine thymic lymphomas in RF and AKR mice: differential expression of c-*myc* and c-*myb*, *Proc. Natl. Acad. Sci. U.S.A.*, 82, 565, 1985.

330. Matsuyama, M., Yamada, C., and Hiai, H., A single dominant susceptible gene determines spontaneous development of thymoma in BUF/Mna rat, *Jpn. J. Cancer Res.*, 77, 1066, 1986.

331. Mally, M.I., Vogt, M., Swift, S.E., and Haas, M., Oncogene expression in murine splenic T cells and in murine T-cell neoplasms, *Virology*, 144, 115, 1985.

332. Huang, F.L. and Cho-Chung, Y.S., Hormone-regulated expression of cellular *ras*[H] oncogene in mammary carcinomas in rats, *Biochem. Biophys. Res. Commun.*, 123, 141, 1984.

333. Yasui, W., Sumiyoshi, H., Yamamoto, T., Oda, N., Kameda, T., Tanaka, T., and Tahara, E., Expression of Ha-*ras* oncogene product in rat gastrointestinal carcinomas induced by chemical carcinogens, *Acta Pathol. Jpn.*, 37, 1731, 1987.

334. Cote, G.J., Lastra, B.A., Cook, J.R., Huang, D.-P., and Chiu, J.-F., Oncogene expression in rat hepatomas and during hepatocarcinogenesis, *Cancer Lett.*, 26, 121, 1985.

335. Cote, G.J. and Chiu, J.-F., The expression of oncogenes and liver-specific genes in Morris hepatomas, *Biochem. Biophys. Res. Commun.*, 143, 624, 1987.

336. Tahiro, F., Morimura, S., Hayashi, K., Makino, R., Kawamura, H., Horikoshi, N., Nemoto, K., Ohtsubo, K., Sugimura, T., and Ueno, Y., Expression of the c-Ha-*ras* and c-*myc* genes in aflatoxin B_1-induced hepatocellular carcinomas, *Biochem. Biophys. Res. Commun.,* 138, 858, 1986.

337. Makino, R., Hayashi, K., Sato, S., and Sugimura, T., Expressions of the c-Ha-*ras* and c-*myc* genes in rat liver tumors, *Biochem. Biophys. Res. Commun.,* 119, 1096, 1984.

338. Corcos, D., Defer, N., Raymodjean, M., Paris, B., Corral, M., Tichonicky, L., and Kruh, J., Correlated increase of the expression of the c-ras genes in chemically induced hepatocarcinomas, *Biochem. Biophys. Res. Commun.,* 122, 259, 1984.

339. Bhave, M.R., Wilson, M.J., and Poirier, L.A., c-H-*ras* and c-K-*ras* gene hypomethylation in the livers and hepatomas of rats fed methyl-deficient, amino acid-defined diets, *Carcinogenesis,* 9, 343, 1988.

340. Galand, P., Jacobovitz, D., and Alexandre, K., Immunohistochemical detection of c-Ha-*ras* oncogene p21 product in pre-neoplastic and neoplastic lesions during hepatocarcinogenesis in rats, *Int. J. Cancer,* 41, 161, 1988.

341. Corral, M., Tichonicky, L., Guguen-Guillouzo, C., Corcos, D., Raymondjean, M., Paris, B., Kruh, J., and Defer, N., Expression of c-*fos* oncogene during hepatocarcinogesis, liver regeneration and in synchronized HTC cells, *Exp. Cell Res.,* 160, 427, 1985.

342. Ito, S., Watanabe, T., Abe, K., Yanaihara, N., Tateno, C., Okuno, Y., Yoshitake, A., and Miyamoto, J., Immunohistochemical demonstration of the c-*myc* oncogene product in rat chemical hepatocarcinogenesis, *Biomed. Res.,* 9, 177, 1988.

343. Corral, M., Paris, B., Guguen-Guillouzo, C., Corcos, D., Kruh, J., and Defer, N., Increased expression of the N-*myc* gene during normal and neoplastic rat liver growth, *Exp. Cell Res.,* 174, 107, 1988.

344. Carr, B.I., Kabbinwar, F., and Slamon, D.J., Hepatocarcinogens induce an increased expression of ras, myc and Abelson oncogene expression in rat liver, in a time- and dose-dependent manner, *Clin. Res.,* 33, 450A, 1985.

345. Yasween, P., Goyette, M., Shank, P.R., and Fausto, N., Expression of c-Ki-*ras*, c-Ha-*ras*, and c-*myc* in specific cell types during hepatocarcinogenesis, *Mol. Cell. Biol.,* 5, 780, 1985.

346. Beer, D.G., Schwarz, M., Sawada, N., and Pitot, H.C., Expression of H-*ras* and c-*myc* protooncogenes in isolated γ-glutamyl transpeptidase-positive rat hepatocytes and in hepatocellular carcinomas induced by diethylnitrosamine, *Cancer Res.,* 46, 2435, 1986.

347. Richmond, R.E., Pereira, M.A., Carter, J.H., Carter, H.W., and Long, R.E., Quantitative and qualitative immunohistochemical detection of myc and src oncogene proteins in normal, nodule, and neoplastic rat liver, *J. Histochem. Cytochem.,* 36, 179, 1988.

348. Corral, M., Defer, N., Paris, B., Raymondjean, M., Corcos, D., Tichonicky, L., Kruh, J., Glaise, D., Kneip, B., and Guguen-Guillouzo, C., Isolation and characterization of complementary DNA clones for genes overexpressed in chemically induced rat hepatomas, *Cancer Res.,* 46, 5119, 1986.

349. Embleton, M.J. and Butler, P.C., Reactivity of monoclonal antibodies to oncoproteins with normal rat liver, carcinogen-induced tumours, and premalignant liver lesions, *Br. J. Cancer,* 57, 48, 1988.

350. Walker, C., Nettesheim, P., Barrett, J.C., and Gilmer, T.M., Expression of a *fms*-related oncogene in carcinogen-induced neoplastic epithelial cells, *Proc. Natl. Acad. Sci. U.S.A.,* 84, 1804, 1987.

351. Thorgeirsson, U.P., Turpeenniemi-Hujanen, T., Talmadge, J.E., and Liotta, L.A., Expression of oncogenes in cancer metastases, in *Cancer Metastases: Experimental and Clinical Strategies,* Alan R. Liss, New York, 1986, 77.

352. Gold, P. and Freedman, S.D., Specific carcinoembryonic antigens of the human digestive system, *J. Exp. Med.,* 122, 468, 1965.

353. Abelev, G.I., Production of embryonal serum α-globulin by hepatomas: review of experimental and clinical data, *Cancer Res.,* 28, 1344, 1968.

354. Abelev, G.I., α-Fetoprotein in oncogenesis and its association with malignant tumors, *Adv. Cancer Res.,* 14, 295, 1971.

355. Wepsic, H.T., Overview of oncofetal antigens in cancer, *Ann. Clin. Lab. Sci.,* 13, 261, 1983.

356. Bartsch, R.A., Joannou, C., Talbot, I.C., and Bailey, D.S., Cloning of mRNA sequences from the human colon: preliminary characterisation of defined mRNAs in normal and neoplastic tissues, *Br. J. Cancer,* 54, 791, 1986.

357. Shiosaka, T., Tanaka, Y., and Kobayashi, Y., Preferentially expressed genes in stomach adenocarcinoma cells, *Br. J. Cancer,* 56, 539, 1987.

358. Scott, M.R.D., Westphal, K.-H., and Rigby, P.W.J., Activation of mouse genes in transformed cells, *Cell,* 34, 557, 1983.

359. Murphy, D., Brickell, P.M., Latchman, D.S., Willison, K., and Rigby, P.W.J., Transcripts regulated during normal embryonic development and oncogenic transformation share a repetitive element, *Cell,* 35, 865, 1983.

360. Brickell, D.S., Latchman, D.S., Murphy, D., Willison, K., and Rigby, P.W.J., Activation of a *Qa/Tla* class I major histocompatibility antigen gene is a general feature of oncogenesis in the mouse, *Nature,* 306, 756, 1983.

361. Winberry, L., Priehs, C., Friderici, K., Thompson, M., and Fluck, M., Expression of proto-oncogenes in normal and papovavirus-transformed or -infected rat fibroblasts, *Virology,* 147, 154, 1985.

362. Melber, K., Krieg, P., Fürstenberger, G., and Marks, F., Molecular cloning of sequences activated during multi-stage carcinogenesis in mouse skin, *Carcinogenesis,* 7, 317, 1986.

363. Toftgard, R., Roop, D.R., and Yuspa, S.H., Proto-oncogene expression during two-stage carcinogenesis in mouse skin, *Carcinogenesis,* 6, 655, 1985.

364. Mountz, J.D., Steinberg, A.D., Klinman, D.M., Smith, H.R., and Mushinski, J.F., Autoimmunity and increased c-*myb* transcription, *Science,* 226, 1087, 1984.

365. Mountz, J.D., Mushinski, J.F., Mark, G.E., and Steinberg, A.D., Oncogene expression in autoimmune mice, *J. Mol. Cell. Immunol.,* 2, 121, 1985.

366. Boumpas, D.T., Mark, G.E., and Tsokos, G.C., Oncogenes and autoimmunity, *Anticancer Res.,* 6, 491, 1986.

367. Rosenberg, Y.J., Malek, T.R., Schaeffer, D.E., Santoro, T.J., Mark, G.E., Steinberg, A.D., and Mountz, J.D., Unusual expression of IL 2 receptors and both the c-*myb* and c-*raf* oncogenes in T cell lines and clones derived from autoimmune MRL-*lpr/lpr* mice, *J. Immunol.,* 134, 3120, 1985.

368. Yokota, S., Yuan, D., Katagiri, T., Eisenberg, R.A., Cohen, P.L., and Ting, J.P.-Y., The expression and regulation of c-*myb* transcription in B6/*lpr* Lyt-2⁻, L3T4⁻ T lymphocytes, *J. Immunol.,* 139, 2810, 1987.

369. Evans, J.L., Boyle, W.J., and Ting, J.P.-Y., Molecular basis of elevated c-*myb* expression in the abnormal L3T4⁻, Lyt-2⁻ T lymphocytes of autoimmune mice, *J. Immunol.,* 139, 3497, 1987.

370. Klinman, D.M., Mushinski, J.F., Honda, M., Ishigatsubo, Y., Mountz, J.D., Raveche, E.S., and Steinberg, A.D., Oncogene expression in autoimmune and normal peripheral blood mononuclear cells, *J. Exp. Med.,* 163, 1986.

371. Husby, G., Williams, R.C., Jr., Watt, R.A., West, S.G., and Tung, K.S.K., Tissue c-*myc* protein expression and immune response in systemic lupus erythematosus, *Clin. Exp. Immunol.,* 69, 493, 1987.

372. Klinman, D.M., Steinberg, A.D., and Mushinski, J.F., Effect of cyclophosphamide therapy on oncogene expression in angioimmunoblastic lymphadenopathy, *Lancet,* 2, 1055, 1986.

373. Mark, G.E., Seeley, T.W., Shows, T.B., and Mountz, J.D., *pks,* a *raf*-related sequence in humans, *Proc. Natl. Acad. Sci. U.S.A.,* 83, 6312, 1986.

374. Cowley, B.D., Jr., Smardo, F.L., Jr., Grantham, J.J., and Calvet, J.P., Elevated c-*myc* protooncogene expression in autosomal recessive polycystic kidney disease, *Proc. Natl. Acad. Sci. U.S.A.,* 84, 8394, 1987.

375. Pachnis, V., Belayew, A., and Tilghman, S.M., Locus unlinked to α-fetoprotein under the control of the murine *raf* and *Rif* genes, *Proc. Natl. Acad. Sci. U.S.A.,* 81, 5523, 1984.

376. Kelly, K., Cochran, B.H., Stiles, C.D., and Leder, P., Cell-specific regulation of the c-*myc* gene by lymphocyte mitogens and platelet-derived growth factor, *Cell,* 35, 603, 1983.

377. Ramsden, M., Cole, G., Smith, J., and Balmain, A., Differential methylation of the c-H-*ras* gene in normal mouse cells and during skin tumour progression, *EMBO J.,* 4, 1449, 1985.

378. Barr, F.G., Rjagopalan, S., MacArthur, C.A., and Lieberman, M.W., Genomic hypomethylation and far-5' sequence alterations are associated with carcinogen-induced activation of the hamster thymidine kinase gene, *Mol. Cell. Biol.,* 6, 3023, 1986.

379. Feinberg, A.P. and Vogelstein, B., Hypomethylation of *ras* oncogenes in primary human cancers, *Biochem. Biophys. Res. Commun.,* 111, 47, 1983.

380. Kaneko, Y., Shibuya, M., Nakayama, T., Hayashida, N., Toda, G., Endo, Y., Oka, H., and Oda, T., Hypomethylation of c-*myc* and epidermal growth factor receptor genes in human hepatocellular carcinoma and fetal liver, *Jpn. J. Cancer Res.,* 76, 1136, 1985.

381. Barbieri, R., Piva, R., Buzzoni, D., Volinia, S., and Gambari, R., Clustering of undermethylated CCGG and GCGC sequences in the 5' region of the Ha-ras-1 oncogene of human leukemic K562 cells, *Biochem. Biophys. Res. Commun.,* 145, 96, 1987.

382. Kris, R.M., Avivi, A., Bar-Eli, M., Alon, Y., Carmi, P., Schlessinger, J., and Raz, A., Expression of Ki-ras oncogene in tumor cell variants exhibiting different metastatic capabilities, *Int. J. Cancer,* 35, 227, 1985.

383. Rotter, V., Wolf, D., Blick, M., and Nicolson, G.L., Expression of *abl* and other oncogenes is independent of metastatic potential in Abelson virus-transformed malignant murine large cell lymphoma, *Clin. Exp. Metastasis,* 3, 77, 1985.

384. Stark, G.R. and Wahl, G.M., Gene amplification, *Annu. Rev. Biochem.,* 53, 447, 1984.

385. Pall, M.L., Gene-amplification model of carcinogenesis, *Proc. Natl. Acad. Sci. U.S.A.,* 78, 2465, 1981.

386. Flintoff, W.F., Livingston, E., Duff, C., and Worton, R.G., Moderate-level gene amplification in methotrexate-resistant Chinese hamster ovary cells is accompanied by chromosomal translocations at or near the site of the amplified DHFR gene, *Mol. Cell. Genet.,* 4, 69, 1984.

387. Schimke, R.T., Gene amplification, drug resistance, and cancer, *Cancer Res.,* 44, 1735, 1984.

388. Zehnbauer, B.A., Small, D., Brodeur, G.M., Seeger, R., and Vogelstein, B., Characterization of N-*myc* amplification units in human neuroblastoma cells, *Mol. Cell. Biol.,* 8, 522, 1988.

389. Wolman, S. and Henderson, A.S., Chromosomal aberrations as markers of oncogene amplification, *Hum. Pathol.,* 20, 308, 1989.

390. Wong, D.T.W., Amplification of the c-*erbB1* oncogene in chemically-induced oral carcinomas, *Carcinogenesis,* 8, 1963, 1987.

391. Caizzi, R. and Bostock, C.J., Gene amplification in methotrexate-resistant mouse cells. IV. Different DNA sequences are amplified in different cell lines, *Nucleic Acids Res.,* 10, 6597, 1982.

392. Wolman, S.R., Lanfrancone, L., Dalla-Favera, R., Ripley, S., and Henderson, A.S., Oncogene mobility in a human leukemia line HL-60, *Cancer Genet. Cytogenet.,* 17, 133, 1985.

393. Sager, R., Gadi, I.K., Stephens, L., and Grabowy, C.T., Gene amplification: an example of accelerated evolution in tumorigenic cells, *Proc. Natl. Acad. Sci. U.S.A.,* 82, 7015, 1985.

394. Alitalo, K., Amplification of cellular oncogenes in cancer cells, *Med. Biol.,* 62, 304, 1984.

395. George, D.L., Amplification of cellular proto-oncogenes in tumours and tumour cell lines, *Cancer Surv.,* 3, 497, 1984.

396. Mäkelä, T.P. and Alitalo, K., Proto-oncogene amplification: role in tumour progression, *Ann. Clin. Res.,* 18, 290, 1986.

397. Alitalo, K., Koskinen, P., Mäkelä, T.P., Saksela, K., Sistonen, L., and Winqvist, R., *myc* oncogenes: activation and amplification, *Biochim. Biophys. Acta,* 907, 1, 1987.

398. Collins, S. and Groudine, M., Amplification of endogenous *myc*-related DNA sequences in a human myeloid leukaemia cell line, *Nature,* 298, 679, 1982.

399. Nowell, P., Finan, J., Dalla Favera, R., Gallo, R.C., ar-Rushdi, A., Romanczuk, H., Selden, J.R., Emanuel, B.S., Rovera, G., and Croce, C.M., Association of amplified oncogene c-*myc* with an abnormally banded chromosome 8 in a human leukaemia cell line, *Nature,* 306, 494, 1983.

400. Graham, S.V., Tindle, R.W., and Birnie, G.D., Variation in *myc* amplification and expression in sublines of HL60 cells, *Leukemia Res.,* 9, 239, 1985.

401. Lee, W.-H., Murphree, A.L., and Benedict, W.F., Expression of the N-*myc* gene in primary retinoblastoma, *Nature,* 309, 458, 1984.

402. Sakai, K., Kanda, N., Shiloh, Y., Donlon, T., Schreck, R., Shipley, J., Dryja, T., Chaum, E., Chaganti, R.S.K., and Latt, S., Molecular and cytologic analysis of DNA amplification in retinoblastoma, *Cancer Genet. Cytogenet.,* 17, 95, 1985.

403. Schwab, M., Alitalo, K., Klempnauer, K.-H., Varmus, H.E., Bishop, J.M., Gilbert, F., Brodeur, G., Goldstein, M., and Trent, J., Amplified DNA with limited homology to *myc* cellular oncogene is shared by human neuroblastoma cell lines and a neuroblastoma tumour, *Nature,* 305, 245, 1983.

404. Montgomery, K.T., Biedler, J.L., Spengler, B.A., and Melera, P.W., Specific DNA sequence amplification in human neuroblastoma cells, *Proc. Natl. Acad. Sci. U.S.A.,* 80, 5724, 1983.

405. Michitsch, R.W., Montgomery, K.T., and Melera, P.W., Expression of the amplified domain in human neuroblastoma cells, *Mol. Cell. Biol.,* 4, 2370, 1984.

406. Trent, J., Meltzer, P., Rosenblum, M., Harsh, G., Kinzler, K., Mashal, R., Feinberg, A., and Vogelstein, B., Evidence for rearrangement, amplification, and expression of c-*myc* in a human glioblastoma, *Proc. Natl. Acad. Sci. U.S.A.,* 83, 470, 1986.

407. Kozbor, D. and Croce, C.M., Amplification of the c-*myc* oncogene in one of five human breast carcinoma cell lines, *Cancer Res.,* 44, 438, 1984.

408. Graham, K.A., Richardson, C.L., Minden, M.D., Trent, J.M., and Buick, R.N., Varying degrees of amplification of the N-*ras* oncogene in the human breast cancer cell line MCF-7, *Cancer Res.,* 45, 2201, 1985.

409. Modjtahedi, N., Lavialle, C., Poupon, M.-F., Landin, R.-M., Cassingena, R., Monier, R., and Brison, O., Increased level of amplification of the c-*myc* oncogene in tumors induced in nude mice by a human breast carcinoma cell line, *Cancer Res.,* 45, 4372, 1985.

410. Yasue, H., Takeda, A., and Ishibashi, M., Amplification of the c-*myc* gene and the elevation of its transcripts in human ovarian tumor lines, *Cell Struct. Funct.,* 12, 121, 1987.

411. Bogenmann, E., Moghadam, H., DeClerck, Y.A., and Mock, A., c-*myc* amplification and expression in newly established human osteosarcoma cell lines, *Cancer Res.,* 47, 3808, 1987.

412. Little, C.D., Nau, M.M., Carney, D.M., Gazdar, A.F., and Minna, J.D., Amplification and expression of the c-*myc* oncogene in human lung cancer cell lines, *Nature,* 306, 194, 1983.

413. Saksela, K., Bergh, J., Lehto, V.-P., Nilsson, K., and Alitalo, K., Amplification of the c-*myc* oncogene in a subpopulation of human small cell lung cancer, *Cancer Res.,* 45, 1823, 1985.

414. Seifter, E.J., Sausville, E.A., and Battey, J., Comparison of amplified and unamplified c-*myc* gene structure and expression in human small cell lung carcinoma cell lines, *Cancer Res.,* 46, 2050, 1986.

415. Saksela, K., Bergh, J., and Nilsson, K., Amplification of the N-*myc* oncogene in an adenocarcinoma of the lung, *J. Cell. Biochem.,* 31, 297, 1986.

416. Saksela, K., Expression of the L-*myc* gene is under positive control by short-lived proteins, *Oncogene,* 1, 291, 1987.

417. Misawa, S., Staal, S.P., and Testa, J.R., Amplification of the c-*myc* oncogene is associated with an abnormally banded region on chromosome 8 or double minute chromosomes in two HL-60 human leukemia sublines, *Cancer Genet. Cytogenet.,* 28, 127, 1987.

418. Nau, M.M., Brooks, B.J., Jr., Carney, D.N., Gazdar, A.F., Battey, J.F., Sausville, E.A., and Minna, J.D., Human small-cell lung cancers show amplification and expression of the N-*myc* gene, *Proc. Natl. Acad. Sci. U.S.A.,* 83, 1092, 1986.

419. Nau, M.M., Brooks, B.J., Battey, J., Sausville, E., Gazdar, A.F., Kirsch, I.R., McBride, O.W., Bertness, V., Hollis, G.F., and Minna, J.D., L-*myc*, a new *myc*-related gene amplified and expressed in human small cell lung cancer, *Nature,* 318, 1985.

420. Taya, Y., Hosogai, K., Hiroyashi, S., Shimosato, Y., Tsuchiya, R., Fushimi, M., Sekiya, T., and Nishimura, S., A novel combination of K-*ras* and *myc* amplification accompanied by point mutational activation of K-*ras* in a human lung cancer, *EMBO J.,* 3, 2943, 1984.

421. Alitalo, K., Schwab, M., Lin, C.C., Varmus, H.E., and Bishop, J.M., Homogeneously staining chromosomal regions contain amplified copies of an abundantly expressed cellular oncogene (c-*myc*) in malignant neuroendocrine cells from a human colon carcinoma, *Proc. Natl. Acad. Sci. U.S.A.,* 80, 1707, 1983.

422. McCoy, M.S., Toole, J.J., Cunningham, J.M., Chang, E.H., Lowy, D.R., and Weinberg, R.A., Characterization of a human colon/lung carcinoma oncogene, *Nature,* 302, 79, 1983.

423. Lin, C.C., Alitalo, K., Schwab, M., George, D., Varmus, H.E., and Bishop, J.M., Evolution of karyotypic abnormalities and c-*myc* oncogene amplification in human colonic carcinoma cell lines, *Chromosoma (Berlin),* 92, 11, 1985.

424. Schwab, M., Klempnauer, K.-H., Alitalo, K., Varmus, H., and Bishop, M., Rearrangement at the 5′ end of amplified c-*myc* in human COLO 320 cells is associated with abnormal transcription, *Mol. Cell. Biol.,* 6, 2752, 1986.

425. Shibuya, M., Yokota, J., and Ueyama, Y., Amplification and expression of a cellular oncogene (c-*myc*) in human gastric adenocarcinoma cells, *Mol. Cell. Biol.,* 5, 414, 1985.

426. Baker, V.V., Shingleton, H.M., Hatch, K.D., and Miller, D.M., Selective inhibition of c-myc expression by the ribonucleic acid synthesis inhibitor mithramycin, *Am. J. Obstet. Gynecol.,* 158, 762, 1988.

427. Kohl, N.E., Kanda, N., Schreck, R.R., Bruns, G., Latt, S.A., Gilbert, F., and Alt, F.W., Transposition and amplification of oncogene-related sequences in human neuroblastomas, *Cell,* 35, 359, 1983.

428. Brodeur, G.M., Seeger, R.C., Schwab, M., Varmus, H.E., and Bishop, J.M., Amplification of N-*myc* in untreated human neuroblastomas correlates with advanced disease stage, *Science,* 224, 1121, 1984.

429. Schwab, M., Varmus, H.E., Bishop, J.M., Grzeschik, K.-H., Naylor, S.L., Sakaguchi, A.Y., Brodeur, G., and Trent, J., Chromosome localization in normal human cells and neuroblastomas of a gene related to c-*myc*, *Nature,* 308, 288, 1984.

430. Emanuel, B.S., Balaban, G., Boyd, J.P., Grossman, A., Negishi, M., Palmiter, A., and Glick, M.C., N-*myc* amplification in multiple homogeneously staining regions in two human neuroblastomas, *Proc. Natl. Acad. Sci. U.S.A.,* 82, 3736, 1985.

431. Schwab, M., Amplification of N-*myc* in human neuroblastomas, *Trends Genet.,* 1, 271, 1985.

432. Ikegaki, N., Bukovsky, J., and Kennet, R.H., Identification and characterization of the *NMYC* gene product in human neuroblastoma cells by monoclonal antibodies with defined specificities, *Proc. Natl. Acad. Sci. U.S.A.,* 83, 5929, 1986.

433. Grady, E.F., Schwab, M., and Rosenau, W., Expression of N-*myc* and c-*src* during the development of fetal human brain, *Cancer Res.,* 47, 2931, 1987.

434. Kohl, N.E., Legouy, E., DePinho, R.A., Nisen, P.D., Smith, R.K., Gee, C.E., and Alt, F.W., Human N-*myc* is closely related in organization and nucleotide sequence to c-*myc*, *Nature,* 319, 73, 1986.

435. Kinzler, K.W., Zehnbauer, B.A., Brodeur, G.M., Seeger, R.C., Trent, J.M., Meltzer, P.S., and Vogelstein, B., Amplification units containing N-*myc* and c-*myc* genes, *Proc. Natl. Acad. Sci. U.S.A.,* 83, 1031, 1986.

436. Shiloh, Y., Korf, B., Kohl, N.E., Sakai, K., Brodeur, G.M., Harris, P., Kanda, N., Seeger, R.C., Alt, F., and Latt, S.A., Amplification and rearrangement of DNA sequences from the chromosomal region 2p24 in human neuroblastomas, *Cancer Res.,* 46, 5297, 1986.

437. Kanda, N., Tsuchida, Y., Hata, J., Kohl, N.E., Alt, F.W., Latt, S.A., and Utakoji, T., Amplification of IMR-32 clones 8, G21, and N-*myc* in human neuroblastoma xenografts, *Cancer Res.,* 47, 3291, 1987.

438. Pelicci, P.-G., Lanfrancone, L., Brathwaite, M.D., Wolman, S.R., and Dalla-Favera, R., Amplification of the c-*myb* gene in a case of human acute myelogenous leukemia, *Science,* 224, 1117, 1984.

439. Alitalo, K., Winqvist, R., Lin, C.C., de la Chapelle, A., Schwab, M., and Bishop, J.M., Aberrant expression of an amplified c-*myb* oncogene in two cell lines from a colon carcinoma, *Proc. Natl. Acad. Sci. U.S.A.,* 81, 4534, 1984.

440. Winqvist, R., Knuutila, S., Leprince, D., Stehelin, D., and Alitalo, K., Mapping of amplified c-*myb* oncogene, sister chromatid exchanges, and karyotypic analysis of the COLO 205 colon carcinoma cell line, *Cancer Genet. Cytogenet.,* 18, 251, 1985.

441. Tobaly-Tapiero, J., Saal, F., Peries, J., and Emanoil-Ravier, R., Amplification and rearrangement of Ki-*ras* oncogene in human teratocarcinoma-derived cell lines, *Biochimie,* 68, 1019, 1986.

442. Wang, L., Vass, W., Gao, C., and Chang, K.S.S., Amplification and enhanced expression of the c-Ki-*ras*2 protooncogene in human embryonal carcinomas, *Cancer Res.,* 47, 4192, 1987.

443. Miyaki, M., Sato, C., Matsui, T., Koike, M., Mori, T., Kosaki, G., Takai, S., Tonomura, A., and Tsuchida, N., Amplification and enhanced expression of cellular oncogene c-Ki-*ras*-2 in a human epidermoid carcinoma of the lung, *Jpn. J. Cancer Res.,* 76, 260, 1985.

444. Nardeux, P.C., Daya-Grosjean, L., Landin, R.M., Andéol, Y., and Suárez, H.G., A c-ras-Ki oncogene is activated, amplified and overexpressed in a human osteosarcoma cell line, *Biochem. Biophys. Res. Commun.*, 146, 395, 1987.

445. Kozma, S.C., Bogaard, M.E., Buser, K., Saurer, S.M., Bos, J.L., Groner, B., and Hynes, N.E., The human c-Kirsten *ras* gene is activated by a novel mutation in codon 13 in the breast carcinoma cell line MDA-MB231, *Nucleic Acids Res.*, 15, 5963, 1987.

446. Filmus, J.E. and Buick, R.N., Stability of c-K-*ras* amplification during progression in a patient with adenocarcinoma of the ovary, *Cancer Res.*, 45, 4468, 1985.

447. Filmus, J., Trent, J.M., Pullano, R., and Buick, R.N., A cell line from a human ovarian carcinoma with amplification of the K-*ras* gene, *Cancer Res.*, 46, 5179, 1986.

448. Hirai, H., Okabe, T., Anraku, Y., Fujisawa, M., Urabe, A., and Takaku, F., Activation of the c-K-*ras* oncogene in a human pancreas carcinoma, *Biochem. Biophys. Res. Commun.*, 127, 168, 1985.

449. Yamada, H., Yoshida, T., Sakamoto, H., Terada, M., and Sugimura, T., Establishment of a human pancreatic adenocarcinoma cell line (PSN-1) with amplifications of both c-*myc* and activated c-Ki-*ras* by a point mutation, *Biochem. Biophys. Res. Commun.*, 140, 167, 1986.

450. Sekiya, T., Fushumi, M., Hirohashi, S., and Tokunaga, A., Amplification of activated c-Ha-*ras*-1 in human melanoma, *Jpn. J. Cancer Res.*, 76, 555, 1985.

451. Heisterkamp, N., Stephenson, J.R., Groffen, J., Hansen, P.F., de Klein, A., Bartram, C.R., and Grosveld, G., Localization of the c-*abl* oncogene adjacent to a translocation break point in chronic myelocytic leukaemia, *Nature*, 306, 239, 1983.

452. Collins, S.J. and Groudine, M.T., Rearrangement and amplification of c-*abl* sequences in the human chronic myelogenous leukemia cell line K-562, *Proc. Natl. Acad. Sci. U.S.A.*, 80, 4813, 1983.

453. Selden, J.R., Emanuel, B.S., Wang, E., Cannizzaro, L., Palumbo, A., Erikson, J., Nowell, P.C., Rovera, G., and Croce, C.M., Amplified C-lambda and c-*abl* genes are on the same marker chromosome in K562 leukemia cells, *Proc. Natl. Acad. Sci. U.S.A.*, 80, 7289, 1983.

454. Leibowitz, D., Cubbon, R., and Bank, A., Increased expression of a novel c-*abl*-related RNA in K562 cells, *Blood*, 65, 526, 1985.

455. Blick, M.B., Andersson, B.S., Gutterman, J.U., Keating, A., and Beran, M., The c-*abl*, bcr, and C-lambda genes are amplified in a cell line but not in the uncultured cells from a patient with chronic myelogenous leukemia, *Leukemia Res.*, 10, 1401, 1986.

456. Daniel, L., Ahmed, C.M.I., Bloodgood, R.S., Kidd, J.R., Castiglione, C.M., Dattagupta, S., and Lebowitz, P., Polymorphism of the human c-*abl* gene: relation to incidence and course of chronic myelogenous leukemia, *Oncogene*, 1, 193, 1987.

457. Downward, J., Yarden, Y., Mayes, E., Scrace, G., Totty, N., Stockwell, P., Ullrich, A., Schelssinger, J., and Waterfield, M.D., Close similarity of epidermal growth factor receptor and v-*erb*-B oncogene protein sequences, *Nature*, 307, 521, 1984.

458. Merlino, G.T., Xu, Y.-H., Ishii, S., Clark, A.J.L., Semba, K., Toyoshima, K., Yamamoto, T., and Pastan, I., Amplification and enhanced expression of the epidermal growth factor receptor gene in A431 human carcinoma cells, *Science*, 224, 417, 1984.

459. Filmus, J., Pollak, M.N., Cairncross, J.G., and Buick, R.N., Amplified, overexpressed and rearranged epidermal growth factor receptor gene in a human astrocytoma cell line, *Biochem. Biophys. Res. Commun.*, 131, 207, 1985.

460. Lebeau, J. and Goubin, G., Amplification of the epidermal growth factor receptor gene in the BT20 breast carcinoma cell line, *Int. J. Cancer*, 40, 189, 1987.

461. King, I.C. and Sartorelli, A.C., The relationship between epidermal growth factor receptors and the terminal differentiation of A431 carcinoma cells, *Biochem. Biophys. Res. Commun.*, 140, 837, 1986.

462. Sakiyama, S., Nakamura, Y., and Yasuda, S., Expression of epidermal growth factor receptor gene in cultured human lung cancer cells, *Jpn. J. Cancer Res.*, 77, 965, 1986.

463. Knowles, A.F., Inhibition of growth and induction of enzyme activities in a clonal human hepatoma cell line (Li-7A): comparison of the effects of epidermal growth factor and an anti-epidermal growth factor receptor antibody, *J. Cell. Physiol.*, 134, 109, 1988.

464. Henn, W., Blin, N., and Zang, K.D., Polysomy of chromosome 7 is correlated with overexpression of the erbB oncogene in human glioblastoma cell lines, *Hum. Genet.*, 74, 104, 1986.

465. Fukushige, S., Murotsu, T., and Matsubara, K., Chromosomal assignment of human genes for gastrin, thyrotropin (TSH)-beta subunit and c-*erb*B-2 by chromosome sorting combined with velocity sedimentation and Southern hybridization, *Biochem. Biophys. Res. Commun.*, 134, 477, 1986.

466. Fukushige, S., Matsubara, K., Yoshida, M., Sasaki, M., Suzuki, T., Semba, K., Toyoshima, K., and Yamamoto, T., Localization of a novel v-*erb*B-related gene, c-*erb*B-2, on human chromosome 17 and its amplification in a gastric cancer cell line, *Mol. Cell. Biol.*, 6, 955, 1986.

467. Barker, P.E., Double minutes in human tumor cells, *Cancer Genet. Cytogenet.*, 5, 81, 1982.

468. Casartelli, C., Cancer and chromosomes — a review, *Rev. Brasil. Genet.,* 5, 595, 1982.
469. Bahr, G., Gilbert, F., Balaban, G., and Engler, W., Homogeneously staining regions and double minutes in a human cell line: chromatin organization and DNA content, *J. Natl. Cancer Inst.,* 71, 657, 1983.
470. Li, Y.S., Double minutes in acute myeloid leukemia, *Int. J. Cancer,* 32, 455, 1983.
471. Gebhart, E., Tulusan, A.H., Maillot, K.V., and Mulz, D., Double minutes — new markers in cells of human solid tumors, *J. Genet. Hum.,* 31, 45, 1983.
472. Arrighi, F.E., Gene amplification in human tumor cells, in *Proc. 13th Int. Cancer Congress, Part C,* Vol. 2, Alan R. Liss, New York, 1983, 259.
473. Nakatani, H., Tahara, E., Sakamoto, H., Terada, M., and Sugimura, T., Amplified DNA sequences in cancers, *Biochem. Biophys. Res. Commun.,* 130, 508, 1985.
474. Yokota, J., Tsunetsugu-Yokota, Y., Battifora, H., Le Fevre, C., and Cline, M.J., Alterations of *myc, myb,* and *ras*[Ha] proto-oncogenes in cancers are frequent and show clinical correlation, *Science,* 231, 261, 1986.
475. Masuda, H., Battifora, H., Yokota, J., Meltzer, S., and Cline, M.J., Tumor specificity of proto-oncogene amplification in human malignant diseases, *Clin. Mol. Med.,* in press.
476. Boehm, T.L.J., Hirth, H.-P., Kornhuber, B., and Drahovsky, D., Oncogene amplifications, rearrangements, and restriction fragment length polymorphisms in human leukemia, *Eur. J. Cancer Clin. Oncol.,* 6, 623, 1987.
477. Boehm, T.L.J. and Drahovsky, D., Oncogene amplification and clonal evolution in acute leukemia, *Eur. J. Cancer Clin. Oncol.,* 23, 871, 1987.
478. U, H.S., Kelley, P., and Lee, W.-H., Abnormalities of the human growth hormone gene and protooncogenes in some human pituitary adenomas, *Mol. Endocrinol.,* 2, 85, 1988.
479. Gebhart, E., Bruderlein, S., Tulusan, A.H., Maillot, K.V., and Birkmann, J., Incidence of double minutes, cytogenetic equivalents of gene amplification, in human carcinoma cells, *Int. J. Cancer,* 34, 369, 1984.
480. Hubbell, H.R., Quinn, L.A., and Dolby, T.W., Cloning of a non-c-*myc* DNA fragment from the double minutes of a human colon carcinoid cell line, *Cancer Genet. Cytogenet.,* 24, 17, 1987.
481. Berthold, F., Current concepts on the biology of neuroblastoma, *Blut,* 50, 65, 1985.
482. Christiansen, H., Franke, F., Bartram, C.R., Adolph, S., Rudolph, B., Harbott, J., Reiter, A., and Lampert, F., Evolution of tumor cytogenetic aberrations and N-*myc* oncogene amplification in a case of disseminated neuroblastoma, *Cancer Genet. Cytogenet.,* 26, 235, 1987.
483. Kaneko, Y., Tsuchida, Y., Maseki, N., Takasaki, N., Sakurai, M., and Saito, S., Chromosome findings in human neuroblastomas xenografted in nude mice, *Jpn. J. Cancer Res.,* 76, 359, 1985.
484. Kaneko, Y., Kanda, N., Maseki, N., Sakurai, M., Tsuchida, Y., Takeda, T., Okabe, I., and Sakurai, M., Different karyotypic patterns in early and advanced stage neuroblastomas, *Cancer Res.,* 47, 311, 1987.
485. Brodeur, G.M., Hayes, F.A., Green, A.A., Casper, J.T., Wasson, J., Wallach, S., and Seeger, R.C., Consistent N-*myc* copy number in simultaneous or consecutive neuroblastoma samples from sixty individual patients, *Cancer Res.,* 47, 4248, 1987.
486. Tonini, G.P., Verdona, G., Garaventa, A., and Cornaglia-Ferraris, P., Antiblastic treatment does not affect N-*myc* gene amplification in neuroblastoma, *Anticancer Res.,* 7, 729, 1987.
487. Kurosawa, H., Yamada, M., and Nakagone, Y., Restriction fragment length polymorphisms of the human N-*myc* gene: relationship to gene amplification, *Oncogene,* 2, 85, 1987.
488. Schwab, M., Ellison, J., Busch, M., Rosenau, W., Varmus, H.E., and Bishop, J.M., Enhanced expression of the human gene N-*myc* consequent to amplification of DNA may contribute to malignant progression of neuroblastoma, *Proc. Natl. Acad. Sci. U.S.A.,* 81, 4940, 1984.
489. Seeger, R.C., Brodeur, G.M., Sather, H., Dalton, A., Siegel, S.E., Wong, K.Y., and Hammond, D., Association of multiple copies of the N-*myc* oncogene with rapid progression of neuroblastomas, *N. Engl. J. Med.,* 313, 1111, 1985.
490. Rosen, N., Reynolds, C.P., Thiele, C.J., Biedler, J.L., and Israel, M.A., Increased N-*myc* expression following progressive growth of human neuroblastoma, *Cancer Res.,* 46, 4139, 1986.
491. Benard, J., Interet pronostique de l'oncogène N-*myc* dans les neuroblastomes, *Bull. Cancer,* 75, 87, 1988.
492. Grady-Leopardi, E.F., Schwab, M., Ablin, A.R., and Rosenau, W., Detection of N-*myc* oncogene expression in human neuroblastoma by *in situ* hybridization and blot analysis: relationship to clinical outcome, *Cancer Res.,* 46, 3196, 1986.
493. Nisen, P.D., Rich, M.A., Gloster, E., Valderrama, E., Saric, O., Shende, A., Lazkowsky, P., and Alt, F.W., N-*myc* oncogene expression in histopathologically unrelated bilateral pediatric renal tumors, *Cancer,* 61, 1821, 1988.
494. Sakai, K., Tanooka, H., Sasaki, M.S., Ejima, Y., and Kaneko, A., Increase in copy number of N-*myc* in retinoblastomas in comparison with chromosome abnormality, *Cancer Genet. Cytogenet.,* 30, 119, 1988.
495. Mitani, K., Kurosawa, H., Suzuki, A., Hayashi, Y., Hanada, R., Yamamoto, K., Komatsu, A., Kobayashi, N., Nakagome, Y., and Yamada, M., Amplification of N-*myc* in a rhabdomyosarcoma, *Jpn. J. Cancer Res.,* 77, 1062, 1986.
496. Norris, M.D., Brian, M.J., Vowels, M.R., and Stewart, B.W., N-*myc* amplification in Wilms' tumor, *Cancer Genet. Cytogenet.,* 30, 187, 1988.

497. Heighway, J. and Hasleton, P.S., c-Ki-*ras* amplification in human lung cancer, *Br. J. Cancer,* 53, 285, 1986.
498. Cline, M.J. and Battifora, H., Abnormalities of protooncogenes in non-small cell lung cancer: correlations with tumor type and clinical characteristics, *Cancer,* 60, 2669, 1987.
499. Wong, A.J., Ruppert, J.M., Eggleston, J., Hamilton, S.R., Baylin, S.B., and Vogelstein, B., Gene amplification of c-*myc* and N-*myc* in small cell carcinoma of the lung, *Science,* 233, 461, 1986.
500. Kawashima, K., Shikama, H., Imoto, K., Izawa, M., Naruke, T., Okabayashi, K., and Nishimura, S., Close correlation between restriction fragment length polymorphism of the L-*MYC* gene and metastasis of human lung cancer to the lymph nodes and other organs, *Proc. Natl. Acad. Sci. U.S.A.,* 85, 2353, 1988.
501. Alitalo, K., Saksela, K., Winqvist, R., Alitalo, R., Keski-Oja, J., Laiho, M., Ilvonen, M., Knuutila, S., and de la Chapelle, A., Acute myelogenous leukaemia with c-myc amplification and double minute chromosomes, *Lancet,* 2, 1035, 1985.
502. Sümegi, J., Hedberg, T., Björkholm, M., Godal, T., Mellstedt, H., Nilsson, M.G., Perlman, C., and Klein, G., Amplification of the c-*myc* oncogene in human plasma-cell leukemia, *Int. J. Cancer,* 36, 367, 1985.
503. Alexander, R.J., Buxbaum, J.N., and Raicht, R.F., Oncogene alterations in primary human colon tumors, *Gastroenterology,* 91, 1503, 1986.
504. Ocadiz, R., Sauceda, R., Cruz, M., Graef, A.M., and Gariglio, P., High correlation between molecular alterations of the c-*myc* oncogene and carcinoma of the uterine cervix, *Cancer Res.,* 47, 4173, 1987.
505. Nakasato, F., Sakamoto, H., Mori, M., Hayashi, K., Shimosato, Y., Nishi, M., Takao, S., Nakatani, K., Terada, M., and Sugimura, T., Amplification of the c-*myc* oncogene in human stomach cancers, *Jpn. J. Cancer Res.,* 75, 737, 1984.
506. Koda, T., Matsushima, S., Sasaki, A., Danjo, Y., and Kakinuma, M., c-*mcy* gene amplification in primary stomach cancer, *Jpn. J. Cancer Res.,* 551, 1985.
507. Seki, T., Fujii, G., Mori, S., Tamaoki, N., and Shibuya, M., Amplification of c-*yes*-1 proto-oncogene in a primary human gastric cancer, *Jpn. J. Cancer Res.,* 76, 907, 1985.
508. Escot, C., Theillet, C., Lidereau, R., Spyratos, F., Champeme, M.-H., Gest, J., and Callahan, R., Genetic alteration of the c-*myc* protooncogene (*MYC*) in human primary breast carcinomas, *Proc. Natl. Acad. Sci. U.S.A.,* 83, 4384, 1986.
509. Varley, J.M., Wainwright, A.M., and Brammar, W.J., An unusual alteration in c-*myc* in tissue from a primary breast carcinoma, *Oncogene,* 1, 431, 1987.
510. Hayashi, K., Kakizoe, T., and Sugimura, T., *In vivo* amplification and rearrangement of the c-Ha-*ras*-1 sequence in a human bladder carcinoma, *Jpn. J. Cancer Res.,* 74, 798, 1983.
511. Yamada, H., Sakamoto, H., Taira, M., Nishimura, S., Shimosato, Y., Terada, M., and Sugimura, T., Amplifications of both c-Ki-*ras* with a point mutation and c-*myc* in a primary pancreatic cancer and its metastatic tumors in lymph nodes, *Jpn. J. Cancer Res.,* 77, 370, 1986.
512. Yamazaki, H., Fukui, Y., Ueyama, Y., Tamaoki, N., Kawamoto, T., Taniguchi, S., and Shibuya, M., Amplification of the structurally and functionally altered epidermal growth factor receptor gene (c-*erb*B) in human brain tumors, *Mol. Cell. Biol.,* 8, 1816, 1988.
513. Ro, J., North, S.M., Gallick, G.E., Hortobagyi, G.N., Gutterman, J.U., and Blick, M., Amplified and overexpressed epidermal growth factor receptor gene in uncultured primary human breast carcinoma, *Cancer Res.,* 48, 161, 1988.
514. Woloschak, G.E., Dewald, G.W., Bahn, R.S., Kyle, R.A., Greipp, P.R., and Ash, R.C., Amplification of RNA and DNA specific for erb B in unbalanced 1;7 chromosomal translocation associated with myelodysplastic syndrome, *J. Cell. Biochem.,* 32, 23, 1986.
515. Sobol, R.E., Astarita, R.W., Hofeditz, C., Masui, H., Fairshter, R., Royston, I., and Mendelsohn, J., Epidermal growth factor receptor expression in human lung carcinomas defined by a monoclonal antibody, *J. Natl. Cancer Inst.,* 79, 403, 1987.
516. Semba, K., Kamata, N., Toyoshima, K., and Yamamoto, T., A v-*erb*B-related protooncogene, c-*erb*B-2, is distinct from the c-*erb*B-1/epidermal growth factor-receptor gene and is amplified in a human salivary gland adenocarcinoma, *Proc. Natl. Acad. Sci. U.S.A.,* 82, 6497, 1985.
517. Yokota, J., Yamamoto, T., Toyoshima, K., Terada, M., Sugimura, T., Battifora, H., and Cline, M.J., Amplification of c-*erb*B-2 oncogene in human adenocarcinomas *in vivo, Lancet,* 1, 765, 1986.
518. King, C.R., Kraus, M.H., and Aaronson, S.A., Amplification of a novel v-*erb*B-related gene in a human mammary carcinoma, *Science,* 229, 974, 1985.
519. Tal, M., Wetzer, M., Josefsberg, Z., Deutch, A., Gutman, M., Assaf, D., Kris, R., Shiloh, Y., Givol, D., and Schlessinger, J., Sporadic amplification of the *HER2/neu* protooncogene in adenocarcinomas of various tissues, *Cancer Res.,* 48, 1517, 1988.
520. van de Vijver, M., van de Bersselaar, R., Develee, P., Cornelisse, C., Peterse, J., and Nusse, R., Amplification of the *neu* (c-*erb*B-2) oncogene in human mammary tumors is relatively infrequent and is often accompanied by amplification of the linked c-*erb*A oncogene, *Mol. Cell. Biol.,* 7, 2019, 1987.
521. Gusterson, B.A., Gullick, W.J., Venter, D.J., Powles, T.J., Elliott, C., Ashley, S., Tidy, A., and Harrison, S., Immunohistochemical localization of c-erbB-2 in human breast carcinomas, *Mol. Cell. Probes,* 2, 383, 1988.

522. Slamon, D.J., Clark, G.M., Wong, S.G., Levin, W.J., Ullrich, A., and McGuire, W.L., Human breast cancer: correlation of relapse and survival with amplification of the HER-2/*neu* oncogene, *Science*, 235, 177, 1987.

523. Cline, M.J., Battifora, H., and Yokota, J., Proto-oncogene abnormalities in human breast cancer: correlations with anatomic features and clinical course of disease, *J. Clin. Oncol.*, 5, 999, 1987.

524. van de Vijver, M.J., Mooi, W.J., Wisman, P., Peterse, J.L., and Nusse, R., Immunohistochemical detection of the *neu* protein in tissue sections of human breast tumors with amplified *neu* DNA, *Oncogene*, 2, 175, 1988.

525. Rovigatti, U., Watson, D.K., and Yunis, J.J., Amplification and rearrangement of Hu-*ets*-1 in leukemia and lymphoma with involvement of 11q23, *Science*, 232, 398, 1986.

526. Mester, J., Wagenaar, E., Sluyser, M., and Nusse, R., Activation of *int*-1 and *int*-2 mammary oncogenes in hormone-dependent and -independent mammary tumors of GR mice, *J. Virol.*, 61, 1073, 1987.

527. Casey, G., Smith, R., McGillivray, D., Peters, G., and Dickson, C., Characterization and chromosome assignment of the human homolog of *int*-2, a potential proto-oncogene, *Mol. Cell. Biol.*, 6, 502, 1986.

528. Zhou, D.J., Casey, G., and Cline, M.J., Amplification of human *int*-2 in breast cancers and squamous carcinomas, *Oncogene*, 2, 279, 1988.

529. Tsutsumi, M., Sakamoto, H., Yoshida, T., Kakizoe, T., Koiso, K., Sugimura, T., and Terada, M., Coamplification of the *hst*-1 and *int*-2 genes in human cancers, *Jpn. J. Cancer Res.*, 79, 428, 1988.

530. McCarthy, D.M., Rasool, F.V., Goldman, J.M., Grahan, S.V., and Birnie, G.D., Genomic alterations involving the c-*myc* proto-oncogene locus during the evolution of a case of chronic granulocytic leukaemia, *Lancet*, ii, 1362, 1984.

531. Riou, G., Barrois, M., Tordjman, I., Dutronquay, V., and Orth, G., Présence de genomes de papillomavirus et amplification des oncogènes c-*myc* et c-Ha-*ras* dans des cancers envahissants du col de l'utérus, *C.R. Acad. Sci.*, 299, 575, 1984.

532. Bernards, R., Dessain, S.K., and Weinberg, R.A., N-*myc* amplification causes down-modulation of MHC class I antigen expression in neuroblastoma, *Cell*, 47, 667, 674, 1986.

533. Slebos, R.J.C., Evers, S.G., Wagenaar, S.S., and Rodenhuis, S., Cellular protooncogenes are infrequently amplified in untreated non-small cell lung cancer, *Br. J. Cancer*, 59, 76, 1989.

534. Cooper, C.S., Tempest, P.R., Beckman, M.P., Heldin, C.-H., and Brookes, P., Amplification and overexpression of the *met* gene in spontaneously transformed NIH3T3 fibroblasts, *EMBO J.*, 5, 2623, 1986.

535. Schwab, M., Alitalo, K., Varmus, H.E., Bishop, J.M., and George, D., A cellular oncogene (c-Ki-*ras*) is amplified, overexpressed, and located within karyotypic abnormalities in mouse adrenocortical tumour cells, *Nature*, 303, 497, 1983.

536. George, D.L., Scott, A.F., de Martinville, B., and Francke, U., Amplified DNA in Y1 mouse adrenal tumor cells: isolation of cDNAs complementary to an amplified c-Ki-*ras* gene and localization of homologous sequences to mouse chromosome 6, *Nucleic Acids Res.*, 12, 2731, 1984.

537. George, D.L., Scott, A.F., Trusko, S., Glick, B., Ford, E., and Dorney, D.J., Structure and expression of amplified cKi-*ras* gene sequences in Y1 mouse adrenal tumor cells, *EMBO J.*, 4, 1199, 1985.

538. Ehrfeld, A., Planas-Bohne, F., and Lücke-Huhle, C., Amplification of oncogenes and integrated SV40 sequences in mammalian cells by the decay of incorporated iodine-125, *Radiat. Res.*, 108, 43, 1986.

539. Lücke-Huhle, C., Pech, M., and Herrlich, P., Selective gene amplification in mammalian cells after exposure to ^{60}Co gamma rays, ^{241}Am alpha particles, or uv light, *Radiat. Res.*, 106, 345, 1986.

540. Quintanilla, M., Brown, K., Ramsden, M., and Balmain, A., Carcinogen-specific mutation and amplification of Ha-*ras* during mouse skin carcinogenesis, *Nature*, 322, 78, 1986.

541. Hayashi, K., Makino, R., and Sugimura, T., Amplification and over-expression of the c-*myc* gene in Morris hepatomas, *Jpn. J. Cancer Res.*, 75, 475, 1984.

542. Schwab, M., Alitalo, K., Varmus, H.E., Bishop, J.M., and George, D., A cellular oncogene (c-Ki-*ras*) is amplified, overexpressed, and located within karyotypic abnormalities in mouse adrenocortical tumour cells, *Nature*, 303, 497, 1983.

543. Yander, G., Halsey, H., Kenna, M., and Augenlicht, L.H., Amplification and elevated expression of c-*myc* in a chemically induced mouse colon tumor, *Cancer Res.*, 45, 4433, 1985.

544. Chaum, E., Ellsworth, R.M., Abramson, D.H., Haik, B.G., Kitchin, F.D., and Chaganti, R.S.K., Cytogenetic analysis of retinoblastoma: evidence for multifocal origin and *in vivo* gene amplification, *Cytogenet. Cell Genet.*, 38, 82, 1984.

545. Shiloh, Y., Shipley, J., Brodeur, G.M., Bruns, G., Korf, B., Donlon, T., Schreck, R.R., Seeger, R., Sakai, K., and Latt, S.A., Differential amplification, assembly, and relocation of multiple DNA sequences in human neuroblastomas and neuroblastoma cell lines, *Proc. Natl. Acad. Sci. U.S.A.*, 82, 3761, 1985.

546. Bevacqua, S.J., Greef, C.W., and Hendrix, M.J.C., Cytogenetic evidence of gene amplification as a mechanism for tumor cell invasion, *Somat. Cell Mol. Genet.*, 14, 83, 1988.

547. Cahilly-Snyder, L., Yang-Feng, T., Francke, U., and George, D.L., Molecular analysis and chromosomal mapping of amplified genes isolated from a transformed mouse 3T3 cell line, *Somat. Cell Mol. Genet.*, 13, 235, 1987.

548. Baskin, F., Grossman, A., Bhagat, S.G., Burns, D., Davis, R.M., Warmoth, L.A., and Rosenberg, R.N., Frequent alterations of specific reiterated DNA sequence abundances in human cancer, *Cancer Genet. Cytogenet.,* 28, 163, 1987.

549. Shafit-Zagardo, B., Maio, J.J., and Brown, F.L., *Kpn*I families of long, interspersed repetitive DNAs in human and other primate genomes, *Nucleic Acids Res.,* 10, 3175, 1982.

550. Simmons, M.C., Maxwell, J., Haliotis, T., Higgins, M.J., Roder, J.C., White, B.N., and Holden, J.J.A., Amplified *Kpn*I repetitive DNA sequences in homogeneously staining regions of a human melanoma cell line, *J. Natl. Cancer Inst.,* 72, 801, 1984.

551. Klingel, R., Mincheva, A., Kahn, T., Gissmann, L., Dippold, W., Meyer zum Büschenfelde, K.-H., and zur Hausen, H., An amplification unit in human melanoma cells showing partial homology with sequences of human papillomavirus type 9 and with nuclear antigen 1 of the Epstein-Barr virus, *Cancer Res.,* 47, 4485, 1987.

552. Colb, M., Yang-Feng, T., Francke, U., Mermer, B., Parkinson, D.R., and Krontiris, T.G., A variable tandem repeat locus mapped to chromosome band 10q26 is amplified and rearranged in leukocyte DNAs of two cancer patients, *Nucleic Acids Res.,* 14, 7929, 1986.

553. Heilbronn, R., Schlehofer, J.R., and zur Hausen, H., Selective killing of carcinogen-treated SV40-transformed Chinese hamster cells by a defective parvovirus, *Virology,* 136, 439, 1984.

554. Gitelman, I., Dexter, D.F., and Roder, J.C., DNA amplification and metastasis of the human melanoma cell line MeWo, *Cancer Res.,* 47, 3851, 1987.

555. Gowda, S.D., Koler, R.D., and Bagby, G.C., Jr., Regulation of c-myc expression during growth and differentiation of normal and leukemic human myeloid progenitor cells, *J. Clin. Invest.,* 77, 271, 1986.

556. Chattopadhyay, S.K., Chang, E.H., Lander, M.R., Ellis, R.W., Scolnick, E.M., and Lowy, D.R., Amplification and rearrangement of *onc* genes in mammalian species, *Nature,* 296, 361, 1982.

557. Srivastava, A., Norris, J.S., Reis, R.J.S., and Goldstein, S., c-Ha-*ras*-1 proto-oncogene amplification and overexpression during the limited replicative life span of normal human fibroblasts, *J. Biol. Chem.,* 260, 6404, 1985.

558. Korsmeyer, S.J. and Waldmann, T.A., Immunoglobulin genes: rearrangement and translocation in human lymphoid malignancy, *J. Clin. Immunol.,* 4, 1, 1984.

559. Knowles, D.M., II, Pelicci, P.-G., and Dalla-Favera, R., Immunoglobulin and T cell receptor beta chain gene DNA probes in the diagnosis and classification of human lymphoid neoplasia, *Mol. Cell. Probes,* 1, 15, 1987.

560. Korsmeyer, S.J., Antigen receptor genes as molecular markers of lymphoid neoplasms, *J. Clin. Invest.,* 79, 1291, 1987.

561. Toyonaga, B. and Mak, T.W., Genes of the T-cell antigen receptor in normal and malignant T cells, *Annu. Rev. Immunol.,* 5, 585, 1987.

562. Cossman, J., Uppenkamp, M., Sundeen, J., Coupland, R., and Raffeld, M., Molecular genetics and the diagnosis of lymphoma, *Arch. Pathol. Lab. Med.,* 112, 117, 1988.

563. Sandberg, A.A., The Chromosomes in *Human Cancer and Leukemia,* Elsevier, Amsterdam, 1981.

564. Rowley, J.D., Nonrandom chromosomal abnormalities in hematologic disorders, of man, *Proc. Natl. Acad. Sci. U.S.A.,* 72, 152, 1975.

565. Mitelman, F. and Levan, G., Clustering of aberrations to specific chromosomes in human neoplasms. II. A survey of 287 neoplasms, *Hereditas,* 82, 167, 1976.

566. Yunis, J.J., Specific fine chromosomal defects in cancer: an overview, *Hum. Pathol.,* 12, 503, 1981.

567. Yunis, J.J., Bloomfield, C.D., and Ensrud, K., All patients with acute nonlymphocytic leukemia may have a chromosomal defect, *N. Engl. J. Med.,* 305, 135, 1981.

568. Rowley, J.D., Identification of the constant chromosome regions involved in human hematologic malignant disease, *Science,* 216, 749, 1982.

569. Yunis, J.J., Oken, M.M., Kaplan, M.E., Ensrud, K.M., Howe, R.R., and Theologides, A., Distinctive chromosomal abnormalities in histologic subtypes of non-Hodgkin's lymphoma, *N. Engl. J. Med.,* 307, 1231, 1982.

570. Mitelman, F., Restricted number of chromosomal regions implicated in aetiology of human cancer and leukaemia, *Nature,* 319, 325, 1984.

571. Fonatsch, C., Cytogenetic markers in hematoproliferative disorders, *Blut,* 51, 315, 1985.

572. Dewald, G.W., Noel, P., Dahl, R.J., and Spurbeck, J.L., Chromosome abnormalities in malignant hematologic disorders, *Mayo Clin. Proc.,* 60, 675, 1985.

573. Le Beau, M.M. and Rowley, J.D., Chromosomal abnormalities in leukemia and lymphoma: clinical and biological significance, *Adv. Hum. Genet.,* 15, 1, 1986.

574. Sandberg, A.A., The chromosomes in human leukemia, *Semin. Hematol.,* 23, 201, 1986.

575. Yunis, J.J. and Brunning, R.D., Prognostic significance of chromosomal abnormalities in acute leukaemias and myelodysplastic syndromes, *Clin. Haematol.,* 15, 597, 1986.

576. De Braekeleer, M., Smith, B., and Lin, C.C., Fragile sites and structural rearrangements in cancer, *Hum. Genet.,* 69, 112, 1985.

577. Le Beau, M.M., Chromosomal fragile sites and cancer-specific breakpoints — a moderating viewpoint, *Cancer Genet. Cytogenet.,* 31, 55, 1988.

578. Cruz-Coke, R., Translocation chromosome map of oncogenes, *J. Med. Genet.,* 24, 111, 1987.
579. Heim, S. and Mitelman, F., Chromosome abnormalities in the myelodysplastic syndromes, *Clin. Haematol.,* 15, 1003, 1986.
580. Klein, G., Specific chromosomal translocations and the genesis of B-cell-derived tumors in mice and men, *Cell,* 32, 311, 1983.
581. Yunis, J.J., The chromosomal basis of human neoplasia, *Science,* 221, 227, 1983.
582. Chaganti, R.S.K., Significance of chromosome change to hematopoietic neoplasms, *Blood,* 62, 515, 1983.
583. Sandberg, A.A., A chromosomal hypothesis of oncogenesis, *Cancer Genet. Cytogenet.,* 8, 277, 1983.
584. Gilbert, F., Chromosomes, genes, and cancer: a classification of chromosome abnormalities in cancer, *J. Natl. Cancer Inst.,* 71, 1107, 1983.
585. Rowley, J.D., Biological implications of consistent chromosome rearrangements in leukemia and lymphoma, *Cancer Res.,* 44, 3159, 1984.
586. Croce, C.M., Tsujimoto, Y., Erikson, J., and Nowell, P., Chromosome translocations and B cell neoplasia, *Lab. Invest.,* 51, 258, 1984.
587. Aisenberg, A.C., New genetics of Burkitt's lymphoma and other non-Hodgkin's lymphomas, *Am. J. Med.,* 77, 1083, 1984.
588. Emanuel, B.S., Chromosomal *in situ* hybridization and the molecular cytogenetics of cancer, *Surv. Synth. Pathol. Res.,* 4, 269, 1985.
589. Showe, L.C. and Croce, C.M., Chromosome translocations in B and T cell neoplasias, *Semin. Hematol.,* 23, 237, 1986.
590. Croce, C.M., Chromosome translocations in human cancer, *Cancer Res.,* 46, 6019, 1986.
591. Heim, S. and Mitelman, F., Nineteen of 26 cellular oncogenes precisely localized in the human genome map to one of the 83 bands involved in primary cancer-specific rearrangements, *Hum. Genet.,* 75, 70, 1987.
592. Haluska, F.G., Tsujimoto, Y., and Croce, C.M., Mechanisms of chromosome translocation in B- and T-cell neoplasia, *Trends Genet.,* 3, 11, 1987.
593. Chevenix-Trench, G., The molecular genetics of human non-Hodgkin's lymphoma, *Cancer Genet. Cytogenet.,* 27, 191, 1987.
594. Champlin, R.E. and Golde, D.W., Chronic myelogenous leukemia: recent advances, *Blood,* 65, 1039, 1985.
595. Gale, R.P. and Canaani, E., The molecular biology of chronic myelogenous leukaemia, *Br. J. Haematol.,* 60, 395, 1985.
596. Konopka, J.B. and Witte, O.N., Activation of the *abl* oncogene in murine and human leukemias, *Biochim. Biophys. Acta,* 823, 1, 1985.
597. Sandberg, A.A., Gemmill, R.M., Hecht, B.K., and Hecht, F., The Philadelphia chromosome: a model of cancer and molecular cytogenetics, *Cancer Genet. Cytogenet.,* 21, 129, 1986.
598. Champlin, R., Gale, R.P., Foon, K.A., and Golde, D.W., Chronic leukemias: oncogenes, chromosomes, and advances in therapy, *Ann. Int. Med.,* 104, 671, 1986.
599. De Klein, A., Oncogene activation by chromosomal rearrangement in chronic myelocytic leukemia, *Mutat. Res.,* 186, 161, 1987.
600. Kurzrock, R., Gutterman, J.U., and Talpaz, M., The molecular genetics of Philadelphia chromosome-positive leukemias, *N. Engl. J. Med.,* 319, 990, 1988.
601. Westbroook, C.A., The ABL oncogene in human leukemias, *Blood Rev.,* 2, 1, 1988.
602. Groffen, J. and Heisterkamp, N., Philadelphia chromosome translocation, *Crit. Rev. Oncogenesis,* 1, 53, 1989.
603. Nowell, P.C. and Hungerford, D.A., A minute chromosome in human chronic granulocytic leukemia, *Science,* 132, 1497, 1960.
604. Caspersson, T., Gahrton, G., Lindsten, J., and Zech, L., Identification of the Philadelphia chromosome as a number 22 by quinacrine mustard fluorescence analysis, *Exp. Cell Res.,* 63, 238, 1970.
605. Rowley, J.D., A new consistent chromosomal abnormality in chronic myelogenous leukaemia identified by quinacrine fluorescence and Giemsa staining, *Nature,* 243, 290, 1973.
606. Misawa, S., Tsuda, S., Taniwaki, M., Takino, T., and Abe, T., High resolution breakpoints of the Philadelphia translocation in patients with chronic myelogenous leukemia, *Jpn. J. Hum. Genet.,* 32, 291, 1987.
607. de Klein, A., van Kessel, A.G., Grosveld, G., Bartram, C.R., Hagemeijer, A., Bootsma, D., Spurr, N.K., Heisterkamp, N., Groffen, J., and Stephenson, J.R., A cellular oncogene is translocated to the Philadelphia chromosome in chronic myelocytic leukaemia, *Nature,* 300, 765, 1982.
608. de Klein, A., van Agthoven, T., Groffen, C., Heisterkamp, N., Groffen, J., and Grosveld, G., Molecular analysis of both translocation products of a Philadelphia-positive CML patient, *Nucleic Acids Res.,* 14, 7071, 1986.
609. Cannizzaro, L.A., The breakpoint in 22q11 in a case of Ph-positive acute lymphocytic leukemia interrupts the immunoglobulin light chain gene cluster, *Cancer Genet. Cytogenet.,* 18, 173, 1985.
610. Silver, A.R.J., Masson, W.K., Breckon, G., and Cox, R., Preliminary molecular studies on two chromosome 2 encoded genes, c-*abl* and beta2M, in radiation-induced murine myeloid leukaemias, *Int. J. Radiat. Biol.,* 53, 57, 1988.
611. Heim, S., Billström, R., Kristoffersson, U., Mandahl, N., Strömbeck, B., and Mitelman, F., Variant Ph translocations in chronic myeloid leukemia, *Cancer Genet. Cytogenet.,* 18, 215, 1985.

612. Maserati, E., Pasquali, F., and Peretti, D., Different break-points in Philadelphia chromosome variant translocations and in constitutional and sporadic translocations, *Ann. Hum. Genet.,* 50, 153, 1986.

613. Verma, R.S. and Macera, M.J., Genomic diversity of Philadelphia-positive chronic myelogenous leukemia, *Leukemia Res.,* 11, 833, 1987.

614. De Braekeleer, M., Breakpoint distribution in variant Philadelphia translocations in chronic myeloid leukemia, *Cancer Genet. Cytogenet.,* 23, 167, 1986.

615. De Braekeleer, M., Variant Philadelphia translocations in chronic myeloid leukemia, *Cytogenet. Cell Genet.,* 44, 215, 1987.

616. Huret, J.L., Tanzer, J., and Henry-Amar, M., Aberrant breakpoints in chronic myelogenous leukaemia; oncogenes and fragile sites, *Hum. Genet.,* 74, 447, 1986.

617. Hagemeijer, A., Bartram, C.R., Smit, E.M.E., van Agthoven, A.J., and Bootsma, D., Is the chromosomal region 9q34 always involved in variants of the Ph¹ translocation?, *Cancer Genet. Cytogenet.,* 13, 1, 1984.

618. Bartram, C.R., Anger, B., Carbonell, F., and Kleihauer, E., Involvement of chromosome 9 in variant Ph¹ translocation, *Leukemia Res.,* 9, 1133, 1985.

619. Mareni, C., Sessarego, M., Coviello, D.A., Origone, P., and Ajmar, F., Involvement of chromosomal region 9q34 in a case of variant Ph¹ translocation t(22;22), *Leukemia Res.,* 10, 1131, 1986.

620. Morris, C.M. and Fitzgerald, P.H., Complexity of an apparently simple variant Ph translocation in chronic myeloid leukemia, *Leukemia Res.,* 11, 163, 1987.

621. Groffen, J., Heisterkamp, N., Stephenson, J.R., van Kessel, A.G., de Klein, A., Grosveld, G., and Bootsma, D., c-*sis* is translocated from chromosome 22 to chromosome 9 in chronic myelocytic leukemia, *J. Exp. Med.,* 158, 9, 1983.

622. Bartram, C.R., de Klein, A., Hagemeijer, A., Grosveld, G., Heisterkamp, N., and Groffen, J., Localization of the human c-*sis* oncogene in Ph¹-positive and Ph¹-negative chronic myelocytic leukemia by *in situ* hybridization, *Blood,* 63, 223, 1984.

623. Romero, P., Blick, M., Talpaz, M., Murphy, E., Hester, J., and Gutterman, J., c-*sis* and c-*abl* expression in chronic myelogenous leukemia and other hematologic malignancies, *Blood,* 67, 839, 1986.

624. Brodsky, I., Hubbell, H.R., Strayer, D.R., and Gillespie, D.H., Implications of retroviral and oncogene activity in chronic myelogenous leukemia, *Cancer Genet. Cytogenet.,* 26, 15, 1987.

625. Bechet, J.M., Bornkamm, G., and Lenoir, G.M., The c-*sis* oncogene is not activated in Ewing's sarcoma, *N. Engl. J. Med.,* 310, 393, 1984.

626. van Kessel, A.G., Turc-Carel, C., de Klein, A., Grosveld, G., Lenoir, G., and Bootsma, D., Translocation of oncogene c-*sis* from chromosome 22 to chromosome 11 in a Ewing sarcoma-derived cell line, *Mol. Cell. Biol.,* 5, 427, 1985.

627. Bolger, G.B., Stamberg, J., Kirsch, I.R., Hollis, G.F., Schwarz, D.F., and Thomas, G.H., Chromosome translocation t(14;22) and oncogene (c-*sis*) variant in a pedigree with familial meningioma, *N. Engl. J. Med.,* 312, 564, 1985.

628. Adolph, S., Bartram, C.R., and Hameister, H., Mapping of the oncogenes *Myc, Sis,* and *int-1* to the distal part of mouse chromosome 15, *Cytogenet. Cell Genet.,* 44, 65, 1987.

629. Sessarego, M., Panarello, C., Coviello, D.A., Boccaccio, P., and Ajmar, F., Karyotype evolution in CML: high frequency of translocations other than the Ph, *Cancer Genet. Cytogenet.,* 25, 73, 1987.

630. Collins, S.J., Breakpoints on chromosome s 9 and 22 in Philadelphia chromosome-positive chronic myelogenous leukemia (CML): amplification of rearranged c-*abl* oncogenes in CML blast crisis, *J. Clin. Invest.,* 78, 1392, 1986.

631. Bernards, A., Rubin, C.M., Westbrook, C.A., Paskind, M., and Baltimore, D., The first intron in the human c-*abl* gene is at least 22 kilobases long and is a target for translocations in chronic myelogenous leukemia, *Mol. Cell. Biol.,* 7, 3231, 1987.

632. Westbrook, C.A., Rubin, C.M., Carrino, J.J., Le Beau, M.M., Bernards, A., and Rowley, J.D., Long-range mapping of the Philadelphia chromosome by pulse-field gel electrophoresis, *Blood,* 71, 697, 1988.

633. Groffen, J., Stephenson, J.R., Heisterkamp, N., de Klein, A., Bartram, C.R., and Grosveld, G., Philadelphia chromosomal breakpoints are clustered within a limited region, bcr, on chromosome 22, *Cell,* 36, 93, 1984.

634. Croce, C.M., Huebner, K., Isobe, M., Fainstain, E., Lifshitz, B., Shtivelman, E., and Canaani, E., Mapping of four distinct *BCR*-related loci to chromosome region 22q11: order of *BCR* loci relative to chronic myelogenous leukemia and acute lymphoblastic leukemia breakpoints, *Proc. Natl. Acad. Sci. U.S.A.,* 84, 7174, 1987.

635. Hirosawa, S., Aoki, N., Shibuya, M., and Onozawa, Y., Breakpoints in Philadelphia chromosome (Ph¹)-positive leukemias, *Jpn. J. Cancer Res.,* 78, 590, 1987.

636. Konopka, J.B., Watanabe, S.M., and Witte, O.N., An alteration of the human c-*abl* protein in K562 leukemia cells unmasks associated tyrosine kinase activity, *Cell,* 37, 1035, 1984.

637. Kloetzer, W., Kurzrock, R., Smith, L., Talpaz, M., Spiller, M., Gutterman, J., and Arlinghaus, R., The human cellular *abl* gene product in the chronic myelogenous leukemia cell line K562 has an associated tyrosine protein kinase, *Virology,* 140, 230, 1985.

638. Konopka, J.B., Watanabe, S.M., Singer, J.W., Collins, S.J., and Witte, O.N., Cell lines and clinical isolates derived from Ph^1-positive chronic myelogenous leukemia patients express c-*abl* proteins with a common structural alteration, *Proc. Natl. Acad. Sci. U.S.A.*, 82, 1810, 1985.

639. Shtivelman, E., Lifshitz, B., Gale, R.P., and Canaani, E., Fused transcript of *abl* and *bcr* genes in chronic myelogenous leukaemia, *Nature*, 315, 550, 1985.

640. Heisterkamp, N., Stam, K., Groffen, J., de Klein, A., and Grosveld, G., Structural organization of the *bcr* gene and its role in the Ph' translocation, *Nature*, 316, 758, 1985.

641. Stam, K., Heisterkamp, N., Grosveld, G., de Klein, A., Verma, R.S., Coleman, M., Dosik, H., and Groffen, J., Evidence of a chimeric *bcr/c-abl* mRNA in patients with chronic myelocytic leukemia and the Philadelphia chromosome, *N. Engl. J. Med.*, 313, 1429, 1985.

642. Grosveld, G., Verwoerd, T., van Agthoven, T., de Klein, A., Ramachandran, K.L., Heisterkamp, N., Stam, K., and Groffen, J., The chronic myelocytic cell line K562 contains a breakpoint in *bcr* and produces a chimeric *bcr/c-abl* transcript, *Mol. Cell. Biol.*, 6, 607, 1986.

643. Ben-Neriah, Y., Daley, G.Q., Mes-Masson, A.-M., Witte, O.N., and Baltimore, D., The chronic myelogenous leukemia-specific P210 protein is the product of the *bcr/abl* hybrid gene, *Science*, 233, 212, 1986.

644. Maxwell, S.A., Kurzrock, R., Parsons, S.J., Talpaz, M., Gallick, G.E., Kloetzer, W.S., Arlinghaus, R.B., Kouttab, N.M., Keating, M.J., and Gutterman, J.U., Analysis of P210$^{bcr-abl}$ tyrosine protein kinase activity in various subtypes of Philadelphia chromosome-positive cells from chronic myelogenous leukemia patients, *Cancer Res.*, 47, 1731, 1987.

645. Lifshitz, B., Fainstein, E., Marcelle, C., Shtivelman, E., Amson, R., Gale, R.P., and Canaani, E., *bcr* genes and transcripts, *Oncogene*, 2, 113, 1988.

646. Collins, S., Coleman, H., and Groudine, M., Expression of *bcr* and *bcr-abl* fusion transcripts in normal and leukemic cells, *Mol. Cell. Biol.*, 7, 2870, 1987.

647. Stam, K., Heisterkamp, N., Reynolds, F.H., Jr., and Groffen, J., Evidence that the *phl* gene encodes a 160,000-dalton phosphoprotein with associated kinase activity, *Mol. Cell. Biol.*, 7, 1955, 1987.

648. Benn, P., Soper, L., Eisenberg, A., Siver, R.T., Coleman, M., Cacciapaglia, B., Bennett, L., Baird, M., Silverstein, M., Berger, C., and Bernhardt, B., Utility of molecular genetic analysis of *bcr* rearrangement in the diagnosis of chronic myeloid leukemia, *Cancer Genet. Cytogenet.*, 29, 1, 1987.

649. Blennerhassett, G.T., Furth, M.E., Anderson, A., Burns, J.P., Chaganti, R.S.K., Blick, M., Talpaz, M., Dev, V.G., Chan, L.C., Wiedemann, L.M., Greaves, M.F., Hagemeijer, A., van der Plas, D., Skuse, G., Wang, N., and Stam, K., Clinical evaluation of a DNA probe assay for the Philadelphia (Ph^1) translocation in chronic myelogenous leukemia, *Leukemia*, 2, 648, 1988.

650. Lee, M.-S., Chang, K.-S., Freireich, E.J., Kantarjian, H.M., Talpaz, M., Trujillo, J.M., and Stass, S.A., Detection of minimal residual *bcr/abl* transcripts by a modified polymerase chain reaction, *Blood*, 72, 893, 1988.

651. Raskind, W.H., Disteche, C.M., Keating, A., and Singer, J.W., Correlation between cytogenetic and molecular findings in human chronic myelogenous leukemia lines EM-2 and EM-3, *Cancer Genet. Cytogenet.*, 25, 271, 1987.

652. Bartram, C.R., Raghavachar, A., Anger, B., Stain, C., and Bettelheim, P., T lymphocytes lack rearrangement of the *bcr* gene in Philadelphia chromosome-positive chronic myelocytic leukemia, *Blood*, 69, 1682, 1987.

653. Konopka, J.B., Clark, S., McLaughlin, J., Nitta, M., Kato, Y., Strife, A., Clarkson, B., and Witte, O.N., Variable expression of the translocated c-*abl* oncogene in Philadelphia-chromosome-positive B-lymphoid cell lines from chronic myelogenous leukemia patients, *Proc. Natl. Acad. Sci. U.S.A.*, 83, 4049, 1986.

654. Canaani, E., Gale, R.P., Steiner-Saltz, D., Berrebi, A., Aghai, E., and Januszewicz, E., Altered transcription of an oncogene in chronic myeloid leukaemia, *Lancet*, i, 593, 1984.

655. Collins, S.J., Kubonishi, I., Miyoshi, I., and Groudine, M.T., Altered transcription of the c-*abl* oncogene in K-562 and other chronic myelogenous leukemia cells, *Science*, 225, 72, 1984.

656. Gale, R.P. and Canaani, E., An 8-kilobase *abl* RNA transcript in chronic myelogenous leukemia, *Proc. Natl. Acad. Sci. U.S.A.*, 81, 5648, 1984.

657. Andrews, D.F., III and Collins, S.J., Heterogeneity in expression of the *bcr-abl* fusion transcript in CML blast crisis, *Leukemia*, 1, 718, 1987.

658. Bartram, C.R., de Klein, A., Hagemeijer, A., Carbonell, F., Kleihauer, E., and Grosveld, G., Additional c-*abl/bcr* rearrangements in a CML patient exhibiting two Ph^1 chromosomes during blast crisis, *Leukemia Res.*, 10, 221, 1986.

659. Bartram, C.R., Janssen, J.W.G., Becher, R., de Klein, A., and Grosveld, G., Persistence of chronic myelomonocytic leukemia despite deletion of rearranged *bcr/c-abl* sequences in blast crisis, *J. Exp. Med.*, 164, 1389, 1986.

660. Kipreos, E.T., Lee, G.J., and Wang, J.Y.J., Isolation of temperature-sensitive tyrosine kinase mutants of v-*abl* oncogene by screening with antibodies for phosphotyrosine, *Proc. Natl. Acad. Sci. U.S.A.*, 84, 1345, 1987.

661. Davis, R.L., Konopka, J.B., and Witte, O.N., Activation of the c-*abl* oncogene by viral transduction or chromosome translocation generates altered c-*abl* proteins with similar *in vitro* kinase properties, *Mol. Cell. Biol.*, 5, 204, 1985.

662. Konopka, J.B. and Witte, O.N., Detection of c-*abl* tyrosine kinase activity *in vitro* permits direct comparison of normal and altered *abl* gene products, *Mol. Cell. Biol,* 5, 3116, 1985.

663. Naldini, L., Stacchini, A., Cirillo, D.M., Aglietta, M., Gavosto, F., and Comoglio, P.M., Phosphotyrosine antibodies identify the p210$^{c\ -abl}$ tyrosine kinase and proteins phosphorylated on tyrosine in human chronic myelogenous leukemia cells, *Mol. Cell. Biol.,* 6, 1803, 1986.

664. Ben-Neriah, Y., Bernards, A., Paskind, M., Daley, G.Q., and Baltimore, D., Alternative 5' exons in c-*abl* mRNA, *Cell,* 44, 577, 1986.

665. Prywes, R., Foulkes, J.G., and Baltimore, D., The minimum transforming region of v-*abl* is the segment encoding protein-tyrosine kinase, *J. Virol.,* 54, 114, 1985.

666. Collins, S.J. and Groudine, M.T., Chronic myelogenous leukemia: amplification of a rearranged c-*abl* oncogene in both chronic phase and blast crisis, *Blood,* 69, 893, 1987.

667. Bartram, C.R., de Klein, A., Hagemeijer, A., van Agthoven, T., van Kessel, A.G., Bootsma, D., Grosveld, G., Ferguson-Smith, M.A., Davies, T., Stone, M., Heisterkamp, N., Stephenson, J.R., and Groffen, J., Translocation of c-*abl* oncogene correlates with the presence of a Philadelphia chromosome in chronic myelocytic leukaemia, *Nature,* 306, 277, 1983.

668. Koeffler, H.P. and Golde, D.W., Chronic myelogenous leukemia: new concepts, *N. Engl. J. Med.,* 304, 1201, 1981.

669. Bartram, C.R., Kleihauer, E., de Klein, A., Grosveld, G., Teyssier, J.R., Heisterkamp, N., and Groffen, J., c-*abl* and *bcr* are rearranged in a Ph^1-negative CML patient, *EMBO J.,* 4, 683, 1985.

670. Morris, C.M., Reeve, A.E., Firzgerald, P.H., Hollings, P.E., Beard, M.E.J., and Heaton, D.C., Genomic diversity correlates with clinical variation in Ph'-negative chronic myeloid leukaemia, *Nature,* 320, 281, 1986.

671. Bartram, C.R., Rearrangement of the c-abl and bcr genes in Ph-negative CML and Ph-positive acute leukemias, *Leukemia,* 2, 63, 1988.

672. Wiedemann, L.M., Karhi, K.K., Shivji, M.K.K., Rayter, S.I., Pegram, S.M., Dowden, G., Bevan, D., Will, A., Galton, D.A.G., and Chan, L.G., The correlation of breakpoint cluster region rearrangement and p210 *phl/abl* expression with morphological analysis of Ph-negative chronic myeloid leukemia and other myeloproliferative disorders, *Blood,* 71, 349, 1988.

673. Bartram, C.R., *bcr* rearrangement without juxtaposition of c-*abl* in chronic myelocytic leukemia, *J Exp. Med.,* 162, 2175, 1985.

674. Ganesan, T.S., Rasool, F., Guo, A.-P., Th'ng, K.H., Dowding, C., Hibbin, J.A., Young, B.D., White, H., Kumaran, T.O., Galton, D.A.G., and Goldman, J.M., Rearrangement of the *bcr* gene in Philadelphia chromosome-negative chronic myeloid leukemia, *Blood,* 68, 957, 1986.

675. Dreazen, O., Klisak, I., Rassool, F., Goldman, J.M., Sparkes, R.S., and Gale, R.P., Do oncogenes determine clinical features in chronic myeloid leukaemia?, *Lancet,* 1, 1402, 1987.

676. Lisker, R., Caras, L., Mutchinik, O., Perez-Chavez, F., and Labardini, J., Late appearing Philadelphia chromosome in 2 patients with chronic myelogenous leukemia, *Blood,* 56, 812, 1980.

677. Hagemeijer, A., Smit, E.M.E., Löwenberg, B., and Abels, J., Chronic myeloid leukemia with permanent disappearance of the Ph^1 chromosome and development of new clonal subpopulations, *Blood,* 53, 1, 1979.

678. Smajda, N., Krulik, M., Audebert, A.A., de Gramont, A., Debray, J., Spontaneous regression of cytogenetic and haematologic anomalies in Ph^1-positive chronic myelogenous leukaemia, *Br. J. Haematol.,* 63, 257, 1986.

679. Yamada, T., Oikawa, T., Kuzumaki, N., Takagi, N., and Sasaki, M., Absence of the hybrid *bcr-abl* mRNA in Ph^1-positive B lymphoblastoid cell lines established from a patient with chronic myelogenous leukemia, *Int. J. Cancer,* 40, 778, 1987.

680. Andrews, D.F., III, Singer, J.W., and Collins, S.J., Effect of recombinant α-interferon on the expression of the *bcr-abl* fusion gene in human chronic myelogenous human leukemia cell lines, *Cancer Res.,* 47, 6629, 1987.

681. Kozbor, D., Giallongo, A., Sierzega, M.E., Konopka, J.B., Witte, O.N., Showe, L.C., and Croce, C.M., Expression of a translocated c-*abl* gene in hybrids of mouse fibroblasts and chronic myelogenous leukaemia cells, *Nature,* 319, 331, 1986.

682. Yamada, T. and Sasaki, M., Differentiation by a tumor promoter of lymphoblastoid cell lines with and without Ph^1 chromosome from a chronic myelogenous leukemia patient, *Jpn. J. Cancer Res.,* 78, 499, 1987.

683. Alitalo, R., Andersson, L.C., Betsholtz, C., Nilsson, K., Westermark, B., Heldin, C.-H., and Alitalo, K., Induction of platelet-derived growth factor gene expression during megakaryoblastic and monocytic differentiation of human leukemia cell lines, *EMBO J.,* 6, 1213, 1987.

684. Alitalo, R., The *bcr-c-abl* tyrosine kinase activity is extinguished by TPA in K562 leukemia cells, *FEBS Lett.,* 222, 293, 1987.

685. Richardson, J.M., Morla, A.O., and Wang, J.Y.J., Reduction in protein tyrosine phosphorylation during differentiation of human leukemia cell line K-562, *Cancer Res.,* 47, 4066, 1987.

686. Daley, G.Q., McLaughlin, J., Witte, O.N., and Baltimore, D., The CML-specific P210 *bcr/abl* protein, unlike v-*abl*, does not transform NIH/3T3 fibroblasts, *Science,* 237, 532, 1987.

687. Burrows, P.D. and Cooper, M.D., The immunoglobulin heavy chain class switch, *Mol. Cell. Biochem.,* 63, 97, 1984.

688. Rabbitts, T.H., Baer, R., Davis, M., Forster, A., Rabbitts, P.H., and Malcolm, S., c-*myc* gene activation and chromosome translocation, *J. Cell Sci.,* Suppl. 1, 95, 1984.

689. Kelly, K. and Siebenlist, U., The role of c-*myc* in the proliferation of normal and neoplastic cells, *J. Clin. Immunol.,* 5, 65, 1985.

690. Wiman, K.G., Clarkson, B., Hayday, A.C., Saito, H., Tonegawa, S., and Hayward, W.S., Activation of a translocated c-*myc* gene: role of structural alterations in the upstream region, *Proc. Natl. Acad. Sci. U.S.A.,* 81, 6798, 1984.

691. Nowell, P.C., Erikson, J., Finan, J., Emanuel, B., and Croce, C.M., Chromosomal translocations, immunoglobulin genes and oncogenes in human B-cell tumours, *Cancer Surv.,* 3, 531, 1984.

692. Waldmann, T.A., Korsmeyer, S.J., Bakhshi, A., Arnold, A., and Kirsch, I.R., Molecular genetic analysis of human lymphoid neoplasms: immunoglobulin genes and the c-*myc* oncogene, *Ann. Int. Med.,* 102, 510, 1985.

693. Klein, G. and Klein, E., *Myc*/Ig juxtaposition by chromosomal translocations: some new insights, puzzles and paradoxes, *Immunol. Today,* 6, 208, 1985.

694. Rabbitts, T.H., The c-*myc* proto-oncogene: involvement in chromosomal abnormalities, *Trends Genet.,* 1, 327, 1985.

695. Klein, G., Constitutive activation of oncogenes by chromosomal translocations in B-cell derived tumors, *AIDS Res.,* 2 (Suppl. 1), 1, 1986.

696. Kirsch, I.R., Morton, C.C., Nakahara, K., and Leder, P., Human immunoglobulin heavy chain genes map to a region of translocations in malignant B lymphocytes, *Science,* 216, 301, 1982.

697. Erikson, J., Finan, J., Nowell, P.C., and Croce, C.M., Translocation of immunoglobulin V_H genes in Burkitt lymphoma, *Proc. Natl. Acad. Sci. U.S.A.,* 79, 5611, 1982.

698. Leder, P., Battey, J., Lenoir, G., Moulding, C., Murphy, W., Potter, H., Stewart, T., and Taub, R., Translocations among antibody genes in human cancer, *Science,* 222, 765, 1983.

699. de la Chapelle, A., Lenoir, G., Boue, J., Boue, A., Gallano, P., Huerre, C., Szajnert, M.-F., Jeanpierre, M., Lalouel, J.-M., and Kaplan, J.-C., Lambda Ig constant region genes are translocated to chromosome 8 in Burkitt's lymphoma with t(8;22), *Nucleic Acids Res.,* 11, 1133, 1983.

700. Mitchell, K.F., Battey, J., Hollis, G.F., Moulding, C., Taub, R., and Leder, P., The effect of translocations on the cellular *myc* gene in Burkitt lymphomas, *J. Cell. Physiol.,* Suppl. 3, 171, 1984.

701. Croce, C.M. and Nowell, P.C., Molecular basis of human B cell neoplasia, *Blood,* 65, 1, 1985.

702. Manolov, G. and Manolova, Y., Marker band in one chromosome 14 from Burkitt lymphomas, *Nature,* 237, 33, 1972.

703. Zech, L., Haglund, U., Nilsson, K., and Klein, G., Characteristic chromosomal abnormalities in biopsies and lymphoid cell lines from patients with Burkitt and non-Burkitt lymphomas, *Int. J. Cancer,* 17, 47, 1976.

704. Dalla Favera, R., Bregni, M., Erikson, J., Patterson, D., Gallo, R.C., and Croce, C.M., Human c-*myc onc* gene is located on the region of chromosome 8 that is translocated in Burkitt lymphoma cells, *Proc. Natl. Acad. Sci. U.S.A.,* 79, 7824, 1982.

705. Taub, R., Kirsch, I., Morton, C., Lenoir, G., Swan, D., Tronick, S., Aaronson, S., and Leder, P., Translocation of the c-*myc* gene into the immunoglobulin heavy chain locus in human Burkitt lymphoma and murine plasmacytoma cells, *Proc. Natl. Acad. Sci. U.S.A.,* 79, 7837, 1982.

706. Dalla Favera, R., Martinotti, S., Gallo, R.C., Erikson, J., and Croce, C.M., Translocation and rearrangements of the c-*myc* oncogene locus in human undifferentiated B-cell lymphomas, *Science,* 219, 963, 1983.

707. Richardson, L.A. and Dickerman, J.D., 8;14 chromosome translocation in a negative bone marrow aspirate from a patient with Burkitt's lymphoma, *Cancer,* 57, 761, 1986.

708. Pelicci, P.-G., Knowles, D.M., II, Arlin, Z.A., Wiczorek, R., Luciw, P., Dina, D., Basilico, C., and Dalla-Favera, R., Multiple monoclonal B cell expansions and c-*myc* oncogene rearrangements in acquired immune deficiency syndrome-related lymphoproliferative disorders, *J. Exp. Med.,* 164, 2049, 1986.

709. Rechavi, G., Ben-Bassat, I., Bekowicz, M., Martinowitz, U., Brok-Simoni, F., Neumann, Y., Vansover, A., Gotlieb-Stematsky, T., and Ramot, B., Molecular analysis of Burkitt's leukemia in two hemophilic brothers with AIDS, *Blood,* 70, 1713, 1987.

710. Potter, M., Genetics of susceptibility to plasmacytoma development in BALB/c mice, *Cancer Surv.,* 3, 247, 1984.

711. Ohno, S., Babonitis, F., Wiener, F., Spira, J., and Klein, G., Nonrandom chromosome changes involving the Ig gene-carrying chromosomes 12 and 6 in pristane-induced mouse plasmacytomas, *Cell,* 18, 1001, 1979.

712. Harris, L.J., D'Eustachio, P., Ruddle, F.H., and Marcu, K.B., DNA sequence associated with chromosome translocations in mouse plasmacytomas, *Proc. Natl. Acad. Sci. U.S.A.,* 79, 6622, 1982.

713. Calame, K., Kim, S., Lalley, P., Hill, R., Davis, M., and Hood, L., Molecular cloning of translocations involving chromosome 15 and the immunoglobulin c_{alpha} gene from chromosome 12 in two murine plasmacytomas, *Proc. Natl. Acad. Sci. U.S.A.,* 79, 6994, 1982.

714. Shen-Ong, G.L.C., Keath, E.J., Piccoli, S.P., and Cole, M.D., Novel *myc* oncogene RNA from abortive immunoglobulin-gene recombination in mouse plasmacytomas, *Cell,* 31, 443, 1982.

715. Huppi, K., Duncan, R., and Potter, M., *Myc-1* is centromeric to the linkage group *Ly-6—Sis—Gdc-*1 on mouse chromosome 15, *Immunogenetics,* 27, 215, 1988.

716. Crews, S., Barth, R., Hood, L., Prehn, J., and Calame, K., Mouse c-myc oncogene is located on chromosome 15 and translocated to chromosome 12 in plasmacytomas, *Science,* 218, 1319, 1982.

717. Sakaguchi, A.Y., Lalley, P.A., and Naylor, S.L., Human and mouse cellular *myc* protooncogenes reside on chromosomes involved in numerical and structural aberrations in cancer, *Somat. Cell Genet.,* 9, 391, 1983.

718. Neuberger, M.S. and Calabi, F., Reciprocal chromosome translocation between c-*myc* and immunoglobulin gamma 2b genes, *Nature,* 305, 240, 1983.

719. Caccia, N.C., Mak, T.W., and Klein, G., c-*myc* involvement in chromosomal translocations in mice and men, *J. Cell. Physiol.,* Suppl. 3, 199, 1984.

720. Potter, M., The *myc* oncogene in mouse plasmacytomagenesis, *Surv. Synthesis Pathol. Res.,* 3, 499, 1984.

721. Harris, L.J., Remmers, E.F., Brodeur, P., Riblet, R., D'Eustachio, P., and Marcu, K.B., c-*myc* gene rearrangements involving gamma immunoglobulin heavy chain gene switch regions in murine plasmacytomas, *Nucleic Acids Res.,* 11, 8303, 1983.

722. Erikson, J., Miller, D.A., Miller, O.J., Abcarian, P.W., Skurla, R.M., Mushinski, J.F., and Croce, C.M., The c-*myc* oncogene is translocated to the involved chromosome 12 in mouse plasmacytoma, *Proc. Natl. Acad. Sci. U.S.A.,* 82, 4212, 1985.

723. Wirschubsky, Z., Ingvarsson, S., Carstenssen, A., Wiener, F., Klein, G., and Sümegi, J., Gene localization on sorted chromosomes: definitive evidence on the relative positioning of genes participating in the mouse plasmacytoma-associated typical translocation, *Proc. Natl. Acad. Sci. U.S.A.,* 82, 6975, 1985.

724. Cory, S., Graham, M., Webb, E., Corcoran, L., and Adams, J.M., Variant (6;15) translocations in murine plamacytomas involve a chromosome 15 locus at least 72 kb from the c-*myc* oncogene, *EMBO J.,* 4, 675, 1985.

725. Banerjee, M., Wiener, F., Spira, J., Babonits, M., Nilsson, M.-G., Sümegi, J., and Klein, G., Mapping of the c-*myc* pvt-1 and immunoglobulin kappa genes in relation to the mouse plasmacytoma-associated variant (6:15) translocation breakpoint, *EMBO J.,* 4, 3183, 1985.

726. Gough, N., Chromosomal translocations and c-*myc* gene: paradigm lost?, *Trends Genet.,* 1, 63, 1985.

727. Jolicoeur, P., Villeneuve, L., Rassart, E., and Kozak, C., Mouse chromosomal mapping of a murine leukemia virus integration region (*Mis-1*) first identified in rat thymic leukemia, *J. Virol.,* 56, 1045, 1985.

728. Dean, M., Kent, R.B., and Sonenshein, G.E., Transcriptional activation of immunoglobulin alpha heavy-chain genes by translocation of the c-*myc* oncogene, *Nature,* 305, 443, 1983.

729. Kindy, M.S., McCormack, J.E., Buckler, A.J., Levine, R.A., and Sonenshein, G.E., Independent regulation of transcription of the two strands of the c-*myc* gene, *Mol. Cell. Biol.,* 7, 2857, 1987.

730. Wiener, F., Babonits, M., Bregula, U., Klein, G., Leonard, A., Wax, J.S., and Potter, M., High resolution banding analysis of the involvement of strain BALB/c- and AKR-derived chromosomes no. 15 in plasmacytoma-specific translocation, *J. Exp. Med.,* 159, 276, 1984.

731. Wiener, F., Ohno, S., Babonits, M., Sumegi, J., Wirschubsky, Z., Klein, G., Mushinski, J.F., and Potter, M., Hemizygous interstitial deletion of chromosome 15 (band D) in three translocation-negative murine plasmacytomas, *Proc. Natl. Acad. Sci. U.S.A.,* 81, 1159, 1984.

732. Fahrlander, P.D., Sümegi, J., Yang, J., Wiener, F., Marcu, K.B., and Klein, G., Activation of the c-*myc* oncogene by the immunoglobulin heavy-chain gene enhancer after multiple switch region-mediated chromosome rearrangements in a murine plasmacytoma, *Proc. Natl. Acad. Sci. U.S.A.,* 82, 3746, 1985.

733. Balachandran, R., Reddy, E.P., Dunn, C.Y., Aaronson, S.A., and Swan, D.C., Immunoblobulin synthesis and gene rearrangements in lymphoid cells transformed by replication-competent Rauscher murine leukemia virus: transformation of B cells at various stages of differentiation, *EMBO J.,* 3, 3199, 1984.

734. Sümegi, J., Spira, J., Bazin, H., Szpirer, J., Levan, G., and Klein, G., Rat c-*myc* oncogene is located on chromosome 7 and rearranges in immunocytomas with t(6;7) chromosomal translocation, *Nature,* 306, 497, 1983.

735. Pear, W.S., Ingvarsson, S., Steffen, D., Münke, M., Francke, U., Bazin, H., Klein, G., and Sümegi, J., Multiple chromosomal rearrangements in a spontaneously arising t(6;7) rat immunocytoma juxtapose c-*myc* and immunoglobulin heavy chain sequences, *Proc. Natl. Acad. Sci. U.S.A.,* 83, 7376, 1986.

736. Tian, S.-S. and Faust, C., Rearrangement of rat immunoglobulin E heavy-chain and c-*myc* genes in the B-cell immunocytoma IR162, *Mol. Cell. Biol.,* 7, 2614, 1987.

737. Cohen, D., The canine transmissible venereal tumor: a unique result of tumor progression, *Adv. Cancer Res.,* 43, 75, 1985.

738. Katzir, N., Rechavi, G., Cohen, J.B., Unger, T., Simoni, F., Segal, S., Cohen, D., and Givol, D., "Retroposon" insertion into the cellular oncogene c-*myc* in canine transmissible venereal tumor, *Proc. Natl. Acad. Sci. U.S.A.,* 82, 1054, 1985.

739. Rogers, J., Retroposons defined, *Nature,* 301, 460, 1983.

740. Rogers, J.H., The origin and evolution of retroposons, *Int. Rev. Cytol.,* 93, 187, 1985.

741. Weiner, A.M., Deininger, P.L., and Efstratiadis, A., Nonviral retroposons: genes, pseudogenes, and transposable elements generated by the reverse flow of genetic information, *Annu. Rev. Biochem.,* 55, 631, 1986.

742. Katzir, N., Arman, E., Cohen, D., Givol, D., and Rechavi, G., Common origin of transmissible venereal tumors (TVT) in dogs, *Oncogene,* 1, 445, 1987.

743. Neel, B.G., Hayward, W.S., Robinson, H.L., Fang, J., and Astrin, S.M., Avian leukosis virus-induced tumors have common proviral integration sites and synthesize discrete new RNAs: oncogenesis by promoter insertion, *Cell,* 23, 323, 1981.

744. Hayward, W.S., Neel, B.G., and Astrin, S.M., Activation of a cellular *onc* gene by promoter insertion in ALV-induced lymphoid leukosis, *Nature,* 290, 475, 1981.

745. Fung, Y.-K.T., Fadly, A.M., Crittenden, L.B., and Kung, H.-J., On the mechanism of retrovirus-induced avian lymphoid leukosis: deletion and integration of the proviruses, *Proc. Natl. Acad. Sci. U.S.A.,* 78, 3418, 1981.

746. Neel, B.G., Gasic, G.P., Rogler, C.E., Skalka, A.M., Ju, G., Hishinuma, F., Papas, T., Astrin, S.M., and Hayward, W.S., Molecular analysis of the c-*myc* locus in normal tissue and in avian leukosis virus-induced lymphomas, *J. Virol.,* 44, 158, 1982.

747. Swift, R.A., Boerkoel, C., Ridgway, A., Fujita, D.J., Dodgson, J.B., and Kung, H.-J., B-lymphoma induction in reticuloendotheliosis virus: characterization of a mutated chicken syncytial virus provirus involved in c-*myc* activation, *J. Virol.,* 61, 2084, 1987.

748. Steffen, D., Proviruses adjacent to c-*myc* in some murine leukemia virus-induced lymphomas, *Proc. Natl. Acad. Sci. U.S.A.,* 81, 2097, 1984.

749. Rappold, G.A., Hameister, H., Cremer, T., Adolph, S., Henglein, B., Freese, U.-K., Lenoir, G.M., and Bornkamm, G.W., c-*myc* and immunoglobulin kappa light chain constant genes are on the 8q$^+$ chromosome of three Burkitt lymphoma lines with t(2;8) translocation, *EMBO J.,* 3, 2951, 1984.

750. Davis, M., Malcolm, S., and Rabbitts, T.H., Chromosome translocation can occur on either side of the c-*myc* oncogene in Burkitt lymphoma cells, *Nature,* 308, 286, 1984.

751. Haluska, F.G., Finver, S., Tsujimoto, Y., and Croce, C.M., The t(8;14) chromosomal translocation occurring in B-cell malignancies results from mistakes in V-D-J joining, *Nature,* 324, 158, 1986.

752. Haluska, F.G., Tsujimoto, Y., and Croce, C.M., The t(8;14) chromosome translocation of the Burkitt lymphoma cell line Daudi occurred during immunoglobulin gene rearrangement and involved the heavy chain diversity region, *Proc. Natl. Acad. Sci. U.S.A.,* 84, 6835, 1987.

753. McIntosh, R.V., Cohen, B.B., Steel, C.M., Read, H., Moxley, M., and Evans, H.J., Evidence for involvement of the immunoglobulin heavy-chain gene locus in the 8:14 translocation of human B lymphomas, *Int. J. Cancer,* 31, 275, 1983.

754. Baas, F., Bikker, H., Geurts van Kessel, A., Melsert, R., Pearson, P.L., de Vijlder, J.J.M., and van Ommen, G.-J.B., The human thyroglobulin gene: a polymorphic marker localized distal to c-MYC on chromosome 8 band q24, *Hum. Genet.,* 69, 138, 1985.

755. Gerondakis, S., Cory, S., and Adams, J.M., Translocation of the c-*myc* cellular oncogene to the immunoglobulin heavy chain locus in murine plasmacytomas is an imprecise reciprocal exchange, *Cell,* 36, 973, 1984.

756. Croce, C.M., Thierfelder, W., Erikson, J., Nishikura, K., Finan, J., Lenoir, G.M., and Nowell, P.C., Transcriptional activation of an unrearranged and untranslocated c-*myc* oncogene by translocation of a C$_{lambda}$ locus in Burkitt lymphoma cells, *Proc. Natl. Acad. Sci. U.S.A.,* 80, 6922, 1983.

757. Denny, C.T., Hollis, G.F., Magrath, I.T., and Kirsch, I.R., Burkitt lymphoma cell line carrying a variant translocation creates new DNA at the breakpoint and violates the hierarchy of immunoglobulin gene rearrangement, *Mol. Cell. Biol.,* 5, 3199, 1985.

758. Malcolm, S., Davis, M., and Rabbitts, T.H., Breakage on chromosome 2 brings the Ck gene to a region 3' of c-*myc* in a Burkitt's lymphoma line carrying a (2;8) translocation, *Cytogenet. Cell Genet.,* 39, 168, 1985.

759. Emanuel, B.S., Selden, J.R., Chaganti, R.S.K., Jhanwar, S., Nowell, P.C., and Croce, C.M., The 2p breakpoint of a 2;8 translocation in Burkitt lymphoma interrupts the V$_{kappa}$ locus, *Proc. Natl. Acad. Sci. U.S.A.,* 81, 2444, 1984.

760. Hollis, G.F., Mitchell, K.F., Battey, J., Potter, H., Taub, R., Lenoir, G.M., and Leder, P., A variant translocation places the immunoglobulin genes 3' to the c-*myc* oncogene in Burkitt's lymphoma, *Nature,* 307, 752, 1984.

761. Taub, R., Kelly, K., Battey, J., Latt, S., Lenoir, G.M., Trantrahavi, U., Tu, Z., and Leder, P., A novel alteration in the structure of an activated c-*myc* gene in a variant t(2;8) Burkitt lymphoma, *Cell,* 37, 511, 1984.

762. Rabbitts, T.H., Forster, A., Hamlyn, P., and Baer, R., Effect of somatic mutation within translocated c-*myc* genes in Burkitt's lymphoma, *Nature,* 309, 592, 1984.

763. Brissenden, J.E., Derynck, R., and Francke, U., Mapping of transforming growth factor alpha gene on human chromosome 2 close to the breakpoint of the Burkitt's lymphoma t(2;8) variant translocation, *Cancer Res.,* 45, 5593, 1985.

764. Otsu, M., Katamine, S., Uno, M., Yamaki, M., Ono, Y., Klein, G., Sasaki, M.S., Yaoita, Y., and Honjo, T., Molecular characterization of novel reciprocal translocation t(6;14) in an Epstein-Barr virus-transformed B cell precursor, *Mol. Cell. Biol.,* 7, 708, 1987.

765. Mathieu-Mahul, D., Caubet, J.F., Bernheim, A., Mauchauffé, M., Palmer, E., Berger, R., and Larsen, C.-J., Molecular cloning of a DNA fragment from human chromosome 14 (14q11) involved in T-cell malignancies, *EMBO J.,* 4, 3427, 1985.

766. Westaway, D., Payne, G., and Varmus, H.E., Proviral deletions and oncogene base substitutions in insertionally mutagenized c-*myc* alleles may contribute to the progression of avian bursal lymphomas, *Proc. Natl. Acad. Sci. U.S.A.,* 81, 843, 1984.

767. Taub, R., Moulding, C., Battey, J., Murphy, W., Vasicek, T., Lenoir, G.M., and Leder, P., Activation and somatic mutation of the translocated c-*myc* gene in Burkitt lymphoma cells, *Cell*, 36, 339, 1984.

768. Rabbitts, T.H., Hamlyn, P.H., and Baer, R., Altered nucleotide sequences of a translocated c-*myc* gene in Burkitt lymphoma, *Nature*, 306, 760, 1983.

769. Murphy, W., Sarid, J., Taub, R., Vasicek, T., Battey, J., Lenoir, G., and Leder, P., A translocated human c-*myc* oncogene is altered in a conserved coding sequence, *Proc. Natl. Acad. Sci. U.S.A.*, 83, 2939, 1986.

770. Szajnert, M.-F., Saule, S., Bornkamm, G.W., Wajcman, H., Lenoir, G.M., and Kaplan, J.-C., Clustered somatic mutations in and around first exon of non-rearranged c-myc in Burkitt lymphoma with t(8:22) translocation, *Nucleic Acids Res.*, 15, 4553, 1987.

771. Gazin, C., Rigolet, M., Briand, J.P., Van Regenmortel, M.H.V., and Galibert, F., Immunochemical detection of proteins related to the human c-*myc* exon 1, *EMBO J.*, 5, 2241, 1986.

772. Caré, A., Cianetti, L., Giampaolo, A., Sposi, N.M., Zappavigna, V., Mavilio, F., Alimena, G., Amadori, S., Mandelli, F., and Peschle, C., Translocation of c-*myc* into the immunoglobulin heavy-chain locus in human acute B-cell leukemia. A molecular analysis, *EMBO J.*, 5, 905, 1986.

773. Cleary, M.L., Meeker, T.C., Levy, S., Lee, E., Trela, M., Sklar, J., and Levy, R., Clustering of extensive somatic mutations in the variable region of an immunoglobulin heavy chain gene from a human B cell lymphoma, *Cell*, 44, 97, 1986.

774. Adams, J.M., Gerondakis, S., Webb, E., Corcoran, L.M., and Cory, S., Cellular *myc* oncogene is altered by chromosome translocation to an immunoglobulin locus in murine plasmacytomas and is rearranged similarly in human Burkitt lymphomas, *Proc. Natl. Acad. Sci. U.S.A.*, 80, 1982, 1983.

775. Perry, R.P., Consequences of *myc* invasion of immunoglobulin loci: facts and speculation, *Cell*, 33, 647, 1983.

776. Fahrlander, P.D., Piechaczyk, M., and Marcu, K.B., Chromatin structure of the murine c-*myc* locus: implications for the regulation of normal and chromosomally translocated genes, *EMBO J.*, 4, 3195, 1985.

777. Dyson, P.J. and Rabbitts, T.H., Chromatin structure around the c-*myc* gene in Burkitt lymphomas with upstream and downstream translocation points, *Proc. Natl. Acad. Sci. U.S.A.*, 82, 1984, 1985.

778. Kakkis, E., Prehn, J., and Calame, K., An active chromatin structure acquired by translocated c-*myc* genes, *Mol. Cell. Biol.*, 6, 1357, 1986.

779. Kakkis, E. and Calame, K., A plasmacytoma-specific factor binds the c-*myc* promoter region, *Proc. Natl. Acad. Sci. U.S.A.*, 84, 7031, 1987.

780. Bentley, D.L. and Groudine, M., Novel promoter upstream of the human c-*myc* gene and regulation of c-*myc* expression in B-cell lymphomas, *Mol. Cell. Biol.*, 6, 3481, 1986.

781. Chung, J., Sinn, E., Reed, R.R., and Leder, P., Trans-acting elements modulate expression of the human c-*myc* gene in Burkitt lymphoma cells, *Proc. Natl. Acad. Sci. U.S.A.*, 83, 7918, 1986.

782. Linial, M., Gunderson, N., and Groudine, M., Enhanced transcription of c-*myc* in bursal lymphoma cells requires continuous protein synthesis, *Science*, 230, 1126, 1985.

783. Marcu, K.B., Harris, L.J., Stanto, L.W., Erikson, J., Watt, R., and Croce, C.M., Transcriptionally active c-*myc* oncogene is contained within NIADR, a DNA sequence associated with chromosome translocations in B-cell neoplasia, *Proc. Natl. Acad. Sci. U.S.A.*, 80, 519, 1983.

784. Erikson, J., ar-Rushdi, A., Drwinga, H.L., Nowell, P.C., and Croce, C.M., Transcriptional activation of the translocated c-*myc* oncogene in Burkitt lymphoma, *Proc. Natl. Acad. Sci. U.S.A.*, 80, 820, 1983.

785. Nishikura, K., ar-Rushdi, A., Erikson, J., Watt, R., Rovera, G., and Croce, C.M., Differential expression of the normal and of the translocated human c-*myc* oncogenes in B cells, *Proc. Natl. Acad. Sci. U.S.A.*, 80, 4822, 1983.

786. Blick, M., Westin, E., Wong-Staal, F., Gallo, R., McCredie, K., and Gutterman, J., Rearrangement and enhanced expression of c-*myc* oncogene in fresh tumor cells obtained from a patient with acute lymphoblastic leukemia, *Leukemia Res.*, 10, 381, 1986.

787. Maguire, R.T., Robins, T.S., Thorgeirsson, S.S., and Heilman, C.A., Expression of cellular *myc* and *mos* genes in undifferentiated B cell lymphomas of Burkitt and non-Burkitt types, *Proc. Natl. Acad. Sci. U.S.A.*, 80, 1947, 1983.

788. Keath, E.J., Kelekar, A., and Cole, M.D., Transcriptional activation of the translocated c-*myc* oncogene in mouse plasmacytomas: similar RNA levels in tumor and proliferating normal cells, *Cell*, 37, 521, 1984.

789. Hann, S.R., King, M.W., Bentley, D.L., Anderson, C.W., and Eisenman, R.N., A non-AUG translational initiation in c-*myc* exon 1 generates an N-terminally distinct protein whose synthesis is disrupted in Burkitt's lymphomas, *Cell*, 52, 185, 1988.

790. Eick, D., Piechaczyk, M., Henglein, B., Blanchard, J.-M., Traub, B., Kofler, E., Wiest, S., Lenoir, G.M., and Bornkamm, G., Aberrant c-*myc* RNAs of Burkitt's lymphoma cells have longer half-lives, *EMBO J.*, 4, 3717, 1985.

791. Guerrasio, A., Avanzi, G.C., Pegoraro, L., Estivill, X., Serra, A., Giubellino, M.C., Fierro, M.T., Novarino, A., Foa, R., and Saglio, G., Rearrangement of the c-*myc* oncogene with heavy-chain immunoglobulin enhancer in tumor DNA from an acute lymphoblastic leukemia patient, *J. Natl. Cancer Inst.*, 78, 845, 1987.

792. Nishikura, K., Erikson, J., ar-Rushdi, A., Huebner, K., and Croce, C.M., The translocated c-*myc* oncogene of Raji Burkitt lymphoma cells is not expressed in human lymphoblastoid cells, *Proc. Natl. Acad. Sci., U.S.A.*, 82, 2900, 1985.

793. Sun, L.K., Showe, L.C., and Croce, C.M., Analysis of the 3′ flanking region of the human c-myc gene in lymphomas with the t(98;22) and t(2;8) translocation, *Nucleic Acids Res.,* 14, 4037, 1986.

794. Showe, L.C., Moore, R.C.A., Erikson, J., and Croce, C.M., *MYC* oncogene involved in a t(8;22) chromosome translocation is not altered in its putative regulatory regions, *Proc. Natl. Acad. Sci. U.S.A.,* 84, 2824, 1987.

795. Prehn, J., Mercola, M., and Calame, K., Translocation affects normal c-*myc* promoter usage and activates fifteen cryptic c-*myc* transcription starts in plasmacytoma M603, *Nucleic Acids Res.,* 12, 8987, 1984.

796. Yang, J., Bauer, S.R., Mushinski, J.F., and Marcu, K.B., Chromosome translocations clustered 5′ of the murine c-*myc* gene qualitatively affect promoter usage: implications for the site of normal c-*myc* regulation, *EMBO J.,* 4, 1441, 1985.

797. Calabi, F. and Neuberger, M.S., Chromosome translocation activates heterogeneously initiated, bipolar transcription of a mouse c-*myc* gene, *EMBO J.,* 4, 667, 1985.

798. Webb, E., Adams, J.M., and Cory, S., Variant (6;15) translocation in a murine plasmacytoma occurs near an immunoglobulin kappa gene but far from the *myc* oncogene, *Nature,* 312, 777, 1984.

799. ar-Rushdi, A., Nishikura, K., Erikson, J., Watt, R., Rovera, G., and Croce, C.M., Differential expression of the translocated and the untranslocated c-*myc* oncogene in Burkitt lymphoma, *Science,* 222, 390, 1983.

800. Croce, C.M., Thierfelder, W., Erikson, J., Nishikura, K., Finan, J., Lenoir, G.M., and Nowell, P.C., Transcriptional activation of an unrearranged and untranslocated c-*myc* oncogene by translocation of a C_{lambda} locus in Burkitt lymphoma cells, *Proc. Natl. Acad. Sci. U.S.A.,* 80, 6922, 1983.

801. Kondoh, N., Oikawa, T., Chiba, I., Ogiso, Y., Mizuno, S., and Kuzumaki, N., Unresponsiveness of both non-rearranged and rearranged c-*myc* to serum stimulation in a mouse plasmacytoma S194, *Leukemia Res.,* 11, 1149, 1987.

802. Feo, S., ar-Rushdi, A., Huebner, K., Finan, J., Nowell, P.C., Clarkson, B., and Croce, C.M., Suppression of the normal mouse c-*myc* oncogene in human lymphoma cells, *Nature,* 313, 493, 1985.

803. Croce, C.M., Erikson, J., Huebner, K., and Nishikura, K., Coexpression of translocated and normal c-*myc* oncogenes in hybrids between Daudi and lymphoblastoid cells, *Science,* 227, 1235, 1985.

804. Rabbitts, T.H., Forster, A., Baer, R., and Hamlyn, P.H., Transcriptional enhancer identified near the human C_{mu} immunoglobulin heavy chain gene is unavailable to the translocated c-*myc* gene in a Burkitt lymphoma, *Nature,* 306, 806, 1983.

805. Hayday, A.C., Gillies, S.D., Saito, H., Wood, C., Wiman, K., Hayward, W.S., and Tonegawa, S., Activation of a translocated human c-*myc* gene by an enhancer in the immunoglobulin heavy-chain locus, *Nature,* 307, 334, 1984.

806. Corcoran, L.M., Cory, S., and Adams, J.M., Transposition of the immunoglobulin heavy chain enhancer to the *myc* oncogene in a murine plasmacytoma, *Cell,* 40, 71, 1985.

807. Kakkis, E., Mercola, M., and Calame, K., Strong transcriptional activation of translocated c-myc genes occurs without a strong nearby enhancer or promoter, *Nucleic Acids Res.,* 16, 77, 1988.

808. Julius, M.A., Street, A.J., Fahrlander, P.D., Yang, J.-Q., Eisenman, R.N., and Marcu, K.B., Translocated c-*myc* genes produce chimeric transcripts containing antisense sequences of the immunoglobulin heavy chain locus in mouse plasmacytomas, *Oncogene,* 2, 469, 1988.

809. Dunnick, W., Shell, B.E., and Dery, C., DNA sequences near the site of reciprocal recombination between a c-*myc* oncogene and an immunoglobulin switch region, *Proc. Natl. Acad. Sci. U.S.A.,* 80, 7269, 1983.

810. Stanton, L.W., Yang, J., Eckhardt, L.A., Harris, L.J., Birshtein, B.K., and Marcu, K.B., Products of a reciprocal chromosome translocation involving the c-*myc* gene in a murine plasmacytoma, *Proc. Natl. Acad. Sci. U.S.A.,* 81, 829, 1984.

811. Showe, L.C., Ballantine, M., Nishikura, K., Erikson, J., Kaji, H., and Croce, C.M., Cloning and sequencing of a c-*myc* oncogene in a Burkitt's lymphoma cell line that is translocated to a germ line alpha switch region, *Mol. Cell. Biol.,* 5, 501, 1985.

812. Nilsen, T.W. and Maroney, P.A., Translational efficiency of c-Myc mRNA in Burkitt lymphoma cells, *Mol. Cell. Biol.,* 4, 2235, 1984.

813. Polack, A., Eick, D., Koch, E., and Bornkamm, G.W., Truncation does not abrogate transcriptional downregulation of the c-*myc* gene by sodium butyrate in Burkitt's lymphoma cells, *EMBO J.,* 6, 2959, 1987.

814. Piechaczyk, M., Yang, J.-Q., Blanchard, J.-M., Jeanteur, P., and Marcu, K.B., Posttranscriptional mechanisms are responsible for accumulation of truncated c-*myc* RNAs in murine plasma cell tumors, *Cell,* 42, 589, 1985.

815. Darveau, A., Pelletier, J., and Sonenberg, N., Differential efficiencies of *in vitro* translation of mouse c-*myc* transcripts differing in the 5′ untranslated region, *Proc. Natl. Acad. Sci. U.S.A.,* 82, 2315, 1985.

816. Butnick, N.Z., Miyamoto, C., Chizzonite, R., Cullen, B.R., Ju, G., and Skalka, A.M., Regulation of the human c-*myc* gene: 5′ noncoding sequences do not affect translation, *Mol. Cell. Biol.,* 5, 3009, 1985.

817. Stanton, L.W., Watt, R., and Marcu, K.B., Translocation, breakage and truncated transcripts of c-*myc* oncogene in murine plasmacytomas, *Nature,* 303, 401, 1983.

818. Battey, J., Moulding, C., Taub, R., Murphy, W., Stewart, T., Potter, H., Lenoir, G., and Leder, P., The human c-*myc* oncogene: structural consequences of translocation into the IgH locus in Burkitt lymphoma, *Cell,* 34, 779, 1983.

819. Stanton, L.W., Fahrlander, P.D., Tesser, P.M., and Marcu, K.B., Nucleotide sequence comparison of normal and translocated murine c-*myc* genes, *Nature,* 310, 423, 1984.

820. Haluska, F.G., Tsujimoto, Y., and Croce, C.M., The t(8;14) breakpoint of the EW 36 undifferentiated lymphoma cell line lies 5′ of MYC in a region prone to involvement in endemic Burkitt's lymphomas, *Nucleic Acids Res.,* 16, 2077, 1988.

821. Zhou, R.-P. and Duesberg, P.H., *myc* protooncogene linked to retroviral promoter, but not to enhancer, transforms embryo cells, *Proc. Natl. Acad. Sci. U.S.A.,* 85, 2924, 1988.

822. Rabbitts, P.H., Forster, A., Stinson, M.A., and Rabbitts, T.H., Truncation of exon 1 from the c-*myc* gene results in prolonged c-*myc* mRNA stability, *EMBO J.,* 4, 3727, 1985.

823. Pachl, C., Schubach, W., Eisenman, R., and Linial, M., Expression of c-*myc* RNA in bursal lymphoma cell lines: identification of c-*myc*-encoded proteins by hybrid-selected translation, *Cell,* 33, 335, 1983.

824. Benjamin, D., Magrath, I.T., Triche, T.J., Schroff, R.W., Jensen, J.P., and Korsmeyer, S.J., Induction of plasmacytoid differentiation by phorbol ester in B-cell lymphoma cell lines bearing 8;14 translocations, *Proc. Natl. Acad. Sci. U.S.A.,* 81, 3547, 1984.

825. Glazer, P.M. and Summers, W.C., Oncogene expression in isogenic, EBV-positive and -negative Burkitt lymphoma cell lines, *Intervirology,* 23, 82, 1985.

826. Mathieu-Mahul, D., Bernheim, A., Berger, R., Mauchauffé, M., Flandrin, G., and Larsen, C.J., Remaniement du proto-oncogène c-myc dans les cellules fraiches d'une leucémie de Burkitt (L3), Nouv. Rev. Fr. Hematol., 27, 157, 1985.

827. Jack, A.S., Gardner, S.J., Mills, K.L., Goyns, M.H., Lee, F.D., and Birnie, G.D., Genomic rearrangements of the c-myc proto-oncogene in human malignant lymphomas, *J. Pathol.,* 149, 25, 1986.

828. Cleary, M.L., Epstein, M.A., Finerty, S., Dorfman, R.F., Bornkamm, G.W., Kirkwood, J.K., Morgan, A.J., and Sklar, J., Individual tumors of multifocal EB virus-induced malignant lymphomas in tamarins arise from different B-cell clones, *Science,* 228, 722, 1985.

829. Perl, A., Wang, N., Williams, J.M., Hunt, M.J., Rosenfeld, S.I., Condemi, J.J., Packman, C.H., and Abraham, G.N., Aberrant immunoglobulin and c-*myc* gene rearrangements in patients with nonmalignant monoclonal cryoglobulinemia, *J. Immunol.,* 139, 3512, 1987.

830. Adams, J.M., Harris, A.W., Pinkert, C.A., Corcoran, L.M., Alexander, W.S., Cory, S., Palmiter, R.D., and Brinster, R.L., The c-*myc* oncogene driven by immunoglobulin enhancers induces lymphoid malignancy in transgenic mice, *Nature,* 318, 533, 1985.

831. Vaux, D.L., Adams, J.M., Alexander, W.S., and Pike, B.L., Immunologic competence of B cells subjected to constitutive c-*myc* oncogene expression in immunoglobulin heavy chain enhancer *myc* transgenic mice, *J. Immunol.,* 139, 3854, 1987.

832. Langdon, W.Y., Harris, A.W., Cory, S., and Adams, J.M., The c-*myc* oncogene perturbs B lymphocyte development in E$_{mu}$-*myc* transgenic mice, *Cell,* 47, 11, 1986.

833. Alexander, W.S., Schrader, J.W., and Adams, J.M., Expression of the c-*myc* oncogene under control of an immunoglobulin enhancer in E$_{mu}$-*myc* transgenic mice, *Mol. Cell. Biol.,* 7, 1436, 1987.

834. Lee, M.-S., Blick, M.B., Pathak, S., Trujillo, J.M., Butler, J.J., Katz, R.L., McLaughlin, P., Hagemeister, F.B., Velasquez, W.S., Goodacre, A., Cork, A., Gutterman, J.U., and Cabanillas, F., The gene located at chromosome 18 band q21 is rearranged in uncultured diffuse lymphomas as well as follicular lymphomas, *Blood,* 70, 90, 1987.

835. Diaz, M.O., Le Beau, M.M., Rowley, J.D., Drabkin, H.A., and Patterson, D., The role of the c-*mos* gene in the 8;21 translocation in human acute myeloblastic leukemia, *Science,* 229, 767, 1985.

836. Revoltella, R.P., Park, M., and Fruscalzo, A., Identification in several human myeloid leukemias or cell lines of a DNA rearrangement next to the c-*mos* 3′-end, *FEBS Lett.,* 189, 97, 1985.

837. Watson, D.K., Sacchi, N., McWilliams-Smith, M.J., O'Brien, S.J., and Papas, T.S., The avian and mammalian *ets* genes: molecular characterization, chromosome mapping, and implication in human leukemia, *Anticancer Res.,* 6, 631, 1986.

838. Le Beau, M.M., Rowley, J.D., Sacchi, N., Watson, D.K., Papas, T.S., and Diaz, M.O., Hu-*ets*-2 is translocated to chromosome 8 in the t(8;21) in acute myelogenous leukemia, *Cancer Genet. Cytogenet.,* 23, 269, 1986.

839. Mise, K., Abe, S., Sato, Y., Miura, Y., and Sasaki, M., Localization of c-Ha-*ras*-1 oncogene in the t(7p–;11p+) abnormality of two cases with myeloid leukemia, *Cancer Genet. Cytogenet.,* 29, 191, 1987.

840. Mitelman, F., Manolov, G., Manolova, Y., Billström, R., Heim, S., Kristoffersson, U., Mandahl, N., Ferro, M.T., and San Roman, C., High resolution chromosome analysis of constitutional and acquired t(15;17) maps c-*erbA* to subband 17q11.2, *Cancer Genet. Cytogenet.,* 22, 95, 1986.

841. Dayton, A.I., Selden, J.R., Laws, G., Dorney, D.J., Finan, J., Tripputi, P., Emanuel, B.S., Rovera, G., Nowell, P.C., and Croce, C.M., A human c-*erbA* oncogene homologue is closely proximal to the chromosome 17 breakpoint in acute promyelocytic leukemia, *Proc. Natl. Acad. Sci. U.S.A.,* 81, 4495, 1984.

842. Le Beau, M.M., Westbrook, C.A., Diaz, M.O., Rowley, J.D., and Oren, M., Translocation of the p53 gene in t(15;17) in acute promyelocytic leukaemia, *Nature,* 316, 826, 1985.

843. Kaneko, Y., Homma, C., Maseki, N., Sakurai, M., Toyoshima, K., and Yamamoto, T., Human c-*erb*B-2 remains on chromosome 17 in band q21 in the 15;17 translocation associated with acute promyelocytic leukemia, *Jpn. J. Cancer Res.,* 78, 16, 1987.

844. Isobe, M., Emanuel, B.S., Givol, D., Oren, M., and Croce, C.M., Localization of gene for human p53 tumour antigen to band 17p13, *Nature,* 320, 84, 1986.

845. Simmers, R.N., Webber, L.M., Shannon, M.F., Garson, O.M., Wong, G., Vadas, M.A., and Sutherland, G.R., Localization of the G-CSF gene on chromosome 17 proximal to the breakpoint in the t(15;17) in acute promyelocytic leukemia, *Blood,* 70, 330, 1987.

846. Nagarajan, L., Louie, E., Tsujimoto, Y., ar-Rushdi, A., Huebner, K., and Croce, C.M., Localization of the human *pim* oncogene (*PIM*) to a region of chromosome 6 involved in translocations in acute leukemias, *Proc. Natl. Acad. Sci. U.S.A.,* 83, 2556, 1986.

847. Okabe, M., Matsushima, S., Morioka, M., Kobayashi, M., Abe, S., Sakurada, K., Kakinuma, M., and Miyazaki, T., Establishment and characterization of a cell line, TOM-1, derived from a patient with Philadelphia chromosome-positive acute lymphocytic leukemia, *Blood,* 69, 990, 1987.

848. Sacchi, N., Watson, D.K., Guerts van Kessel, A.H.M., Hagemeijer, A., Kersey, J., Drabkin, H.D., Patterson, D., and Papas, T.S., Hu-*ets*-1 and Hu-*ets*-2 genes are transposed in acute leukemias with (4;11) and (8;21) translocations, *Science,* 231, 379, 1986.

849. Diaz, M.O., Le Beau, M.M., Pitha, P., and Rowley, J.D., Interferon and c-*ets*-1 genes in the translocation (9;11)(p22;q23) in human acute monocytic leukemia, *Science,* 231, 265, 1986.

850. Luster, A.D., Jhanwar, S.C., Chaganti, R.S.K., Kersey, J.H., and Ravetch, J.V., Interferon-inducible gene maps to a chromosomal band associated with a (4;11) translocation in acute leukemia cells, *Proc. Natl. Acad. Sci. U.S.A.,* 84, 2868, 1987.

851. Le Beau, M.M., Diaz, M.O., and Rowley, J.D., Metallothionein gene cluster is split by chromosome 16 rearrangements in myelomonocytic leukaemia, *Nature,* 313, 709, 1985.

852. Simmers, R.N., Sutherland, G.R., West, A., and Richards, R.I., Fragile sites at 16q22 are not at the breakpoint of the chromosomal rearrangement in AmMoL, *Science,* 236, 92, 1987.

853. Larson, R.A., Kondo, K., Vardiman, J.W., Butler, A.E., Golomb, H.M., and Rowley, J.D., Evidence for a 15;17 translocation in every patient with acute promyelocytic leukemia, *Am. J. Med.,* 76, 827, 1984.

854. Kanda, N., Fukushige, S., Murotsu, T., Yoshida, M.C., Tsuchiya, M., Asano, S., Kaziro, Y., and Nagata, S., Human gene coding for granulocyte-colony stimulating factor is assigned to the q21-q22 region of chromosome 17, *Somat. Cell Mol. Genet.,* 13, 679, 1987.

855. Le Beau, M.M., Lemons, R.L., Carrino, J.J., Pettenati, M.J., Souza, L.M., Diaz, M.O., and Rowley, J.D., Chromosomal localization of the human *G-CSF* gene to 17q11 proximal to the breakpoint of the t(15:17) in acute promyelocytic leukemia, *Leukemia,* 1, 795, 1987.

856. van Tuinen, P., Johnson, K.R., Ledbetter, S.A., Nussbaum, R.L., Rovera, G., and Ledbetter, D.H., Localization of myeloperoxidase to the long arm of human chromosome 17: relationship to the 15;17 translocation of acute promyelocytic leukemia, *Oncogene,* 1, 319, 1987.

857. Weil, S.C., Rosner, G.L., Reid, M.S., Chisholm, R.L., Lemons, R.S., Swanson, M.S., Carrino, J.J., Diaz, M.O., and Le Beau, M.M., Translocation and rearrangement of myeloperoxidase gene in acute promyelocytic leukemia, *Science,* 240, 790, 1988.

858. Look, A.T., The emerging genetics of acute lymphoblastic leukemia: clinical and biologic implications, *Semin. Oncol.,* 12, 92, 1985.

859. Williams, D.L., Harber, J., Murphy, S.B., Look, A.T., Kalwinsky, D.K., Rivera, G., Melvin, S.L., and Dahl, G.V., Chromosomal translocations play a unique role in influencing prognosis in childhood acute lymphoblastic leukemia, *Blood,* 68, 205, 1986.

860. Bloomfield, C.D., Brunning, R.D., Smith, K.A., and Nesbit, M.E., Prognostic significance of the Philadelphia chromosome in acute lymphocytic leukemia, *Cancer Genet. Cytogenet.,* 1, 229, 1980.

861. Dreazen, O., Klisak, I., Jones, G., Ho, W.G., Sparkes, R.S., and Peter, R., Multiple molecular abnormalities in Ph¹ chromosome positive acute lymphoblastic leukaemia, *Br. J. Haematol.,* 67, 319, 1987.

862. Erikson, J., Griffin, C.A., ar-Rushdi, A., Valtieri, M., Hoxie, J., Finan, J., Emanuel, B.S., Rovera, G., Nowell, P.C., and Croce, C.M., Heterogeneity of chromosome 22 breakpoint in Philadelphia-positive (PH⁺) acute lymphocytic leukemia, *Proc. Natl. Acad. Sci. U.S.A.,* 83, 1807, 1986.

863. De Klein, A., Hagemeijer, A., Bartram, C.R., Houwen, R., Hoefsloot, L., Carbonell, F., Chan, L., Barnett, M., Greaves, M., Kleihauer, E., Heisterkamp, N., Groffen, J., and Grosveld, G., *bcr* rearrangement and translocation of the c-*abl* oncogene in Philadelphia positive acute lymphoblastic leukemia, *Blood,* 68, 1369, 1986.

864. Kurzrock, R., Shtalrid, M., Gutterman, J.U., Koller, C.A., Walters, R., Trujillo, J.M., and Talpaz, M., Molecular analysis of chromosome 22 breakpoints in adult Philadelphia-positive acute lymphoblastic leukaemia, *Br. J. Haematol.,* 65, 55, 1987.

865. Hirsch-Ginsberg, C., Childs, C., Chang, K.-S., Beran, M., Cork, A., Reuben, J., Freireich, E.J., Chang, L.C.M., Bollum, F.J., Trujillo, J., and Stass, S.A., Phenotypic and molecular heterogeneity in Philadelphia chromosome-positive acute leukemia, *Blood,* 71, 186, 1988.

866. Clark, S.S., McLaughlin, J., Crist, W.M., Champlin, R., and Witte, O.N., Unique forms of the *abl* tyrosine kinase distinguish Ph¹-positive CML from Ph¹-positive ALL, *Science,* 235, 85, 1987.

867. Kurzrock, R., Shtalrid, M., Romero, P., Kloetzer, W.S., Talpas, M., Trujillo, J.M., Blick, M., Beran, M., and Gutterman, J.U., A novel c-*abl* protein in Philadelphia-positive acute lymphoblastic leukaemia, *Nature,* 325, 631, 1987.

868. Chan, L.C., Karhi, K.K., Rayter, S.I., Heisterkamp, N., Eridan, S., Powles, R., Lawler, S.D., Groffen, J., Foulkes, J.G., Greaves, M.F., and Wiedemann, L.M., A novel *abl* protein expressed in Philadelphia chromosome positive acute lymphoblastic leukaemia, *Nature,* 325, 635, 1987.

869. Walker, L.C., Ganesan, T.S., Dhut, S., Gibbons, B., Lister, T.A., Rothbard, J., and Young, B.D., Novel chimaeric protein expressed in Philadelphia positive acute lymphoblastic leukaemia, *Nature,* 329, 851, 1987.

870. Eridani, S., Gorman, P., Sheer, D., Duncombe, A.S., Glass, U.H., and Shivji, M.K.K., Monosomy 7 and Ph-positive acute lymphoblastic leukaemia: cytogenetic and molecular aspects, *Leukaemia Res.,* 11, 965, 1987.

871. Rubin, C.M., Carrino, J.J., Dickler, M.N., Leibowitz, D., Smith, S.D., and Westbrook, C.A., Heterogeneity of genomic fusion of *BCR* and *ABL* in Philadelphia chromosome-positive acute lymphoblastic leukemia, *Proc. Natl. Acad. Sci. U.S.A.,* 85, 2795, 1988.

872. ar-Rushdi, A., Negrini, M., Kurzrock, R., Huebner, K., and Croce, C.M., Fusion of the *bcr* and the c-*abl* genes in Ph'-positive acute lymphoblastic leukemia with no rearrangement in the breakpoint cluster region, *Oncogene,* 2, 353, 1988.

873. Naumovski, L., Morgan, R., Hecht, F., Link, M.P., Glader, B.E., and Smith, S.D., Philadelphia chromosome-positive acute lymphoblastic leukemia cell lines without classical breakpoint cluster region rearrangement, *Cancer Res.,* 48, 2876, 1988.

874. Williams, D.L., Look, A.T., Melvin, S.L., Roberson, P.K., Dahl, G., Flake, T., and Stass, S., New chromosomal translocations correlate with specific immunophenotypes of childhood acute lymphoblastic leukemia, *Cell,* 36, 101, 1984.

875. Peschle, C., Mavilio, F., Sposi, N.M., Giampaolo, A., Care, A., Bottero, L., Bruno, M., Mastroberardino, G., Gastaldi, R., Testa, M.G., Alimena, G., Amadori, S., and Mandelli, F., Translocation and rearrangement of c-*myc* into immunoglobulin alpha heavy chain locus in primary cells from acute lymphocytic leukemia, *Proc. Natl. Acad. Sci. U.S.A.,* 81, 5514, 1984.

876. Savage, P.D., Hanson, C.A., and Kersey, J.H., Identification of a restriction fragment length polymorphism involving the oncogene ETS-1 on chromosome 11q23, *Blood,* 70, 327, 1987.

877. Goyns, M.H., Hann, I.M., Stewart, J., Gegonne, A., and Birnie, G.D., The c-*ets*-1 proto-oncogene is rearranged in some cases of acute lymphoblastic leukaemia, *Br. J. Cancer,* 56, 611, 1987.

878. Denny, C.T., Hollis, G.F., Hecht, F., Morgan, R., Link, M.P., Smith, S.D., and Kirsch, I.R., Common mechanism of chromosome inversion in B- and T-cell tumors: relevance to lymphoid development, *Science,* 234, 197, 1986.

879. Bloomfield, C.D. and de la Chapelle, A., Chromosome abnormalities in acute nonlymphocytic leukemia: clinical and biologic significance, *Semin. Oncol.,* 14, 372, 1987.

880. Westbrook, C.A., Le Beau, M.M., Diaz, M.O., Groffen, J., and Rowley, J.D., Chromosomal localization and characterization of c-*abl* in the t(6;9) of acute nonlymphocytic leukemia, *Proc. Natl. Acad. Sci. U.S.A.,* 82, 8742, 1985.

881. Drabkin, H.A., Diaz, M., Bradley, C.M., Le Beau, M.M., Rowley, J.D., and Patterson, D., Isolation and analysis of the 21q+ chromosome in the acute myelogenous leukemia 8;21 translocation: evidence that c-*mos* is not translocated, *Proc. Natl. Acad. Sci. U.S.A.,* 82, 464, 1985.

882. Rosendorff, J., Bowcock, A.M., Kuyl, J.M., Mendelow, B., Pinto, M.R., and Bernstein, R., Localization of the human c-*mos* gene by *in situ* hybridization in two cases of acute nonlymphocytic leukemia type M2, *Cancer Genet. Cytogenet.,* 24, 137, 1987.

883. Chevenix-Trench, G., Behm, F.G., and Westin, E.H., Somatic rearrangement of the c-*myc* oncogene in primary human diffuse large-cell lymphoma, *Int. J. Cancer,* 38, 513, 1986.

884. Aisenberg, A.C., Wilkes, B.M., and Jacobson, J.O., The *bcl*-2 gene is rearranged in many diffuse B-cell lymphomas, *Blood,* 71, 969, 1988.

885. Weiss, L.M., Warnke, R.A., Sklar, J., and Cleary, M.L., Molecular analysis of the t(14;18) chromosomal translocation in malignant lymphomas, *N. Engl. J. Med.,* 317, 1185, 1987.

886. Tsujimoto, Y., Finger, L.R., Yunis, J., Nowell, P.C., and Croce, C.M., Cloning of the chromosome breakpoint of neoplastic B cells with the t(14;18) chromosome translocation, *Science,* 226, 1097, 1984.

887. Yunis, J.J., Frizzera, G., Oken, M.M., McKenna, J., Theologides, A., and Arnesen, M., Multiple recurrent genomic defects in follicular lymphoma: a possible model for cancer, *N. Engl. J. Med.,* 316, 79, 1987.

888. Lee, M.-S., Chang, K.-S., Cabanillas, F., Freireich, E.J., Trujillo, J.M., and Stass, S.A., Detection of minimal residual cells carrying the t(14;18) by DNA sequence amplification, *Science,* 237, 175, 1987.

889. Tsujimoto, Y., Cossman, J., Jaffe, E., and Croce, C.M., Involvement of the *bcl*-2 gene in human follicular lymphoma, *Science,* 228, 1440, 1985.

890. Seto, M., Jaeger, U., Hockett, R.D., Graninger, W., Bennet, S., Goldman, P., and Korsmeyer, S.J., Alternative promoters and exons, somatic mutation and deregulation of the *Bcl*-2-*Ig* fusion gene in lymphoma, *EMBO J.,* 7, 123, 1988.

891. Tsujimoto, Y., Bashir, M.M., Givol, I., Cossman, J., Jaffe, E., and Croce, C.M., DNA rearrangements in human follicular lymphoma can involve the 5′ of the 3′ region of the *bcl-2* gene, *Proc. Natl. Acad. Sci. U.S.A.,* 84, 1329, 1987.

892. Ohno, H., Fukuhara, S., Takahashi, R., Mihara, K., Sugiyama, T., Doi, S., Uchino, H., and Toyoshima, K., *c-yes* and *c-bcl-2* genes located on 18q21.3 in a follicular lymphoma cell line carrying a t(14;18) chromosomal translocation, *Int. J. Cancer,* 39, 785, 1987.

893. Cleary, M.L., Smith, S.D., and Sklar, J., Cloning and structural analysis of cDNAs for *bcl-2* and a hybrid *bcl-2*/immunoglobulin transcript resulting from the t(14;18) translocation, *Cell,* 47, 19, 1986.

894. Gurfinkel, N., Unger, T., Givol, D., and Mushinski, J.F., Expression of the *bcl-2* gene in mouse B lymphocytic cell lines is differentiation stage specific, *Eur. J. Immunol.,* 17, 567, 1987.

895. Raffeld, M., Wright, J.J., Lipford, E., Cossman, J., Longo, D.L., Bakhshi, A., and Korsmeyer, S.J., Clonal evolution of t(14;18) follicular lymphomas demonstrated by immunoglobulin genes and the 18q21 major breakpoint region, *Cancer Res.,* 47, 2537, 1987.

896. Minden, M.D., Toyonaga, B., Ha, K., Yanagi, Y., Chin, B., Gelfand, E., and Mak, T., Somatic rearrangement of T-cell antigen receptor gene in human T-cell malignancies, *Proc. Natl. Acad. Sci. U.S.A.,* 82, 1224, 1985.

897. Rabbitts, T.H., Lefranc, M.P., Stinson, M.A., Sims, J.E., Schroder, J., Steinmetz, M., Spurr, N.L., Solomon, E., and Goodfellow, P.N., The chromosomal location of T-cell receptor genes and a T cell rearranging gene: possible correlation with specific translocations in human T cell leukaemia, *EMBO J.,* 4, 1461, 1985.

898. Waldmann, T.A., Davis, M.M., Bongiovanni, K.F., and Korsmeyer, S.J., Rearrangements of genes for the antigen receptor on T cells as markers of lineage and clonality in human lymphoid neoplasms, *N. Engl. J. Med.,* 313, 776, 1985.

899. Cossman, J., Uppenkamp, M., Sundeen, J., Coupland, R., and Raffeld, M., Molecular genetics and the diagnosis of lymphoma, *Arch. Pathol. Lab. Med.,* 112, 117, 1988.

900. Hood, L., Kronenberg, M., and Hunkapiller, T., T cell antigen receptors and the immunoglobulin supergene family, *Cell,* 40, 225, 1985.

901. Murre, C., Waldmann, R.A., Morton, C.C., Bongiovanni, K.F., Waldmann, T.A., Shows, T.B., and Seidman, J.G., Human gamma-chain genes are rearranged in leukamic T cells and map to the short arm of chromosome 7, *Nature,* 316, 549, 1985.

902. Finger, L.R., Harvey, R.C., Moore, R.C.A., Showe, L.C., and Croce, C.M., A common mechanism of chromosomal translocation in T- and B-cell neoplasia, *Science,* 234, 982, 1986.

903. Foroni, L., Foldi, J., Matutes, E., Catovsky, D., O'Connor, N.J., Baer, R., Forster, A., Rabbitts, T.H., and Luzzatto, L., α, β, and γ T-cell receptor genes: rearrangements correlate with haematological phenotype in T cell leukemias, *Br. J. Haematol.,* 67, 307, 1987.

904. Mathieu-Mahul, D., Sigaux, F., Zhu, C., Bernheim, A., Mauchauffé, M., Daniel, M.-T., Berger, R., and Larsen, C.-J., A t(8;14)(q24;q11) translocation in a T-cell leukemia (L1-ALL) with c-*myc* and TcR-alpha chain locus rearrangements, *Int. J. Cancer,* 38, 835, 1986.

905. Shima, E.A., Le Beau, M.M., McKeithan, T.W., Minowada, J., Showe, L.C., Mak, T.W., Minden, M.D., Rowley, J.D., and Diaz, M.O., Gene encoding the alpha chain of the T-cell receptor is moved immediately downstream of c-*myc* in a chromosomal 8;14 translocation in a cell line from a human T-cell leukemia, *Proc. Natl. Acad. Sci. U.S.A.,* 83, 3439, 1986.

906. Erikson, J., Finger, L., Sun, L., ar-Rushdi, A., Nishikura, K., Minowada, J., Finan, J., Emanuel, B.S., Nowell, P.C., and Croce, C.M., Deregulation of c-*myc* by translocation of the alpha-locus of the T-cell receptor in T-cell leukemias, *Science,* 232, 884, 1986.

907. McKeithan, T.W., Shima, E.A., Le Beau, M.M., Minowada, J., Rowley, J.D., and Diaz, M.O., Molecular cloning of the breakpoint junction of a human chromosomal 8;14 translocation involving the T-cell receptor alpha-chain gene and sequences on the 3′ side of *MYC*, *Proc. Natl. Acad. Sci. U.S.A.,* 83, 6636, 1986.

908. Saglio, G., Emanuel, B.S., Guerrasio, A., Giubellino, M.C., Serra, A., Lusso, P., Cambrin, G.R., Mazza, U., Malavasi, F., Pegoraro, L., and Foa, R., 3′ c-*myc* rearrangement in a human leukemic T-cell line, *Cancer Res.,* 46, 1413, 1986.

909. Raimondi, S.C., Pui, C.-H., Behm, F.G., and Williams, D.L., 7q32-q36 translocation in childhood T cell leukemia: cytogenetic evidence for involvement of the T cell receptor beta-chain gene, *Blood,* 69, 131, 1987.

910. Russo, G., Isobe, M., Pegararo, L., Finan, J., Nowell, P.C., and Croce, C.M., Molecular analysis of a t(7;14)(q35;q32) translocation in a T cell leukemia of a patient with ataxia telangiectasia, *Cell,* 53, 137, 1988.

911. Ino, T., Kurosawa, Y., Yoshida, M.C., and Hirano, M., DNA segment containing $C_{beta 1}$, a gene for the constant region of the beta chain of the T-cell antigen receptor, Iwas inserted into chromosome 6 in cells from one patient with human T-cell leukemia, *Proc. Natl. Acad. Sci. U.S.A.,* 84, 4264, 1987.

912. Le Beau, M.M., McKeithan, T.W., Shima, E.A., Goldman-Leikin, R.E., Chan, S.J., Bell, G.I., Rowley, J.D., and Diaz, M.O., T-cell receptor alpha-chain gene is split in a human T-cell leukemia cell line with a t(11;14)(p15;q11), *Proc. Natl. Acad. Sci. U.S.A.,* 83, 9744, 1986.

913. Gahrton, G. and-Robert, K.-H., Chromosomal aberrations in chronic B-cell lymphocytic leukemia, *Cancer Genet. Cytogenet.,* 6, 171, 1982.

914. Gahrton, G., Juliusson, G., Robèrt, K.H., and Zech, L., Specific chromosomal markers in B- and T-cell chronic lymphocytic leukemia, *Tumour Biol.,* 6, 1, 1985.

915. Butturini, A. and Gale, R.P., Oncogenesis in chronic lymphocytic leukemia, *Leukemia Res.,* 12, 89, 1988.

916. Gale, R.P. and Foon, K.A., Chronic lymphocytic leukemia: recent advances in biology and treatment, *Ann. Int. Med.,* 103, 101, 1985.

917. Knuutila, S., Elonen, E., Teerenhovi, L., Rossi, L., Leskinen, R., Bloomfield, C.D., and de la Chapelle, A., Trisomy 12 in B cells of patients with B-cell chronic lymphocytic leukemia, *N. Engl. J. Med.,* 314, 865, 1986.

918. Fell, H.P., Smith, R.G., and Tucker, P.W., Molecular analysis of the t(2;14) translocation of childhood chronic lymphocytic leukemia, *Science,* 232, 491, 1986.

919. McKeithan, T.W., Rowley, J.D., Shows, T.B., and Diaz, M.O., Cloning of the chromosome translocation breakpoint junction of the t(14;19) in chronic lymphocytic leukemia, *Proc. Natl. Acad. Sci. U.S.A.,* 84, 9257, 1987.

920. Tsujimoto, Y., Yunis, J., Onorato-Showe, L., Erikson, J., Nowell, P.C., and Croce, C.M., Molecular cloning of the chromosomal breakpoint of B-cell lymphomas and leukemias with the t(11;14) chromosome translocation, *Science,* 224, 1403, 1984.

921. Erikson, J., Finan, J., Tsujimoto, Y., Nowell, P.C., and Croce, C.M., The chromosome 14 breakpoint in neoplastic B cells with the t(11;14) translocation involves the immunoglobulin heavy chain locus, *Proc. Natl. Acad. Sci. U.S.A.,* 81, 4144, 1984.

922. Tsujimoto, Y., Jaffe, E., Cossman, J., Gorham, J., Nowell, P.C., and Croce, C.M., Clustering of breakpoints on chromosome 11 in human B-cell neoplasms with the t(11;14) translocation, *Nature,* 315, 340, 1985.

923. Gattoni-Celli, S., Hsiao, W.-L., and Weinstein, I.B., Rearranged c-*mos* locus in a MOPC 21 murine myeloma cell line and its persistence in hybridomas, *Nature,* 306, 795, 1983.

924. Hollis, G.F., Gazdar, A.F., Bertness, V., and Kirsch, I.R., Complex translocation disrupts c-*myc* regulation in a human plasma cell myeloma, *Mol. Cell. Biol.,* 8, 124, 1988.

925. Diaz, M.O., Le Beau, M.M., Harden, A., and Rowley, J.D., Trisomy 8 in human hematologic neoplasia and the c-*myc* and c-*mos* oncogenes, *Leukemia Res.,* 9, 1437, 1985.

926. Atkin, N.B., Lack of reciprocal translocations in carcinomas, *Cancer Genet. Cytogenet.,* 21, 275, 1986.

927. Drabkin, H.A., Bradley, C., Hart, I., Bleskan, J., Li, F.P., and Patterson, D., Translocation of c-*myc* in the hereditary renal cell carcinoma associated with a t(3;8)(p14.2;q24.13) chromosomal translocation, *Proc. Natl. Acad. Sci. U.S.A.,* 82, 6980, 1985.

928. Teyssier, J.R., Henry, I., Dozier, C., Ferre, D., Adnet, J.J., and Pluot, M., Recurrent deletion of the short arm of chromosome 3 in human renal cell carcinoma: shift of the c-*raf* 1 locus, *J. Natl. Cancer Inst.,* 77, 1187, 1986.

929. Yoshimoto, K., Shiraishi, M., Hirohashi, S., Morinaga, S., Shimosato, Y., Sugimura, T., and Sekiya, T., Rearrangement of the c-*myc* gene in two giant cell carcinomas of the lung, *Jpn. J. Cancer Res.,* 77, 731, 1986.

930. Morse, B., Rotherg, P.G., South, V.J., Spandorfer, J.M., and Astrin, S.M., Insertional mutagenesis of the *myc* locus by a LINE-1 sequence in a human breast carcinoma, *Nature,* 333, 87, 1988.

931. Linnenbach, A.J., Huebner, K., Reddy, E.P., Herlyn, M., Parmiter, A.H., Nowell, P.C., and Koprowski, H., Structural alteration in the *MYB* protooncogene and deletion within the gene encoding alpha-type protein kinase C in human melanoma cell lines, *Proc. Natl. Acad. Sci. U.S.A.,* 85, 74, 1988.

932. Aurias, A., Rimbaut, C., Buffe, D., Dubousset, J., and Mazabraud, A., Chromosomal translocation in Ewing's sarcoma, *N. Engl. J. Med.,* 309, 496, 1983.

933. Turc-Carel, C., Philip, I., Berger, M.P., and Lenoir, G.M., Chromosomal translocations in Ewing's sarcoma, *N. Engl. J. Med.,* 309, 497, 1983.

934. Whang-Peng, J., Triche, T.J., Knutsen, T., Miser, J., Douglass, E.C., and Israel, M.A., Chromosome translocation in peripheral neuroepithelioma, *N. Engl. J. Med.,* 311, 584, 1984.

935. Griffin, C.A., McKeon, C., Israel, M.A., Gegonne, A., Ghysdael, J., Stehelin, D., Douglass, E.C., Green, A.A., and Emanuel, B.S., Comparison of constitutional and tumor-associated 11;22 translocations: nonidentical breakpoints on chromosomes 11 and 22, *Proc. Natl. Acad. Sci. U.S.A.,* 83, 6122, 1986.

936. Douglass, E.C., Valentine, M., Green, A.A., Hayes, F.A., and Thompson, E.I., t(11;22) and other chromosomal rearrangements in Ewing's sarcoma, *J. Natl. Cancer Inst.,* 77, 1211, 1986.

937. Thiele, C.J., Whang-Peng, J., Kao-Shan, C.-S., Miser, J., and Israel, M., Translocation of c-*sis* protooncogene in peripheral neuroepithelioma, *Cancer Genet. Cytogenet.,* 24, 119, 1987.

938. Williams, M.E., Innes, D.J., Jr., Borowitz, M.J., Lovell, M.A., Swerdlow, S.H., Hurtubise, P.E., Brynes, R.K., Chan, W.C., Byrne, G.E., Jr., Whitcomb, C.C., and Thomas, C.Y., IV, Immunoglobulin and T cell receptor gene rearrangements in human lymphoma and leukemia, *Blood,* 69, 79, 1987.

939. Cheng, G.Y., Minden, M.D., Toyonaga, B., Mak, T.W., and McCulloch, E.A., T cell receptor and immunoglobulin gene rearrangements in acute myeloblastic leukemia, *J. Exp. Med.,* 163, 414, 1986.

940. Boehm, T.L.J., Werle, A., and Drahovsky, D., Immunoglobulin heavy chain and T-cell receptor gamma and beta chain gene rearrangements in acute myeloid leukemias, *Mol. Biol. Med.,* 4, 51, 1987.

941. Rechavi, G., Givol, D., and Canaani, E., Activation of a cellular oncogene by DNA rearrangement: possible involvement of an IS-like element, *Nature,* 300, 607, 1982.

942. Cohen, J.B., Unger, T., Rechavi, G., Canaani, E., and Givol, D., Rearrangement of the oncogene c-*mos* in mouse myeloma NSI and hybridomas, *Nature,* 306, 797, 1983.

943. Moav, B., Horowitz, M., Cohen, J.B., Rechavi, G., Eliyahu, E., Oren, M., and Givol, D., Structure and activity of the translocated c-*myc* in mouse plasmacytoma XRPC-24, *Gene,* 48, 297, 1986.

944. Mushinski, J.F., Potter, M., Bauer, S.R., and Reddy, E.P., DNA rearrangement and altered RNA expression of the c-*myb* oncogene in mouse plasmacytoid lymphosarcomas, *Science,* 220, 795, 1983.

945. Mushinski, J.F., Bauer, S.R., Potter, M., and Reddy, E.P., Increased expression of *myc*-related oncogene mRNA characterizes most BALB/c plasmacytomas induced by pristane or Abelson murine leukemia virus, *Proc. Natl. Acad. Sci. U.S.A.,* 80, 1073, 1983.

946. Takahashi, R., Mihara, K., Maeda, S., Yamaguchi, T., Chen, H.-L., Aoyama, N., Murao, S.-I., Hatanaka, M., and Sugiyama, T., Secondary activation of c-*abl* may be related to the nucleolar organizer region in an *in vitro* cultured rat leukemia cell line (K3D), *Proc. Natl. Acad. Sci. U.S.A.,* 83, 1079, 1986.

947. Tempest, P.R., Cooper, C.S., and Major, G.N., The activated human *met* gene encodes a protein tyrosine kinase, *FEBS Lett.,* 209, 357, 1986.

948. Plasterk, R.H.A. and van de Putte, P., Genetic switches by DNA inversions in prokaryotes, *Biochim. Biophys. Acta,* 782, 111, 1984.

949. Gheysen, G., Van Montagu, M., and Zambryski, P., Integration of *Agrobacterium tumefaciens* transfer DNA (T-DNA) involved rearrangements of target plant DNA sequences, *Proc. Natl. Acad. Sci. U.S.A.,* 84, 6169, 1987.

950. Neri, G., Some questions on the significance of chromosome alterations in leukemias and lymphomas: a review, *Am. J. Med. Genet.,* 18, 871, 1984.

951. Reid, M.M., Tantravahi, R., Grier, H.E., O'Toole, S., Miller, B.A., Lipton, J.M., Weinstein, H.J., and Nathan, D.G., Detection of leukemia-related karyotypes in granulocyte/macrophage colonies from a patient with acute myelomonocytic leukemia, *N. Engl. J. Med.,* 308, 1324, 1983.

952. Williams, D.L., Look, A.T., Melvin, S.L., Roberson, P.K., Dahl, G., Flake, T., and Stass, S., New chromosomal translocations correlate with specific immunophenotypes of childhood acute lymphoblastic leukemia, *Cell,* 36, 101, 1984.

953. Billström, R., Nilsson, P.-G., and Mitelman, F., Cytogenetic analysis in 941 consecutive patients with haematologic disorders, *Scand. J. Haematol.,* 37, 29, 1986.

954. Bartholdi, M.F., Ray, F.A., Cram, L.S., and Kraemer, P.M., Karyotype instability of Chinese hamster cells during *in vivo* tumor progression, *Somat. Cell Mol. Genet.,* 13, 1, 1987.

955. Sistonen, L. and Alitalo, K., Activation of c-*ras* oncogenes by mutations and amplification, *Ann. Clin. Res.,* 18, 297, 1986.

956. Kahn, S., Yamamoto, F., Almoguera, C., Winter, E., Forrester, K., Jordano, J., and Perucho, M., The c-K-*ras* gene and human cancer, *Anticancer Res.,* 7, 639, 1987.

957. Barbacid, M., *ras* genes, *Annu. Rev. Biochem.,* 56, 779, 1987.

958. Bos, J.L., The *ras* gene family and human carcinogenesis, *Mutat. Res.,* 195, 255, 1988.

959. Krontiris, T.G., DiMartino, N.A., Colb, M., and Parkinson, D.R., Unique allelic restriction fragments of the human Ha-*ras* locus in leukocyte and tumor DNAs of cancer patients, *Nature,* 313, 369, 1985.

960. Krontiris, T.G., DiMartino, N.A., Colb, M., Mitcheson, H.D., and Parkinson, D.R., Human restriction fragment length polymorphisms and cancer risk assessment, *J. Cell. Biochem.,* 30, 319, 1986.

961. Lidereau, R., Escot, C., Theillet, C., Champeme, M.-H., Brunet, M., Gest, J., and Callahan, R., High frequency of rare alleles of the human c-Ha-*ras*-1 proto-oncogene in breast cancer patients, *J. Natl. Cancer Inst.,* 77, 697, 1986.

962. Radice, P., Pierotti, M.A., Borrello, M.G., Illeni, M.T., Rovini, D., and Della Porta, G., HRAS1 proto-oncogene polymorphisms in human malignant melanoma: TaqI defined alleles significantly associated with the disease, *Oncogene,* 2, 91, 1987.

963. Hayward, N.K., Keegan, R., Nancarrow, D.J., Little, M.H., Smith, P.J., Gardiner, R.A., Seymour, G.J., Kidson, C., and Lavin, M.F., c-Ha-ras-1 alleles in bladder cancer, Wilms' tumour and malignant melanoma, *Hum. Genet.,* 78, 115, 1988.

964. Thein, S.L., Oscier, D.G., Flint, J., and Wainscoat, J.S., Ha-*ras* hypervariable alleles in myelodysplasia, *Nature,* 321, 84, 1986.

965. Sutherland, C., Shaw, H.M., Roberts, C., Grace, J., Stewart, M.M., McCarthy, W.H., and Kefford, R.F., Harvey-*ras* oncogene restriction fragment alleles in familial melanoma kindreds, *Br. J. Cancer,* 54, 787, 1986.

966. Gerhard, D.S., Dracopoli, N.C., Bale, S.J., Houghton, A.N., Watkins, P., Payne, C.E., Greene, M.H., and Housman, D.E., Evidence against Ha-*ras*-1 involvement in sporadic and familial melanoma, *Nature,* 325, 73, 1987.

967. Bos, J.L., Verlaan-de Vries, M., Jansen, A.M., Veeneman, G.H., van Boom, J.H., and van der Eb, A.J., Three different mutations in codon 61 of the human N-*ras* gene detected by synthetic oligonucleotide hybridization, *Nucleic Acids Res.,* 12, 9155, 1984.

968. Bos, J.L., Toksoz, D., Marshall, C.J., Verlaan-de Vries, M., Veeneman, G.H., van der Eb, A.J., van Boom, J.H., Janssen, J.W.G., and Steenvoorden, A.C.M., Amino-acid substitutions at codon 13 of the N-*ras* oncogene in human acute myeloid leukaemia, *Nature,* 315, 726, 1985.

969. Valenzuela, D.M. and Groffen, J., Four human carcinoma cell lines with novel mutations in position 12 of c-K-*ras* oncogene, *Nucleic Acids Res.*, 14, 843, 1986.

970. Bos, J.L., Verlaan-de Vries, M., Marshall, C.J., Veeneman, G.H., van Boom, J.H., and van der Eb, A.J., A human gastric carcinoma contains a single mutated and an amplified normal allele of the Ki-*ras* oncogene, *Nucleic Acids Res.*, 14, 1209, 1986.

971. Forrester, K., Almoguera, C., Han, K., Grizzle, W.E., and Perucho, M., Detection of high incidence of K-*ras* oncogenes during human colon tumorigenesis, *Nature*, 327, 298, 1987.

972. Forrester, K., Almoguera, C., Jordano, J., Grizzle, W.E., and Perucho, M., High incidence of c-K-*ras* oncogenes in human colon cancer detected by the RNAse A mismatch cleavage method, *J. Tumor Marker Oncol.*, 2, 113, 1987.

973. Shibata, D., Martin, W.J., and Arnheim, N., Analysis of DNA sequences in forty-year-old paraffin-embedded thin-tissue sections: a bridge between molecular biology and classical histology, *Cancer Res.*, 48, 4564, 1988.

974. Kumar, R. and Barbacid, M., Oncogene detection at the single cell level, *Oncogene*, 3, 647, 1988.

975. Wong, G., Arnheim, N., Clark, R., McCabe, R., Innis, M., Aldwin, L., Nitecki, D., and McCormick, F., Detection of activated M$_r$ 21,000 protein, the product of *ras* oncogenes, using antibodies with specificity for amino acid 12, *Cancer Res.*, 46, 6029, 1986.

976. Wick, M.R., Immunohistologic detection of *ras* oncogene products, *Arch. Pathol. Lab. Med.*, 113, 13, 1989.

977. Goldfarb, M., Shimizu, K., Perucho, M., and Wigler, M., Isolation and preliminary characterization of a human transforming gene from T24 bladder carcinoma cells, *Nature*, 296, 404, 1982.

978. Pulciani, S., Santos, E., Lauver, A.V., Long, L.K., Robbins, K.C., and Barbacid, M., Oncogenes in human tumor cell lines: molecular cloning of a transforming gene from human bladder carcinoma cells, *Proc. Natl. Acad. Sci. U.S.A.*, 79, 2845, 1982.

979. Shih, C. and Weinberg, R.A., Isolation of a transforming sequence from a human bladder carcinoma cell line, *Cell*, 29, 161, 1982.

980. Parada, L.F., Tabin, C.J., Shih, C., and Weinberg, R.A., Human EJ bladder carcinoma oncogene is homologue of Harvey sarcoma virus *ras* gene, *Nature*, 297, 474, 1982.

981. Santos, E., Tronick, S.R., Aaronson, S.A., Pulciani, S., and Barbacid, M., T24 human bladder carcinoma oncogene is an activated form of the normal human homologue of BALB- and Harvey-MSV transforming genes, *Nature*, 298, 343, 1982.

982. Tabin, C.J., Bradley, S.M., Bargmann, C.I., Weinberg, R.A., Papageorge, A.G., Scolnick, E.M., Dhar, R., Lowy, D.R., and Chang, E.H., Mechanism of activation of a human oncogene, *Nature*, 300, 143, 1982.

983. Reddy, E.P., Reynolds, R.K., Santos, E., and Barbacid, M., A point mutation is responsible for the acquisition of transforming properties by the T24 human bladder carcinoma oncogene, *Nature*, 300, 149, 1982.

984. Taparowsky, E., Suard, Y., Fasano, O., Shimizu, K., Goldfarb, M., and Wigler, M., Activation of the T24 bladder carcinoma transforming gene is linked to a single amino acid change, *Nature*, 300, 762, 1982.

985. Capon, D.J., Chen, E.Y., Levinson, A.D., Seeburg, P.H., and Goeddel, D.V., Complete nucleotide sequences of the T24 human bladder carcinoma oncogene and its normal homologue, *Nature*, 301, 33, 1983.

986. Reddy, E.P., Nucleotide sequence analysis of the T24 human bladder carcinoma oncogene, *Science*, 220, 1061, 1983.

987. Santos, E., Reddy, E.P., Pulciani, S., Feldmann, R.J., and Barbacid, M., Spontaneous activation of a human proto-oncogene, *Proc. Natl. Acad. Sci. U.S.A.*, 80, 4679, 1983.

988. Sekiya, T., Prassolov, V.S., Fushumi, M., and Nishimura, S., Transforming activity of the c-Ha-*ras* oncogene having two point mutations in codons 12 and 61, *Jpn. J. Cancer Res.*, 76, 851, 1985.

989. Kagimoto, M., Miyoshi, J., Tashiro, K., Naito, Y., Sasaki, Y., Sueishi, K., Tanaka, K., and Imamura, T., Isolation and characterization of an activated c-H-*ras*-1 gene from a squamous-cell lung carcinoma cell line, *Int. J. Cancer*, 35, 809, 1985.

990. Deng, G., Lu, Y., Chen, S., Miao, J., Lu, G., Li, H., Cai, H., Xu, X., E, Z., and Liu, P., Activated c-Ha-*ras* oncogene with a guanidine to thymine transversion at the twelfth codon in a human stomach cancer cell line, *Cancer Res.*, 47, 3195, 1987.

991. Der, C.J. and Cooper, G.M., Altered gene products are associated with activation of cellular *ras*up6 k genes in human lung and colon carcinomas, *Cell*, 32, 201, 1983.

992. Yuasa, Y., Srivastava, S.K., Dunn, C.Y., Rhim, J.S., Reddy, E.P., and Aaronson, S.A., Acquisition of transforming properties by alternative point mutations within c-*bas*/*has* human proto-oncogene, *Nature*, 303, 775, 1983.

993. Shimizu, K., Birnbaum, D., Ruley, M.A., Fasano, O., Suard, Y., Edlund, L., Taparowsky, E., Goldfarb, M., and Wigler, M., Structure of the Ki-*ras* gene of the human lung carcinoma cell line Calu-1, *Nature*, 304, 497, 1983.

994. Capon, D.J., Seeburg, P.H., McGrath, J.P., Hayflick, J.S., Edman, U., Levinson, A.D., and Goeddel, D.V., Activation of Ki-*ras*2 gene in human colon and lung carcinomas by two different point mutations, *Nature*, 304, 507, 1983.

995. Greenhalgh, D.A. and Kinsella, A.R., c-Ha-*ras* not c-Ki-*ras* activation in three colon tumour cell lines, *Carcinogenesis*, 6, 1533, 1985.

996. O'Hara, B.M., Oskarsson, M., Tainsky, M.A., and Blair, D.G., Mechanism of activation of human *ras* genes cloned from a gastric adenocarcinoma and pancreatic carcinoma cell line, *Cancer Res.,* 46, 4695, 1986.

997. Yuasa, Y., Oto, M., Sato, C., Miyaki, M., Iwama, T., Tonomura, A., and Namba, M., Colon carcinoma K-*ras* 2 oncogene of a familial polyposis coli patient, *Jpn. J. Cancer Res.,* 77, 901, 1986.

998. Nakano, H., Yamamoto, F., Neville, C., Evans, D., Mizuno, T., and Perucho, M., Isolation of transforming sequences of two human lung carcinomas: structural and functional analysis of the activated c-K-*ras* oncogenes, *Proc. Natl. Acad. Sci. U.S.A.,* 81, 71, 1984.

999. Yamamoto, F. and Perucho, M., Activation of a human c-K-*ras* oncogene, *Nucleic Acids Res.,* 12, 8873, 1984.

1000. Taparowsky, E., Shimizu, K., Goldfarb, M., and Wigler, M., Structure and activation of the human N-*ras* gene, *Cell,* 34, 581, 1983.

1001. Yuasa, Y., Gol, R.A., Chang, A., Chiu, I.-M., Reddy, E.P., Tronick, S.R., and Aaronson, S.A., Mechanism of activation of an N-*ras* oncogene of SW-1271 human lung carcinoma cells, *Proc. Natl. Acad. Sci. U.S.A.,* 81, 3670, 1984.

1002. Brown, R., Marshall, C.J., Pennie, S.G., and Hall, A., Mechanism of activation of an N-*ras* gene in the human fibrosarcoma cell line HT1080, *EMBO J.,* 3, 1321, 1984.

1003. Padua, R.A., Barrass, N.C., and Currie, G.A., Activation of N-*ras* in a human melanoma cell line, *Mol. Cell. Biol.,* 5, 582, 1985.

1004. Yuasa, Y., Reddy, E.P., Rhim, J.S., Tronick, S.R., and Aaronson, S.A., Activated N-*ras* in a human rectal carcinoma cell line associated with clonal homozygosity in *myb* locus-restriction fragment polymorphism, *Jpn. J. Cancer Res.,* 77, 639, 1986.

1005. Brady, G., Funk, A., Mattern, J., Schütz, G., and Brown, R., Use of gene transfer and a novel cosmid rescue strategy to isolate transforming sequences, *EMBO J.,* 4, 2583, 1985.

1006. Doniger, J., Notario, V., and DiPaolo, J.A., Carcinogens with diverse mutagenic activities initiate neoplastic guinea pig cells that acquire the same N-*ras* point mutation, *J. Biol. Chem.,* 262, 3813, 1987.

1007. Doniger, J. and DiPaolo, J.A., Coordinate N-*ras* mRNA up-regulation with mutational activation in tumorigenic guinea pig cells, *Nucleic Acids Res.,* 16, 969, 1988.

1008. O'Toole, C.M., Povey, S., Hepburn, P., and Franks, L.M., Identity of some human bladder cancer cell lines, *Nature,* 301, 429, 1983.

1009. Muschel, R.J., Khoury, G., Lebowitz, P., Koller, R., and Dhar, R., The human c-*ras*$_1$^{H} oncogene: a mutation in normal and neoplastic tissue from the same patient, *Science,* 219, 853, 1983, and 220, 336, 1983.

1010. Lebkowski, J.S., DuBridge, R.B., Antell, E.A., Greisen, K.S., and Calos, M.P., Transfected DNA is mutated in monkey, mouse, and human cells, *Mol. Cell. Biol.,* 4, 1951, 1984.

1011. Newbold, R.F. and Overell, R.W., Fibroblast immortality is a prerequisite for transformation by EJ c-Ha-*ras* oncogene, *Nature,* 304, 648, 1983.

1012. Feinberg, A.P., Vogelstein, B., Droller, M.J., Baylin, S.B., and Nelkin, B.D., Mutation affecting the 12th amino acid of the c-Ha-*ras* oncogene product occurs infrequently in human cancer, *Science,* 220, 1175, 1983.

1013. Sekiya, T., Fushumi, M., Hori, H., Hirohashi, S., Nishimura, S., and Sugimura, T., Molecular cloning and the total nucleotide sequence of the human c-Ha-*ras*-1 gene activated in a melanoma from a Japanese patient, *Proc. Natl. Acad. Sci. U.S.A.,* 81, 4771, 1984.

1014. Spandidos, D.A., Oncogene activation in malignant transformation: a study of H-*ras* in human breast cancer, *Anticancer Res.,* 7, 991, 1987.

1015. Leon, J., Kamino, H., Steinberg, J.J., and Pellicer, A., H-*ras* activation in benign and self-regressing skin tumors (keratoacanthomas) in both humans and an animal model system, *Mol. Cell. Biol.,* 8, 786, 1988.

1016. Liu, E., Hjelle, B., and Bishop, J.M., Transforming genes in chronic myelogenous leukemia, *Proc. Natl. Acad. Sci. U.S.A.,* 85, 1952, 1988.

1017. Santos, E., Martin-Zanca, D., Reddy, E.P., Pierotti, M.A., Della Porta, G., and Barbacid, M., Malignant activation of a K-*ras* oncogene in lung carcinoma but not in normal tissue of the same patient, *Science,* 223, 661, 1984.

1018. Milici, A., Blick, M., Murphy, E., and Gutterman, J.U., c-K-*ras* codon 12 GGT-CGT point mutation an infrequent inven in human lung cancer, *Biochem. Biophys. Res. Commun.,* 140, 699, 1986.

1019. Feig, L.A., Bast, R.C., Jr., Knapp, R.C., and Cooper, G.M., Somatic activation of *ras*^{K} gene in a human ovarian carcinoma, *Science,* 223, 698, 1984.

1020. Tsuda, H., Hirohashi, S., Shimosato, Y., Ino, Y., Yoshida, T., and Terada, M., Low incidence of point mutation of c-Ki-*ras* and N-*ras* oncogenes, in human hepatocellular carcinomas, *Jpn. J. Cancer Res.,* 80, 196, 1989.

1021. Bos, J.L., Fearon, E.R., Hamilton, S.R., Verlaan-de Vries, M., van Boom, J.H., van der Eb, A.J., and Vogelstein, B., Prevalence of *ras* gene mutations in human colorectal cancers, *Nature,* 327, 293, 1987.

1022. Yanez, L., Groffen, J., and Valenzuela, D.M., c-K-*ras* mutations in human carcinomas occur preferentially in codon 12, *Oncogene,* 1, 315, 1987.

1023. Rodenhuis, S., van de Wetering, M.L., Mooi, W.J., Evers, S.G., van Zandwijk, N., and Bos, J.L., Mutational activation of the K-*ras* oncogene, *N. Engl. J. Med.,* 317, 929, 1987.

1024. Almoguera, C., Shibata, D., Forrester, K., Martin, J., Arnheim, N., and Perucho, M., Most human carcinomas of the exocrine pancreas contain mutant c-K-*ras* genes, *Cell,* 53, 549, 1988.

1025. Nishida, J., Hirai, H., and Takaku, F., Activation mechanism of the N-*ras* oncogene in human leukemias detected by synthetic oligonucleotide probes, *Biochem. Biophys. Res. Commun.,* 147, 870, 1987.

1026. Gambke, C., Hall, A., and Moroni, C., Activation of an N-*ras* gene in acute myeloblastic leukemia through somatic mutation in the first exon, *Proc. Natl. Acad. Sci. U.S.A.,* 82, 879, 1985.

1027. Janssen, J.W.G., Steenvoordenk, A.C.M., Lyons, J., Anger, B., Böhlke, J.U., Bos, J.L., Seliger, H., and Bartram, C.R., *RAS* gene mutations in acute and chronic myelocytic leukemias, chronic myeloproliferative disorders, and myelodysplastic syndromes, *Proc. Natl. Acad. Sci. U.S.A.,* 84, 9228, 1987.

1028. Needleman, S.W., Devine, S.E., and Kraus, M.H., 12th codon mutation resulting in c-N-*ras* activation in acute myelogenous leukemia, *Leukemia,* 2, 91, 1988.

1029. Liu, E., Hjelle, B., Morgan, R., Hecht, F., and Bishop, J.M., Mutations of the Kirsten-*ras* proto-oncogene in human preleukaemia, *Nature,* 330, 186, 1987.

1030. Janssen, J.W.G., Lyons, J., Steenvoorden, A.C.M., Seliger, H., and Bartram, C.R., Concurrent mutations in two different ras genes in acute myelocytic leukemias, *Nucleic Acids Res.,* 15, 5669, 1987.

1031. Toksoz, D., Farr, C.J., and Marshall, C.J., *ras* gene activation in a minor proportion of the blast population in acute myeloid leukemia, *Oncogene,* 1, 409, 1987.

1032. Senn, H.-P., Tran-Thang, C., Wodnar-Filipowicz, A., Jiricny, J., Fopp, M., Gratwohl, A., Signer, E., Weber, W., and Moroni, C., Mutation analysis of the N-*ras* proto-oncogene in active and remission phase of human acute leukemias, *Int. J. Cancer,* 41, 59, 1988.

1033. Pedersen-Bjergaard, J., Janssen, J.W.G., Lyons, J., Philip, P., and Bartram, C.R., Point mutation or the *ras* protooncogenes and chromosome aberrations in acute nonlymphocytic leukemia and preleukemia related to therapy with alkylating agents, *Cancer Res.,* 48, 1812, 1988.

1034. Bos, J.L., Verlaan-de Vries, M., van der Eb, A.J., Janssen, J.W.G., Delwel, R., Löwenberg, B., and Colly, L.P., Mutations in N-*ras* predominate in acute myeloid leukemia, *Blood,* 69, 1237, 1987.

1035. Wodnar-Filipowicz, A., Senn, H.-P., Jiricny, J., Signer, E., and Moroni, C., Glycine-cysteine substitution at codon 13 of the N-*ras* proto-oncogene in a human T cell non-Hodgkin's lymphoma, *Oncogene,* 1, 457, 1987.

1036. Hirai, H., Okada, M., Mizoguchi, H., Mano, H., Kobayashi, Y., Nishida, J., and Takaku, F., Relationship between an activated N-*ras* oncogene and chromosomal abnormality during leukemic progression from myelodysplastic syndrome, *Blood,* 71, 256, 1988.

1037. Nitta, N., Ochiai, M., Nagao, M., and Sugimura, T., Amino-acid substitution at codon 13 of the N-*ras* oncogene in rectal cancer in a Japanese patient, *Jpn. J. Cancer Res.,* 78, 12, 1987.

1038. Nishida, J., Kobayashi, Y., Hirai, H., and Takaku, F., A point mutation at codon 13 of the N-*ras* oncogene in a human stomach cancer, *Biochem. Biophys. Res. Commun.,* 146, 247k 1987.

1039. Guerrero, I., Villasante, A., Corces, V., and Pellicer, A., Activation of a c-K-*ras* oncogene by somatic mutation in mouse lymphomas induced by gamma radiation, *Science,* 225, 1159, 1984.

1040. Zarbl, H., Sukumar, S., Arthur, A.V., Martin-Zanca, D., and Barbacid, M., Direct mutagenesis of Ha-*ras*-1 oncogenes by *N*-nitroso-*N*-methylurea during initiation of mammary carcinogenesis in rats, *Nature,* 315, 382, 1985.

1041. Guerrero, I., Villasante, A., Corces, V., and Pellicer, A., Loss of the normal N-*ras* allele in a mouse thymic lymphoma induced by a chemical carcinogen, *Proc. Natl. Acad. Sci. U.S.A.,* 82, 7810, 1985.

1042. Wiseman, R.W., Stowers, S.J., Miller, E.C., Anderson, M.W., and Miller, J.A., Activating mutations of the c-Ha-*ras* protooncogene in chemically induced hepatomas of the male B6C3 F_1 mouse, *Proc. Natl. Acad. Sci. U.S.A.,* 83, 5825, 1986.

1043. Reynolds, S.H., Stowers, S.J., Patterson, R.M., Maronpot, R.R., Aaronson, S.A., and Anderson, M.W., Activated oncogenes in B6C3F1 mouse liver tumors: implications for risk assessment, *Science,* 237, 1309, 1987.

1044. Tahira, T., Hayashi, K., Ochiai, M., Tsuchida, N., Nagao, M., and Sugimura, T., Structure of the c-Ki-*ras* gene in a rat fibrosarcoma induced by 1,8-dinitropyrene, *Mol. Cell. Biol.,* 6, 1349, 1986.

1045. Sukumar, S., Perantoni, A., Reed, C., Rice, J.M., and Wenk, M.L., Activated K-*ras* and N-*ras* oncogenes in primary renal mesenchymal tumors induced in F344 rats by methyl(methoxymethyl)nitrosamine, *Mol. Cell. Biol.,* 6, 2716, 1986.

1046. Dandekar, S., Sukumar, S., Zarbl, H., Young, L.J.T., and Cardiff, R.D., Specific activation of the cellular Harvey-*ras* oncogene in dimethylbenzanthracene-induced mouse mammary tumors, *Mol. Cell. Biol.,* 6, 4104, 1986.

1047. Bizub, D., Wood, A.W., and Skalka, A.M., Mutagenesis of the Ha-*ras* oncogene in mouse skin tumors induced by polycyclic aromatic hydrocarbons, *Proc. Natl. Acad. Sci. U.S.A.,* 83, 6048, 1986.

1048. Strickland, J.E., Greenhalgh, D.A., Koceva-Chyla, A., Hennings, H., Restrepo, C., Balaschak, M., and Yuspa, S.H., Development of murine epidermal cell lines which contain an activated *ras*^Ha oncogene and form papillomas in skin grafts on athymic nude mouse hosts, *Cancer Res.,* 48, 165, 1988.

1049. Harper, J.R., Reynolds, S.H., Greenhalgh, D.A., Strickland, J.E., Lacal, J.C., and Yuspa, S.H., Analysis of the *ras*^H oncogene and its p21 product in chemically induced skin tumors and tumor-derived cell lines, *Carcinogenesis,* 8, 1821, 1987.

1050. Hochwalt, A.E., Solomon, J.J., and Garte, S.J., Mechanism of H-*ras* oncogene activation in mouse squamous carcinoma induced by an alkylating agent, *Cancer Res.,* 48, 556, 1988.

1051. Varmus, H.E., The molecular genetics of cellular oncogenes, *Annu. Rev. Genet.,* 18, 553, 1984.

1052. Topal, M.D., DNA repair, oncogenes and carcinogenesis, *Carcinogenesis,* 9, 691, 1988.

1053. Stowers, S.J., Glover, P.L., Reynolds, S.H., Boone, L.R., Maronpot, R.R., and Anderson, M.W., Activation of the K-*ras* protooncogene in lung tumors from rats and mice chronically exposed to tetranitromethane, *Cancer Res.,* 47, 3212, 1987.

1054. Rhim, J.S., Fujita, J., Arnstein, P., and Aaronson, S.A., Neoplastic conversion of human keratinocytes by adenovirus 12-SV40 virus and chemical carcinogens, *Science,* 232, 385, 1986.

1055. Bargmann, C.I., Hung, M.-C., and Weinberg, R.A., Multiple independent activations of the *neu* oncogene by a point mutation altering the transmembrane domain of p185, *Cell,* 45, 649, 1986.

1056. Perantoni, A.O., Rice, J.M., Reed, C.D., Watanabe, M., and Wenk, M.L., Activated *neu* oncogene sequences in primary tumors of the peripheral nervous system induced in rats by transplacental exposure to ethylnitrosourea, *Proc. Natl. Acad. Sci. U.S.A.,* 84, 6317, 1987.

1057. Hurlin, P.J., Morphological transformation, focus formation, and anchorage independence induced in diploid human fibroblasts by expression of a transfected H-*ras* oncogene, *Cancer Res.,* 47, 5752, 1987.

1058. DeFeo-Jones, D., Tatchell, K., Robinson, L.C., Sigal, I.S., Vass, W.C., Lowy, D.R., and Scolnick, E.M., Mammalian and yeast *ras* gene products: biological function in their heterologous systems, *Science,* 228, 179, 1985.

1059. Lobanenkov, V.V., Plumb, M., Goodwin, G.H., and Grover, P.L., The effect of neighbouring bases on G-specific DNA cleavage mediated by treatment with the *anti*-diol epoxide of benzo(a)pyrene *in vitro*, *Carcinogenesis,* 7, 1689, 1986.

1060. Schäfer, R., Griegel, S., Dubbert, M.-A., and Willecke, K., Unstable transformation of mouse 3T3 cells by transfection with DNA from normal human lymphocytes, *EMBO J.,* 3, 659, 1984.

1061. Schäfer, Griegel, S., Schwarte, I., Geisse, S., Traub, O., and Willecke, K., Transforming activity of DNA fragments from normal human lymphocytes results from spontaneous activation of a c-Ha-*ras1* gene, *Mol. Cell. Biol.,* 5, 3617, 1985.

1062. Fasano, O., Aldrich, T., Tamanoi, F., Taparowski, E., Furth, M., and Wigler, M., Analysis of the transforming potential of the human H-*ras* gene by random mutagenesis, *Proc. Natl. Acad. Sci. U.S.A.,* 81, 4008, 1984.

1063. Pincus, M.R., van Renswoude, J., Harford, J.B., Chang, E.H., Carty, R.P., and Klausner, R.D., Prediction of the three-dimensional structure of the transforming region of the EJ/T24 human bladder oncogene product and its normal cellular homologue, *Proc. Natl. Acad. Sci. U.S.A.,* 80, 5253, 1983.

1064. Pincus, M.R. and Brandt-Rauf, P.W., Structural effects of substitutions on the p21 proteins, *Proc. Natl. Acad. Sci. U.S.A.,* 82, 3596, 1985.

1065. McCormick, F., Clark, B.F.C., la Cour, T.F.M., Kjeldgaard, M., Norskov-Lauritsen, L., and Nyborg, J., A model for the tertiary structure of p21, the product of the *ras* oncogene, *Science,* 230, 78, 1985.

1066. de Vos, A.M., Tong, L., Milburn, M.V., Matias, P.M., Jancarik, J., Noguchi, S., Nishimura, S., Miura, K., Ohtsuka, E., and Kim, S.-H., Three dimensional structure of an oncogene protein: catalytic domain of human c-H-*ras* p21, *Science,* 239, 888, 1988.

1067. Tong, L., de Vos, A.M., Milburn, M.V., Jancarik, J., Noguchi, S., Nishimura, S., Miura, K., Ohtsuka, E., and Kim, S.-H., Structural differences between a *ras* oncogene protein and the normal protein, *Nature,* 337, 90, 1989.

1068. McGrath, J.P., Capon, D.J., Goeddel, D.V., and Levinson, A.D., Comparative biochemical properties of normal and activated human *ras* p21 proteins, *Nature,* 310, 644, 1984.

1069. Seeburg, P.H., Colby, W.W., Capon, D.J., Goeddel, D.V., and Levinson, A.D., Biological properties of human c-Ha-*ras*1 genes mutated at codon 12, *Nature,* 312, 71, 1984.

1070. Der, C.J., Finkel, T., and Cooper, G.M., Biological and biochemical properties of human ras[H] genes mutated at codon 61, *Cell,* 44, 167, 1986.

1071. Colby, W.W., Hayflick, J.S., Clark, S.G., and Levinson, A.D., Biochemical characterization of polypeptides encoded by mutated human Ha*ras*1 genes, *Mol. Cell. Biol.,* 6, 730, 1986.

1072. Srivastava, S.K., Yuasa, Y., Reynolds, S.H., and Aaronson, S.A., Effects of two major activating lesions on the structure and conformation of human *ras* oncogene products, *Proc. Natl. Acad. Sci. U.S.A.,* 82, 38, 1985.

1073. Tanaka, T., Slamon, D.J., and Cline, M.J., Efficient generation of antibodies to oncoproteins by using synthetic peptide antigens, *Proc. Natl. Acad. Sci. U.S.A.,* 82, 3400, 1985.

1074. Gibbs, J.B., Sigal, I.S., and Scolnick, E.M., Biochemical properties of normal and oncogenic *ras* p21, *Trends Biochem. Sci.,* 10, 350, 1985.

1075. Chipperfield, R.G., Jones, S.S., Lo, K.-M., and Weinberg, R.A., Activation of Ha-*ras* p21 by substitution, deletion, and insertion mutations, *Mol. Cell. Biol.,* 5, 1809, 1985.

1076. Gibbs, J.B., Ellis, R.W., and Scolnick, E.M., Autophosphorylation of v-Ha-*ras* p21 is modulated by amino acid residue 12, *Proc. Natl. Acad. Sci. U.S.A.,* 81, 2674, 1984.

1077. Feramisco, J.R., Gross, M., Kamata, T., Rosenberg, M., and Sweet, R.W., Microinjection of the oncogenic form of the human H-*ras* (T24) protein results in rapid proliferation of quiescent cells, *Cell*, 38, 109, 1984.

1078. Gibbs, J.B., Sigal, I.S., Poe, M., and Scolnick, E.M., Intrinsic GTPase activity distinguishes normal and oncogenic *ras* p21 molecules, *Proc. Natl. Acad. Sci. U.S.A.*, 81, 5704, 1984.

1079. Miyoshi, J., Kagimoto, M., Soeda, E., and Sakaki, Y., The human c-Ha-*ras*2 is a processed pseudogene inactivated by numerous base substitutions, *Nucleic Acids Res.*, 12, 1821, 1984.

1080. Andersen, P.R., Tronick, S.R., and Aaronson, S.A., Structural organization and biological activity of molecular clones of the integrated genome of a BALB/c mouse sarcoma virus, *J. Virol.*, 40, 431, 1981.

1081. Manne, V., Bekesi, E., and Kung, H-F., Ha-*ras* proteins exhibit GTPase activity: point mutations that activate Ha-*ras* gene products result in decreased GTPase activity, *Proc. Natl. Acad. Sci. U.S.A.*, 82, 376, 1985.

1082. Sweet, R.W., Yokohama, S., Kamata, T., Feramisco, J.R., Rosenberg, M., and Gross, M., The product of *ras* is a GTPase and T24 oncogenic mutant is deficient in this activity, *Nature*, 311, 273, 1984.

1083. Lacal, J.C., Srivastava, S.K., Anderson, P.S., and Aaronson, S.A., *ras* p21 protein with high or low GTPase activity can efficiently transform NIH/3T3 cells, *Cell*, 44, 609, 1986.

1084. Walter, M., Clark, S.G., and Levinson, A.D., The oncogenic activation of human p21[ras] by a novel mechanism, *Science*, 233, 649, 1986.

1085. Trahey, M., Milley, R.J., Cole, G.E., Innis, M., Paterson, H., Marshall, C.J., Hall, A., and McCormick, F., Biochemical and biological properties of the human N-*ras* p21 protein, *Mol. Cell. Biol.*, 7, 541, 1987.

1086. Clark, R., Wong, G., Arnheim, N., Nitecki, D., and McCormick, F., Antibodies specific for amino acid 12 of the *ras* oncogene product inhibit GTP binding, *Proc. Natl. Acad. Sci. U.S.A.*, 82, 5280, 1985.

1087. Feramisco, J.R., Clark, R., Wong, G., Arnheim, N., Milley, R., and McCormick, F., Transient reversion of *ras* oncogene-induced cell transformation by antibodies specific for amino acid 12 of *ras* protein, *Nature*, 314, 639, 1985.

1088. Feig, L.A., Pan, B.-T., Roberts, T.M., and Cooper, G.M., Isolation of *ras* GTP-binding mutants using an *in situ* colony-binding assay, *Proc. Natl. Acad. Sci. U.S.A.*, 83, 4607, 1986.

1089. Der, C.J., Pan, B.-T., and Cooper, G.M., *ras*[H] mutants deficient in GTP binding, *Mol. Cell. Biol.*, 6, 3291, 1986.

1090. Clanton, D.J., Lu, Y., Blair, D.G., and Shih, T.Y., Structural significance of the GTP-binding domain of *ras* p21 studied by site-directed mutagenesis, *Mol. Cell. Biol.*, 7, 3092, 1987.

1091. Trahey, M. and McCormick, F., A cytoplasmic protein stimulates normal N-*ras* p21 GTPase, but does not affect oncogenic mutants, *Science*, 238, 542, 1987.

1092. Lumpkin, C.K., Knepper, J.E., Butel, J.S., Smith, J.R., and Pereira-Smith, O.M., Mitogenic effects of the proto-oncogene and oncogene forms of c-H-*ras* DNA in human diploid fibroblasts, *Mol. Cell. Biol.*, 6, 2990, 1986.

1093. Tarpley, W.G., Hopkins, N.K., and Gorman, R.R., Reduced hormone-stimulated adenylate cyclase activity in NIH-3T3 cells expressing the EJ human bladder *ras* oncogene, *Proc. Natl. Acad. Sci. U.S.A.*, 83, 3703, 1986.

1094. Benjamin, C.W., Tarpley, W.G., and Gorman, R.R., Loss of platelet-derived growth factor-stimulated phospholipase activity in NIH-3T3 cells expressing the EJ-*ras* oncogene, *Proc. Natl. Acad. Sci. U.S.A.*, 84, 546, 1987.

1095. Ulsh, L.S. and Shih, T.Y., Metabolic turnover of human c-*ras*[H] p21 protein of EJ bladder carcinoma and its normal cellular and viral homologs, *Mol. Cell. Biol.*, 4, 1647, 1984.

1096. Saltarelli, D., Fischer, S., and Gacon, G., Modulation of adenylate cyclase by guanine nucleotides and Kirsten sarcoma virus mediated transformation, *Biochem. Biophys. Res. Commun.*, 127, 318, 1985.

1097. Hiwasa, T. and Sakiyama, S., Altered properties of cAMP-dependent protein kinase in H-*ras*-transformed NIH3T3 cells, *Biochem. Biophys. Res. Commun.*, 139, 787, 1986.

1098. Hiwasa, T., Sakiyama, S., Noguchi, S., Ha, J.-M., Miyazawa, T., and Yokoyama, S., Degradation of a cAMP-binding protein is inhibited by human c-Ha-*ras* gene products, *Biochem. Biophys. Res. Commun.*, 146, 731, 1987.

1099. Fleischman, L.F., Chahwala, S.B., and Cantley, L., *ras*-transformed cells: altered levels of phosphatidylinositol-4,5-bisphosphate and catabolites, *Science*, 231, 407, 1986.

1100. Wolfman, A. and Macara, I.G., Elevated levels of diacylglycerol and decreased phorbol ester sensitivity in *ras*-transformed fibroblasts, *Nature*, 325, 359, 1987.

1101. Wakelam, M.J.O., Houslay, M.D., Davies, S.A., Marshall, C.J., and Hall, A., The role of N-*ras* p21 in the coupling of growth factor receptors to inositol phospholipid turnover, *Biochem. Soc. Trans.*, 15, 45, 1987.

1102. Seuwen, K., Lagarde, A., and Pouysségur, J., Deregulation of hamster fibroblast proliferation by mutated *ras* oncogenes is not mediated by constitutive activation of phosphoinositide-specific phospholipase C, *EMBO J.*, 7, 161, 1988.

1103. Matyas, G.R., Aaronson, S.A., Brady, R.O., and Fishman, P.H., Alteration of glycolipids in *ras*-transfected NIH 3T3 cells, *Proc. Natl. Acad. Sci. U.S.A.*, 84, 6065, 1987.

1104. Finkel, T., Der, C.J., and Cooper, G.M., Activation of *ras* genes in human tumors does not affect localization, modification, or nucleotide binding properties of p21, *Cell*, 37, 151, 1984.

1105. Willumsen, B.M., Norris, K., Papageorge, A.G., Hubbert, N.L., and Lowy, D.R., Harvey murine sarcoma virus p21 *ras* protein: biological and biochemical significance of the cysteine nearest the carboxy terminus, *EMBO J.*, 3, 2581, 1984.

1106. Gross, M., Sweet, R.W., Sathe, G., Yokoyama, S., Fasano, O., Goldfarb, M., Wigler, M., and Rosenberg, M., Purification and characterization of human H-*ras* proteins expressed in *Escherichia coli*, *Mol. Cell. Biol.*, 5, 1015, 1985.

1107. Hiwasa, T., Sakiyama, S., Yokoyama, S., Ha, J.-M., Fujita, J., Noguchi, S., Bando, Y., Kominami, E., and Katunuma, N., Inhibition of cathepsin L-induced degradation of epidermal growth factor receptors by c-Ha-*ras* gene products, *Biochem. Biophys. Res. Commun.*, 151, 78, 1988.

1108. McKay, I.A., Malone, P., Marshall, C.J., and Hall, A., Malignant transformation of murine fibroblasts by a human c-Ha-*ras*-1 oncogene does not require a functional epidermal growth factor receptor, *Mol. Cell. Biol.*, 6, 3382, 1986.

1109. Flier, J.S., Mueckler, M.M., Usher, P., and Lodish, H.F., Elevated levels of glucose transport and transporter messenger RNA are induced by *ras* or *src* oncogenes, *Science*, 235, 1492, 1987.

1110. Yamasaki, H., Hollstein, M., Mesnil, M., Martel, N., and Aguelon, A.-M., Selective lack of intercellular communication between transformed and nontransformed cells as a common property of chemical and oncogene transformation of BALB/c 3T3 cells, *Cancer Res.*, 47, 5658, 1987.

1111. Warburton, M.J., Ferns, S.A., and Hynes, N.E., Collagen processing in ras-transfected mouse mammary epithelial cells, *Biochem. Biophys. Res. Commun.*, 137, 161, 1986.

1112. Liotta, L.A., Tumor invasion and metastases — role of the extracellular matrix, *Cancer Res.*, 46, 1, 1986.

1113. Li, Y., Seyama, T., Godwin, A.K., Winokur, T.S., Lebovitz, R.M., and Lieberman, M.W., MT*ras*T24, a metallothionein-*ras* fusion gene, modulates expression in cultured rat liver cells of two genes associated with *in vivo* liver cancer, *Proc. Natl. Acad. Sci. U.S.A.*, 85, 344, 1988.

1114. Wyllie, A.H., Rose, K.A., Morris, R.G., Steel, C.M., Foster, E., and Spandidos, D.A., Rodent fibroblast tumours expressing human *myc* and *ras* genes: growth, metastasis and endogenous oncogene expression, *Br. J. Cancer*, 56, 251, 1987.

1115. Chang, E.H., Furth, M.E., Scolnick, E.M., and Lowy, D.R., Tumorigenic transformation of mammalian cells induced by a normal human gene homologous to the oncogene of Harvey murine sarcoma virus, *Nature*, 297, 479, 1982.

1116. Spandidos, D.A. and Wilkie, N.M., Malignant transformation of early passage rodent cells by a single mutated human oncogene, *Nature*, 310, 469, 1984.

1117. Sager, R., Tanaka, K., Lau, C.C., Ebina, Y., and Anisowicz, A., Resistance of human cells to tumorigenesis induced by cloned transforming genes, *Proc. Natl. Acad. Sci. U.S.A.*, 80, 7601, 1983.

1118. Taparowsky, E.J., Heaney, M.L., and Parsons, J.T., Oncogene-mediated multistep transformation of C3H10T1/2 cells, *Cancer Res.*, 47, 4125, 1987.

1119. Schwab, M., Varmus, H.E., and Bishop, J.M., Human N-*myc* gene contributes to neoplastic transformation of mammalian cells in culture, *Nature*, 316, 160, 1985.

1120. Land, H., Chen, A.C., Morgenstern, J.P., Parada, L.F., and Weinberg, R.A., Behavior of *myc* and *ras* oncogenes in transformation of rat embryo fibroblasts, *Mol. Cell. Biol.*, 6, 1917, 1986.

1121. Lee, W.M.F., Schwab, M., Westaway, D., and Varmus, H.E., Augmented expression of normal c-*myc* is sufficient for cotransformation of rat embryo cells with a mutant *ras* gene, *Mol. Cell. Biol.*, 5, 3345, 1985.

1122. Kohl, N.E. and Ruley, H.E., Role of c-*myc* in the transformation of REF52 cells by viral and cellular oncogenes, *Oncogene*, 2, 41, 1987.

1123. Suárez, H.G., Nardeux, P.C., Andéol, Y., and Sarasin, A., Multiple activated oncogenes in human tumors, *Oncogene Res.*, 1, 201, 1987.

1124. Jenkins, J.R., Rudge, K., and Currie, G.A., Cellular immortalization by a cDNA clone encoding the transformation-associated phosphoprotein p53, *Nature*, 312, 651, 1984.

1125. Kelekar, A. and Cole, M.D., Immortalization by c-*myc*, H-*ras*, and E1a oncogenes induces differential cellular gene expression and growth factor responses, *Mol. Cell. Biol.*, 7, 3899, 1987.

1126. Pater, A. and Pater, M.M., Transformation of primary human embryonic kidney cells to anchorage independence by a combination of BK virus DNA and the Harvey-*ras* oncogene, *J. Virol.*, 58, 680, 1986.

1127. Muschel, R.J., Nakahara, K., Chu, E., Pozzatti, R., and Liotta, L.A., Karyotypic analysis of diploid or near diploid metastatic Harvey *ras* transformed rat embryo fibroblasts, *Cancer Res.*, 46, 4104, 1986.

1128. Cerni, C., Moigneau, E., and Cuzin, F., Transfer of "immortalizing" oncogenes into rat fibroblasts induces both high rates of sister chromatid exchange and appearance of abnormal karyotypes, *Exp. Cell Res.*, 168, 439, 1987.

1129. Perucho, M. and Massague, J., Reversible induction of transforming growth factor-alpha by human *ras* oncogenes, *J. Tumor Marker Oncol.*, 1, 81, 1986.

1130. Buick, R.N., Filmus, J., and Quaroni, A., Activated H-*ras* transforms rat intestinal epithelial cells with expression of α-TGF, *Exp. Cell Res.*, 170, 300, 1987.

1131. Geiser, A.G., Der, C.J., Marshall, C.J., and Stanbridge, E.J., Suppression of tumorigenicity with continued expression of the c-Ha-*ras* oncogene in EJ bladder carcinoma-human fibroblast hybrid cells, *Proc. Natl. Acad. Sci. U.S.A.*, 83, 5209, 1986.

1132. Griegel, S., Traub, O., Willecke, K., and Schäfer, R., Suppression and re-expression of transformed phenotype in hybrids of Ha-*ras*-1-transformed Rat-1 cells and early-passage rat embryonic fibroblasts, *Int. J. Cancer*, 38, 697, 1986.

1133. Willecke, K., Griegel, S., Martin, W., Traub, O., and Schäfer, R., The Ha-ras-induced transformed phenotype of Rat-1 cells can be suppressed in hybrids with rat embryonic fibroblasts, *J. Cell. Biochem.*, 34, 23, 1987.

1134. Hillova, J., Hill, M., Belehradek, J., Jr., Mariage-Samson, R., and Brada, Z., Loss of the oncogene from human H-*ras*-1-transfected NIH/3T3 cells grown in the presence of excess of methionine, *J. Natl. Cancer Inst.*, 77, 721, 1986.

1135. Olson, E.N., Spizz, G., and Tainsky, M.A., The oncogenic forms of N-*ras* or H-*ras* prevent skeletal myoblast differentiation, *Mol. Cell. Biol.*, 7, 2104, 1987.

1136. Payne, P.A., Olson, E.N., Hsiau, P., Roberts, R., Perryman, M.B., and Schneider, M.D., An activated c-Ha-*ras* allele blocks the induction of muscle-specific genes whose expression is contingent on mitogen withdrawal, *Proc. Natl. Acad. Sci. U.S.A.*, 84, 8956, 1987.

1137. Bell, J.C., Jardine, K., and McBurney, M.W., Lineage-specific transformation after differentiation of multipotential murine stem cells containing a human oncogene, *Mol. Cell. Biol.*, 6, 617, 1986.

1138. Hsiao, W.-L.W., Gattoni-Celli, S., and Weinstein, I.B., Oncogene-induced transformation of C3H 1oT1/2 cells is enhanced by tumor promoters, *Science*, 226, 552, 1984.

1139. Hsiao, W.-L.W., Wu, T., and Weinstein, I.B., Oncogene-induced transformation of a rat embryo fibroblast cell line is enhanced by tumor promoters, *Mol. Cell. Biol.*, 6, 1943, 1986.

1140. Hsiao, W.-L. W., Lopez, C.A., Wu, T., and Weinstein, I.B., A factor present in fetal calf serum enhances oncogene-induced transformation of rodent fibroblasts, *Mol. Cell. Biol.*, 7, 3380, 1987.

1141. Wickremasinghe, R.G., Piga, A., Campana, D., Yaxley, J.C., and Hoffbrand, A.V., Rapid down-regulation of protein kinase C and membrane association in phorbol ester-treated leukemia cells, *FEBS Lett.*, 190, 50, 1985.

1142. Harewood, K.R., Wilson, D.S., Higdon, R.C., Tsaparikos, K.E., and Brunson, K.W., Regulated expression of the human mutant *ras* gene after transfection of BALB/c mouse embryo fibroblast cells, *J. Natl. Cancer Inst.*, 80, 122, 1988.

1143. Greenberg, A.H., Egan, S.E., Jarolim, L., Gingras, M.-C., and Wright, J.A., Natural killer cell regulation of implantation and early lung growth of H-*ras*-transformed 10T1/2 fibroblasts in mice, *Cancer Res.*, 47, 4801, 1987.

1144. Vousden, K.H., Eccles, S.A., Purvies, H., and Marshall, C.J., Enhanced spontaneous metastasis of mouse carcinoma cells transfected with an activated c-Ha-*ras*-1 gene, *Int. J. Cancer*, 37, 425, 1986.

1145. Thorgeirsson, U.P., Turpeeniemi-Hujanen, T., Williams, J.E., Westin, E.H., Heilmen, C.A., Talmadge, J.E., and Liotta, L.A., NIH/3T3 cells transfected with human tumor DNA containing activated *ras* oncogenes express the metastatic phenotype in nude mice, *Mol. Cell. Biol.*, 5, 259, 1985.

1146. Egan, S.E., McClarty, G.A., Jarolim, L., Wright, J.A., Spiro, I., Hager, G., and Greenberg, A.H., Expression of H-*ras* correlates with metastatic potential: evidence for direct regulation of the metastatic phenotype in 10T1/2 NIH 3T3 cells, *Mol. Cell. Biol.*, 7, 830, 1987.

1147. Jarani, J., Fligiel, S.E.G., and Wilson, B., Motility of ras[H] oncogene transformed NIH-3T3 cells, *Invasion Metast.*, 6, 335, 1986.

1148. Bradley, M.O., Kraynak, A.R., Storer, R.D., and Gibbs, J.B., Experimental metastasis in nude mice of NIH 3T3 cells containing various *ras* genes, *Proc. Natl. Acad. Sci. U.S.A.*, 83, 5277, 1986.

1149. Verrelle, P., Lascaut, V., Poupon, M.-F., and Hillova, J., DNA transfection affects the metastatic capacity of tumour cells, *Anticancer Res.*, 7, 181, 1987.

1150. Caignard, A., Kitagawa, Y., Sato, S., and Nagao, M., Activated K-*ras* in tumorigenic and non-tumorigenic cell variants from a rat colon adenocarcinoma, induced by dimethylhydrazine, *Jpn. J. Cancer Res.*, 79, 244, 1988.

1151. Elvin, P., Kerr, I.B., McArdle, C.S., and Birnie, G.D., Isolation and preliminary characterisation of cDNA clones representing mRNAs associated with tumour progression and metastasis in colorectal cancer, *Br. J. Cancer*, 57, 36, 1988.

1152. Muschel, R.J., Williams, J.E., Lowy, D.R., and Liotta, L.A., Harvey *ras* induction of metastatic potential depends upon oncogene activation of the type of recipient cell, *Am. J. Pathol.*, 121, 1, 1985.

1153. Wieman, J., Zucker, S., Wilkie, D., and Lysik, R.M., Purification of a hemolytic factor from ras oncogene transformed fibroblasts, *Biochem. Biophys. Res. Commun.*, 140, 365, 1986.

1154. Bernstein, S.C. and Weinstein, R.A., Expression of the metastatic phenotype in cells transfected with human metastatic tumor DNA, *Proc. Natl. Acad. Sci. U.S.A.*, 82, 1726, 1985.

1155. Roth, J.A., Ames, R.S., Restrepo, C., Scuderi, P., Scannon, P.J., and Lee, H.M., Cells transformed by a human oncogene (c-Ha-*ras*) and human tumors express a common cell surface antigen, *Proc. Am. Assoc. Cancer Res.*, 26, 294, 1985.

1156. Roth, J.A., Ames, R.S., Restrepo, C., and Scuderi, P., Monoclonal antibody 45-2D9 recognizes a cell surface glycoprotein on a human c-Ha-ras transformed cell line (45-342) and a shared epitope on human tumors, *J. Immunol.*, 137, 2385, 1986.

1157. Roth, J.A., Ames, R.S., Byers, V., Lee, H.M., and Scannon, P.J., Monoclonal antibody 45-2D9 conjugated to the A chain of ricin is specifically toxic to c-Ha-ras-transfected NIH 3T3 cells expressing gp74, *J. Immunol.*, 136, 2305, 1986.

1158. Lanza, L.A., Wilson, D.J., Ikejiri, B., Roth, J.A., and Grimm, E.A., Human oncogene-transfected tumor cells display differential susceptibility to lysis by lymphokine-activated killer cells (LAK) and natural killer cells, *J. Immunol.*, 137, 2716, 1986.

1159. Sklar, M.D., Increased resistance to *cis*-diamminedichloroplatinum(II) in NIH 3T3 cells transformed by *ras* oncogenes, *Cancer Res.*, 48, 793, 1988.

1160. Sklar, M.D., The *ras* oncogenes increase the intrinsic resistance of NIH 3Tw cells to ionizing radiation, *Science,* 239, 645, 1988.

1161. Spandidos, D.A., The human T24-*ras*1 oncogene: a study of the effects of overexpression of the mutated *ras* gene product in rodent cells, *Anticancer Res.*, 6, 259, 1986.

1162. Katz, E. and Carter, B.J., Effect of adeno-associated virus on transformation of NIH 3T3 cells by *ras* gene and on tumorigenicity of an NIH 3T3 transformed cell line, *Cancer Res.*, 46, 3023, 1986.

1163. Stoler, A. and Bouck, N., Identification of a single chromosome in the normal genome essential for suppression of hamster cell transformation, *Proc. Natl. Acad. Sci. U.S.A.*, 82, 570, 1985.

1164. Koi, M. and Barrett, J.C., Loss of tumor-suppressive function during chemically induced neoplastic progression of Syrian hamster embryo cells, *Proc. Natl. Acad. Sci. U.S.A.*, 83, 5992, 1986.

1165. Vogelstein, B., Fearon, E.R., Kern, S.E., Hamilton, S.R., Preisinger, A.C., Nakamura, Y., and White, R., Allelotype of colorectal carcinomas, *Science,* 244, 207, 1989.

1166. Klein, G., The approaching era of tumor suppressor genes, *Science,* 238, 1539, 1987.

1167. Friend, S.H., Dryja, T.P., and Weinberg, R.A., Oncogenes and tumor-suppressing genes, *N. Engl. J. Med.,* 318, 618, 1988.

1168. Skuse, G.R. and Rowley, P.T., Tumor suppressor genes and inherited predisposition to malignancy, *Semin. Oncol.*, 16, 128, 1989.

1169. Opper, M., Schuler, G., and Mechler, B.M., Hereditary suppression of *lethal (2) giant larvae* malignant tumor development in *Drosophila* by gene transfer, *Oncogene,* 1, 91, 1987.

1170. Gateff, E. and Mechler, B.M., Tumor-suppressor genes of *Drosophila melanogaster*, *Crit. Rev. Oncogenesis,* 1, 1989.

1171. Schaefer, R., Iyer, J., Iten E., and Nirkko, A.C., Partial reversion of the transformed phenotype in *HRAS*-transfected tumorigenic cells by transfer of a human gene, *Proc. Natl. Acad. Sci. U.S.A.*, 85, 1590, 1988.

1172. Dallapiccola, B., Cytogenetics of Mendelian mutations associated with cancer proneness, *Cancer Genet. Cytogenet.*, 26, 85, 1987.

1173. Phillips, R.A. and Gallie, B.L., Retinoblastoma: importance of recessive mutations in tumorigenesis, *J. Cell. Physiol.*, Suppl. 3, 79, 1984.

1174. Green, A.R., Recessive mechanisms of malignancy, *Br. J. Cancer,* 58, 115, 1988.

1175. Donis-Keller, H., Green, P., Helms, C., Cartinhour, S., Weiffenbach, B., Stephens, K., Keith, T.P., Bowden, D.W., Smith, D.R., Lander, K.S., Gravius, T., Brown, V.A., Rising, M.B., Parker, C., Powers, J.A., Watt, D.E., Kauffman, E.R., Bricker, A., Phipps, P., Muller-Kahle, H., Fulton, T.R., Ng, S., Schumm, J.W., Braman, J.C., Knowlton, R.G., Barker, D.F., Crooks, S.M., Lincoln, S.E., Daly, M.J., and Abrahamson, J., A genetic linkage map of the human genome, *Cell,* 51, 319, 1987.

1176. McAlpine, P.J., Van Cong, N., Boucheix, C., Pakstis, A.J., Doute, R.C., and Shows, T.B., The 1987 catalog of mapped genes and report of the nomenclature committee, *Cytogenet. Cell Genet.*, 46, 29, 1987.

1177. Bloomfield, C.D., Trent, J.M., and van den Berghe, H., Report of the committee on structural chromosome changes in neoplasia, *Cytogenet. Cell Genet.*, 46, 344, 1987.

1178. Ivankovic, S., Chemical and viral agents in prenatal experimental carcinogenesis, *Biol. Res. Pregnancy,* 3, 99, 1982.

1179. Mesrobian, H.-G.J., Wilms tumor: past, present, future, *J. Virol.*, 140, 231, 1988.

1180. Yunis, J.J. and Ramsay, N.K.C., Familial occurrence of the aniridia-Wilms' tumor syndrome with deletion 11p13-14.1, *J. Pediat.*, 96, 1027, 1980.

1181. Kaneko, Y., Egues, M.C., and Rowley, J.D., Interstitial deletion of short arm of chromosome 11 limited to Wilms' tumor cells in a patient without aniridia, *Cancer Res.*, 41, 4577, 1981.

1182. Huerre, C., Despoisse, S., Gilgenkrautz, S., Lenoir, G.M., and Junien, C., c-Ha-*ras*1 is not deleted in aniridia-Wilms' tumour association, *Nature,* 305, 638, 1983.

1183. de Martinville, B. and Francke, U., The c-Ha-*ras*1, insulin and beta-globin loci map outside the deletion associated with aniridia-Wilms' tumour, *Nature,* 305, 641, 1983.

1184. Grundy, P., Koufos, A., Morgan, K., Li, F.P., Meadows, A.T., and Cavenee, W.K., Familial predisposition to Wilms' tumour does not map to the short arm of chromosome 11, *Nature,* 336, 374, 1988.

1185. Huff, V., Compton, D.A., Chao, L.-Y., Strong, L.C., Geiser, C.F., and Saunders, G.F., Lack of linkage of familial Wilms' tumour to chromosomal band 11p13, *Nature,* 336, 377, 1988.

1186. Slater, R.M., de Kraker, J., Voute, P.A., and Delemarre, J.F.M., A cytogenetic study of Wilms' tumor, *Cancer Genet. Cytogenet.*, 14, 95, 1985.

1187. Dao, D.D., Schroeder, W.T., Chao, L.-Y., Kikuchi, H., Strong, L.C., Riccardi, V.M., Pathak, S., Nichols, W.W., Lewis, W.H., and Saunders, G.F., Genetic mechanisms of tumor-specific loss of 11p DNA sequences in Wilms tumor, *Am. J. Hum. Genet.*, 41, 202, 1987.

1188. Schroeder, W.T., Chao, L.-Y., Dao, D.D., Strong, L.C., Pathak, S., Riccardi, V., Lewis, W.H., and Saunders, G.F., Nonrandom loss of maternal chromosome 11 alleles in Wilms tumors, *Am. J. Hum. Genet.*, 40, 413, 1987.

1189. Orkin, S.H., Goldman, D.S., and Sallan, S.E., Development of homozygosity for chromosome 11p markers in Wilms' tumour, *Nature*, 309, 172, 1984.

1190. Solomon, E., Recessive mutation in aetiology of Wilms' tumour, *Nature*, 309, 111, 1984.

1191. Koufos, A., Hansen, M.F., Lampkin, B.C., Workman, M.L., Copeland, N.G., Jenkins, N.A., and Cavenee, W.K., Loss of alleles at loci of human chromosome 11 during genesis of Wilms' tumour, *Nature*, 309, 170, 1984.

1192. Fisher, J.H., Miller, Y.E., Sparkes, R.S., Bateman, J.B., Kimmel, K.A., Carey, T.E., Rodell, T., Shoemaker, S.A., and Scoggin, C.H., Wilms' tumor-aniridia association: segregation of affected chromosome in somatic cell hybrids, identification of cell surface antigen associated with deleted area, and regional mapping of c-Ha-ras-1 oncogene, insulin gene, and beta globin gene, *Somat. Cell Mol. Genet.*, 10, 455, 1984.

1193. Przepiorka, D., Baylin, S.B., McBride, O.W., Testa, J.R., de Bustros, A., and Nelkin, B.D., The human calcitonin gene is located on the short arm of chromosome 11, *Biochem. Biophys. Res. Commun.*, 120, 493, 1984.

1194. Pimentel, E., Hormones as tumor markers, *Cancer Detect. Prevent.*, 6, 87, 1983.

1195. Chaganti, R.S.K., Jhanwar, S.C., Antonarakis, S.E., and Hayward, W.S., Germ-line chromosomal localization of genes in chromosome 11p linkage: parathyroid hormone, β-globin, c-Ha-ras-1, and insulin, *Somat. Cell Mol. Genet.*, 11, 197, 1985.

1196. Zabel, B.U., Kronenberg, H.M., Bell, G.I., and Shows, T.B., Chromosome mapping of genes on the short arm of human chromosome 11: parathyroid hormone gene is at 11p15 together with the genes for insulin, c-Harvey-ras 1, and β-hemoglobin, *Cytogenet. Cell Genet.*, 39, 200, 1985.

1197. Glaser, T., Lewis, W.H., Bruns, G.A.P., Watkins, P.C., Rogler, C.E., Shows, T.B., Powers, V.E., Willard, H.F., Goguen, J.M., Simola, K.O.J., and Housman, D.E., The beta-subunit of follicle-stimulating hormone is deleted in patients with aniridia and Wilms' tumour, allowing a further definition of the WAGR locus, *Nature*, 321, 882, 1986.

1198. Michalopoulos, E.E., Bevilacqua, P.J., Stokoe, N., Powers, V.E., Willard, H.F., and Lewis, W.H., Molecular analysis of gene deletion in aniridia-Wilms tumor association, *Hum. Genet.*, 70, 157, 1985.

1199. Davis, L.M., Stallard, R., Thomas, G.H., Couillin, P., Junien, C., Nowak, N.J., and Shows, T.B., Two anonymous DNA segments distinguish the Wilms' tumor and aniridia loci, *Science*, 241, 840, 1988.

1200. Reeve, A.E., Eccles, M.R., Wilkins, R.J., Bell, G.I., and Millow, L.J., Expression of insulin-like growth factor-II transcripts in Wilms' tumour, *Nature*, 317, 258, 1985.

1201. Scrable, H.J., Witte, D.P., Lampkin, B.C., and Cavenee, W.K., Chromosomal localization of the human rhabdomyosarcoma locus by mitotic recombination mapping, *Nature*, 329, 645, 1987.

1202. Hayward, N.K., Little, M.H., Mortimer, R.H., Clouston, W.M., and Smith, P.J., Generation of homozygosity at the c-Ha-*ras*-1 locus on chromosome 11p in an adrenal adenoma from an adult with Wiedemann-Beckwith syndrome, *Cancer Genet. Cytogenet.*, 30, 127, 1988.

1203. Vogel, F., Genetics of retinoblastoma, *Hum. Genet.*, 52, 1, 1979.

1204. Sparkes, R.S., Cytogenetics of retinoblastoma, *Cancer Surv.*, 3, 479, 1984.

1205. Sparkes, R.S., The genetics of retinoblastoma, *Biochim. Biophys. Acta*, 780, 95, 1985.

1206. Potluri, V.R., Helson, L., Ellsworth, R.M., Reid, T., and Gilbert, F., Chromosomal abnormalities in human retinoblastoma: a review, *Cancer*, 58, 663, 1986.

1207. Squire, J., Phillips, R.A., Boyce, S., Godbout, R., Rogers, B., and Gallie, B.L., Isochromosome 6p, a unique chromosomal abnormality in retinoblastoma: verification by standard staining techniques, new densitometric methods, and somatic cell hybridization, *Hum. Genet.*, 66, 46, 1984.

1208. Lee, W.-H., Bookstein, R., and Lee, E.Y.-H.P., Studies on the human retinoblastoma susceptibility gene, *J. Cell. Biochem.*, 38, 213, 1988.

1209. Knudson, A.G., Meadows, A.T., Nichols, W.W., and Hill, R., Chromosomal deletion and retinoblastoma, *N. Engl. J. Med.*, 295, 1120, 1976.

1210. Wilson, M.G., Ebbin, A.J., Towner, J.W., and Spencer, W.H., Chromosomal anomalies in patients with retinoblastoma, *Clin. Genet.*, 12, 1, 1977.

1211. Balaban, G., Gilbert, F., Nichols, W., Meadows, A.T., and Shields, J., Abnormalities of chromosome #13 in retinoblastomas from individuals with normal constitutional karyotypes, *Cancer Genet. Cytogenet.*, 6, 213, 1982.

1212. Benedict, W.F., Banerjee, A., Mark, C., and Murphree, A.L., Nonrandom chromosomal changes in untreated retinoblastomas, *Cancer Genet. Cytogenet.*, 10, 311, 1983.

1213. Turleau, C., de Grouchy, J., Chavin-Colin, F., Junien, C., Séger, J., Schlienger, P., Leblanc, A., and Haye, C., Cytogenetic forms of retinoblastoma: their incidence in a survey of 66 patients, *Cancer Genet. Cytogenet.*, 16, 321, 1985.

1214. Bunin, G.R., Emanuel, B.S., Meadows, A.T., Buckley, J.D., Woods, W.G., and Hammond, G.D., Frequency of 13q abnormalities among 203 patients with retinoblastoma, *J. Natl. Cancer Inst.*, 81, 370, 1989.

1215. Benedict, W.F., Murphree, A.L., Banerjee, A., Spina, C.A., Sparkes, M.C., and Sparkes, R.S., Patient with 13 chromosome deletion: evidence that the retinoblastoma gene is a recessive cancer gene, *Science,* 219, 973, 1983.

1216. Murphree, A.L. and Benedict, W.F., Retinoblastoma: clues to human oncogenesis, *Science,* 223, 1028, 1984.

1217. Hansen, M.F., Koufos, A., Gallie, B.L., Phillips, R.A., Fodstad, O., Brogger, A., Gedde-Dahl, T., and Cavenee, W.K., Osteosarcoma and retinoblastoma: a shared chromosomal mechanism revealing recessive predisposition, *Proc. Natl. Acad. Sci. U.S.A.,* 82, 6216, 1985.

1218. Buchanan, J.A. and Cavenee, W.K., Genetic markers for assessment of retinoblastoma predisposition, *Disease Markers,* 5, 141, 1987.

1219. Horowitz, J.M., Yandell, D.W., Park, S.-H., Canning, S., Whyte, P., Buchkovich, K., Harlow, E., Weinberg, R.A., and Dryja, T.P., Point mutational inactivation of the retinoblastoma antioncogene, *Science,* 243, 937, 1989.

1220. Knudson, A.G., Jr., Hereditary cancer, oncogenes, and antioncogenes, *Cancer Res.,* 45, 1437, 1985.

1221. Cavenee, W.K., Dryja, T.P., Phillips, R.A., Benedict, W.F., Godbout, R., Gallie, B.L., Murphree, A.L., Strong, L.C., and White, R.L., Expression of recessive alleles by chromosome mechanisms in retinoblastoma, *Nature,* 305, 779, 1983.

1222. Dryja, T.P., Cavenee, W., White, R., Rapaport, J.M., Petersen, R., Albert, D.M., and Bruns, G.A.P., Homozygosity of chromosome 13 in retinoblastoma, *N. Engl. J. Med.,* 310, 550, 1984.

1223. Dryja, T.P., Rapaport, J.M., Joyce, J.M., and Petersen, R.A., Molecular detection of deletions involving band q14 of chromosome 13 in retinoblastomas, *Proc. Natl. Acad. Sci. U.S.A.,* 83, 7391, 1986.

1224. Cavenee, W.K., Hansen, M.F., Nordenskjold, M., Kock, E., Maumenee, I., Squire, J.A., Phillips, R.A., and Gallie, B.L., Genetic origin of mutations predisposing to retinoblastoma, *Science,* 228, 501, 1985.

1225. Friend, S.H., Bernards, R., Rogelj, S., Weinberg, R.A., Rapaport, J.M., Albert, D.M., and Dryja, T.P., A human DNA segment with properties of the gene that predisposes to retinoblastoma and osteosarcoma, *Nature,* 323, 643, 1986.

1226. Friend, S.H., Horowitz, J.M., Gerber, M.R., Wang, X.-F., Bogenmann, E., Li, F.P., and Weinberg, R.A., Deletions of a sequence in retinoblastomas and mesenchymal tumors: organization of the sequence and its encoded protein, *Proc. Natl. Acad. Sci. U.S.A.,* 84, 9059, 1987.

1227. Weichselbaum, R.R., Beckett, M., and Diamond, A., Some retinoblastomas, osteosarcomas, and soft tissue sarcomas may share a common etiology, *Proc. Natl. Acad. Sci. U.S.A.,* 85, 2106, 1988.

1228. Horsthemke, B., Greger, V., Barnert, H.J., Höpping, W., and Passarge, E., Detection of submicroscopic deletions and a DNA polymorphism at the retinoblastoma locus, *Hum. Genet.,* 76, 257, 1987.

1229. Wiggs, J., Nordenskjöld, M., Yandell, D., Rapaport, J., Gronding, V., Janson, M., Werelius, B., Petersen, B., Craft, A., Riedel, K., Liberfarb, R., Walton, D., Wilson, W., and Dryja, T.P., Prediction of the risk of hereditary retinoblastoma, using DNA polymorphisms within the retinoblastoma gene, *N. Engl. J. Med.,* 318, 151, 1988.

1230. Mukai, S., Rapaport, J.M., Shields, J.A., Augsburger, J.J., and Dryja, T.P., Linkage of genes for human esterase D and hereditary retinoblastoma, *Am. J. Ophthalmol.,* 97, 681, 1984.

1231. Connolly, M.J., Payne, R.H., Johnson, G., Gallie, B.L., Allderdice, P.W., Marshall, W.H., and Lawton, R.D., Familial, *EsD*-linked, retinoblastoma with reduced penetrance and variable expressivity, *Hum. Genet.,* 65, 122, 1983.

1232. Duncan, A.M.V., Morgan, C., Gallie, B.L., Phillips, R.A., and Squire, J., Re-evaluation of the sublocalization of esterase D and its relation to the retinoblastoma locus by *in situ* hybridization, *Cytogenet. Cell Genet.,* 44, 153, 1987.

1233. Squire, J.S., Dryja, T.P., Dunn, J., Goddard, A., Hofmann, T., Musarella, M., Willard, H.F., Becker, A.J., Gallie, B.L., and Phillips, R.A., Cloning of the esterase D gene: a polymorphic gene probe closely linked to the retinoblastoma locus on chromosome 13, *Proc. Natl. Acad. Sci. U.S.A.,* 83, 6573, 1986.

1234. Lee, E.Y.-H.P. and Lee, W.H., Molecular cloning of the human esterase D gene, a genetic marker of retinoblastoma, *Proc. Natl. Acad. Sci. U.S.A.,* 83, 6337, 1986.

1235. Cavenee, W.K., Murphree, A.L., Shull, M.M., Benedict, W.F., Sparkes, R.S., Kock, E., and Nordenskjold, M., Prediction of familial predisposition to retinoblastoma, *N. Engl. J. Med.,* 314, 1201, 1986.

1236. Benedict, W.F., Srivastan, E.S., Mark, C., Banerjee, A., Sparkes, R.S., and Murphree, A.L., Complete or partial homozygosity of chromosome 13 in primary retinoblastoma, *Cancer Res.,* 47, 4189, 1987.

1237. Lee, W.-H., Bookstein, R., Hong, F., Young, L.-J., Shew, J.-Y., and Lee, E.Y.-H.P., Human retinoblastoma susceptibility gene: cloning, identification, and sequence, *Science,* 235, 1394, 1987.

1238. Lee, W.-H., Shew, J.-Y., Hong, F.D., Sery, T.W., Donoso, L.A., Young, L.-J., Bookstein, R., and Lee, E.Y.-H.P., The retinoblastoma susceptibility gene encodes a nuclear phosphoprotein associated with DNA binding activity, Nature, 329, 642, 1987.

1239. Huang, H.-J.S., Yee, J.-K., Shew, J.-Y., Chen, P.-L., Bookstein, R., Friedman, T., Lee, E.Y.-H.P., and Lee, W.-H., Suppression of the neoplastic phenotype by replacement of the RB gene in human cancer cells, *Science,* 242, 1563, 1988.

1240. Zang, K.D., Cytologic and cytogenetic studies on human meningioma, *Cancer Genet. Cytogenet.*, 6, 249, 1982.

1241. Dumanski, J.P., Carlbom, E., Collins, V.P., and Nordenskjöld, M., Deletion mapping of a locus on human chromosome 22 involved in the oncogenesis of meningioma, *Proc. Natl. Acad. Sci. U.S.A.*, 84, 9275, 1987.

1242. Seizinger, B.R., de la Monte, S., Atkins, L., Gusella, J.F., and Martuza, R.L., Molecular genetic approach to human meningioma: loss of genes on chromosome 22, *Proc. Natl. Acad. Sci. U.S.A.*, 84, 5419, 1987.

1243. Okazaki, M., Nishimo, I., Tateishi, H., Motomura, K., Yamamoto, M., Miki, T., Hakayama, T., Takai, S., Honjo, T., and Mori, T., Loss of genes on the long arm of chromosome 22 in human meningiomas, *Mol. Biol. Med.*, 5, 15, 1988.

1244. Seizinger, B.R., Martuza, R.L., and Gusella, J.F., Loss of genes on chromosome 22 in tumorigenesis of human acoustic neuroma, *Nature,* 322, 644, 1986.

1245. Whang-Peng, J., Kao-Shan, C.S., Lee, E.C., Bunn, P.A., Carney, D.N., Gazdar, A.F., and Minna, J.D., Specific chromosome defect associated with human small-cell lung carcinoma: deletion 3p(14-23), *Science,* 215, 191, 1982.

1246. Naylor, S.L., Johnson, B.E., Minna, J.D., and Sakaguchi, A.Y., Loss of heterozygosity of chromosome 3p markers in small-cell lung cancer, *Nature,* 329, 451, 1987.

1247. Kok, K., Osinga, J., Carritt, B., Davis, M.B., van der Hout, A.H., van der Veen, A.Y., Landsvater, R.M., de Leij, L.F.M.H., Berendsen, H.H., Postmus, P.E., Poppema, S., and Buys, C.H.C.M., Deletion of a DNA sequence at the chromosomal region 3p21 in all major types of lung cancer, *Nature,* 330, 578, 1987.

1248. Harbour, J.W., Lai, S.-L., Whang-Peng, J., Gazdar, A.F., Minna, J.D., and Kaye, F.J., Abnormalities in structure and expression of the human retinoblastoma gene in SCLC, *Science,* 241, 353, 1988.

1249. Shiraishi, M., Morinaga, S., Noguchi, M., Shimosato, Y., and Sekiya, T., Loss of genes on the short arm of chromosome 11 in human lung carcinomas, *Jpn. J. Cancer Res.,* 78, 1302, 1987.

1250. Becker, D. and Sahin, A.A., Loss of heterozygosity at chromosomal regions 3p and 13q in non-small-cell carcinoma of the lung represents low-frequency events, *Genomics,* 4, 97, 1989.

1251. Bodmer, W.F., Bailey, C.J., Bodmer, J., Bussey, H.J.R., Ellis, A., Gorman, P., Lucibello, F.C., Murday, V.A., Rider, S.H., Scambler, P., Sheer, D., Solomon, E., and Spurr, N.K., Localization of the gene for familial adenomatous polyposis on chromosome 5, *Nature,* 328, 614, 1987.

1252. Solomon, E., Voss, R., Hall, V., Bodmer, W.F., Jass, J.R., Jeffreys, A.J., Lucibello, F.C., Patel, I., and Rider, S.H., Chromosome 5 allele loss in human colorectal carcinomas, *Nature,* 328, 616, 1987.

1253. Okamoto, M., Sasaki, M., Sugio, K., Sato, C., Iwama, T., Ikeuchi, T., Tonomura, A., Sasazuki, T., and Miyaki, M., Loss of constitutional heterozygosity in colon carcinoma from patients with familial polyposis coli, *Nature,* 331, 273, 1988.

1254. Wildrick, D.M. and Boman, B.M., Chromosome 5 allele loss at the glucocorticoid receptor locus in human colorectal carcinomas, *Biochem. Biophys. Res. Commun.,* 150, 591, 1988.

1255. Baker, S.J., Fearon, E.R., Nigro, J.M., Hamilton, S.R., Preisinger, A.C., Jessup, J.M., van Tuinen, P., Ledbetter, D.H., Barker, D.F., Nakamura, Y., White, R., and Vogelstein, B., Chromosome 17 deletions and p53 gene mutations in colorectal carcinomas, *Science,* 244, 217, 1989.

1256. Monpezat, J.-P., Delattre, O., Bernard, A., Grunwald, D., Remvikos, Y., Muleris, M., Salmon, R.J., Frelat, G., Dutrillaux, B., and Thomas, G., Loss of alleles on chromosome 18 and on the short arm of chromosome 17 in polyploid colorectal carcinomas, *Int. J. Cancer,* 41, 404, 1988.

1257. Bernstein, R., Philip, P., and Ueshima, Y., Abnormalities of chromosome 7 resulting in monosomy 7 or in deletion of the long arm (7q-), *Cancer Genet. Cytogenet.,* 11, 300, 1984.

1258. Le Beau, M.M., Westbrook, C.A., Diaz, M.O., and Rowley, J.D., c-src is consistently conserved in the chromosomal deletion (20q) observed in myeloid disorders, *Proc. Natl. Acad. Sci. U.S.A.,* 82, 6692, 1985.

1259. Pollak, C. and Hagemeijer, A., Abnormalities of the short arm of chromosome 9 with partial loss of material in hematological disorders, *Leukemia,* 1, 541, 1987.

1260. Blatt, C. and Sachs, L., Deletion of a homeobox gene in myeloid leukemias with a deletion in chromosome 2, *Biochem. Biophys. Res. Commun.,* 156, 1265, 1988.

1261. Tinegate, H., Gaunt, L., and Hamilton, P.J., The 5q- syndrome: an underdiagnosed form of macrocytic anaemia, *Br. J. Haematol.,* 54, 103, 1983.

1262. Wisniewski, L.P. and Hirschhorn, K., Acquired partial deletions of the long arm of chromosome 5 in hematologic disorders, *Am. J. Hematol.,* 15, 295, 1983.

1263. Benitez, J., Martinez Frejo, C., Toledo, C., Sanchez Fayos, J., and Ramos, C., Leukemic transformation in patients with the 5q- alteration: analysis of the behavior of the 5q- clones in preleukemic to leukemic phases, *Cancer Genet. Cytogenet.,* 26, 199, 1987.

1264. Groffen, J., Heisterkamp, N., Spurr, N., Dana, S., Wasmuth, J.J., and Stephenson, J.R., Chromosomal localization of the human c-*fms* oncogene, *Nucleic Acids Res.,* 11, 6331, 1983.

1265. Le Beau, M.M., Westbrook, C.A., Diaz, M.O., Larson, R.A., Rowley, J.D., Gasson, J.C., Golden, D.W., and Sherr, C.J., Evidence for the involvement of *GM-CSF* and *FMS* in the deletion (5q) in myeloid disorders, *Science,* 231, 984, 1986.

1266. Bartram, C.R., Böhlke, J.V., Adolph, S., Hameister, H., Ganser, A., Anger, B., Heisterkamp, N., and Groffen, J., Deletion of c-*fms* sequences in the 5q- syndrome, *Leukemia,* 1, 146, 1987.

1267. Sherr, C.J., Rettenmier, C.W., Sacca, R., Roussel, M.F., Look, A.T., and Stanley, E.R., The c-*fms* proto-oncogene product is related to the receptor for the mononuclear phagocyte growth factor, CSF-1, *Cell*, 41, 665, 1985.

1268. Nienhuis, A.W., Bunn, H.F., Turner, P.H., Gopal, T.V., Nash, W.G., O'Brien, S.J., and Sherr, C.J., Expression of the human c-*fms* proto-oncogene in hematopoietic cells and its deletion in the 5q- syndrome, *Cell*, 42, 421, 1985.

1269. Pettenati, M.J., Le Beau, M.M., Lemons, R.S., Shima, E.A., Kawasaki, E.S., Larson, R.A., Sherr, C.J., Diaz, M.O., and Rowley, J.D., Assignment of *CSF-1* to 5q33.1: evidence for clustering of genes regulating hematopoiesis and for their involvement in the deletion of the long arm of chromosome 5 in myeloid disorders, *Proc. Natl. Acad. Sci. U.S.A.*, 84, 2970, 1987.

1270. Le Beau, M.M., Epstein, N.D., O'Brien, S.J., Nienhuis, A.W., Yang, Y.-C., Clark, S.C., and Rowley, J.D., The interleukin 3 gene is located on human chromosome 5 and is deleted in myeloid leukemias with a deletion of 5q, *Proc. Natl. Acad. Sci. U.S.A.*, 84, 5913, 1987.

1271. Yarden, Y., Escobedo, J.A., Kuang, W.-J., Yang-Feng, T.L., Daniel, T.O., Tremble, P.M., Chen, E.Y., Ando, M.E., Harkins, R.N., Francke, U., Fried, V.A., Ullrich, A., and Williams, L.T., Structure of the receptor for platelet-derived growth factor helps define a family of closely related growth factor receptors, *Nature*, 323, 226, 1986.

1272. Kobilka, B.K., Dixon, R.A.F., Frielle, T., Dohlman, H.G., Bolanowski, M.A., Sigal, I.S., Yang-Feng, T.L., Francke, U., Caron, M.G., and Lefkowitz, R.J., cDNA for the human β_2-adrenergic receptor: a protein with multiple membrane-spanning domains and encoded by a gene whose chromosomal location is shared with that of the receptor for platelet-derived growth factor, *Proc. Natl. Acad. Sci. U.S.A.*, 84, 46, 1987.

1273. Goyert, S.M., Ferrero, E., Rettig, W.J., Yenamandra, A.K., Obata, F., and Le Beau, M.M., The CD14 monocyte differentiation antigen maps to a region encoding growth factor and receptors, *Science*, 239, 497, 1988.

1274. Babu, V.R., Van Dyke, D.L., and Jackson, C.E., Chromosome 20 deletion in human multiple endocrine neoplasia types 2A and 2B: a double-blind study, *Proc. Natl. Acad. Sci. U.S.A.*, 81, 2525, 1984.

1275. Butler, M.G., Repaske, D.R., Joseph, G.M., and Phillips, J.A., III, High resolution chromosome and DNA analysis in multiple endocrine neoplasia type II syndrome, *Cancer Genet. Cytogenet.*, 24, 129, 1987.

1276. Mathew, C.G.P., Chin, K.S., Easton, D.F., Thorpe, K., Carter, C., Liou, G.I., Fong, S.-L., Bridges, C.D.B., Haak, H., Nieuwenhuijzen Kruseman, A.C., Schifter, S., Hansen, H.H., Telenius, H., Telenius-Berg, M., and Ponder, B.A.J., A linked genetic marker for multiple endocrine neoplasia type 2A on chromosome 10, *Nature*, 328, 527, 1987.

1277. Simpson, N.E., Kidd, K.K., Goodfellow, P.J., McDermid, H., Myers, S., Kidd, J.R., Jackson, C.E., Duncan, A.M.V., Farrer, L.A., Brasch, K., Castiglione, C., Genel, M., Gertner, J., Greenberg, C.R., Gusella, J.F., Holden, J.J.A., and White, B.N., Assignment of multiple endocrine neoplasia type 2A to chromosome 10 by linkage, *Nature*, 328, 528, 1987.

1278. Landsvater, R.M., Mathew, C.G.P., Smith, B.A., Marcus, E.M., te Meerman, G.J., Lips, C.J.M., Geerdink, R.A., Nakamura, Y., Ponder, B.A.J., and Buys, C.H.C.M., Development of multiple endocrine neoplasia type 2A does not involve substantial deletions of chromosome 10, *Genomics*, 4, 246, 1989.

1279. Larsson, C., Skogseid, B., Oberg, K., Nakamura, Y., and Nordenskjöld, M., Multiple endocrine neoplasia type 1 gene maps to chromosome 11 and is lost in insulinoma, *Nature*, 332, 85, 1988.

1280. Koufos, A., Hansen, M.F., Copeland, N.G., Jenkins, N.A., Lampkin, B.C., and Cavenee, W.K., Loss of heterozygosity in three embryonal tumours suggests a common pathogenetic mechanism, *Nature*, 316, 330, 1985.

1281. Fearon, E.R., Feinberg, A.P., Hamilton, S.H., and Vogelstein, B., Loss of genes on the short arm of chromosome 11 in bladder cancer, *Nature*, 318, 377, 1985.

1282. Zbar, B., Brauch, H., Talmadge, C., and Lineham, M., Loss of alleles of loci on the short arm of chromosome 3 in renal cell carcinoma, *Nature*, 327, 721, 1987.

1283. Lundberg, C., Skoog, L., Cavenee, W.K., and Nordenskjöld, M., Loss of heterozygosity in human ductal breast tumors indicates a recessive mutation on chromosome 13, *Proc. Natl. Acad. Sci. U.S.A.*, 84, 2372, 1987.

1284. Lee, E.Y.-H.P., To, H., Shew, J.-Y., Bookstein, R., Scully, P., and Lee, W.-H., Inactivation of the retinoblastoma susceptibility gene in human breast cancers, *Science*, 241, 218, 1988.

1285. Rogler, C.E., Sherman, M., Su, C.Y., Shafritz, D.A., Summers, J., Shows, T.B., Henderson, A., and Kew, M., Deletion in chromosome 11p associated with a hepatitis integration site in hepatocellular carcinoma, *Science*, 230, 319, 1985.

1286. Wada, M., Yokota, J., Mizoguchi, H., Sugimura, T., and Terada, M., Infrequent loss of chromosomal heterozygosity in human stomach cancer, *Cancer Res.*, 48, 2988, 1988.

1287. Le Beau, M.M., Chromosomal fragile sites and cancer-specific rearrangements, *Blood*, 67, 849, 1986.

1288. Schroeder, T.M., Genetically determined chromosome instability syndromes, *Cytogenet. Cell. Genet.*, 33, 119, 1982.

1289. de Nuñez, M., Penchaszadeh, V., and Pimentel, E., Chromosome fragility in patients with sporadic unilateral retinoblastoma, *Cancer Genet. Cytogenet.*, 11, 139, 1984.

1290. Gainer, H.S.C. and Kinsella, A.R., Analysis of spontaneous, carcinogen-induced and promoter-induced chromosomal instability in patients with hereditary retinoblastoma, *Int. J. Cancer*, 32, 449, 1983.

1291. Suckling, R.D., Fitzgerald, P.H., Stewart, J., and Wells, E., The incidence and epidemiology of retinoblastoma in New Zealand: a 30-year survey, *Br. J. Cancer*, 46, 729, 1982.

1292. Hecht, F. and Hecht, B.K., Autosomal fragile sites and cancer, *Am. J. Hum. Genet.*, 36, 718, 1984.

1293. Yunis, J.J. and Soreng, A.L., Constitutive fragile sites and cancer, *Science*, 226, 1199, 1984.

1294. Ishikawa, J., Maeda, S., Takahashi, R., Kamidono, S., and Sugiyama, T., Lack of correlation between rare Ha-*ras* alleles and urothelial cancer in Japan, *Int. J. Cancer*, 40, 474, 1987.

1295. Lee, J.H., Kavanagh, J.J., Wharton, J.T., Wildrick, D.M., and Blick, M., Allele loss at the c-Ha-*ras* 1 locus in human ovarian cancer, *Cancer Res.*, 49, 1220, 1988.

1296. Riou, G., Barrois, M., Sheng, Z.-M., Duvillard, P., and Lhomme, C., Somatic deletions and mutations of c-Ha-*ras* gene in human cervical cancers, *Oncogene*, 3, 329, 1988.

1297. Fujita, J., Kraus, M.H., Onoue, H., Srivastava, S.K., Ebi, Y., Kitamura, Y., and Rhim, J.S., Activated H-*ras* oncogenes in human kidney tumors, *Cancer Res.*, 48, 5251, 1988.

LIST OF ABBREVIATIONS

AAF	2-Acetylamino-fluorene
AAV	Adeno-associated virus
ABR	Abnormally banded region
ADP	Adenosine diphosphate
ADPRT	ADP-ribosyl transferase
AEV	Avian erythroblastosis virus
AFP	α-Fetoprotein
AIDS	Acquired immune deficiency syndrome
AILA	Angioimmunoblastic lymphadenopathy
ALV	Avian leukemia virus
AMCV	Avian myelocytomatosis virus
AML	Acute myelocytic leukemia
AMML	Acute myelomonocytic leukemia
AMOL	Acute monocytic leukemia
AMP	Adenosine 3':5'-monophosphate
AMV	Avian myeloblastosis virus
ANLL	Acute nonlymphocytic leukemia
APML	Acute promyelocytic leukemia
ARV	Avian reticuloendothelial virus
ASV	Avian sarcoma virus
ATL	Adult T-cell leukemia
ATLV	Adult T-cell leukemia virus
ATPase	Adenosine triphosphatase
ATP	Adenosine triphosphate
AV	Avian virus
AWTA	Aniridia-Wilms' tumor association
Ab	Antibody
Ag	Antigen
BCGF	B-cell growth factor
BEVI	Baboon endogenous viral infection
BHK	Baby hamster kidney
BKV	BK virus
BLV	Bovine leukemia virus
BMK	Baby mouse kidney
BP	Benzo-*a*-pyrene
BPV	Bovine papilloma virus
BSF	B-cell stimulating factor
BaEV	Baboon endogenous virus
bp	Base pairs
cAMP	Cyclic AMP
cDNA	Complementary DNA
CEA	Carcinoembryonic antigen
CEF	Chick embryo fibroblasts
cGMP	Cyclic GMP
CHO	Chinese hamster ovary
CLL	Chronic lymphocytic leukemia
CML	Chronic myelogenous leukemia
CMP	Cytosine monophosphate
CMV	Cytomegalovirus

CSF	Colony stimulating factor
CTVT	Canine transmissible venereal tumor
cs	Cold sensitive
DENA	Diethylnitrosamine
DES	Diethylstilbestrol
DIA	Differentiation-inducing activity
DIF	Differentiation-inducing factor
DMBA	7,12-Dimethylbenz(*a*)anthracene
DMSO	Dimethylsulfoxide
DM	Double minute chromosome
DNA	Deoxyribonucleic acid
DNase	Deoxyribonuclease
EA	Eary antigen
EBNA	EBV-associated nuclear antigen
EBV	Epstein-Barr virus
EF	Elongation factor
EGF	Epidermal growth factor
ELISA	Enzyme-linked immune sorbance assay
E1	Early region 1
ENU	1-Ethyl-1-nitrosourea
EPBF	Embryonal promoter-binding factor
ERV	Endogenous retrovirus
FAIDS	Feline AIDS
FBJ-MuSV	Finkel-Biskis-Jenkins MuSV
FGF	Fibroblast growth factor
FSBA	*p*-Fluorosulfonylbenzoyl 5′-adenosine
FSH	Follicle-stimulating hormone
FSV	Fujinami avian sarcoma virus
FeLV	Feline leukemia virus
FeSV	Feline sarcoma virus
F-MuLV	Friend murine leukemia virus
GA	Gardner-Arnstein strain
GABA	γ-Aminobutyric acid
GAD	Glutamic acid decarboxylase
GC	Guanosine-cytosine
GDP	Guanosine diphosphate
GMP	Guanosine monophosphate
GM-CSF	Granulocyte-macrophage colony stimulating factor
GPDH	Glucose-6-phosphate dehydrogenase
GR	Gardner-Rasheed strain
GRE	Glucocorticoid regulatory element
GTPase	Guanosine triphosphatase
GTP	Guanosine triphosphate
GaLV	Gibbon ape leukemia virus
HBLV	Human B-lymphotropic virus
HBV	Hepatitis B virus
HBsAg	Hepatitis B virus surface antigen
HCMV	Human cytomegalovirus
HEK	Human embryo kidney
HIV	Human immunodeficiency virus
HLA	Human leukocyte antigen

HMBA	Hexamethylene bisacetamide
HMG	High mobility group
HPRT	Hypoxanthine phosphoribosyl transferase
HPV	Human papilloma virus
HRE	Hormone regulatory element
HSP	Heat shock protein
HSR	Homogeneously staining region
HSV	Herpes simplex virus
HTLV	Human T-cell lymphotropic virus
HVT	Herpes virus of turkeys
HZ	Hardy-Zuckerman strain
HuERS	Human endogenous retroviruses
IAP	Intracisternal A particle
IDF	Inhibitory diffusible factor
IFN	Interferon
IGF	Insulin-like growth factor
IL	Interleukin
IS	Insertion sequence
ITR	Inverted terminal repeat sequence
Ig	Immunoglobulin
kDa	Kilodalton
K-MuLV	Kirsten murine leukemia virus
K-MuSV	Kirsten murine sarcoma virus
kb	Kilobase
kbp	Kilobase pair
LAS	Lymphadenopathy syndrome
LAV	Lymphadenopathy-associated virus
LDH	Lactate dehydrogenase
LDL	Low-density lipoprotein
LINE	Long interspersed repetitive sequence
LMP	Latent membrane protein
LPS	Lipopolysaccharide
LPV	Lymphotropic papovavirus
LTR	Long terminal repeat
MA	Membrane antigen
MCA	3-Methyl-cholanthrene
MCF	Mink cell focus
MCFV	Mink cell focus virus
MCMV	Mouse cytomegalovirus
MDCK	Madin-Darby canine kidney
MDV	Marek's disease virus
MEL	Mouse erythroleukemia
MEN	Multiple endocrine neoplasia
MGI	Macrophage-granulocyte inducer
MHC	Major histocompatibility complex
MHSV	Malignant histiocytosis virus
MMTV	Mouse mammary tumor virus
MNNG	N-Methyl-N'-nitroso-guanidine
MPF	Maturation-promoting factor
MPLV	Myeloproliferative leukemia virus
MPMV	Mason-Pfizer monkey virus

MPO	Myeloperoxidase
mRNA	Messenger RNA
mol wt	Molecular weight
MuLV	Murine leukemia virus
MuSV	Murine sarcoma virus
NAD	Nicotinamide adenine dinucleotide
NGF	Nerve growth factor
NHBE	Normal human bronchial epithelial cells
NK	Natural killer
NMU	Nitrosomethylurea (*N*-methyl-*N*-nitrosourea)
NRK	Normal rat kidney
ODC	Ornithine decarboxylase
ORF	Open reading frame
PCNA	Proliferating cell nuclear antigen
PCR	Polymerase chain reaction
PDGF	Platelet-derived growth factor
PFK	Phosphofructokinase
PGE	Prostaglandin E
PHA	Phytohemagglutinin
PHC	Primary hepatocellular carcinoma
PI-FeSV	Parodi-Irgens FeSV
PMA	Phorbol 12-myristate 13-acetate
PTH	Parathyroid hormone
Rad-MuLV	Radiation murine leukemia virus
RAV	RSV-associated virus
REF	Rat embryo fibroblasts
REV	Reticuloendotheliosis virus
RFLP	Restriction fragment length polymorphism
RNA	Ribonucleic acid
RNAse	Ribonuclease
RNP	Ribonucleoprotein
rRNA	Ribosomal RNA
RSV	Rous sarcoma virus
RadLV	Radiation leukemia virus
SAIDS	Simian AIDS
SCE	Sister chromatid exchange
SDS	Sodium dodecyl sulfate
SFFV	Spleen focus-forming virus
SFV	Shope fibroma virus
SINE	Short interspersed repetitive sequence
SIV	Simian immunodeficiency virus
SLE	Systemic lupus erythematosus
SMRV	Squirrel monkey retrovirus
SM	Susan McDonough strain
SNV	Spleen necrosis virus
SRV	Simian AIDS retrovirus
SSAV	Simian sarcoma-associated virus
SSV	Simian sarcoma virus
STLV	Simian T-cell leukemia virus
ST	Snyder-Theilen strain
SV-40	Simian virus 40

TAA	Tumor associated antigen
TGF	Transforming growth factor
TNF	Tumor necrosis factor
TPA	12-*O*-Tetradecanoyl-phorbol 13-acetate
tRNA	Transfer RNA
TSA	Tumor surface antigen
TSH	Thyroid-stimulating factor
TSTA	Tumor-specific transplantation antigen
ts	Temperature sensitive
UMS	Upstream mouse sequence
UV	Ultraviolet
VCA	Viral capsid antigen
VTR	Variable tandem repeat
VVGF	Vaccinia virus growth factor
WHV	Woodchuck hepatitis virus

INDEX

A

S